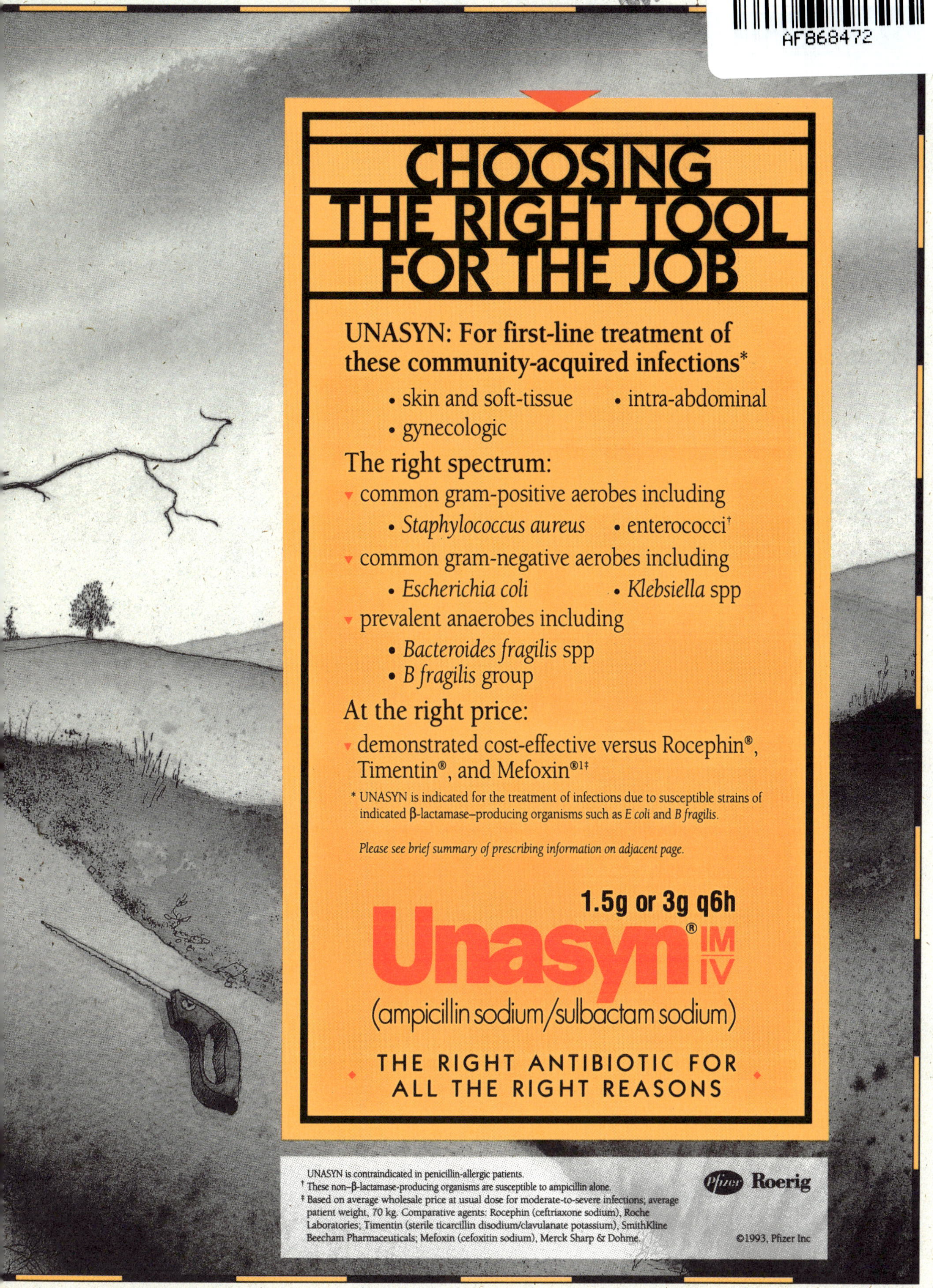
CHOOSING THE RIGHT TOOL FOR THE JOB
UNASYN: For first-line treatment of these community-acquired infections*
• skin and soft-tissue • intra-abdominal
• gynecologic
The right spectrum:
common gram-positive aerobes including
• Staphylococcus aureus • enterococci†
common gram-negative aerobes including
• Escherichia coli • Klebsiella spp
prevalent anaerobes including
• Bacteroides fragilis spp
• B fragilis group
At the right price:
demonstrated cost-effective versus Rocephin®, Timentin®, and Mefoxin®1‡
* UNASYN is indicated for the treatment of infections due to susceptible strains of indicated β-lactamase–producing organisms such as E coli and B fragilis.
Please see brief summary of prescribing information on adjacent page.
1.5g or 3g q6h
Unasyn® IM IV
(ampicillin sodium/sulbactam sodium)
THE RIGHT ANTIBIOTIC FOR ALL THE RIGHT REASONS
UNASYN is contraindicated in penicillin-allergic patients.
† These non–β-lactamase-producing organisms are susceptible to ampicillin alone.
‡ Based on average wholesale price at usual dose for moderate-to-severe infections; average patient weight, 70 kg. Comparative agents: Rocephin (ceftriaxone sodium), Roche Laboratories; Timentin (sterile ticarcillin disodium/clavulanate potassium), SmithKline Beecham Pharmaceuticals; Mefoxin (cefoxitin sodium), Merck Sharp & Dohme.
Pfizer Roerig
©1993, Pfizer Inc

Current Opinion in GENERAL SURGERY

CONTENTS

Critical care and trauma
Donald S Gann and J David Richardson

Liver, biliary tract, and pancreas
John R T Monson, Josef E Fischer, and Howard A Reber

Endocrine
Norman W Thompson

Laparoscopy and endoscopy
Bruce V MacFadyen, Jr

Colorectal
Richard L Nelson

Surgical oncology and tumor immunology
Timothy J Eberlein

Esophageal, gastric, and small intestine
Robert J Ginsberg, Thomas A Miller, and Irvin M Modlin

Vascular surgery
Robert W Hobson II

Other titles in the Current Opinion series

Anaesthesiology
Biotechnology
Cardiology
Cell Biology
Cosmetic Dentistry
Dermatology
Endocrinology & Diabetes
Gastroenterology
Genetics & Development
Hematology
Immunology
Infectious Diseases
Lipidology
Nephrology & Hypertension
Neurobiology
Neurology & Neurosurgery
Obstetrics & Gynecology
Oncology
Ophthalmology
Orthopedics
Otolaryngology & Head and Neck Surgery
Pediatrics
Periodontology
Psychiatry
Rheumatology
Structural Biology
Surgical Infections
Urology

Available soon

Critical Care
General Dentistry
Pulmonary Medicine
Public Health

Philadelphia office

Editor: Joseph Barron   Typesetting: William Donnelly
Acquisitions Editor: Leslie Ryan   Subscriptions: Sean McGlinchey
Advertising: Fred Wood

20 North Third Street, Philadelphia, PA 19106-2199
Tel 215 574 2266   Fax 215 574 3533

London office

Subscriptions: Roy Dunn   Advertising: Simon Lang

34–42 Cleveland Street, London W1P 5FB
Tel (0)71 323 0323   Fax (0)71 580 1938

Current Opinion in General Surgery subscription information

Current Opinion in General Surgery is published annually by Current Science (Philadelphia, PA). Each volume consists of approximately 300 pages.

1994 Subscription rates	USA and Canada* $US (+ postage)	Rest of World $US (+ postage)	United Kingdom £UK (+ postage)	Europe† £UK (+ postage)	Rest of World £UK (+ postage)	Japan Yen (+ postage)
Personal	129.95 (4.00)	129.95 (16.00)	84.95 (5.00)	84.95 (6.00)	84.95 (10.00)	27,930 (1,470)
Institutional	259.95 (4.00)	259.95 (16.00)	169.95 (5.00)	169.95 (6.00)	169.95 (10.00)	55,930 (1,470)
Students/residents‡	74.95 (4.00)	74.95 (16.00)	39.95 (5.00)	39.95 (6.00)	39.95 (10.00)	13,930 (1,470)

*Canadian residents must add GST.
†Subscribers within the EC may be liable to a European tax.
‡Students/residents must give the name of their institution or school, plus the name of the residency director or department chairman, to qualify for the discounted rate. Students/residents rate is available for a maximum of 2 years.

Orders should be placed with a bookseller or subscription agent, or sent to Current Science: *In the USA and Canada:* Current Science, 20 North Third Street, Philadelphia, PA 19106-2199, USA or call TOLL FREE 1-800-552-5866 (in PA 215 574-2266; fax: 215 574-2270). *In Japan:* Nankodo Co Ltd 42-6 Hongo 3-chome, Bunkyo Ku, Tokyo 113, Japan. *Rest of the world:* Current Science, 34-42 Cleveland Street, London W1P 5FB, UK. Second class postage paid at Rahway, NJ. Postmaster send address corrections to Current Science, 20 North Third Street, Philadelphia, PA 19106-2199 USA.

ISBN 1-85922-671-X
ISSN 1065–6243

Printed in Hong Kong by Paramount Printing Group, Ltd.

Contents

John M. Daly	Editorial	1

Critical care and trauma

Edited by Donald S. Gann and J. David Richardson

Donald S. Gann and J. David Richardson	Critical care and trauma: editorial overview	3
Charles J. Shanley and Robert H. Bartlett	The management of acute respiratory failure	7
Kazue Ozawa, Keiichiro Mori, and Taisuke Morimoto	Evaluation of hepatic function	17
Kenneth A. Kudsk and Gayle Minard	Management of nutrition in the critically ill patient	24
Timothy C. Flynn	Peripheral vascular injury	30
David H. Livingston	New diagnostic techniques in trauma	35
Matthew L. Moront and Martin R. Eichelberger	Advances in the treatment of pediatric trauma	41

Endocrine

Edited by Norman W. Thompson

Norman W. Thompson	Endocrine: editorial overview	51
Brian M. Stephenson, Malcolm H. Wheeler, and Orlo H. Clark	The role of total thyroidectomy in the management of differentiated thyroid cancer	53
Kerstin Sandelin, Catharina Larsson, and Ruth Anne Decker	Genetic aspects of multiple endocrine neoplasia types 1 and 2	60
Romano Delcore and Stanley R. Friesen	The place for curative surgical procedures in the treatment of sporadic and familial Zollinger-Ellison syndrome	69

Colorectal

Edited by Richard L. Nelson

Richard L. Nelson	Colorectal: editorial overview	77
Jack S. Mandel	Screening for colorectal cancer	79
Bernard J. Cummings	Adjuvant radiation for rectal cancer: when and with what?	85
Carina G. Biggs and Garth H. Ballantyne	Sensitivity versus cost effectiveness in postoperative follow-up for colorectal cancer	94
J. Denis, R. Ganansia, and T. Puy-Montbrun	Rare anorectal pathologic conditions	103

Continued

Esophageal, gastric, and small intestine

Edited by Robert J. Ginsberg, Thomas A. Miller, and Irvin M. Modlin

Robert J. Ginsberg, Thomas A. Miller, and Irvin M. Modlin	Esophageal, gastric, and small intestine: editorial overview	109
Nasser K. Altorki	Extended resections in the management of esophageal carcinoma	113
Carlos A. Pellegrini	The role of minimal-access surgery in esophageal disease	117
Mohammed T. Al-Assi and David Y. Graham	Peptic ulcer disease, *Helicobacter pylori*, and the surgeon: changing of the guard	120
Martin S. Karpeh, Jr. and Murray F. Brennan	Progress in the management of gastric cancer	125
Gary P. Lawton and Irvin M. Modlin	Recent advances in the localization and surgical management of duodenal gastrinomas	131
Marc D. Basson	Mucosal healing and adaptation in the small intestine	138

Liver, biliary tract, and pancreas

Edited by John R.T. Monson, Josef E. Fischer, and Howard A. Reber

John R.T. Monson, Josef E. Fischer, and Howard A. Reber	Liver, biliary tract, and pancreas: editorial overview	147
Peter McCulloch	Nonsurgical treatment of liver metastases	151
John W. Braasch	Surgery for sclerosing cholangitis	156
Keith D. Lillemoe	Current status of surgery for Klatskin tumors	161
Jay Grosfeld	Is there a place for the Kasai procedure in biliary atresia?	168
Charles J. Yeo	Pancreatic pseudocysts, ascites, and fistulas	173
F. Charles Brunicardi and Christopher R. Shackleton	Whole-organ versus islet pancreatic transplantation	179
Jennifer B. Meko and Jeffrey A. Norton	Endocrine tumors of the pancreas	186

Laparoscopy and endoscopy

Edited by Bruce V. MacFadyen, Jr.

Bruce V. MacFadyen, Jr.	Laparoscopy and endoscopy: editorial overview	195
Moses J. Fallas and Edward H. Phillips	Laparoscopic inguinal herniorrhaphy	198
David E. Pitcher, Daniel T. Martin, and Karl A. Zucker	Laparoscopic and endoscopic management of common bile duct stones	203
David M. Ota, Heidi Nelson, and Jane C. Weeks	Controversies regarding laparoscopic colectomy for malignant diseases	208

Continued

Surgical oncology and tumor immunology

Edited by Timothy J. Eberlein

Timothy J. Eberlein	Surgical oncology and tumor immunology: editorial overview	215
Yvedt L. Matory	The diagnosis and treatment of breast cancer	217
Raphael E. Pollock	Limb-sparing therapy for soft tissue sarcomas	224
Alan P. Meagher and John H. Pemberton	Alternative surgical procedures for primary rectal carcinoma	230
James C. Yang	Cellular immunotherapy of cancer	238
Michael T. Lotze	Molecular biology and clinical applications to cancer	245

Vascular surgery

Edited by Robert W. Hobson II

Robert W. Hobson II	Vascular surgery: editorial overview	255
Kenneth Ouriel	Thrombolytic therapy for acute arterial occlusion	257
Robert W. Hobson II	Randomized clinical trial results define operative indications in symptomatic and asymptomatic carotid endarterectomy patients	265
Virginia S. Newman and Richard H. Dean	Ischemic nephropathy as an indication for renal artery reconstruction in renovascular hypertension	272
	Index to subjects	277

Editorial

John M. Daly, MD

Lewis Atterbury Stimson Professor of Surgery
Chairman, Department of Surgery
Cornell University Medical College
Surgeon-in-Chief, The New York Hospital
New York, New York, USA

Current Opinion in General Surgery 1994:1–2

This edition of *Current Opinion in General Surgery* has been modified and expanded to reflect the diverse and encompassing roles of general surgeons in patient management. A major section on "Laparoscopy and endoscopy" has been added, consonant with the increasing use of these techniques in patient care. In addition, a new section on "Vascular surgery" provides current reviews on arterial and venous abnormalities. The book's design continues to provide the reader with focused, up-to-date reviews of critical areas in surgery. The authors' "opinions" are founded on the scientific literature, which has been abstracted and cited as both "references and recommended reading." The authors and section editors have aptly noted areas of controversy where individuals of good will disagree on the interpretation of the facts laid before them.

Charles Shanley and Robert Bartlett (pp 7–16) present the physiologic basis for mechanical ventilatory support for acute respiratory failure and the potential for extracorporeal life support and liquid ventilation. Kazue Ozawa, Keiichiro Mori, and Taisuke Morimoto (pp 17–23) review redox theory as it applies to the evaluation of hepatic reserve, which is critical to predicting the metabolic and functional results after hepatic resection in cirrhotic patients. Kenneth Kudsk and Gayle Minard (pp 24–29) describe the background and use of specific nutrients and anabolic agents in trauma and critically ill patients. Timothy Flynn (pp 30–34) focuses on the issue that "less may be better" in civilian vascular trauma, describing "hard" and "soft" signs of vascular injury and the use of duplex scanning. David Livingston (pp 35–40) notes the usefulness of transesophageal echocardiography, laparoscopy, and thoracoscopy in trauma patients. Matthew Moront and Michael Eichelberger (pp 41–49) review a systematic approach to pediatric trauma, which is particularly important for general surgeons in areas where pediatric surgeons are not immediately available.

In the "Endocrine" section, Brian Stephenson, Malcolm Wheeler, and Orlo Clark (pp 53–59) describe the role of total thyroidectomy in differentiated cancer, which appears quite safe in experienced hands. Kerstin Sandelin, Catharina Larsson, and Ruth Decker (pp 60–68) review the molecular biologic basis of the multiple endocrine neoplasia syndromes permitting identification of individuals by DNA screening. Finally, Romano Delcore and Stanley Friesen (pp 69–76) describe the use of "curative" surgical procedures for those with Zollinger-Ellison Syndrome.

In the "Colorectal" section, Jack Mandel (pp 79–84) reviews the use of sigmoidoscopy and fecal occult blood testing to reduce mortality. Recent identification of the genetic defect associated with familial, nonpolyposis large bowel cancer will help to focus screening efforts. Adjuvant radiation therapy for rectal cancer is reviewed by Bernard Cummings (pp 85–93), and Carina Biggs and Garth Ballantyne (pp 94–102) note the benefits and deficiencies inherent in the follow-up of patients with colorectal cancer. Rare anorectal conditions are described by J. Denis, R. Ganansia, and T. Puy-Montbrun (pp 103–107).

In the gastrointestinal sections, Nasser Altorki (pp 113–116) reviews the results of radical en bloc resection for esophageal cancer. Carlos Pellegrini (pp 117–119) describes the use of laparoscopy and thoracoscopy in esophageal abnormalities. Mohammed Al-Assi and David Graham (pp 120–124) review current information on *Helicobacter pylori* and its important role in peptic ulcer disease. Martin Karpeh and Murray Brennan (pp 125–130) describe newer methods of staging gastric cancer patients. Duodenal gastrinomas are reviewed by Gary Lawton and Irvin Modlin (pp 131–137), and Marc Basson (pp 138–146) describes the autocrine and juxtacrine growth factors that affect mucosal healing and small bowel adaptation. Peter McCulloch (pp 151–155) reviews nonresectional approaches to liver metastases. John Braasch (pp 156–160) describes the use of bypass stenting and transplantation for sclerosing cholangitis, while Keith Lillemoe (pp 161–167) focuses on diagnosis, staging, and therapy for Klatskin tumors, noting that surgical resection is possible in 35% to 45% of patients. The Kasai procedure for biliary atresia is suggested by Jay Grosfeld (pp 168–172) for most children with liver transplantation who are older than 3 to 4 months, who fail the procedure, or who have cirrhosis. Charles Yeo (pp 173–178) nicely describes pancreatic pseudocysts and fistulas and the use of octreotide in the management of ascites and fistulas. Pancreatic whole-organ and islet transplantation are reviewed by F. Charles Brunicardi and Christopher Shackleton (pp 179–185) while Jennifer Meko and Jeffrey Norton (pp 186–194) describe the diagnostic and therapeutic approaches to pancreatic endocrine tumors.

In the new section on "Laparoscopy and endoscopy," Moses Fallas and Edward Phillips (pp 198–202) review inguinal herniorrhaphy by various approaches. Management of common bile duct stones by both endoscopic and laparoscopic techniques is described by David Pitcher, Daniel Martin, and Karl Zucker (pp 203–207). David Ota, Heidi Nelson, and Jane Weeks (pp 208–213) describe the rationale, techniques, and complications of laparoscopic colectomy and note the need for prospective randomized studies.

In the "Surgical oncology and tumor immunology" section, Yvedt Matory (pp 217–223) gives an up-to-date review of breast cancer management. Raphael Pollock (pp 224–229) provides the rationale for multidisciplinary management of soft tissue sarcomas to utilize limb sparing whenever possible. Alan Meagher and John Pemberton (pp 230–237) describe local-regional alternatives to radical surgery for localized rectal cancer. Finally, James Yang (pp 238–244) reviews the cellular immunotherapy of cancer, and Michael Lotze (pp 245–254) describes the molecular biologic approaches to cancer. These last two reviews provide timely documentation of basic-science approaches to cancer therapy.

In the new section on "Vascular surgery," Kenneth Ouriel (pp 257–264) focuses on thrombolytic therapy of acute arterial occlusion. Robert Hobson (pp 265–271) reviews the results of randomized trials of carotid endarterectomy, and Virginia Newman and Richard Dean (pp 272–276) describe the need for renal artery reconstruction in renovascular hypertension.

This second edition provides up-to-date reviews of new, critical areas of patient management for general surgeons. The editorial overviews provide an unbiased synthesis of recent literature combined with experience in a given area. Expert opinion based on recent scientific literature form the basis for clinical decision-making.

Critical care and trauma*

Editorial overview

Donald S. Gann, MD, and J. David Richardson, MD

University of Maryland School of Medicine, Baltimore, Maryland, and
University of Louisville School of Medicine, Louisville, Kentucky, USA

*The articles on critical care in this section were edited by Dr. Gann and those on trauma, by Dr. Richardson.

Current Opinion in General Surgery 1994:3–5

Critical care

Successful care of the critically ill surgical patient frequently demands an understanding and application of fundamental principles of pathophysiology. Consequently, progress in surgical critical care often depends on the application of increasingly sophisticated principles of pathophysiology to problems of diagnosis or therapy. It is often the case, however, that when one looks at a successful application of a particular sophisticated principle in retrospect, that application appears elegant in its simplicity. The present collection of topics in critical care serve, in my view, to illustrate this point. In each case, significant changes in the care of the critically ill surgical patients have already been or are on the verge of being undertaken.

In their examination of acute respiratory failure, Charles Shanley and Robert Bartlett (pp 7–16) focus initially on the use of systemic mixed venous oxygen concentration as the most reliable indicator of adequate oxygen delivery. When optimization of this critical variable becomes the goal of respiratory support, alternative approaches to such support become evident. Some relatively novel forms of support cannot be demonstrated to improve oxygen delivery and may lead to injuriously high inspiratory pressures. The development of extracorporeal oxygenation and more recently extracorporeal removal of carbon dioxide demonstrates innovative approaches that appear to lead increasingly to clinical success without barotrauma. This review also discusses the intriguing possibilities offered by pharmacologic therapy for this problem.

Until recently, there was little progress in the evaluation of hepatic function. As Kazue Ozawa, Keiichiro Mori, and Taisuke Morimoto (pp 17–23) point out, the increasing reliance on endoscopic approaches to bleeding esophageal varices has greatly reduced the frequency of emergency portosystemic shunts and thus has reduced the pressure for better preoperative evaluation of liver function. With recent increases in hepatic surgery, however, especially on patients with underlying cirrhosis, and with the increasing frequency of hepatic transplantation, more sophisticated approaches to the evaluation of hepatic function have become important. In their review, the authors consider a number of approaches to such evaluation, based on measurements of cytokine, various clotting factors, specific proteins and metabolic events involving evaluation of metabolism of methionine or vasopressin, or use of dynamic magnetic resonance spectroscopy. Other methods are more invasive or appear to add little to currently available routine studies. Having painted this background, the authors then introduce a simple approach to the evaluation of the redox state of the mitochondrion by measurement of the arterial ketone body ratio, which consists of a simple pair of biochemical measurements. They show that this measure will reflect the ability to synthesize ATP to carry out gluconeogenesis (perhaps the most important single function of the liver), and that it can be used to assess hepatic function after transplantation or to evaluate reserve by measurement of the ketone body response to a glucose load. They make a strong case, in my opinion, for the routine use of these measurements in the setting of hepatic transplantation.

The review of nutritional management by Kenneth Kudsk and Gayle Minard (pp 24–29) takes a fresh look at what many would regard as a routine subject. The authors point out that the use of parenteral nutrition may not reduce the incidence of sepsis in every setting and in fact may enhance it in some. They consider a number of modifications of nutritional management that may have promise. The case for enteral rather than parenteral feeding when possible has been made elsewhere but is reviewed here. The authors direct more attention to the use of specific nutrients, including ω-3 fatty acids, arginine, and glutamine, as well as growth

 ISBN 1-85922-671-X ISSN 1065–6243

hormone or insulin-like growth factor 1 induced by it, to modify metabolism. Initial results in these areas appear quite promising and again may be expected to alter routine therapy in the relatively near future.

In each of these cases, innovation has followed a closer look at the meaning of a measurement or the goal of an intervention. In no case is the approach suggested likely to be the final word on the subject. However, the general theme involving the application of basic science principles to clinical problems seems to set the stage for current and future advances in surgical critical care.

Trauma

The article by Timothy Flynn (pp 30–34) is an excellent overview of the current literature and thoughts on peripheral vascular injury. The evolution in thought about the diagnosis and treatment of suspected vascular injury has been interesting to follow over the past several decades. Once vascular reconstructive techniques became common during the Korean War era, increasingly aggressive diagnostic techniques were used to detect injury. Operative exploration of wounds in proximity of major vessels became the watchword of surgical practice. Several studies, particularly from Dallas, indicated that arteriography was a safe method of excluding blood vessel injuries, and in most trauma centers, the use of angiography to exclude vessel injuries has become standard practice.

Whether angiography or vascular exploration is used to diagnose blood vessel injuries, operative treatment will generally not be required. The use of angiography or exploration has resulted in actual treatment rates of roughly 5% to 20% in most series. Because most patients do not have injuries, the desire to decrease the use of unnecessary procedures (including arteriography) is laudable. Why then has this area remained so controversial? I would suggest several possible reasons.

One possible source of confusion revolves around the entry or exclusion for operation and angiography. Most of the papers on this subject provide few data on which patients undergo angiography. Clearly, if every extremity-penetrating wound has an angiogram without careful judgment as to the likelihood of a vascular wound, the rate of positivity will be quite low.

Similarly, many authors state that all patients with "hard signs" should have a vascular exploration without an angiogram. Does this mean that every hematoma mandates operation, regardless of size or location? What does bleeding from a wound mean? Is profuse arterial hemorrhage a clear harbinger of vascular injury, or does some trickling from the muscle denote nothing serious? Experienced surgeons can usually discern the difference, but inexperienced house officers or emergency-room physicians may be unsure and opt for an "aggressive" approach. In our experience, operations done for hematoma *per se* disclosed no injury in the majority of cases. Our unit tends to perform angiography for many patients with "hard" signs, and we often observe the patient if the results are negative. Thus, we recently reviewed a series of arteriographies for suspected vascular trauma and found a positive rate of 35%. I would submit that publication of these rates is not very meaningful because of the extreme variability in criteria for exclusion or inclusion. Hence, a major source of misunderstanding and controversy.

The second source of controversy has centered on the reports from Jacksonville, Florida [1–3], in which an approach that could be termed *nihilistic* has been advocated. Actually, these authors have stated their treatment policy better than most authors and indicate they operate on patients who have hard signs of vascular injury. However, these authors have then championed a position of not performing angiography on other patients because of the low yield they obtained. They then expanded this concept to the observation of vascular injuries that were clinically occult. The usefulness of this approach depends in large part on one's view of the world, similar to the analogy of a glass being half full or half empty depending on one's perspective. I submit their data can be interpreted in a similar fashion. As Flynn notes, Frykberg *et al.* [4] reported 6 pseudoaneurysms that required operative treatment during a 3-month period of observation of 46 patients with "clinically occult injuries." In my view, pseudoaneurysms are dangerous and may cause death, limb loss, or major disability. They are more easily repaired early than late, and therefore, I advocate aggressive repair. In my view of this problem, a 15% operative rate for a potentially lethal problem is unacceptable. Clearly, others have a different interpretation of the data. (Perhaps the glass is half full!) Hence, the controversy continues.

As Flynn indicates, a method of noninvasive diagnosis of vascular injuries is needed, lest we squander valuable resources in excluding injuries that had a low probability of being present. Increased reliance on clinical judgment in conjunction with the appropriate use of technology will allow us to husband our resources more effectively. Moreover, authors who are espousing new approaches to the management of vascular injuries must be careful that their approach is carefully delineated and that problems with these new approaches are honestly reported.

The theme of making a diagnosis and potentially treating intra-abdominal or intrathoracic injuries in a less invasive fashion dominates the review on new diagnostic techniques in trauma by David Livingston (pp 35–40). Sounding a theme similar to that of Flynn on vascular injury, Livingston reviews the current advances in transesophageal echocardiography, laparoscopy, and thoracoscopy in making diagnosis less invasive and, with the latter two modalities, in potentially offering treatment.

It seems clear that laparoscopy will be useful for certain types of patients, although the specter of missed injuries still looms large in the series reported to date. There will almost certainly be some patients who would be better treated by laparoscopy to evaluate certain types of penetrating injuries, such as flank injury, particularly if those patients would otherwise be candidates for exploratory celiotomy. What the role will be for patients with blunt trauma is less clear. Certain groups, such as our own, have used this modality in patients who would otherwise be candidates for operation, such as those who have stabilized and have a positive diagnostic peritoneal lavage. What is needed is a rapid means of assessing a patient by some type of small peritoneoscope or laparoscope in the emergency department. Technology that might allow such evaluation through a small incision, such as would be used for diagnostic peritoneal lavage, is being tested. If these modalities are successful, they would be of great aid in the rapid evaluation and triage of the patient with multiple injuries.

Thoracoscopy will undoubtedly find a larger role in the evaluation and treatment of some types of traumatic injury, particularly those with penetrating mechanisms. The precise role for this therapy remains unknown, but it is clear that if used early, thoracoscopy can remove a clotted hemothorax. In our unreported experience, the problem has been to select the proper patient for treatment early enough that it can be successful. Further studies are needed to elucidate the precise role of this modality.

The final section, by Matthew Moront and Martin Eichelberger (pp 41–49), deals with the management of pediatric trauma. One of the difficult issues confronting many trauma centers and systems is the question of who should care for the injured child. There are great differences throughout the United States in the provision of trauma care for injured children. In many places, care is provided by children's hospitals with dedicated pediatric surgeons who are interested in the provision of trauma care. Other children's hospitals do not even have emergency rooms and are not staffed with the multidisciplinary team necessary to provide triage and treatment. In certain locales, children are treated in the same hospital as adults, often by the same physicians. In many areas, moreover, the small number of injured children has made the designation of separate institutions for treating the children impractical and often impossible. As the nation attempts to move toward more inclusive trauma care systems, the assurance of adequate trauma care for injured children is of paramount importance. Surgeons who treat adults primarily but occasionally treat children must be familiar with the important differences in physiologic responses to injuries and in the treatment of the specific injuries inherent in the successful management of pediatric trauma. To that end, Moront and Eichelberger's paper is very important.

References

1. MENZOLAN JO, DOYLE JE, LOGERFO FW, CANTELMO N, WEITZMAN AF, SEQUIERA JC: **Evaluation and Management of Vascular Injuries of the Extremities.** *Arch Surg* 1983, **118**:93–95.
2. DENNIS JW, FRYKBERG ER, CRUMP JM, VINES FS, ALEXANDER RH: **New Perspectives on the Management of Penetrating Trauma in Proximity to Major Limb Arteries.** *J Vasc Surg* 1990, **11**:84–93.
3. FRYKBERG ER, CRUMP JM, DENNIS JW, VINES FS, ALEXANDER RH: **Nonoperative Observation of Clinically Occult Arterial Injuries: A Prospective Evaluation.** *Surgery* 1991, **109**:85–96.
4. FRYKBERG ER, DENNIS JW, BISHOP K, LANEVE L, ALEXANDER RH: **The Reliability of Physical Examination in the Evaluation of Penetrating Extremity Trauma for Vascular Injury: Results at One Year.** *J Trauma* 1991, **31**:502–511.

Donald S. Gann, MD, University of Maryland School of Medicine, Department of Surgery, 22 South Greene Street, Baltimore, MD 21201, USA.

J. David Richardson, MD, University of Louisville School of Medicine, Department of Surgery, Louisville, KY 40292, USA.

The management of acute respiratory failure

Charles J. Shanley, MD, and Robert H. Bartlett, MD

University of Michigan Medical Center, Ann Arbor, Michigan, USA

The mortality rate of severe respiratory failure in most centers remains 60% to 90% with conventional pulmonary support techniques. Recent advances in the physiologic management of patients with acute respiratory failure include optimizing systemic oxygen delivery as reflected by continuous mixed-venous saturation monitoring, avoidance of the damaging effects of high inflation pressures and volumes during mechanical ventilation, and the increasing application of extracorporeal life support techniques for refractory respiratory failure. The future promises the routine clinical application of novel support techniques including implantable intracorporeal gas exchange devices and perfluorocarbon liquid ventilation.

Current Opinion in General Surgery 1994:7–16

Despite recent advances in pulmonary supportive therapy, acute respiratory failure remains a common and highly lethal problem. Considerable progress has been made in defining the basic biochemical, molecular, and cellular mechanisms responsible for the pathophysiologic changes seen in the acute respiratory failure (ARF). For detailed discussion of this rapidly expanding field of basic research, the reader is referred to several excellent recent reviews [1••,2–6]. The following discussion focuses on recent clinical advances in the management of acute respiratory failure.

Oxygen kinetics and venous saturation monitoring

Central to the intelligent management of respiratory failure is a clear understanding of systemic oxygen kinetics (Table 1) [7•]. In the steady state, systemic oxygen delivery (DO_2) is approximately four to five times greater than oxygen consumption (VO_2). Therefore, 20% to 25% of systemically delivered oxygen is extracted from arterial blood, and the remainder returns to the heart in mixed-venous blood. If arterial blood is 100% saturated, then normal mixed-venous blood will be approximately 75% to 80% saturated. Acute changes in either DO_2 or VO_2 result in reflex changes in cardiac output to maintain the normal DO_2/VO_2 ratio. Whenever the DO_2/VO_2 ratio is persistently less than 4 to 1, peripheral oxygen extraction increases, the difference between arterial (a) and venous (v) oxygen content (*ie*, $a-vDO_2$) widens, and mixed-venous oxygen saturation (SvO_2) falls in order to maintain aerobic metabolism. It becomes quite clear that the status of the overall DO_2/VO_2 relationship is reflected most accurately in the amount of oxygen remaining in mixed-venous blood (*ie*, SvO_2). Continuous SvO_2 monitoring by means of a fiberoptic pulmonary artery catheter is central to the modern management of ARF [8–10].

Carefully controlled laboratory investigation has clearly shown that VO_2 is independent of DO_2 as long as the DO_2/VO_2 ratio exceeds approximately 2:1 [7•,11•,12••,13]. Whenever the DO_2/VO_2 ratio falls below this critical value, a "physiologic" state of supply-dependent VO_2 occurs. This biphasic DO_2/VO_2 relationship exists at any "steady-state" level of VO_2. Supply-dependent VO_2 leads to anaerobic metabolism with the "pathologic" manifestations of lactic acidosis, hemodynamic instability, and eventually, if uncorrected, death. These relationships are shown diagrammatically in Figure 1.

The question of whether a state of "pathologic supply dependency" exists in critically ill patients with sepsis or adult respiratory distress syndrome (ARDS) remains controversial [14•,15•]. Proponents of the pathologic supply dependency theory contend that a pathologic defect in peripheral oxygen extraction exists in ARDS and sepsis. The "extraction defect" theoretically results in widespread tissue hypoxia and anaerobic metabolism. Although this is an elegant hypothesis, the supporting data are largely clinical and indirect, based on limited numbers of observations, fraught with methodologic and statistical inaccuracies, and perhaps most importantly, not substantiated by carefully controlled laboratory investigation [16•]. It has been our bias that supply-dependent oxygen consumption is indeed a pathologic manifestation of the normal

Abbreviations

ARDS—adult respiratory distress syndrome; **ARF**—acute respiratory failure; **CPPV**—controlled positive pressure ventilation; **$ECCO_2R$**—extracorporeal carbon dioxide removal; **ECLS**—extracorporeal life support; **IVOX**—intravascular oxygenator; **LFPPV**—low frequency positive pressure ventilation; **PC-IRV**—pressure controlled inverse ratio ventilation; **PEEP**—positive end-expiratory pressure; **PIP**—peak inspiratory pressure.

 ISBN 1-85922-671-X ISSN 1065–6243

Table 1. Oxygen kinetics formulas and terms

Formulas

$CaO_2 = (Hgb \times SaO_2 \times 1.36) + (.0031 \times PaO_2)$
$CvO_2 = (Hgb \times SvO_2 \times 1.36) + (.0031 \times PvO_2)$
$a - vDO_2 = (CaO_2 - CvO_2)$
$O_2ER = VO_2/DO_2 = (a - vDO_2)/(CaO_2)$
$DO_2 = QT \times CaO2$
$VO_2 = QT \times (a - vDO2)$
$DO_2/VO_2 = (CaO^2)/(a - vDO^2)$

Terms

CaO_2—arterial oxygen content, expressed in mL O_2/dL blood
CvO_2—mixed-venous oxygen content, expressed in mL O_2/dL blood
Hgb—hemoglobin concentration, expressed in mg/dL blood
PaO_2—arterial partial pressure of oxygen, expressed in mm Hg
PvO_2—mixed-venous partial pressure of oxygen, expressed in mm Hg
$a - vDO_2$—arteriovenous oxygen difference, expressed in mL O_2/dL blood
O_2ER—oxygen extraction ratio
DO_2—systemic oxygen delivery, expressed in mL $O_2/min/m^2$
VO_2—systemic oxygen consumption, expressed in mL $O_2/min/m^2$
QT—cardiac index, expressed mL/min/m^2

physiologic response to inadequate oxygen delivery [7•,11•,12••,13].

While the DO_2/VO_2 debate wears on, it has become quite clear that efforts to optimize systemic DO_2 are clearly warranted in critically ill patients. Recently, in a prospective study of 67 adult critically ill patients (54% with ARDS), Yu *et al.* [17••] reported a significant increase in mortality, an increase in the rate of subsequent development of ARDS, and a trend toward an increase in the rate of subsequent development of multiple organ failure in patients who were unable to achieve "supranormal" levels of DO_2 (*ie*, >600 mL/min/m^2). Although it is marred by a number of methodologic and statistical flaws, this study, as well as other recently published prospective series in ARDS [18], septic [19] and severely traumatized patients [20], is important because it emphasizes the need to focus upon optimizing DO_2 in critically ill patients. In addition, these studies suggest that failure to do so may actually increase morbidity and mortality.

The difficulty in interpreting studies of this type relates to the fact that the term *supranormal* DO_2 is meaningless unless one also reports a paired, independently measured VO_2 value for each value of DO_2. For instance, it may be that the "supranormal" DO_2 values were in fact normal if the individual patients were hypermetabolic at the time. Conversely, "normal" DO_2 values may have been profoundly "subnormal" if VO_2 was elevated, or "supranormal" if VO_2 was depressed (Fig. 1). This problem is resolved if one defines "optimal" DO_2 not as an arbitrary value but rather as that level of DO_2 that optimizes the DO_2/VO_2 ratio as reflected by the SvO_2 [8–10,16•] (Fig. 1).

The primary goal in the management of ARF must be to optimize SvO_2 and hence the DO_2/VO_2 ratio [7•]. DO_2 can be optimized by improving oxygenation, correcting anemia, and optimizing cardiac output. Techniques utilized to minimize VO_2 include treatment of infection, sedation, skeletal muscle paralysis, and active cooling if necessary. All interventions are carefully and logically titrated to ensure an optimal DO_2/VO_2 ratio based on continuously measured SvO_2.

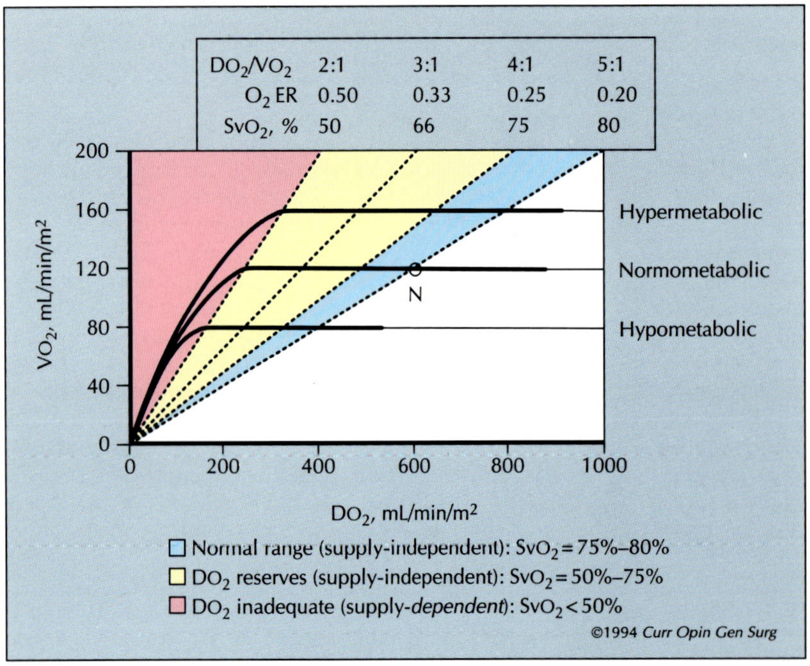

Fig. 1. Theoretic relationship of systemic oxygen consumption (VO_2) to oxygen delivery (DO_2) under various steady-state conditions of VO_2. DO_2/VO_2 ratios are represented by *isobars* corresponding to mixed-venous oxygen saturation (SvO_2). For completeness, the corresponding values for the oxygen extraction ratio (O_2 ER) are reported as well. Values assume 100% arterial saturation and no anatomic or functional arteriovenous fistula.

Mechanical ventilation

The optimal approach to gas exchange support in acute respiratory failure remains controversial. Most conventional techniques have utilized some form of controlled positive pressure ventilation (CPPV). Because CPPV is only supportive therapy, it is desirable that it not contribute to the ongoing pathophysiology of respiratory failure. The basic mechanisms responsible for ventilator-induced lung injury were recently reviewed by Parker *et al.* [21••]. Ventilation with high peak inspiratory pressure (PIP) clearly increases pulmonary microvascular permeability [22–25]. However, the large tidal volumes that usually accompany high PIP may contribute more to mechanical disruption of the alveolar-capillary membrane than high airway pressures *per se*. Hernandez *et al.* [26] were able to completely eliminate pressure induced increases in pulmonary microvascular permeability in rabbits using inspiratory volume limitation with a full-body plaster cast. Furthermore, recent electron microscopic studies by Fu *et al.* [27••] demonstrated that inflation to high lung volumes increases stress failure of pulmonary capillary walls regardless of the transmural pulmonary capillary pressure. Gattinoni *et al.* [28] as well as Shapiro and Bartlett [29] have suggested that when conventional tidal volumes (*ie* 10–15 mL/kg) are applied to the small residual component of functional lung in ARF, regional alveolar overdistention may result, thus exacerbating lung injury. Completely safe tidal volumes and PIP have not yet been identified. A common-sense approach to CPPV would be to manipulate tidal volume, inspiratory flow rate and inspiratory time to keep PIP as low as possible, certainly less than 40 cm H_2O.

The ideal level of positive end-expiratory pressure (PEEP) also remains controversial. PEEP prevents alveolar collapse at end-expiration, increases functional residual capacity, improves compliance, and reduces transpulmonary shunt. Comparisons of static pressure-volume curves and computed tomograms have suggested that the ideal level of PEEP may be closely related to the lower inflection point or knee of the pressure-volume curve as shown schematically in Figure 2 [28]. The inspiratory inflection point represents rapid recruitment of collapsed alveoli and hence improved compliance during inflation. The expiratory inflection point represents derecruitment or collapse of alveoli that fall below the critical closing pressure. Maintaining PEEP at least as high as the expiratory inflection point would thus appear to be a rational aim. Computed tomography has clearly demonstrated the dependent nature of radiographic densities in acute lung injury with preferential obliteration of air spaces in dependent regions of the lung [30]. Furthermore, Gattinoni *et al.* [31••] recently demonstrated that the application of PEEP leads to alveolar recruitment by opposing the compressive atelectasis that develops secondary to the hydrostatic pressure of overlying edematous lung tissue. These data also suggest that the maximal PEEP that should be applied to a supine patient to prevent compressive atelectasis should not exceed the ventral-dorsal height of the lung in centimeters (*ie*, the maximal hydrostatic gradient). However, increasing PEEP also increases mean intrathoracic pressure, thus reducing venous return and cardiac output and compromising systemic DO_2. Therefore, the application of PEEP should also be titrated based on continuous SvO_2 monitoring.

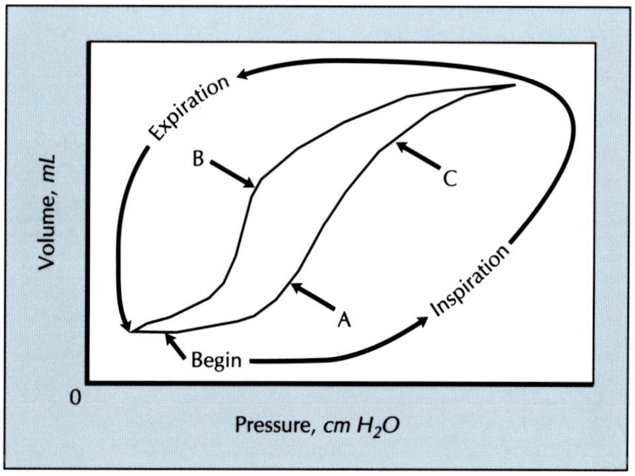

Fig. 2. Ventilatory pressure-volume relationships in adult respiratory distress syndrome are represented with an exaggerated hysteresis loop. Inflection *point A* represents the sudden recruitment of a large volume of collapsed alveoli during inflation. *Point B* represents the corresponding collapse of a large volume of alveoli during expiration as airway pressure falls below the critical closing pressure. *Point C* represents the upper inflection point of the curve where further increases in pressure result in minimal further increases in volume but may result in lung damage by regional overdistention of normal alveolar units. (*From* Swami and Keogh [82]; with permission.)

Pressure controlled inverse ratio ventilation (PC-IRV) has become popular in the treatment of ARF [32]. During PC-IRV, PIP is held constant, and the inspiratory/expiratory (I/E) ratio is lengthened by prolonging inspiratory time to more than half the respiratory cycle. Inspiratory gas flow decelerates as the airway pressure equilibrates during the prolonged inspiratory phase. These relationships are shown in Figure 3. By prolonging inspiration, PC-IRV allows more effective recruitment of collapsed alveoli and improved oxygenation at lower levels of PIP and PEEP. Proposed mechanisms include the development of intrinsic PEEP (autoPEEP) secondary to the shortened expiratory phase [33] and improved alveolar recruitment due to higher mean alveolar pressure maintained over a greater fraction of the respiratory cycle [34]. Increased mean airway pressure may also reduce cardiac output and oxygen delivery; hence, SvO_2 monitoring is essential during PC-IRV. Furthermore, PC-IRV is an unnatural breathing pattern and is not compatible with spontaneous respiration. PC-IRV generally requires heavy sedation and skeletal muscle paralysis. Its routine use is therefore limited. Finally, a reduction in mortality over conventional CPPV has not been demonstrated [32,35].

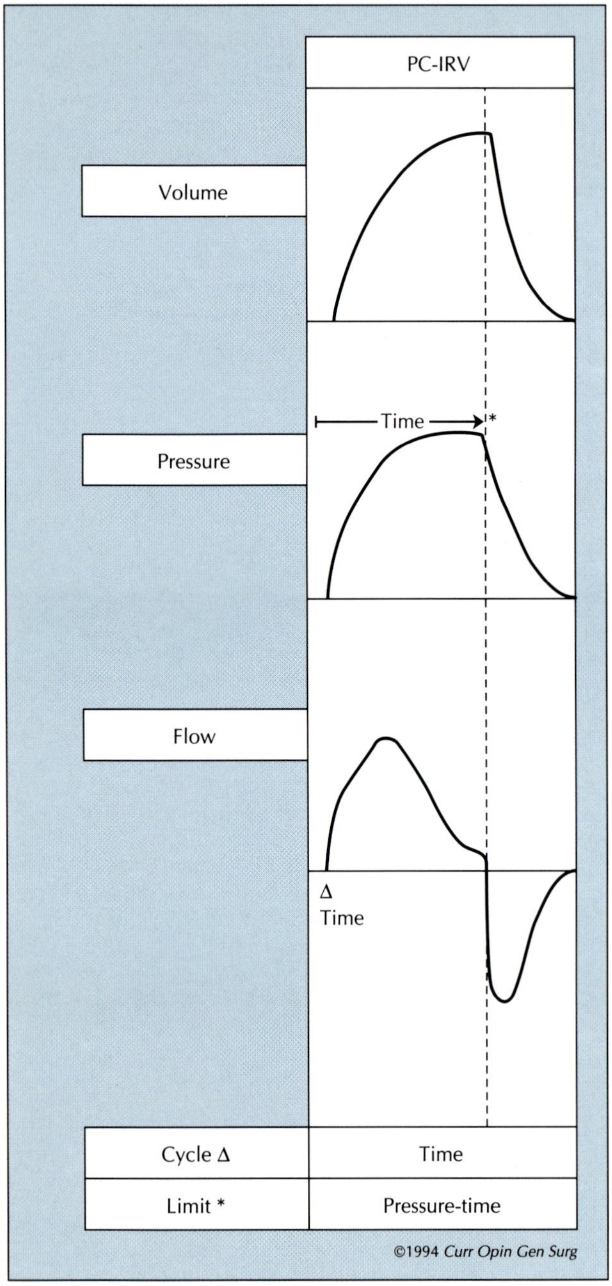

Fig. 3. Volume, pressure, flow, and inspiratory/expiratory ratio of pressure controlled inverse ratio ventilation (PC-IRV). *Cycle* refers to what initiates gas flow (*ie*, time-cycled). *Limit* refers to what stops gas flow (*ie*, pressure-time limited).

New approaches to mechanical ventilation include the use of continuous positive airway pressure, airway pressure release ventilation, high frequency jet ventilation, and intratracheal pulmonary ventilation. By maintaining increased airway pressure throughout the respiratory cycle, continuous positive airway pressure increases lung volumes while decreasing the work of breathing during spontaneous respiration. Airway pressure release ventilation employs a release valve which intermittently discharges airway pressure from higher to lower levels of continuous positive airway pressure, thus enhancing carbon dioxide clearance. Theoretic advantages of airway pressure release ventilation are that lung volumes are maintained and high PIP avoided while permitting spontaneous respiration with decreased work of breathing [36,37]. Its usefulness in the treatment of severe acute respiratory failure has not been determined. High frequency jet ventilation refers to the delivery of very small tidal volumes (< 100 mL) at very rapid rates (60–2000/min). Peak airway pressures are reduced, and alveolar ventilation is enhanced. No improvement in outcome has yet been demonstrated with high frequency jet ventilation, but improved gas exchange using ultra high frequency jet ventilation (3–6 Hz) has been demonstrated in at least one preliminary report [37–41]. Tracheal insufflation or intratracheal pulmonary ventilation refers to insufflation of fresh ventilating gas near the carina using a small catheter thereby reducing dead space ventilation and improving carbon dioxide clearance. This technique has been used successfully in newborn infants and is currently undergoing clinical trials [42•].

Adjunctive treatment modalities include the use of prone positioning, permissive hypercapnia, and aggressive diuresis to decrease extravascular lung water. Prone positioning improves oxygenation by diverting pulmonary blood flow from atelectatic posterior lung segments to better inflated anterior lung segments. Permissive hypercapnia refers to the use of pressure limited, low tidal volume ventilation to avoid high PIP while allowing arterial P_{CO_2} to rise [43]. Hickling *et al.* [44] recently reported a retrospective study of 50 patients with severe acute lung injury in whom PIP was limited to 30 cm H_2O, often necessitating the use of tidal volumes as low as 5 mL/kg. Arterial P_{CO_2} was allowed to rise, and PEEP was titrated to maintain adequate oxygenation. The overall survival rate was 84% in this series, and although this was an uncontrolled study, these results suggest that permissive hypercapnia can be used successfully in severe ARF [45]. Finally, aggressive diuresis and fluid restriction to reduce extravascular lung water has been shown prospectively to reduce ventilatory requirements, ventilator days, and days in intensive care [46••]. We have found continuous arteriovenous or venovenous hemofiltration to be particularly helpful in this regard.

Extracorporeal life support

Extracorporeal life support (ECLS) refers to the use of prolonged extracorporeal circulation achieved via extrathoracic vascular cannulation to provide support for patients with reversible cardiac or pulmonary failure. It is important to realize that ECLS is a supportive and not a therapeutic intervention. By providing for normal perfusion and gas exchange, ECLS theoretically helps to avoid the damaging effects of positive pressure ventilation for a period of days to weeks while allowing time for the injured lungs to heal.

Extracorporeal life support is accomplished by draining venous blood, providing adequate oxygenation or carbon dioxide removal, or both, with an artificial mem-

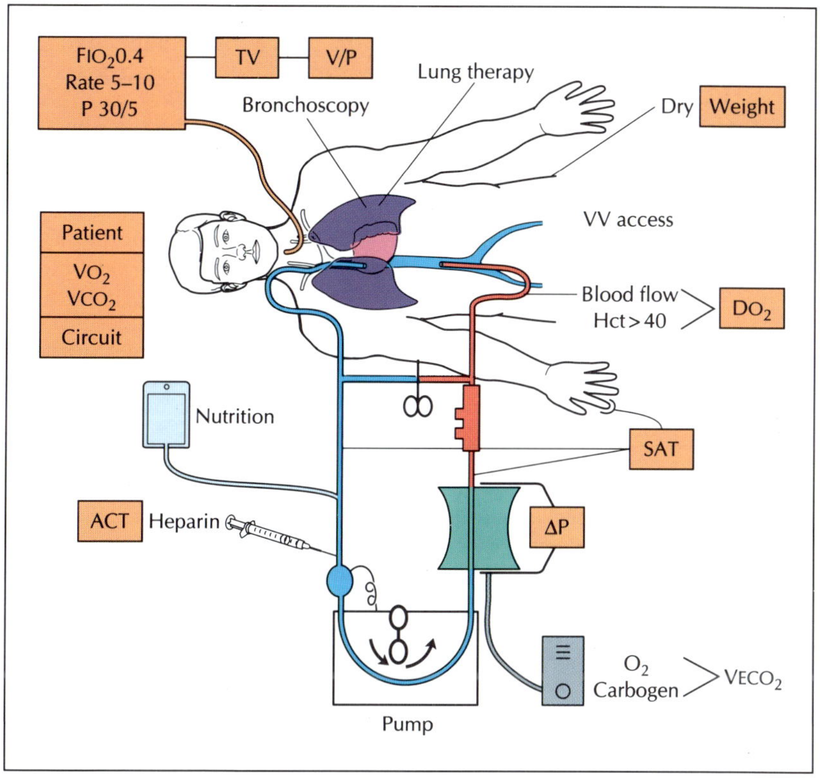

Fig. 4. Current patient management techniques during extracorporeal life support (ECLS) for acute respiratory failure. For venovenous ECLS, venous blood is drained via the right internal jugular vein, passes through a servoregulated pump, and then is perfused through a membrane oxygenator of sufficient size to provide total gas exchange. Perfusate blood then flows through a heat exchanger and is returned to the patient via the femoral vein. During venoarterial ECLS, oxygenated blood is returned via the right common carotid artery. Hemodynamic and metabolic parameters that are continuously monitored are contained within *boxes.* Mixed-venous drainage is represented in *blue*; perfusate blood is represented in *red.* ACT—activated clotting time; DO_2—oxygen delivery; FIO_2-inspired oxygen fraction; Hct—hematocrit; Δ P—pressure drop across membrane oxygenator; SAT—percent saturation of hemoglobin by oxygen; TV—tidal volume; VCO_2—carbon dioxide production; $VECO_2$—oxygenator outlet carbon dioxide concentration; VO_2—oxygen consumption; V/P—volume/pressure compliance; VV—venovenous. (*From* Anderson *et al.* [58••]; with permission.)

brane lung, and then returning the blood via a systemic artery ("venoarterial") or vein ("venovenous"). Detailed discussion of the various techniques, applications and results of ECLS have been the subject of several recent reviews [47•,48•]. Current ECLS management techniques are summarized in Figure 4. Suffice it to say that recent technical advances, such as safe and reliable surface-heparinized equipment and percutaneous vascular access, have ushered in an entirely new era in prolonged extracorporeal circulation [49,50,51••,52–54]. The overall results of ECLS for respiratory failure recorded in the registry of the Extracorporeal Life Support Organization as of July 1993, are summarized in Table 2.

Neonatal extracorporeal membrane oxygenation has been the most common clinical application of ECLS and is clearly the treatment of choice for neonatal respiratory failure refractory to conventional ventilator management. The use of ECLS in older children and adults was essentially abandoned in the United States in the late 1970s after a prospective, randomized trial, sponsored by the National Institutes of Health, of extracorporeal membrane oxygenation versus conventional treatment in adult respiratory failure demonstrated 90% mortality in both treatment and control groups [55]. Gattinoni *et al.* [56] first introduced the technique of extracorporeal carbon dioxide removal ($ECCO_2R$) combined with low frequency positive pressure ventilation (LFPPV) in 1986. Since that time, $ECCO_2R$ and LFPPV have been enthusiastically used in the management of adult respiratory failure refractory to conventional treatment; an overall survival rate of 47% was achieved in 264 patients treated in several European centers [57•].

Encouraged by these results, we initiated a phase I clinical trial of ECLS for cardiorespiratory failure in

Table 2. Results of extracorporeal life support for primary respiratory failure*

	University of Michigan		International registry	
Patient group	Cases, *n*	Survival, %	Cases, *n*	Survival, %
Neonate (0 to 14 days old)	428	87	8020	81
Pediatric (15 days to 17.9 years old)	64	47	567	48
Adults (>18 years old)	42	48	90	30
Total	534		8677	

**Data courtesy of* Registry of the Extracorporeal Life Support Organization, as of July 1993.

older children and adults. Results in the first 40 patients demonstrated an overall survival rate of 47% in patients with a 90% mortality risk (46% survival for ARDS patients) [58••]. Selection criteria used to identify patients with a 90% mortality risk included failure to respond to optimal medical management including time-cycled, pressure-limited ventilation, optimal PEEP based on $S\bar{v}O_2$, aggressive diuresis to dry weight, and efforts to maximize the DO_2/VO_2 ratio as reflected by continuous $S\bar{v}O_2$ monitoring. Additional inclusion criteria included a transpulmonary shunt of more than 30% on a fraction of inspired oxygen (FIO_2) greater than 0.6, static compliance of less than 0.5 mL/cm H_2O/kg, and diffuse bilateral (four quadrant) infiltrates on chest roentgenogram.

On the other hand, Morris *et al.* [59] recently reported a phase II prospective, randomized, trial comparing protocol driven ventilator management (PC-IRV) to LFPPV-$ECCO_2R$ for ARDS. There was no statistically significant difference in overall survival between the two groups, although the survival rate in the conventional treatment group was 42%, suggesting that conventional ventilator management techniques have improved for severe ARDS. The survival rate in the LFPPV-$ECCO_2R$ group was only 33% in this study, and although this was not statistically significant, the authors failed to undertake a preliminary phase I trial demonstrating safety and efficacy of ECLS at their institution. Conventional wisdom, as well as published data, would suggest a substantial learning curve exists for the use of such complex technology [48•,60]. In addition, recent advances such as percutaneous cannulation and heparin-bonded circuitry may dramatically reduce the risks of ECLS [49,50,51••,52–54]. Finally, the results reported by Anderson *et al.* [58••] suggest that low-flow $ECCO_2R$ may not be the best technique for *all* patients with severe respiratory failure being considered for ECLS.

Debate abounds as to the appropriateness of using costly, invasive, and as yet unproven technology in an era when cost-containment priorities have superseded responsibility for improving patient care. It is instructive to remember that in 1970, a neonate with severe respiratory failure secondary to meconium aspiration syndrome had a mortality risk of more than 90%; today, that same child (and his or her parents) can expect a nearly 100% chance of survival with appropriate application of ECLS techniques. Furthermore, late follow-up studies have demonstrated reduced overall costs and improved long term function in neonates treated with ECLS for acute respiratory failure [48•]. While the ultimate clinical utility of ECLS in the management of adult respiratory failure remains unknown, lessons from the past would suggest that these techniques are worthy of continued thoughtful study.

Liquid ventilation

Theoretically, liquid ventilation with perfluorocarbon has several potential advantages over conventional gas ventilation in the setting of acute respiratory failure. First, atelectasis and surfactant depletion are characteristic of the ARDS. Alveolar surface tension is markedly reduced with perfluorocarbon ventilation, suggesting that liquid ventilation may be more effective than gas ventilation in alveolar recruitment and hence may actually improve pulmonary compliance in ARDS. Furthermore, because pulmonary surfactant is immiscible in perfluorocarbon, further surfactant depletion is not promoted during liquid ventilation. Second, in ARDS the majority of pulmonary blood flow is diverted to dependent, consolidated lung units thus increasing transpulmonary shunt. During perfluorocarbon ventilation, pulmonary blood flow is redistributed to nondependent, well-ventilated lung units; this may result in improved ventilation-perfusion matching and decreased transpulmonary shunt. Finally, the alveolar hemorrhage and inflammatory exudate characteristic of ARDS not only contribute to gas exchange abnormalities but also promote lung injury and fibrosis. Lung lavage with perfluorocarbon during liquid ventilation may theoretically assist in removal of this inflammatory exudate and hemorrhage and thus improve gas exchange and attenuate lung injury and fibrosis. Shaffer *et al.* [61•] recently published an excellent review of this topic.

Recent experimental studies have demonstrated quite clearly that perfluorocarbon ventilation can provide adequate gas exchange in both normal and injured lungs. Using a closed-circuit volumetric technique to measure gas exchange and a flow-limited, time-cycled liquid ventilator, Hirschl *et al.* [62] have shown that systemic oxygen consumption and carbon dioxide production do not change during total liquid ventilation with oxygenated perfluorocarbon compared to conventional gas ventilation. Furthermore, in a model of severe respiratory failure, Tutuncu *et al.* [63,64] demonstrated long-term, dose-dependent improvement in gas exchange and reduction in mean airway pressure following intratracheal administration of perfluorocarbon in combination with conventional gas ventilation. In a similar model, Lachman *et al.* [65] noted that total perfluorocarbon liquid ventilation provided for improved gas exchange at lower mean airway pressures than conventional gas ventilation in a model of severe respiratory failure. Furthermore, Tooley *et al.* [66] demonstrated significant improvement in alveolar recruitment and static compliance during perfluorocarbon ventilation of atelectatic normal and surfactant depleted lungs. Finally, using a combined inflammatory (oleic acid) and surfactant-depleted (saline bronchoalveolar lavage) model of lethal respiratory failure requiring extracorporeal life support, Hirschl *et al.* [67] demonstrated improved gas exchange, decreased transpulmonary shunt, and improved compliance during total perfluorocarbon liquid ventilation compared to conventional gas ventilation. In addition, histopathologic examination of the excised lungs demonstrated marked reduction in alveolar hemorrhage, fluid accumulation and inflammatory cellular infiltrate in liquid ventilated animals when compared to conventional gas ventilated animals. Based on these data it seems quite clear that liquid ventilation, whether used alone or in combination with other pulmonary support techniques, has a promising future in the management of ARF.

Intravascular oxygenation

A potentially important recent advance in the management of severe respiratory failure has been the development of an intravascular oxygenator (IVOX) first described by Mortensen [68] and Mortensen and Berry [69]. The IVOX is a cigar-shaped bundle of 600 to 1000 microporous, polypropylene hollow fibers with a surface area ranging from 0.21 to 0.52 m^2 for the 7- to 10-mm diameter devices available for clinical use. IVOX is actually an intracorporeal hollow fiber membrane oxygenator implanted surgically into the vena cava. Oxygen is drawn (at subatmospheric pressure to avoid air embolism), through the device, which is capable of up to 81 mL/min of oxygen transfer and 67 mL/min of carbon dioxide transfer, according to previous animal studies [70].

Although the IVOX device has generated tremendous excitement, clinical results have been somewhat disappointing. Until recently, published data on the use of the IVOX in severe respiratory failure have been limited to case reports and small series of highly selected patients without appropriate controls, making attempts to ascribe benefit to this technique purely conjecture [71–74]. Nonetheless, High *et al.* [73] reported on five patients with severe ARDS treated with IVOX of whom only one survived. Interestingly, the authors measured oxygen and carbon dioxide exchange across the native lung simultaneously and were able to demonstrate that the IVOX was able to transfer a maximum of only 28% of overall metabolic gas exchange requirements. Recognizing these limitations, Zwischenberger *et al.* [71] utilized the technique of permissive hypercapnia to increase mixed-venous carbon dioxide concentration and hence the gradient for carbon dioxide transfer. This enhances carbon dioxide clearance by the IVOX device, allowing for further reduction in airway pressure, but it necessitates concomitant efforts to minimize the adverse effects of systemic acidosis.

Mortensen [75••] recently reported preliminary results from a phase I clinical trial, approved by the US Food and Drug Administration of the IVOX in 36 patients with severe respiratory failure from 18 centers. The data suggest that the risks and hazards of the IVOX are minimal, and while overall survival was only 30%, gas exchange was improved in 86%, and requirements for mechanical ventilator support were reduced in 83% of these patients. Thus, despite the lack of prospective, randomized data showing a definite advantage over conventional pulmonary support techniques, and in the face of disappointing overall survival statistics, the IVOX does provide predictable supplemental gas exchange and reduction in mechanical ventilatory support. The ultimate clinical utility of this device in the management of severe respiratory failure remains to be defined.

Pharmacologic therapy

Recent advances in the pharmacologic therapy of ARF include the use of nitric oxide and exogenous surfactant. In a preliminary study, Rossant *et al.* [76] demonstrated significantly decreased pulmonary artery pressures, decreased transpulmonary shunt, and improved oxygenation (PaO_2/FIO_2) without adverse systemic effects following administration of inhaled nitrous oxide in nine patients with severe ARDS. It seems clear from both clinical and animal studies that abnormalities of pulmonary surfactant play a significant role in the pathophysiology of ARDS [77–80]. Results from a prospective, randomized clinical trial evaluating the efficacy of aerosolized exogenous surfactant in patients with ARDS have suggested improved gas exchange and a trend toward decreased mortality [81]. The ultimate clinical utility of exogenous surfactant therapy in ARF remains to be determined.

Conclusions

Current state-of-the-art management of ARF depends on a thorough understanding of the physiology of systemic oxygen kinetics, with an emphasis on optimizing systemic oxygen delivery based on continuous mixed-venous saturation monitoring. Every effort must be made to minimize the damaging effects of high inflation pressures and regional overdistention of normal alveoli through the use of pressure-limited mechanical ventilation. Aggressive diuresis with strict attention to fluid balance should be used to minimize extravascular lung water. The use of PEEP to facilitate alveolar recruitment requires a thorough understanding of pulmonary mechanics and cutaneous mixed-venous saturation monitoring. For patients with refractory respiratory failure, the timely application of ECLS techniques in a qualified center may prove to be lifesaving. Finally, the future promises the increasing application of pharmacologic therapy for ARF as well as novel pulmonary support techniques including perfluorocarbon liquid ventilation and implantable gas exchange devices.

References and recommended reading

Papers of particular interest, published within the annual period of review, have been highlighted as:

- • Of special interest
- •• Of outstanding interest

1. •• DEMLING RH: **Adult Respiratory Distress Syndrome: Current Concepts.** *New Horizons* 1993, **1**:388–401.

A state-of-the-art review of concepts regarding the biochemical, molecular, and cellular mechanisms and mediators as well as the pathophysiology of ARDS. Excellent summary diagrams as well as a fairly complete list of important references.

2. WINDSOR AC, MULLEN PG, FOWLER AA, SUGERMAN HJ: **Role of the Neutrophil in Adult Respiratory Distress Syndrome.** *Br J Surg* 1993, **80**:10–17.
3. ST JOHN RC, DORINSKY PM: **Immunologic Therapy for ARDS, Septic Shock, and Multiple-Organ Failure.** *Chest* 1993, **103**:932–943.
4. BONE PM, BALK R, SLOTMAN G: **Adult Respiratory Distress Syndrome: Sequence and Importance of Development of Multiple Organ Failure.** *Chest* 1992, **101**:320–326.

5. BITTERMAN PB: **Pathogenesis of Fibrosis in Acute Lung Injury**. *Am J Med* 1992, 92:39S–43S.

6. DEITCH EA: **Multiple Organ Failure: Pathophysiology and Potential Future Therapy**. *Ann Surg* 1992, **216**:117–134.

7. • BARTLETT RH: **Critical Care**. In *Surgery: Scientific Principles and Practice*, edn 1. Edited by Greenfield LJ, Mulholland MW, Oldham KT, Zelenock GB. Philadelphia: JB Lippincott; 1993:195–222.

An excellent review of the basic physiology of systemic oxygen kinetics as it pertains to the clinical management of critically ill patients, with an emphasis on ARF.

8. BARTLETT RH: **Oxygen Kinetics and the Art of Physiological Monitoring**. *J Crit Care* 1993, **8**:77–79.

9. ZWISCHENBERGER JB, CILLEY RE, KIRSH MM, DECHERT RE, BARTLETT RH: **Does Continuous Monitoring of Mixed-Venous Oxygen Saturation Accurately Reflect Oxygen Delivery and Consumption Following Coronary Bypass Grafting?** *Surg Forum* 1986, **37**:66–68.

10. WHITE KM: **Completing the Hemodynamic Picture: SVO2**. *Heart Lung* 1985, **14**:272–280.

11. • SINARD JM, VYAS D, HULTQUIST K, HARB J, BARTLETT RH: **Effects of Moderate Hypothermia on O2 Consumption at Various O2 Deliveries in a Sheep Model**. *J Appl Physiol* 1992, 72:2428–2434.

In an ovine model, hypothermia was utilized to decrease Vo_2 in six sheep on total cardiopulmonary bypass. Do_2 was regulated by varying extracorporeal blood flow. Compared with normothermia, a similar biphasic relationship between Do_2 and Vo_2 was observed during hypothermia; however the critical Do_2 below which Vo_2 became supply-dependent was reduced in hypothermia.

12. •• HIRSCHL RB, HEISS KF, CILLEY RE, HULTQUIST KA, HOUSNER J, BARTLETT RH: **Oxygen Kinetics in Experimental Sepsis**. *Surgery* 1992, **112**:37–44.

In a canine model of septic peritonitis, Do_2 was regulated with controlled pericardial tamponade, and Vo_2 was measured independently by closed-circuit spirometry. Vo_2 remained independent of Do_2 as long as the Do_2/Vo_2 ratio remained greater than 2.4 ($Svo_2 > 42\%$). Below a Do_2/Vo_2 ratio of 2.4, Vo_2 became supply-dependent. This study is extremely important because it refutes through carefully controlled laboratory investigation the concept of continuous "pathologic" supply dependency in sepsis and ARDS.

13. CILLEY RE, SCHARENBERG AM, BONGIORNO PF, GUIRE MS, BARTLETT RH: **Low Oxygen Delivery Produced by Anemia, Hypoxia and Low Cardiac Output**. *J Surg Res* 1993, **51**:425–433.

14. • CAIN SM: **Oxygen Supply Dependency in the Critically Ill: A Continuing Conundrum**. *Adv Exp Med Biol* 1992, **317**:35–45.

An excellent review of the subject of pathologic supply dependency by a noted expert in the field of oxygen kinetics.

15. • KNOX JB: **Oxygen Consumption–Oxygen Delivery Dependency in Adult Respiratory Distress Syndrome**. *New Horizons* 1993, **1**:381–387.

An excellent review of the current status of the clinical Do_2/Vo_2 debate as it pertains to ARDS. Data reported favor the pathologic supply dependency hypothesis. Unfortunately, only clinical papers are discussed, and a large body of well-controlled experimental data to the contrary is ignored.

16. • BARTLETT RH, DECHERT RE: **Oxygen Kinetics: Pitfalls in Clinical Research**. *J Crit Care* 1990, **5**:77–80.

An excellent discussion of some of the methodologic and statistical problems which haunt clinical studies of the Do_2/Vo_2 relationship.

17. •• YU M, LEVY MM, SMITH P, TAKIGUCHI SA, MIYASAKI A, MYERS SA: **Effect of Maximizing Oxygen Delivery on Morbidity and Mortality Rates in Critically Ill Patients: A Prospective, Randomized, Controlled Study**. *Crit Care Med* 1993, **21**:830–838.

A prospective, randomized study of 67 critically ill patients randomly assigned either to treatment (supranormal Do_2 defined as >600 mL/min/m^2) or to control (normal Do_2 defined as 450 to 500 mL/min/m^2). There was no statistically significant difference in outcome between treatment and control groups; however, subgroup analysis revealed a significant increase in mortality and incidence of subsequent development of multiple organ failure in patients who failed to achieve supranormal Do_2. Unfortunately, paired, independently measured Vo_2 or Svo_2 values were not reported, making interpretation of normalcy difficult. However, this study is important because it points to the importance of monitoring and optimizing Do_2 in critically ill patients.

18. APPEL PL, SHOEMAKER WC: **Relationship of Oxygen Consumption and Oxygen Delivery in Surgical Patients With ARDS**. *Chest* 1992, **102**:906–911.

19. TUCHSCHMIDT J, FRIED J, ASTIZ M, RACKOV E: **Elevation of Cardiac Output and Oxygen Delivery Improves Outcome in Septic Shock**. *Chest* 1992, **102**:216–220.

20. BISHOP MH, SCHOEMAKER WC, APPEL PL, WO CJ, ZWICK C, KRAM HB, MEADE P, KENNEDY F, FLEMING AW: **Relationship Between Supranormal Circulatory Values, Time Delays, and Outcome in Severely Traumatized Patients**. *Crit Care Med* 1993, **21**:56–63.

21. •• PARKER JC, HERNANDEZ LA, PEEVY KJ: **Mechanisms of Ventilator Induced Lung Injury**. *Crit Care Med* 1993, **21**:131–143.

An inclusive review of the subject of ventilator-induced lung injury with an emphasis on carefully controlled clinical and laboratory investigation. Provides much of the scientific basis for the current state of the art in the use of mechanical ventilation. Superbly written, well-illustrated, and worthy of repeated careful study by anyone caring for patients with respiratory failure.

22. DREYFUSS D, GASSET G, SOLER P: **Intermittent Positive Pressure Hyperventilation With High Inflation Pressures Produce Pulmonary Microvascular Injury in Rats**. *Am Rev Respir Dis* 1985, **132**:880–884.

23. PARKER JC, TOWNSLEY MI, RIPPE B: **Increased Microvascular Permeability in Dogs Due to High Peak Airway Pressures**. *J Appl Physiol* 1984, **57**:1809–1816.

24. KOLOBOW TA, MORETTI MP, FUMAGALI R: **Severe Impairment of Lung Function Induced by High Peak Airway Pressure During Mechanical Ventilation: An Experimental Study**. *Am Rev Respir Dis* 1987, **135**:312–315.

25. TSUNO K, PRATO P, KOLOBOW T: **Acute Lung Injury From Mechanical Ventilation at High Peak Airway Pressures**. *J Appl Physiol* 1990, 69:956–961.

26. HERNANDEZ LA, PEEVY KJ, MOISE AA, PARKER JC: **Chest Wall Restriction Limits High Airway Pressure-Induced Lung Injury in Young Rabbits**. *J Appl Physiol* 1989, *66*:2364–2368.

27. •• FU Z, COSTELLO ML, KOICHI T, RENATO P, ELLIOTT AR, MATHIEU-COSTELLO O, WEST JB: **High Lung Volume Increases Stress Failure in Pulmonaries**. *J Appl Physiol* 1993, **73**:123–133.

Light and electron microscopic studies of *in situ* perfused rabbit lungs demonstrating increased stress failure of the pulmonary capillary endothelium and epithelium following inflation to high lung volumes. Elucidates the microvascular mechanisms responsible for the increased permeability noted following ventilation with increased peak inspiratory pressures. This study sheds considerable light on the concept of "volutrauma" and emphasizes the importance of avoiding alveolar overdistention in regions of normal lung during mechanical ventilation for ARF.

28. GATTINONI L, PESENTI A, AVALLI L, ROSSI F, BOMBINO M: **Pressure-Volume Curve of Total Respiratory System in Acute Respiratory Failure: A Computed Tomographic Study**. *Am Rev Respir Dis* 1987, **136**:730–736.

29. SHAPIRO MB, BARTLETT RH: **Pulmonary Compliance and Mechanical Ventilation**. *Arch Surg* 1992, **127**:485–486.

30. GATTINONI L, PELOSI P, VITALE G, PESENTI A, D'ANDREA L, MASHERONI D: **Body Position Changes Redistribute Lung Computed Tomographic Density in Patients With Acute Respiratory Failure**. *Anesthesiology* 1991, 74:15–29.

31. •• GATTINONI L, D'ANDREA L, PELOSI P, VITALE G, PESENTI A, FUMAGALLI R: **Regional Effects and Mechanism of Positive End-Expiratory Pressure in Early Adult Respiratory Distress Syndrome**. *JAMA* 1993, **269**:2122–2127.

A superb clinical study of the mechanism of alveolar recruitment following the application of PEEP in patients with ARF. Computed tomographic scans were obtained and gas/tissue density studies performed at different levels of PEEP in mechanically ventilated patients with ARF. PEEP appears to recruit alveoli simply by counteracting the hydrostatic pressure of overlying edematous lung tissue, which usually leads to compressive atelectasis of dependent lung units.

32. MARCY TW, MARINI JJ: **Inverse Ratio Ventilation in ARDS: Rationale and Implementation**. *Chest* 1991, **100**:494–504.

33. EAST TD, BOHM SH, WALLACE CJ, CLEMMER TP, WEAVER LK, ORME JR JR, MORRIS AH: **A Successful Computerized Protocol for Clinical Management of Pressure Control Inverse Ratio Ventilation in ARDS Patients**. *Chest* 1992, **101**:697–710.

34. MANTHOUS CA, SCHMIDT GA: **Inverse Ratio Ventilation in ARDS. Improved Oxygenation Without AutoPEEP**. *Chest* 1993, **103**:953–954.

35. MACNAUGHTON PD, EVANS TW: **Management of Adult Respiratory Distress Syndrome**. *Lancet* 1992, **339**:469–472.

36. FALKENHAIN SK, REILLEY TE, GREGORY JS: **Improvement in Cardiac Output During Airway Pressure Release Ventilation**. *Crit Care Med* 1992, **20**:1358–1360.

37. JOUSELA I, LINKO K, MAKELAINEN A: **A Comparison of Continuous Positive Pressure Ventilation, Combined High Frequency Ventilation and Airway Pressure Release Ventilation on Experimental Lung Injury**. *Intensive Care Med* 1992, **18**:299–303.

38. GLUCK E, HEARD S, PATEL C, MOHR J, CALKINS J: **Use of Ultrahigh Frequency Ventilation in Patients With ARDS: A Preliminary Report**. *Chest* 1993, **103**:1413–1420.

39. QUAN SF, OTTO CW: **Ultrahigh Frequency Ventilation: Nouvelle Ventilation or Just Old Hash? [Editorial; Comment]**. *Chest* 1993, **103**:1313–1314.

40. Lichtwarck-Aschoff M, Nielsen JB, Sjostrand UH, Edgren EL: **An Experimental Randomized Study of Five Different Ventilatory Modes in a Piglet Model of Severe Respiratory Distress.** *Intensive Care Med* 1992, **18**:339–347.

41. Hurst JM, Branson RD, Davis K, Barrette RR, Adams KS: **Comparison of Conventional Ventilation and High Frequency Jet Ventilation.** *Ann Surg* 1990, **211**:486–491.

42. Wilson JM, Thompson JR, Schnitzer JJ, Bower LK, Lillehei CW,
• Perlman ND, Kolobow T: **Intratracheal Pulmonary Ventilation and Congenital Diaphragmatic Hernia: A Report of 2 Cases.** *J Pediatr Surg* 1993, **28**:484–487.
This is the first clinical report of the use of intratracheal pulmonary ventilation and is worthy of study if only for that reason. Both the technique and the theoretic basis for the use of intratracheal pulmonary ventilation are discussed. It appears that intratracheal pulmonary ventilation is likely to find its greatest usefulness in neonates in whom the conducting airways constitute a significant fraction of the tidal volume.

43. Reynolds EM, Ryan DP, Doody DP: **Permissive Hypercapnia and Pressure-Controlled Ventilation as Treatment of Severe Adult Respiratory Distress Syndrome in a Pediatric Burn Patient.** *Crit Care Med* 1993, **21**:944–947. [Corrected and republished article originally printed in *Crit Care Med* 1993, **21**:468–471.]

44. Hickling KG, Henderson SJ, Jackson R: **Low Mortality Associated With Low Volume Pressure Limited Ventilation With Permissive Hypercapnia in Severe Adult Respiratory Distress Syndrome.** *Intensive Care Med* 1990, **16**:372–377.

45. Hickling KG: **Ventilatory Management of ARDS: Can It Affect Outcome?** *Intensive Care Med* 1990, **16**:219–226.

46. Mitchell JP, Schuller D, Calandrino FS, Schuster DP: **Improved
•• Outcome Based on Fluid Management in Critically Ill Patients Requiring Pulmonary Artery Catheterization.** *Am Rev Respir Dis* 1992, **145**:990–998.
A prospective, randomized trial of patients with pulmonary edema to determine whether a fluid management protocol which emphasized aggressive diuresis and fluid restriction to reduce indicator-dilution determined extravascular lung water. In patients randomized to the extravascular long water reduction protocol, extravascular lung water decreased and ventilator and days spent in intensive care were significantly reduced. This study provides prospective data to support a policy of aggressive attempts to minimize extravascular lung water in patients with ARF through the liberal use of diuretics and fluid restriction.

47. Shanley CJ, Bartlett RH: **Extracorporeal Life Support: Techniques,
• Indications and Results.** In *Current Surgical Therapy.* Edited by Cameron JL. St. Louis: Mosby Yearbook/BC Decker; 1993:1062–1066.
An excellent review of the basic physiology and techniques of ECLS as well as the current status and results of ECLS for cardiorespiratory failure.

48. Custer JR, Bartlett RH: **Recent Research in Extracorporeal Life Sup-
• port.** *ASAIO Trans* 1992, **38**:754–770.
An inclusive review of the current literature pertaining to ECLS with an emphasis on ECLS for ARF.

49. Fjalldal O, Torfason B, Onundarson PT, Thorsteinsson A, Vigfusson G, Stefansson T, Magnusson V: **Prolonged Total Extracorporeal Lung Assistance Without Systemic Heparinization.** *Acta Anaesthesiol Scand* 1993, **37**:115–120.

50. Willms D, Dembitsky W: **Prolonged Extracorporeal Support for ARDS Using Surface-Heparinized Equipment.** *Chest* 1992, **102**:968–970.

51. Knoch M, Kollen B, Dietrich G, Muller E, Mottaghy K, Lennartz
•• H: **Progress in Veno-venous Long-Term Bypass Techniques for the Treatment of ARDS: Controlled Clinical Trial With the Heparin-Coated Bypass Circuit.** *Int J Artif Organs* 1992, **15**:103–108.
A prospective, randomized trial of 18 patients undergoing venovenous $ECCO_2R$-LFPPV for ARF. This study compared conventional to heparin-coated circuit components and demonstrated significantly less transfusion requirements, fewer bleeding complications, and improved survival in patients randomly assigned to the heparin-coated circuits. This study is important because it suggests that the use heparin-coated circuit components could significantly reduce the risk of hemorrhagic complications and may actually decrease mortality.

52. Rossaint R, Slama K, Lewandowski K, Streich R, Henin P, Hopfe T, Barth H, Nienhaus M, Weidemann H, Lemmens P: **Extracorporeal Lung Assist With Heparin-Coated Systems.** *Int J Artif Organs* 1992, **15**:29–34.

53. Brunet F, Mira JP, Belghith M, Lanore JJ, Schlumberger S, Toulon P, Dhainaut JF: **Effects of Aprotinin on Hemorrhagic Complications in ARDS Patients During Prolonged Extracorporeal CO2 Removal.** *Intensive Care Med* 1992, **18**:364–367.

54. Shanley CJ, Hultquist KA, Rosenberg DM, McKenzie JM, Shah NL, Bartlett RH: **Prolonged Extracorporeal Circulation Without Heparin: Evaluation of the Medtronic Minimax Oxygenator.** *ASAIO Trans* 1992, **38**:M311–M316.

55. Zapol WM, Snider MT, Hill JD, Fallat RJ, Bartlett RH, Edmunds LH, Morris AH, Peirce EC, Thomas AN, Proctor HJ, Drinker PA, Pratt PC, Bagniewski A, Miller RJ Jr: **Extracorporeal Membrane Oxygenation in Severe Acute Respiratory Failure: A Randomized Prospective Study.** *JAMA* 1979, **242**:2193–2196.

56. Gattinoni L, Pesenti A, Mascheroni D, Mardolin R, Fumagali R, Rossi F, Iapichino G, Romangoli G, Uzeil L, Agostino A, Kolobow T, Damia G: **Low Frequency Positive Pressure Ventilation With Extracorporeal CO2 Removal in Severe Acute Respiratory Failure.** *JAMA* 1986, **256**:881–886.

57. Gattinoni L: **Extracorporeal Support for Acute Respiratory Failure.**
• *Curr Opin Anesthesiology* 1992, 4:261–265.
This article represents the European experience and is the largest collective review of the use of $ECCO_2R$-LFPPV for ARF. The overall survival rate of 47% is impressive given the high mortality rate of this condition and emphasizes the need for continued careful study of this technology.

58. Anderson HL, Steimle C, Shapiro M, Delius R, Chapman R, Hirschl R,
•• Bartlett RH: **Extracorporeal Life Support for Adult Cardiorespiratory Failure.** *Surgery* 1993, **114**:161–173.
This study represents the first phase I (safety and efficacy) trial of ECLS for adult cardiorespiratory failure and represents the largest single-institution experience with adult ECLS in the United States. The 47% survival rate reported for 30 patients with ARF carrying a 90% mortality risk is very encouraging. This study clearly sets the stage for a multi-institution prospective randomized trial of ECLS for adult respiratory failure.

59. Morris AH, Wallace CJ, Menlove RL: **A Randomized Trial of PCIRV and LFPPV-ECCO2R for ARDS.** *Am Rev Respir Dis* 1993, in press.

60. Bartlett RH, Anderson HL: **Extracorporeal Membrane Oxygenation Revisited, Revisited [Letter; comment].** *Ann Thorac Surg* 1992, **53**:738–739.

61. Shaffer TH, Wolfson MR, Clark LC Jr: **Liquid Ventilation.** *Pediatr*
• *Pulmonol* 1992, **14**:102–109.
An excellent review of the status of perfluorocarbon liquid ventilation.

62. Hirschl RB, Glover B, McCracken M, Wolfson MR, Shaffer TH, Bartlett RH: **Oxygen Consumption and Carbon Dioxide Production During Liquid Ventilation.** *J Ped Surg* 1993, **28**:513–519.

63. Tutuncu AS, Akpir K, Mulder P, Faithfull NS, Erdmann W, Lachmann B: **Gas Exchange and Lung Mechanics During Long-Term Mechanical Ventilation With Intratracheal Perfluorocarbon Administration in Respiratory Distress Syndrome.** *Adv Exp Med Biol* 1992, **317**:401–407.

64. Tutuncu AS, Lachmann B, Faithfull NS, Erdmann W: **Dose-Dependent Improvement of Gas Exchange by Intratracheal Perflubron (Perfluoroctylbromide) Instillation in Adult Animals With Acute Respiratory Failure.** *Adv Exp Med Biol* 1992, **317**:397–400.

65. Lachmann B, Tutuncu AS, Bos JA, Faithfull NS, Erdmann W: **Perflubron (Perfluorooctylbromide) Instillation Combined With Mechanical Ventilation: An Alternative Treatment of Acute Respiratory Failure in Adult Animals.** *Adv Exp Med Biol* 1992, **317**:409–412.

66. Tooley R, Hirschl RB, Parent A, Bartlett RH: **Perfluorocarbon Ventilation Improves Alveolar Recruitment and Pulmonary Compliance in the Setting of Acute Respiratory Failure.** *FASEB J* 1993, **7**:A230.

67. Hirschl RB, Parent A, Tooley R, McKracken M, Johnston K, Schaffer T, Wolfson M, Bartlett RH: **Liquid Ventilation Improves Pulmonary and Gas Exchange During Extracorporeal Life Support.** *FASEB J* 1993, **7**:A229.

68. Mortensen JD: **An Intravenacaval Blood Gas Exchange Device (IVCBGED).** *ASAIO Trans* 1987, **33**:570–573.

69. Mortensen JD, Berry G: **Conceptual and Design Features of a Practical, Clinically Effective Intravenous Mechanical Blood Oxygen/Carbon Dioxide Exchange Device (IVOX).** *Int J Artif Organs* 1989, **12**:384–389.

70. Bagley B, Bagley A, Henrie J, Froerer C, Brohamer J, Burkhart J, Mortensen JD: **Quantitative Gas Transfer In and Out of Circulating Venous Blood by Means of an Intravenacaval Oxygenator.** *ASAIO Trans* 1991, **37**:413–415.

71. Zwischenberger JB, Cox CS, Graves D, Bidani A **Intravascular Membrane Oxygenation and Carbon Dioxide Removal-A New Application for Permissive Hypercapnia?** *Thorac Cardiovasc Surg* 1992, **40**:115–120.

72. Jurmann MJ, Demertzis S, Schaefers HJ, Wahlers T, Haverich A: **Intravascular Oxygenation for Advanced Respiratory Failure.** *ASAIO J* 1992, **38**:120–124.

73. High KM, Snider MT, Richard R, Russell GB, Stene JK, Campbell DB, Aufiero TX, Thieme GA: **Clinical Trials of an Intravenous Oxygenator**

in Patients With Adult Respiratory Distress Syndrome. *Anesthesiology* 1992, 77:856–863.

74. Conrad SA, Eggerstedt JM, Morris VF, Romero MD: **Prolonged Intracorporeal Support of Gas Exchange With an Intravenacaval Oxygenator.** *Chest* 1993, **103**:158–161.

75. •• Mortensen JD: **Intravascular Oxygenator: A New Alternative Method for Augmenting Blood Gas Transfer in Patients With Acute Respiratory Failure.** *Artif Organs* 1992, **16**:75–82.

Presents preliminary results of a phase I clinical trial of the IVOX in the management of adult ARF. Gas exchange was improved in 86% of the patients studied, but the IVOX is clearly not sufficient to provide total gas exchange support.

76. Rossaint R, Falke KJ, Lopez F, Slama K, Pison U, Zapol WM: **Inhaled Nitric Oxide for the Adult Respiratory Distress Syndrome.** *N Engl J Med* 1993, **328**:399–405.

77. Patton CD, Schulman ES: **Surfactant: Clinical Applications.** *Am Fam Physician* 1992, **46**:233–236.

78. Gregory GA, Phibbs RH: **Surfactant Replacement for Respiratory Failure: Lessons From the Neonate [Editorial; comment].** *Anesth Analg* 1993, **76**:465–466.

79. Seeger W, Gunther A, Walmrath HD, Grimminger F, Lasch HG: **Alveolar Surfactant and Adult Respiratory Distress Syndrome: Pathogenetic Role and Therapeutic Prospects.** *Clin Investig* 1993, **71**:177–190.

80. Pison U, Obertacke U, Seeger W, Hawgood S: **Surfactant Protein A (SP-A) Is Decreased in Acute Parenchymal Lung Injury Associated With Polytrauma.** *Eur J Clin Invest* 1992, **22**:712–718.

81. Lewis JF, Jobe AH: **Surfactant and the Adult Respiratory Distress Syndrome.** *Am Rev Respir Dis* 1993, **147**:218–233. [published erratum appears in *Am Rev Respir Dis* 1993, **147**:1068].

82. Swami A, Keogh BF: **The Pulmonary Physician and Critical Care: 2. The Injured Lung: Conventional and Novel Respiratory Therapy.** *Thorax* 1992, **47**:555–562.

Charles J. Shanley, MD, and Robert H. Bartlett, MD, 1500 East Medical Center Drive, 2918 Taubman Center, Box 0331, Ann Arbor, MI 48109-0331, USA.

Evaluation of hepatic function

Kazue Ozawa, MD,* Keiichiro Mori, MD,† and Taisuke Morimoto, MD†

*Shiga University of Medical Science, Shiga, and †Kyoto University, Kyoto, Japan

Nine articles published since January 1992 on new methods of evaluating hepatic function are reviewed. These articles described the clinical significance of blood levels of cytokines, fibrin- or fibrinogen-related antigens, vitronectin, and endothelin, and of magnetic resonance spectroscopy, methionine metabolism, vasopressin clearance, vascular compliance, and radioreceptor imaging in gastroenterology. None of the methods have yet been applied to surgery. In addition, the redox theory, the evaluation of hepatic mitochondrial redox potential by arterial ketone body ratio and its clinical application, is introduced, and recent publications on the assessment of graft viability in liver transplantation and preoperative hepatic functional reserve in liver surgery based on the theory are reviewed.

Current Opinion in General Surgery 1994:17–23

Rarely does the normal liver critically deteriorate after an operation—this resiliency results from its large functional reserve. Surgical intervention in patients with liver disease, by contrast, usually carries considerable risk; hence, methods of evaluating preoperative hepatic function or functional reserve have been developed. Among them are the well-known Child-Turcott classification [1] and its modification, the Child-Pugh criteria [2], which determine surgical indication for portosystemic shunt in patients with esophageal varices. Because recent progress in endoscopic treatments has enabled surgeons to ligate or sclerose the varices, thus reducing their clinical significance in surgical treatment for portal hypertension, the preoperative assessment of hepatic function has focused on liver surgery, especially the difficult cirrhotic liver resection.

In this article, we review new tests or indicators for evaluating hepatic function that have been published since January 1992 and will be applicable to the surgical candidate. In addition, we introduce and discuss the noninvasive evaluation of hepatic mitochondrial redox potential, based on the arterial ketone body ratio (AKBR) and the redox theory.

New hepatic function tests

The parameters and tests reviewed here were published in the field of gastroenterology and have yet to be applied to surgery. Because these methods depend on recent progress in the medical and biologic sciences, however, they contribute to the preoperative evaluation of hepatic function in surgery.

Cytokines

Cytokines are bioactive polypeptides that show a wide spectrum of regulation in the inflammatory, metabolic, hematopoietic, and immunologic processes. Because the liver is an important site of synthesis and clearance for several cytokines, liver diseases may induce changes in blood cytokine levels. Tilg *et al.* [3•] studied serum levels, four kinds of cytokines, interleukin-1β, interleukin-6, tumor necrosis factor-α (TNF-α), and interferon gamma, and one acute-phase reactant of C-reactive protein in 264 patients with various chronic liver diseases. The results showed significant elevation of levels of interleukin-1β, interleukin-6, TNF, interferon gamma, and C-reactive protein in patients with chronic liver disease, regardless of etiology of the underlying liver disease. Moreover, the cirrhotic group of chronic liver disease patients had significantly higher serum interleukin-1β, interleukin-6, TNF-α, and C-reactive protein levels than did the noncirrhotic group. The authors discussed the possibility that the phenomenon of enhanced endogenous cytokines in chronic liver disease is a consequence of chronic liver failure that leads to enhanced endogenous endotoxin levels and decreased cytokine clearance. As expected, surgical patients are risky candidates when they show preoperatively high levels of proinflammatory cytokines, especially interleukin-1β and TNF-α.

Abbreviations

AKBR—arterial ketone body ratio; **ASGP-R**—asialoglycoprotein receptor; **RTI**—redox tolerance index; **TNF-α**—tumor necrosis factor-α.

 ISBN 1-85922-671-X ISSN 1065–6243

Fibrin-related and fibrinogen-related antigens

Because patients with liver disease show various types of coagulopathy, Kruskal *et al.* [4•] measured the levels and proportions of the total fibrin- and fibrinogen-related antigens in 50 patients with liver disease and 25 healthy control subjects. Fibrin- and fibrinogen-related antigens were extracted from serum and were subjected to sodium dodecylsulfate–polyacrylamide gel electrophoresis. Their proportions and levels were determined by densitometry and radioimmunoassay, respectively. Total fibrin- and fibrinogen-related antigens and D-dimer levels were significantly higher in patients with liver cirrhosis and hepatocellular carcinoma than in patients with acute viral hepatitis and in control subjects.

Although the methods to determine fibrin- and fibrinogen-related antigens are somewhat complicated, they may provide a new approach to coagulopathy in chronic liver disease.

Vitronectin

Vitronectin is a cell-adhesive glycoprotein distributed in the connective tissue and plasma. Inuzuka *et al.* [5•] measured plasma vitronectin concentrations in 136 patients with various liver diseases and 24 healthy control subjects. In patients with cirrhosis and hepatocellular carcinoma, plasma vitronectin levels were significantly lower than those of control subjects. Furthermore, the plasma vitronectin level was positively correlated with the levels of serum cholinesterase, albumin, plasma α_2 plasmin inhibitor–plasmin complex and the prothrombin time and results of the hepaplastin test. The authors concluded that the plasma vitronectin level could be a good clinical indicator of the severity of chronic liver disease.

Endothelin

Endothelin is a 21-amino-acid polypeptide that possesses a strong vasoconstricting effect. The plasma endothelin level is elevated in various diseases, such as renal failure, cardiogenic shock, sepsis, hypertension, acute myocardial infarction, and subarachnoid hemorrhage. Uchihara *et al.* [6•] compared plasma endothelin concentrations in 35 patients with chronic liver diseases, with those of 14 control subjects. The plasma endothelin levels were significantly higher in patients with cirrhosis with ascites than in patients with chronic hepatitis, patients with cirrhosis without ascites, and control subjects. In patients with cirrhosis, the plasma endothelin concentration showed a significant negative correlation with creatinine clearance. Furthermore, the plasma endothelin levels were significantly higher in patients with endotoxemia than in those without. Decompensated cirrhosis may be revealed by an elevated plasma endothelin level, which is related to kidney dysfunction and endotoxemia.

Dynamic ^{31}P spectroscopy after fructose loading

Magnetic resonance spectroscopy is a potential means of directly assessing the metabolism *in vivo*, noninvasively, and in real time. Dufour *et al.* [7•] studied the responses through ^{31}P magnetic resonance spectroscopy to a fructose load in nine patients with nonalcoholic cirrhosis and in six healthy subjects. After intravenous injection of fructose, the formation of monophosphate esters and utilization of inorganic phosphate were significantly lower in cirrhotic patients than in normal volunteers. Furthermore, these changes were correlated with results in the galactose-elimination capacity test. For these reasons, dynamic ^{31}P magnetic resonance spectroscopy is a noninvasive and clinically feasible test to analyze the pathophysiologic metabolic disorder in liver cirrhosis.

Methionine metabolism

Because about half of the methionine, an essential amino acid, is metabolized by the liver, cirrhotic patients sometimes show deterioration in methionine clearance. Marchesini *et al.* [8•] compared methionine plasma clearance in 12 patients with cirrhosis with that of six control subjects during steady-state conditions obtained by a primed, continuous methionine infusion. Methionine plasma clearance was significantly lower in cirrhotic patients than in control subjects, and fasting methionine levels were significantly correlated with methionine clearance. In addition, in cirrhotic patients, methionine plasma clearance was significantly correlated with galactose elimination capacity and with the Child-Pugh score.

Impaired methionine metabolism and hypermethioninemia may be an indicator of liver cell dysfunction, although this can be replaced by the conventional parameters such as galactose elimination capacity and the Child-Pugh score.

Vasopressin clearance

Patients with decompensated cirrhosis frequently show water imbalance and elevated plasma levels of antidiuretic hormone. Solis-Herruzo *et al.* [9•] measured metabolic clearance rate and half-time of arginine vasopressin in 43 cirrhotic patients and 10 control subjects. After intravenous infusion of arginine vasopressin, the metabolic clearance rate was significantly reduced, and the half-time of arginine vasopressin was significantly increased in patients with cirrhosis, particularly in accordance with the severity of cirrhosis. Changes in metabolic clearance rate and half-time of arginine vasopressin were correlated with the liver dysfunction score, prothrombin activity, and levels of serum albumin and bilirubin, but not with the parameters of kidney function. Impaired antidiuretic hormone catabolism may be another factor leading to fluid retention and to dilutional hyponatremia in cirrhosis and may reflect the degree of liver dysfunction.

Vascular compliance

Low arterial resistance and high cardiac index are the main explanations for systemic hemodynamic changes in cirrhosis. Because little is known about venous compliance in cirrhotic patients, Hadengue *et al.* [10•] measured total effective vascular compliance during acute volume expansion in 19 patients with cirrhosis and in four patients with mild chronic hepatitis as the control. Total effective vascular compliance was higher in patients with decompensated cirrhosis (n=8) than in those with compensated cirrhosis (n=11) and in control patients. The authors concluded that in patients with cirrhosis and severe liver failure, venous compliance is elevated and probably accounts for the blunted systemic and kidney effects of volume expansion. The methods used in this study were invasive and troublesome for surgical application, although the findings clarified interesting aspects of pathophysiology of the hemodynamic changes in cirrhosis.

Pharmacokinetic analysis of radioreceptor imaging of the liver

Asialoglycoprotein receptor (ASGP-R) is a hepatocyte surface receptor specific for galactose-terminated glycoprotein. Kudo *et al.* [11•] studied the three-compartment pharmacokinetic analysis of ^{99m}Tc–diethylenetriamine penta-acetic acid–galactosyl human serum albumin, which is a newly developed analogue ligand to ASGP-R, in 51 patients with chronic liver disease, 18 patients with acute liver disease, and six control subjects without liver disease. The concentrations of ASGP-R were significantly correlated with the clinical severity in chronic and acute liver disease and were also correlated with conventional liver function tests in both liver disease groups. The ASGP-R concentration may be a sensitive parameter of functioning hepatocyte mass in acute and chronic liver disease.

This radioreceptor imaging analysis is quite new, but whether it can provide additional information to the conventional indicators, including the galactose elimination capacity test, is uncertain.

Before applying any of these new hepatic function tests to the preoperative evaluation of the surgical patient, we have to consider several important points: 1) the conceptual originality of the test, 2) its methodologic feasibility, 3) the degree of invasiveness to the patient, and 4) the economic problem. For example, ^{31}P magnetic resonance spectroscopy, methionine clearance test, and ASGP-R analysis may not be superior to the galactose elimination capacity test or other clearance tests, because their results correlated with those of conventional tests, as noted earlier. In addition, the assessment of total effective vascular compliance is rather invasive to the surgical patient. Another important point is that the surgical risk to patients in child class B must be defined in detail because although child class A patients can safely tolerate even major hepatic resection, child class C patients frequently are risky candidates even for minor laparotomy. Hence, when clinicians select from among the new tests available for preoperative evaluation of hepatic function, they should consider these points of view.

Redox theory

Background

The regulation of mitochondrial ATP synthesis is a major determinant in the great number of metabolic reactions taking place in the cells because ATP synthesis by the mitochondria meets the demands for functional ATPase in normal cells. The overall process of electron transfer from respiratory chain substrates to molecular oxygen is in nonequilibrium to ensure adequate flow of electron and net ATP formation. This nonequilibriated character of oxidative phosphorylation derives from the NADH supplied from the tricarboxylic acid cycle and also from the final reduction of molecular oxygen to water. Thus, the ratio of NAD^+ to NADH with a concomitant NADH oxidation may be a very likely mode of regulation of the regeneration of ATP.

In the liver mitochondria, high endogenous levels of the enzyme β-hydroxybutyrate dehydrogenase make measuring liver mitochondrial NAD^+/NADH ratio and the ATP synthesizing ability possible. In a clinical study, the oxidized flavoprotein/reduced pyridine nucleotide (FP/PN) ratio in frozen liver tissue was compared with the ketone body ratio (acetoacetate/β-hydroxybutyrate) in the arterial blood taken simultaneously during operation in patients with liver damage: AKBR was closely correlated with hepatic tissue redox state [12••].

Another breakthrough came in experimental studies on liver damage in animal models, in which, under the suppression of ketogenesis by sufficient glucose load, a high degree of correlation existed between AKBR and hepatic energy charge. Through various trials, we demonstrated that after large-dose administration of glucose, AKBR is also closely correlated with mitochondrial redox state and hepatic energy charge.

The Oxi_{max} of AKBR shows the maximal capacity of mitochondrial NAD^+/NADH to increase during glucose oxidation of hepatocytes. In hepatic surgery and experimental models, a positive correlation was shown to exist between the changes in hepatic energy charge and the Oxi_{max} of AKBR. Based on these findings, we proposed the redox theory [13,14,15••,16]. The redox theory states that the decrease in energy charge, which occurs when the redox state of the liver mitochondria shifts from oxidation to reduction due to impairment, can be estimated from the AKBR. Investigation of these results has shown that normal hepatocytes maintain a much higher NAD^+/NADH ratio than is generally observed after glucose load in damaged hepatocytes.

Figure 1 shows the changes in metabolic stability, energy charge, energy substrates, and insulin/glucagon ratio to the Oxi_{max} of AKBR. When the AKBR increases above 1.0, the liver mitochondria oxidize glucose, and the hepatic energy charge is maintained above 0.80, while the biosynthesizing ability of the liver is enhanced. However, the ATP synthesizing ability of the mitochondria is enhanced maximally in the range of 1.0 to 0.7 of AKBR, probably because of the high secretion of Ca^{2+}–mobilizing hormones. With further decrease of the Oxi_{max} of AKBR to below 0.7, mitochondrial ATP synthesis decreases. With the decrease in hepatic energy charge, the biosynthetic pathways are inhibited. These findings suggest that the metabolism is stable at AKBR of 1.0, quasistable between 0.7 and 0.4, and unstable below 0.4.

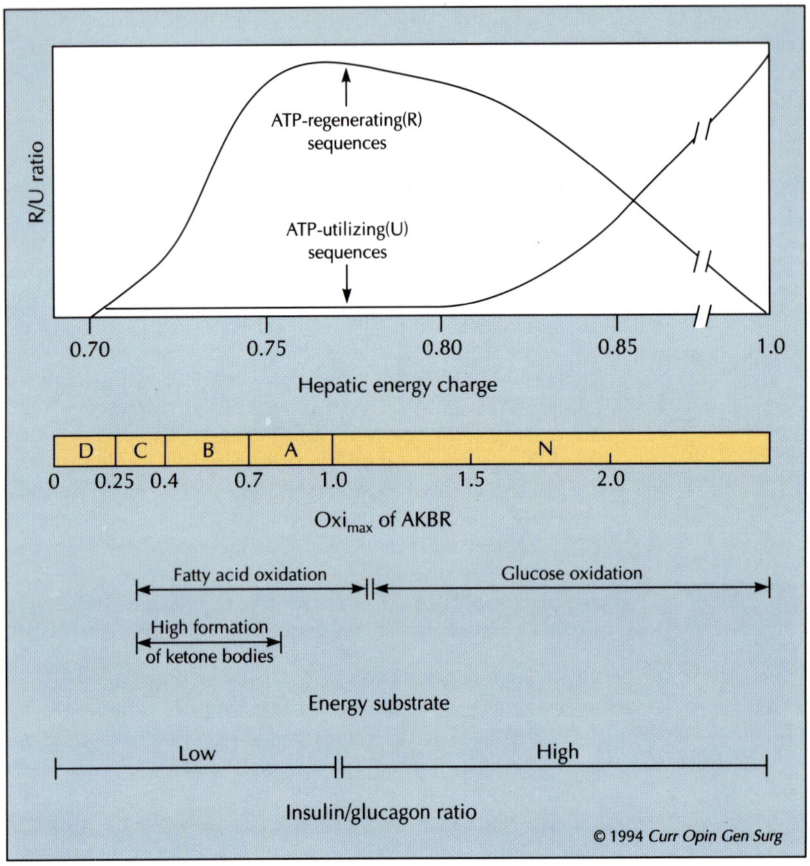

Fig. 1. Changes in metabolic stability, hepatic energy charge, energy substrates, and insulin/glucagon ratio in relation to Oxi_{max} of arterial ketone body ratio (AKBR). Oxi_{max} of AKBR shows the maximal capacity of mitochondrial $NAD^+/NADH$ to increase during glucose oxidation of hepatocytes. Energy charge=(ATP + 0.5 ADP)/(ATP + ADP + AMP). *A, B, C, D,* and *N* indicate patients grouped according to AKBR.

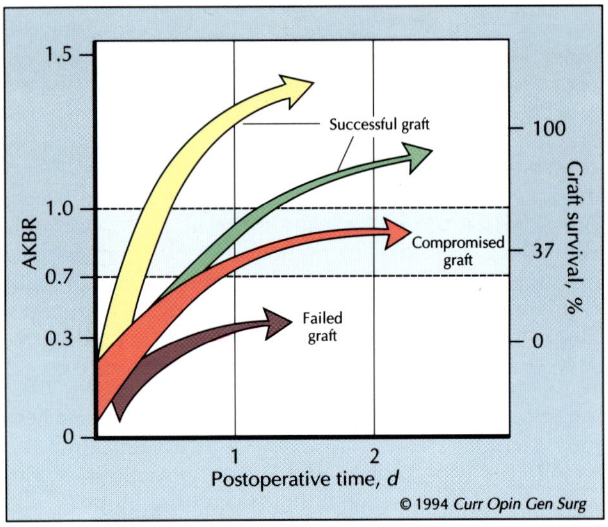

Fig. 2. Relationship between arterial ketone body ratio (AKBR) and graft survival in 615 patients.

Finally, let us consider the relation of AKBR to the cellular metabolism of other organs. When the AKBR decreases markedly to below 0.4, unphysiologic amounts of lactate accumulate in the blood because of impaired gluconeogenesis and cause a decrease in the pyruvate/lactate ratio. This leads to a decrease in the cytosolic $NAD^+/NADH$ of other organs in the body. The reduction of the cytosolic redox state in all organs induces wide-ranging derangements of the cellular energy metabolism, which is one of the most important factors leading to multiple organ failure. Lactic acidosis further deteriorates the ADP control transfer function by inhibiting both the efficiency and the rate of oxidative phosphorylation. This process leads to a loss of metabolic control, that is, a loss of ATP, and cell ion gradient, and ends in the death of membrane integrity and cells. Thus, the fact that the mitochondrial $NAD^+/NADH$ has a reciprocal effect on the kinase of liver pyruvate dehydrogenase renders this regulatory system an exceedingly sensitive mechanism of metabolic control. It is here that the significance of the redox theory becomes apparent.

Clinical application to liver transplantation

The investigation of AKBR in experimental liver transplantation revealed that the AKBR immediately recovered after reflow of the transplanted graft without preservation, whereas it could not recover in the preservation-damaged graft. Based on these results, the significance of AKBR has been investigated in the field of clinical liver transplantation. Joint research with several liver transplantation institutes abroad has shown that the rapid increase in AKBR after reperfusion of the graft is essential for successful liver transplantation, that AKBR is a good indicator for the assessment of the function of the transplanted graft, that the pattern of the

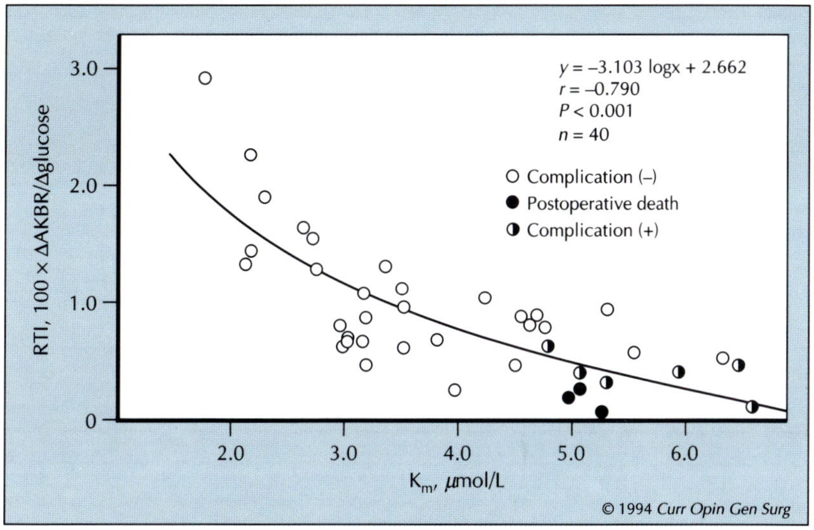

Fig. 3. Correlation between redox tolerance index (RTI) values and K_m of cytochrome *c* oxidase. AKBR—arterial ketone body ratio.

changes in AKBR can predict the outcome of the liver transplantation, that AKBR of the cadaveric donor can indicate the graft function and predict the short-term prognosis of the graft (Fig. 2), and that AKBR should be maintained at high levels in the donor to obtain a liver graft with high liver viability [17–20,21•,22••,23•].

Since June 1991, based on these results showing the high clinical significance of AKBR in the field of cadaveric liver transplantation, we have performed our living, related, partial liver transplantation protocol in children with end-stage liver disease, using grafts obtained from their parents. The AKBR of the donors was maintained in the normal range in all cases, and the AKBR of the recipients recovered to normal range within 48 hours after reperfusion of the transplanted graft. A postoperative decrease in the AKBR predicts certain trouble for the transplanted graft, such as portal or hepatic arterial thrombosis and hepatic vein occlusion, that may be lethal for the recipient. Thus, the clinical significance of AKBR has been demonstrated not only in cadaveric liver transplantation but also in pediatric cases receiving living, related liver transplantation [24,25,26••,27•].

Redox tolerance test

In an attempt to quantify the deterioration of hepatic mitochondrial energy metabolism, we recently developed a new test, called the *redox tolerance test*, to evaluate preoperative hepatic functional reserve based on the redox theory [28]. The indicator in the redox tolerance test or redox tolerance index (RTI) represents a 100-fold cumulative enhancement of AKBR to that of the glucose level (100 × ΔAKBR/ Δglucose) during a 75-g oral glucose tolerance test. The RTIs in patients with hepatocellular carcinoma, more than 90% of whom also had chronic hepatitis or cirrhosis, were significantly lower than those in patients with other hepatic tumors. We then analyzed the predictive value of RTI for assessing surgical risk in hepatectomy. Subjects were divided into three classes (class I, RTI > 1.0, or normal; class II, 0.5 < RTI < 1.0, or deteriorated; and class III, RTI < 0.5, or critical). Postoperative mortality was significantly different among the three classes in 127 hepatic resections. Furthermore, of 97 patients with hepatocellular carcinoma, major hepatic resections in class III patients resulted in significantly higher postoperative morbidity and mortality rates.

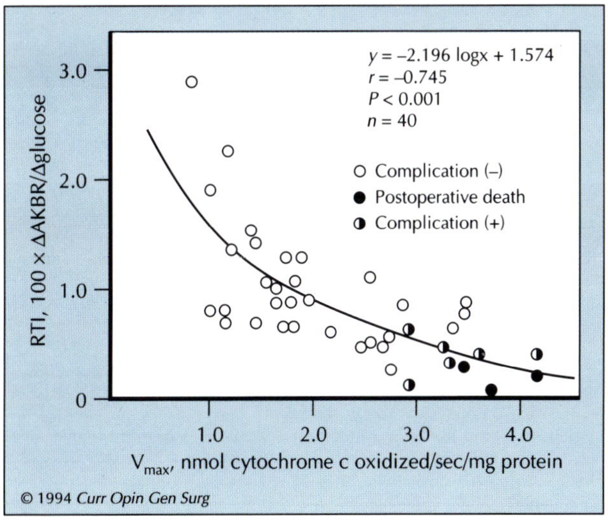

Fig. 4. Correlation between redox tolerance index (RTI) and V_{max} of cytochrome *c* oxidase. AKBR—arterial ketone body ratio.

We recently succeeded in demonstrating a direct relationship between the RTI and changes in enzyme activity of hepatic mitochondria in hepatectomy cases [29••]. Several previous reports from our laboratory showed that the amount of cytochrome a ($+a_3$) in the hepatic mitochondria is of predictive value for surgical risk in hepatectomy [30], and that the cytochrome *c* oxidase activity, which can be assayed by needle-biopsied material, correlates with the cytochrome *a* ($+a_3$) activity. Furthermore, V_{max} and K_m, parameters of the enzyme kinetics of cytochrome oxidase, can serve as one of the prognostic indicators of liver resection [31].

Therefore, we analyzed the RTI in 40 patients in relation to cytochrome *c* oxidase activity and hepatic energy charge. The RTI values in the liver cirrhosis group (n=20) and the chronic hepatitis group (n=12) were significantly lower than those in the normal liver group (n=8). Eight of 11 cases with RTIs below 0.5 (72.7%) showed postoperative complications. Subjects were divided into two groups: group A, RTI ≥ 0.5 and group B, RTI < 0.5. The V_{max} and K_m values of the cytochrome *c* oxidase in group B were significantly higher than those in group A. There were significant decreases in the concentrations of ATP and total adenine nucleotides and the energy charge level in group B compared with those of group A. The RTI values were negatively correlated with the K_m and V_{max} the values (Figs. 3 and 4, respectively). The RTI in the redox tolerance test can noninvasively estimate the cytochrome *c* oxidase activity of hepatic mitochondrial function and can be a useful determinant of the perioperative strategy for liver surgery.

References and recommended reading

Papers of particular interest, published within the annual period of review, have been highlighted as:

- • Of special interest
- •• Of outstanding interest

1. CHILD CG III, TURCOTTE JG: **Surgery and Portal Hypertension.** In *The Liver and Portal Hypertension.* Edited by Child CG III. Philadelphia: WB Saunders; 1964:50.

2. PUGH RNH, MURRAY-LYON M, DAWSON JL, PIETRONI MC, WILLIAMS R: **Transection of the Oesophagus for Bleeding Oesophageal Varices.** *Br J Surg* 1973, **60**:646–648.

3. • TILG H, WILMER A, VOGEL W, HEROLD M, NÖLCHEN B, JUDMAIER G, HUBER C: **Serum Levels of Cytokines in Chronic Liver Diseases.** *Gastroenterology* 1992, **103**:264–274.

Reports that serum levels of four kinds of cytokines, interleukin-1β, interleukin-6, TNF-α, and interferon gamma, were elevated in patients with chronic liver diseases. This phenomenon may be a consequence of chronic liver failure that leads to enhanced endogenous endotoxin levels and decreased cytokine clearance.

4. • KRUSKAL JB, ROBSON SC, FRANKS JJ, KIRSCH RE: **Elevated Fibrin-related and Fibrinogen-related Antigens in Patients With Liver Disease.** *Hepatology* 1992, **16**:920–923.

Reports that total fibrin- and fibrinogen-related antigens and D-dimer levels were significantly higher in patients with liver cirrhosis and hepatocellular carcinoma than those in patients with acute viral hepatitis and in control subjects.

5. • INUZUKA S, UENO T, TORIMURA T, TAMAKI S, SAKATA R, SATA M, YOSHIDA H, TANIKAWA K: **Vitronectin in Liver Disorders: Biochemical and Immunohistochemical Studies.** *Hepatology* 1992, **15**:629–636.

Reports that plasma vitronectin levels were significantly higher in patients with cirrhosis and hepatocellular carcinoma than in control subjects. The authors concluded that plasma vitronectin level could be a good clinical indicator of the severity of chronic liver disease.

6. • UCHIHARA M, IZUMI N, SATO C, MARUNO F: **Clinical Significance of Elevated Plasma Endothelin Concentration in Patients With Cirrhosis.** *Hepatology* 1992, **16**:95–99.

Reports that plasma endothelin levels were significantly higher in patients with cirrhosis with ascites than in patients with chronic hepatitis, patients with cirrhosis without ascites, and control subjects. Decompensated cirrhosis may be revealed by the elevated plasma endothelin level, which is related to kidney dysfunction and endotoxemia.

7. • DUFOUR JF, STOUPIS C, LAZEYRAS F, VOCK P, TERRIER F, REICHEN J: **Alterations in Hepatic Fructose Metabolism in Cirrhotic Patients Demonstrated by Dynamic ^{31}Phosphorus Spectroscopy.** *Hepatology* 1992, **15**:835–842.

Magnetic resonance spectroscopy showed that after intravenous injection of fructose, the formation of monophosphate esters and utilization of inorganic phosphate were significantly lower in cirrhotic patients than in normal volunteers. Dynamic ^{31}P magnetic resonance spectroscopy is a noninvasive test for the analysis of the pathophysiologic metabolic disorder in liver cirrhosis.

8. • MARCHESINI G, BUGIANESI E, BIANCHI G, FABBRI A, MARCHI E, ZOLI M, PISI E: **Defective Methionine Metabolism in Cirrhosis: Relation to Severity of Liver Disease.** *Hepatology* 1992, **16**:149–155.

Reports that methionine plasma clearance was significantly lower in cirrhotic patients than in control subjects, and that fasting methionine levels were significantly correlated with methionine clearance.

9. • SOLIS-HERRUZO JA, GONZALEZ-GAMARRA A, CASTELLANO G, MUÑOZ-YAGÜE MT: **Metabolic Clearance Rate of Arginine Vasopressin in Patients With Cirrhosis.** *Hepatology* 1992, **16**:974–979.

After intravenous infusion of arginine vasopressin, the metabolic clearance rate was significantly reduced, and the half-time of arginine vasopressin was significantly increased in patients with cirrhosis, particularly in accordance with the severity of cirrhosis.

10. • HADENGUE A, MOREAU R, GAUDIN C, BACQ Y, CHAMPIGNEULLE B, LEBREC D: **Total Effective Vascular Compliance in Patients With Cirrhosis: A Study of the Response to Acute Blood Volume Expansion.** *Hepatology* 1992, **15**:809–815.

Reports that total effective vascular compliance was higher in patients with decompensated cirrhosis than in those with compensated cirrhosis and in control patients.

11. • KUDO M, TODO A, IKEKUBO K, YAMAMOTO K, VERA DR, STADALNIK RC: **Quantitative Assessment of Hepatocellular Function Through In Vivo Radioreceptor Imaging With Technetium 99m Galactosyl Human Serum Albumin.** *Hepatology* 1993, **17**:814–819.

Pharmacokinetic analysis of ASGP-R showed that concentrations of ASGP-R were significantly correlated with the clinical severity of both chronic and acute liver disease and were also correlated with conventional liver function tests in both liver disease groups.

12. •• OZAWA K, CHANCE B, TANAKA A, IWATA S, KITAI T, IKAI I: **Linear Correlation Between Acetoacetate/β-hydroxybutyrate in Arterial Blood and Oxidized Flavoprotein/reduced Pyridine Nucleotide in Freeze-trapped Human Liver Tissue.** *Biochim Biophys Acta* 1992, **1138**:350–352.

Presents the linear correlation between AKBR and the oxidized flavoprotein/reduced pyridine nucleotide ratio in freeze-trapped human liver specimens obtained intraoperatively by the collaborative investigation conducted by the Kyoto and Pennsylvania University groups. The correlation indicated that the redox state of liver mitochondria regulates the first step of the mitochondrial electron transporting system.

13. OZAWA K, AOYAMA H, YASUDA K, SHIMAHARA Y, NAKATANI T, TANAKA J, YAMAMOTO M, KAMIYAMA Y, TOBE T: **Metabolic Abnormalities Associated With Postoperative Organ Failure: A Redox Theory.** *Arch Surg* 1983, **118**:1245–1251.

14. OZAWA K: **Biological Significance of Mitochondrial Redox Potential in Shock and Multiple Organ Failure: Redox Theory.** In *Molecular and Cellular Aspects of Shock and Trauma.* Edited by Lefer AM, Schumer W. New York: Alan R. Liss; 1983:39–66.

15. •• OZAWA K: *Liver Surgery Approached Through the Mitochondria: The Redox Theory in Evolution.* Basel: Karger; 1992.

Summarizes the principles of the redox theory, founded on basic research on the liver mitochondria, and its application to the clinical field, especially in liver surgery, including hepatectomy and liver transplantation.

16. OZAWA K: *Towards the Aggressive Surgery of Liver Cancer Based on the Redox Theory.* Tokyo: Nakayama Institute of Cancer Research; 1992.

17. TAKI Y, GUBERNATIS G, YAMAOKA Y, OELLERICH M, YAMAMOTO Y, RINGE B, OKAMOTO R, BUNZENDAHL H, BENEKING M, BURDELSKI M, BORNSCHEUER A, OZAWA K, PICHLMAYR R: **Significance of Arterial Ketone Body Ratio Measurement in Human Liver Transplantation.** *Transplantation* 1990, **49**:535–539.

18. ASONUMA K, TAKAYA S, SELBY R, OKAMOTO R, YAMAMOTO Y, YOKOYAMA T, TODO S, OZAWA K, STARZL TE: **The Clinical Significance of the Arterial Ketone Body Ratio as an Early Indicator of Graft Viability in Human Liver Transplantation.** *Transplantation* 1991, **51**:164–171.

19. OZAKI N, GUBERNATIS G, RINGE B, OELLERICH M, WASHIDA M, YAMAOKA Y, OZAWA K, PICHLMAYR R: **Arterial Ketone Body Ratio as an Indicator for Viability of Donor Livers.** *Transplant Proc* 1991, **23**:2487–2489.

20. OZAKI N, RINGE B, BUNZENDAHL H, TAKI Y, GUBERNATIS G, OELLERICH M, KUSE ER, KIUCHI T, YAMAUCHI K, TAKADA Y, YAMAGUCHI T, OZAWA K, PICHLMAYR R: **Ketone Body Ratio as an Indicator of Early Graft Survival in Clinical Liver Transplantation.** *Clin Transplantation* 1991, 5:48–54.

21. • TAKADA Y, OZAKI N, RINGE B, MORI K, GUBERNATIS G, OELLERICH M, YAMAGUCHI T, KIUCHI T, SHIMAHARA Y, YAMAOKA Y, SAKURAI K, OZAWA K, PICHLMAYR R: **Receiver Operating Characteristic (ROC) Analysis of the Ability of Arterial Ketone Body Ratio to Predict Graft Outcome After Liver Transplantation: Its Sensitivity and Specificity.** *Transpl Int* 1992, **5**:23–26.

Reports the high sensitivity and specificity of arterial ketone body ratio to predict graft outcome in clinical liver transplantation and compares this system with other routine liver function tests.

22. YAMAOKA Y, WASHIDA M, MANAKA D, GUBERNATIS G, RINGE B, OZAKI
•• N, YAMAGUCHI T, TAKADA Y, OELLERICH M, OZAWA K, PICHLMAYR R: **Arterial Ketone Body Ratio as a Predictor of Donor Liver Viability in Human Liver Transplantation.** *Transplantation* 1993, **55**:92–95.

Reports the significance of AKBR in cadaveric donors for liver transplantation. Indicates that grafts obtained from donors with high AKBRs are viable after liver transplantation, whereas those obtained from donors with low AKBRs have an increased risk of primary nonfunction in the early postoperative phase.

23. EGAWA H, SHAKED A, KONISHI Y, MCDIARMID SV, VARGAS J, SHIMAHARA
• Y, COLONNA J, MORI K, YAMAMOTO N, OZAWA K, BUSUTTIL RW: **Arterial Ketone Body Ratio in Pediatric Liver Transplantation.** *Transplantation* 1993, **55**:522–526.

Indicates that the rapid recovery of AKBR in pediatric liver transplantation results in a high survival rate, that AKBR decreased in the cases of early hepatic arterial thrombosis but gradually recovered, and that AKBR recovery was unlikely in cases of primary nonfunctioning graft.

24. MORIMOTO T, TERASAKI M, HIGASHIYAMA H, TANAKA K, UEMOTO S, TANAKA A, SHIMAHARA Y, MORI K, KIM HJ, KAMIYAMA Y, YAMAOKA Y, KUMADA K, OZAWA K: **Clinical Application of Arterialization of Portal Vein in Living Related Donor Partial Liver Transplantation.** *Transpl Int* 1992, **5**:151–154.

25. TAKADA Y, SHIMAHARA Y, MANAKA D, UEMOTO S, MORI K, TANAKA K, YAMAOKA Y, KUMADA K, OZAWA K: **Decrease in Arterial Ketone Body Ratio Indicating Graft Dysfunction After Liver Transplantation.** *Eur J Surg* 1992, **158**:317–319.

26. OZAWA K, UEMOTO S, TANAKA K, KUMADA K, YAMAOKA Y, KOBAYASHI
•• N, INAMOTO T, SHIMAHARA Y, MORI K, HONDA K, KAMIYAMA Y, KIM HJ, MORIMOTO T, TANAKA A: **An Appraisal of Pediatric Liver Transplantation From Living Relatives.** *Ann Surg* 1992, **216**:547–553.

The first report by the Kyoto group on the ethical grounds, concept, technique, and outcome in the protocol of living, related, partial liver transplantation in children with end-stage liver disease.

27. SHIMAHARA Y, AWANE M, YAMAOKA Y, TANAKA A, MORIMOTO T, MORI
• K, HIGASHIYAMA H, YAMAGUCHI T, KUMADA K, TAKADA Y, TANAKA K, UEMOTO S, OZAWA K: **Analysis of the Risk and Operative Stress for Donors in Living-Related Partial Liver Transplantation.** *Transplantation* 1992, **54**:983–988.

Reports findings on the operative stress placed on donors participating living, related liver transplantation performed by the Kyoto group. Indicates the safety of the donor operation in this protocol.

28. MORI K, OZAWA K, YAMAMOTO Y, MAKI A, SHIMAHARA Y, KOBAYASHI N, YAMAOKA Y, KUMADA K: **Response of Hepatic Mitochondrial Redox State to Oral Glucose Load: Redox Tolerance Test as a New Predictor of Surgical Risk in Hepatectomy.** *Ann Surg* 1990, **211**:439–446.

29. UEDA J, MORI K, SAKAI Y, TANAKA A, KATAYAMA T, MAKI A, SHIMAHARA
•• Y, YAMAOKA Y, OZAWA K: **Noninvasive Evaluation of Cytochrome *c* Oxidase Activity of the Liver: Its Prognostic Value for Hepatic Resection.** *Arch Surg*, in press.

Reports on the RTI as a parameter in the redox tolerance test, which assesses the preoperative hepatic functional reserve based on the redox theory. The RTI was shown to be directly correlated with changes in cytochrome *c* oxidase activity of the liver in patients with cirrhosis, in patients with chronic hepatitis, and in patients with normal livers. The RTI can noninvasively estimate the cytochrome *c* oxidase activity of hepatic mitochondrial function.

30. OZAWA K, YAMAOKA Y, KITAMURA O, NANBU H, KAMIYAMA Y, TAKEDA H, TAKASAN H, HONJO I: **Clinical Application of Cytochrome $a(+a_3)$ Assay of Mitochondria From Liver Specimens: An Aid in Determining Metabolic Tolerance of Liver Remnant for Hepatic Resection.** *Ann Surg* 1974, **180**:868–876.

31. SAKAI Y, TANAKA A, IKAI I, MAKI A, TAKAYASU T, YAMAOKA Y, OZAWA K, ORII Y: **Cytochrome *c* Oxidase Activity in Human Liver Specimens: An Index of Prognosis for Hepatic Resection.** *Arch Surg* 1990, **125**:632–635.

Kazue Ozawa, MD, Vice President, Shiga University of Medical Science, Seta-Tsukinowa-cho, Otsu, Shiga, 520-21 Japan.

Management of nutrition in the critically ill patient

Kenneth A. Kudsk, MD, and Gayle Minard, MD

The University of Tennessee, Memphis, Tennessee, USA

Many recent clinical studies focus on the critically ill or injured hypermetabolic patient and investigate nutritional factors and regimens that can potentially reduce septic complications and improve clinical outcome. In addition to better defining the amount and type of nutrients appropriate for this population, these studies provide insight into important variables such as route of nutrient administration, supplementation of formulas with immune-enhancing (or nonimmunosuppressive) nutrients, and anabolic agents that promote increased nitrogen retention and lean body mass accumulation.

Current Opinion in General Surgery 1994:24–29

The introduction of total parenteral nutrition (TPN) revolutionized the specialized nutrition support of hospitalized patients, a population at risk for progressive malnutrition as a result of injury, disease, or infection. TPN effectively reduces progressive lean body mass catabolism due to starvation either from gastrointestinal tract loss or the inability to eat, but it has not proven to be a panacea in the critically ill hypermetabolic patient. There is some concern that TPN might actually increase septic complications in certain patients. For example, the Veterans Administration Cooperative Study on perioperative nutrition [1••] demonstrated an increase in septic complications in mild and moderately malnourished patients randomly assigned to receive preoperative TPN for 7 to 15 days compared with control subjects who received no supplemental nutrition preoperatively. Significant reduction in nonseptic complications was demonstrated only in those patients with preexistent severe malnutrition.

Nutrient requirements in critical illness

Traditionally, the following Harris-Benedict equations have been used to estimate basal energy expenditure (BEE):

Men: BEE (kilocalories) = 66.47 + (13.75 × weight in kilograms) + (5 × height in centimeters) – (6.76 × age in years)

Women: BEE (kilocalories) = 655.10 + (9.56 × weight in kilograms) + (1.85 × height in centimeters) – (4.68 × age in years).

These formulas fall short of the energy needs of the critically ill; therefore, corrective factors for activity and stress have been derived to control for the increase in metabolism in these patients. Recently, indirect calorimetry has provided improved ability to monitor metabolic rate by measuring oxygen consumption and carbon dioxide production. Hwang *et al.* [2] prospectively studied 30 fasting, critically ill patients with sepsis or multiple trauma on mechanical ventilation 3 to 5 days after injury. The measured energy expenditure was correlated with several scoring systems of injury and disease to determine whether a relationship existed between actual metabolic needs and individual scores. In the 15 septic patients, the measured energy expenditure correlated best with the septic severity score (SSS), which measures seven key organ systems of the body and correlates well with hospital stay and prognosis (Table 1). The measured energy expenditure averaged 42.2 ± 2.6 kcal/kg with an excellent correlation between a low of approximately 25 kcal/kg for an SSS of 20 to a high of 50 to 60 kcal/kg for an SSS of 35 to 45.

The measured energy expenditure of multiple trauma patients correlated best with the injury severity score (ISS), a quantitative measure of diffuse body injury, averaging 34.9 ± 1.6 kcal/kg with a progressive increase from approximately 25 kcal/kg for patients with an ISS greater than 20 to a high of 40 kcal/kg for patients with an ISS of 40 to 50.

As a result of these studies, the authors suggested two new correction factors to better predict energy expenditure for septic or traumatized patients: 1) sepsis factor = 0.97 + 0.0125 × SSS, and 2) multiple trauma factor = 1.04 + 0.0077 × ISS. Multiplication of the BEE obtained from the Harris-Benedict calculation by these new stress factors in addition to the 1.2 activity factor more accurately assessed needs than the standard

Abbreviations

BEE—basal energy expenditure; **IGF-1**—insulin-like growth factor 1; **ISS**—injury severity score; **SSS**—septic severity score; **TPN**—total parenteral nutrition.

 ISBN 1-85922-671-X ISSN 1065–6243

Table 1. Levels of dysfunction in seven organ systems for determining septic severity score*†

	Rating of dysfunction				
System	1	2	3	4	5
Lung	O_2 by mask	Intubated; no PEEP	PEEP, 0%–10%	PEEP > 10%; Po_2 > 50 mm Hg	Maximal PEEP; Po_2 < 50 mm Hg
Kidney	CL, 1.5–2.5 mg/dL	CL, 2.6–3.5 mg/dL	CL > 3.6 mg/dL; adequate urine volume	CL > 3.6 mg/dL; urine volume, 20–50 mL/h	CL > 3.6 mg/dL; urine volume, 20 mL/h
Coagulation	Ecchymoses; PT, PTT, and platelet count normal	PTT, 45–65 s; PT, 12–14 s	Platelets, 20,000–100,000/µL; PTT > 50 s; PT > 14 s	Platelets, 20,000/µL; elevated PT and PTT	Increased FSP and euglobulin, bleeding
Cardiovascular	Slight hypotension	Livedo; moderate hypotension	Vasopressors, moderate doses	Vasopressors, large doses	Profound BP decrease despite vasopressors
Liver	LDH and SGOT increased; bilirubin normal	Bilirubin, 1.5–2.5 mg/dL	Bilirubin, 2.6–4.0 mg/dL	Bilirubin, 4.9–8.0 mg/dL	Precoma bilirubin > 8.0 mg/dL
Gastrointestinal tract	Mild ileus	Moderate ileus	Severe ileus	Bleeding due to erosive gastritis	Mesentric venous thrombosis
Neurologic	Obtunded	Disoriented	Irrational	Hyporeactive	Coma

**From* Stevens [15]; with permission.
†Score equals the sum of the squares of the three highest dysfunction ratings.
BP–blood pressure; CL–creatinine level; FSP–fibrin split products; LDH–lactate dehydrogenase; PEEP–positive end-expiratory pressure; PT–prothrombin time; PTT–partial thromboplastin time; SGOT–serum glutamic-oxaloacetic transaminase.

stress factor of 1.5 currently used. This is a highly relevant study that can be used to modify nutrient delivery based on initial injury and developing postoperative and posttrauma complications. The study shows great promise but needs prospective validation.

Route of nutrient administration

The gastrointestinal tract is receiving increasing attention as an important immunologic barrier. The well-fed intestine is a metabolically active organ that passively and actively maintains barriers against intraluminal toxins and bacteria. Peristalsis, secretory IgA, the mucin layer, and the cells of the villi appear to have protective and supportive roles in maintaining this function. Various other immunologic mechanisms support this barrier, for example the Kupffer's cells of the liver serve as a secondary defense against bacterial invasion. While the phenomenon of "bacterial translocation" remains hypothetical and unsubstantiated under clinical conditions, investigators speculate that various barrier-protective mechanisms fail after such insults as starvation, shock, and infection. It also appears that delivery of nutrients to severely injured patients via the gastrointestinal tract reduces septic complications compared with nutrients delivered intravenously.

Kudsk *et al.* [3••] randomly assigned 98 patients with significant intra-abdominal injuries requiring celiotomy to either enteral or parenteral feeding within 24 hours of surgery. Postpyloric access via jejunostomy was obtained in both groups. Patients were not excluded because of excessive blood loss, need for reoperation within 72 hours, or an unusually high abdominal trauma index. (The abdominal trauma index is a scoring system that quantitates the number and severity of intra-abdominal organ injuries and the risk of subsequent sepsis.) Enterally fed patients developed significantly fewer pneumonias, intra-abdominal abscesses, and catheter-related sepsis than patients receiving TPN despite the delivery of significantly more nutrition to the TPN group. Infected TPN patients also developed significantly more infections per patient than infected enteral patients. This improvement in infectious complications occurred primarily in the most severely injured patients with an ISS greater than 20 or an abdominal trauma index greater than 25 (Fig. 1).

Moore *et al.* [4] performed a meta-analysis of eight prospective, randomized trials comparing early enteral versus early parenteral nutrition in 230 high-risk general surgery and trauma patients using standard enteral and parenteral formulation. The authors demonstrated tolerance of these patients to early enteral nutrition and a reduced number of septic complications in the enterally fed patients compared with those given TPN.

These recent studies point out the importance of planning for specialized nutrition support at the time of surgery. Intragastric feeding following severe injury or major abdominal procedures is rarely possible because of the gastric atony which may last at least 4 days following surgery. Postpyloric access either by placement of a jejunostomy tube, transgastric jejunostomy, or advancement of a nasoenteric tube beyond the ligament of Treitz assures the opportunity to deliver nutrients into the small intestine for nutritional support of the patient and perhaps maintenance of the gastrointesti-

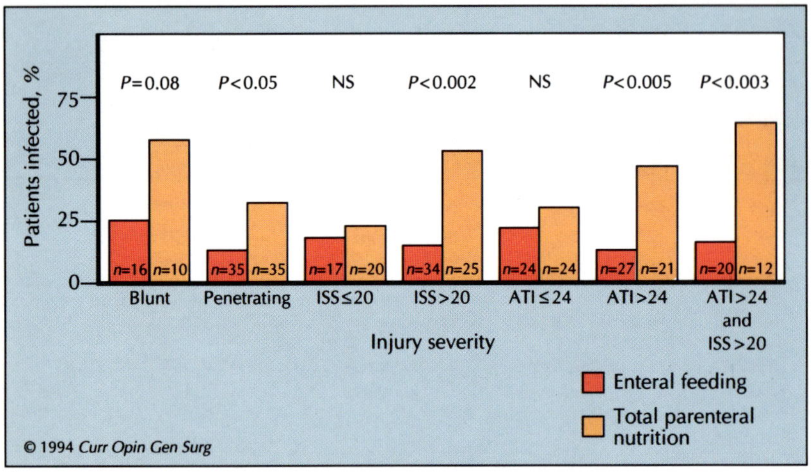

Fig. 1. Septic morbidity compared with injury severity. Patients sustaining penetrating trauma suffered significantly fewer infections when randomly assigned to receive enteral feeding. Statistical significance was nearly achieved in the blunt-trauma patients. Significant benefit with enteral feeding was found in those patients with a high injury severity score (ISS) and a high abdominal trauma index (ATI). NS—not significant.

nal immunologic barrier. If not obtained at the time of surgery, postpyloric access can be difficult, expensive, and perhaps dangerous to achieve in critically ill and injured patients.

Specialty nutrients

Both cellular and humoral immunity appear to be depressed in critically ill patients, and experimental evidence suggests that specific nutrients in the diet may enhance or depress the immune responsiveness of the host. Glutamine, arginine, nucleotides, and ω-3 and ω-6 polyunsaturated fatty acids have gathered the most attention, and several recent clinical studies provide evidence that combinations of these specific nutrients can potentially influence patient outcome.

ω-3 and ω-6 Fatty acids

Contemporary nutritional therapy recommends a lower calorie to nitrogen ratio in sepsis and severe stress than that used in unstressed patients. Both lipid and carbohydrate calories can serve as nonprotein caloric sources to enhance nitrogen retention by the body, but the most beneficial ratio of these nutrients during critical illness remains unknown. Some fat must be administered to avoid deficiency caused by inadequate amounts of essential polyunsaturated fatty acids. Clinical effects of fatty acid deficiency reflect the importance of these lipid components on cell membranes of platelets, healing wounds, the skin, and the lymphoid tissue. As much as 50% of standard lipid supplements consist of ω-6 fatty acids (primarily linoleic acid). These ω-6 fatty acids appear to be immunosuppressive in animal models by decreasing the function of cytotoxic T lymphocytes, reducing cytokine secretions, inhibiting leukocyte migration, and depressing clearance of foreign bodies by the reticuloendothelial system. These ω-6 fatty acids function as precursors prostaglandins and leukotrienes of the two and four series, which are potent vasoconstrictors as well as inducers of platelet aggregation. The less commonly used ω-3 fatty acids found in fish and canola oil are precursors of the three-series prostanoids and five-series leukotrienes. As a group, ω-3 fatty acids are less inflammatory and less immunosuppressive than the ω-6 fatty acids but still eliminate the clinical effects of essential fatty acid deficiency.

Arginine

Arginine is an otherwise nonessential amino acid that can become depleted following injury. In animal models, depletion of arginine reduces wound healing and decreases Kupffer's cell function while supplementation stimulates T-lymphocyte proliferation in response to mitogens or cytokines, as well as increasing macrophage and natural killer cell function and stimulating interleukin-2 production.

Nucleotides

The normal maturation of lymphocytes requires dietary nucleotides; therefore, deprivation reduces T-cell and macrophage function and decreases survival of laboratory animals in response to sepsis from such organisms as *Staphylococcus aureus* and *Candida albicans* [5]. Deficiency states of nucleotides also enhance survival of cardiac allografts.

Glutamine

Glutamine, the most abundant amino acid in the body, appears to be a conditionally essential amino acid important in the levels of secretory IgA and function of lymphocytes and macrophages. Animal models of deprivation have demonstrated decreases in these immunologic parameters. In addition to the immunologic function, glutamine provides an energy source for other rapidly growing cells including the intestinal mucosa. Intracellular glutamine depletion characteristically occurs under hypercatabolic conditions despite the increased production by skeletal muscle.

Clinical studies using specialty nutrients

Recently, a number of immune-enhancing enteral formulas have become available to clinicians. Several randomized prospective studies suggest significantly improved outcome with their use.

Daly *et al.* [6] randomly assigned 85 postoperative patients with upper gastrointestinal malignancies to receive either a standard enteral formula or a diet supplemented with arginine, RNA, and ω-3 fatty acids. Mean nitrogen intake and nitrogen balance were significantly greater in the supplemented group. *In vitro* lymphocyte mitogenesis, which was depressed on the first postoperative day, regained normal levels only in the treatment group. Significantly fewer patients with the supplemented diet sustained either infectious or wound healing complications, and supplemented patients had significantly shorter hospital stays. These results are consistent with those of a previous study by Gottschlich *et al.* [7] in which burn patients were randomly assigned to a high-protein diet enriched with arginine and ω-3 fatty acids versus one of two standard enteral diets. Length of stay per percentage body burn and wound infections were significantly lower in the supplemented group. Mortality, incidence of pneumonia, and total number of infectious episodes were higher in the standard-fed group although these differences were not statistically significant.

Another randomized prospective study compared septic and critically ill patients fed a standard enteral diet or a diet enriched in arginine, nucleotides, and ω-3 fatty acids [5]. Patients who completed the study and received the supplemented diet had a significant reduction in length of hospital stay and fewer infections. Unfortunately, this study has been published only in abstract form.

Glutamine also appears to be a conditionally essential amino acid in times of stress but is unstable in solution over time, limiting its commercial availability in TPN or liquid enteral products. Ziegler *et al.* [8••] supplemented TPN solutions with fresh glutamine prior to administration to 45 allogenic bone marrow transplant recipients randomly assigned to receive either the glutamine solution or a standard TPN solution. A significant improvement in nitrogen balance occurred in the supplemented group along with a significant reduction in clinical infection and incidence of microbial colonization. Hospital stay also appeared to be shortened for the patients receiving glutamine supplementation.

One solution for the instability problems of glutamine is the use of dipeptides as a nutrient source [9,10••]. Alanyl-L-glutamine and glutamine-dipeptides are stable in solution but rapidly disassociate *in vivo* within 3 to 4 minutes. While clinical experience with these solutions is limited, van der Hulst *et al.* [11] randomly assigned 20 patients to receive parenteral nutrition enriched with glycyl-L-glutamine or standard parenteral nutrition. Permeability of the gastrointestinal tract to lactulose and mannitol increased in the unsupplemented population but remained unchanged in the glutamine-supplemented group. No dramatic changes in mucosal thickness were noted on biopsy in the glutamine-supplemented patients; however, the standard TPN group had a statistically significant decrease in villus height.

Arginine also enhances immune function and promotes wound healing. In a randomized double-blind study, 30 elderly (>65 years of age) healthy human volunteers received daily supplements of 30 g/d of arginine aspartate, while 15 received placebo [12]. Studies of lymphocyte blastogenesis, mixed lymphocyte response, fibroplasia, and epithelialization were performed after 2 weeks of supplementation. Arginine supplementation increased collagen deposition as measured by hydroxyproline accumulation in polytetrafluoroethylene catheters implanted subcutaneously into the right deltoid muscle. Epithelialization of a 2×2 cm partial-thickness wound was not affected by arginine administration, but peripheral blood lymphocyte responses to phytohemagglutinin, pokeweed mitogen, and concanavalin A, as well as mixed lymphocyte responses, were significantly greater with arginine supplementation. While these responses are intriguing in this elderly, well-nourished population, applicability to the critically ill or critically injured patient is speculative only, as the authors admit. Interestingly, arginine also stimulated an important anabolic hormone, insulin-like growth factor 1 (IGF-1), which is an important factor in growth hormone activity.

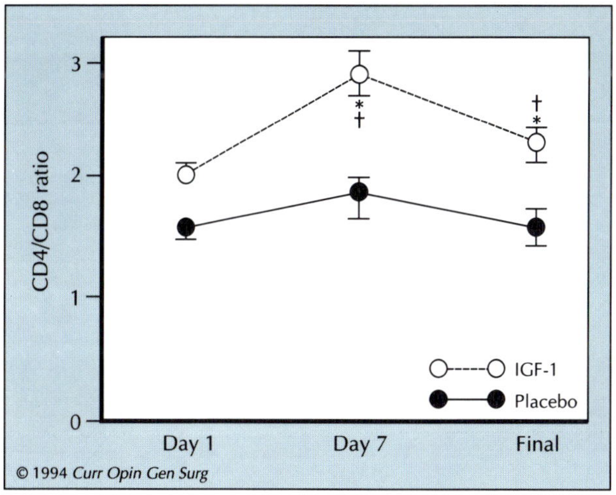

Fig. 2. Effect of insulin-like growth factor 1 (IGF-1) on CD4/CD8 ratio, compared with placebo. There was a significant increase in the CD4/CD8 ratio in treated patients at day 7 and on the final day of a study of 14 patients with severe closed-head injury. *$P<0.005$ between IGF-1 and placebo groups; †$P<0.005$.

Anabolic hormones

With the availability of recombinant DNA technology, several potent anabolic agents have become available and have been studied as a means to increase lean body mass. Growth hormone stimulates nitrogen retention by the body, exerting some of its effects via IGF-1, a somatomedin synthesized by the liver in response to circulating growth hormone levels. In addition, recent studies demonstrated effects of growth hormones on visceral protein synthesis, immunologic function, and other nutritional parameters.

Vara-Thorbeck *et al.* [13] randomly assigned 38 patients requiring elective gastrectomy, colectomy, or ab-

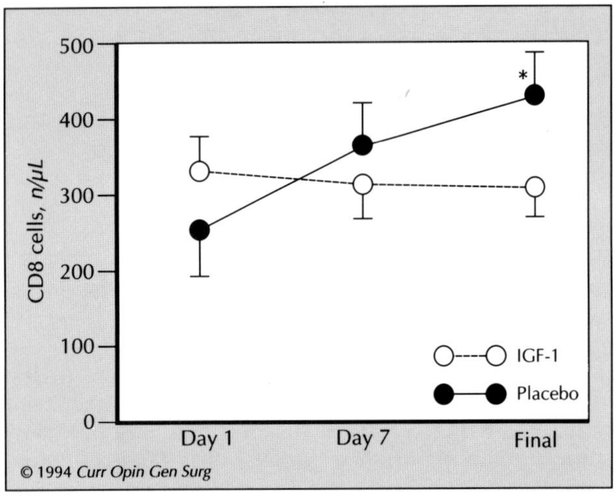

Fig. 3. Effect of insulin-like growth factor 1 (IGF-1) on CD8 cells. IGF-1 treatment reduced the number of circulating CD8 cells following severe closed-head injury in a study of 14 patients. $^*P<0.005$ from baseline.

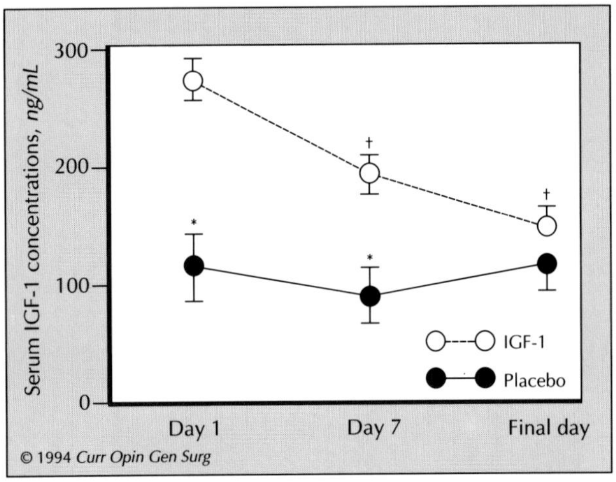

Fig. 4. Effect of continuous infusion of insulin-like growth factor 1 (IGF-1) on serum levels of growth hormone. In a study of 14 patients with severe closed-head injury, serum IGF-1 concentrations decreased over time in the treated patients but remained above baseline values on all days of the experiment. IGF-1 serum values were significantly higher in the treatment group than in the placebo group on days 1 and 7. $^*P<0.003$ between IGF-1– and placebo-treated groups; $^\dagger P<0.005$ from baseline.

dominoperineal resection for malignancy or peptic ulcer disease to receive parenteral nutrition with or without human growth hormone in the postoperative period. Both groups received parenteral nutrition for an average of 11±3 days while growth hormone treatment with 4 IU subcutaneous injections of human growth hormone was carried out for 7 days. In these ambulatory surgical patients, human growth hormone therapy resulted in more positive nitrogen balance and significant increases in IGF-1 (somatomedin-C). In addition, by day 12 after operation, transferrin, albumin, and total proteins were significantly greater in the growth hormone treated patients.

Kudsk *et al.* [14] studied 14 severely injured closed-head injured patients. Patients were randomly assigned to receive either aggressive intravenous nutrition alone or aggressive intravenous nutrition with a continuous infusion of IGF-1 at 0.1 mg/kg/d for 2 weeks while effects on CD4 (helper cells) and CD8 (suppressor cells) values as well as nitrogen balance were measured. Although this small population study did not demonstrate statistical significance in nitrogen balance, there was inhibition of the normal increase in CD8 cells that occurs following closed-head injury and, as a result, a significant increase in the CD4 to CD8 ratio with IGF-1 therapy (Fig. 2) primarily due to fewer CD8 cells in the group treated with IGF-1 (Fig. 3). Unfortunately, continuous IGF-1 infusion results in decreasing serum levels of growth hormones over 2 weeks of therapy (Fig. 4). This may be due to a reduction in binding proteins that are dependent upon circulating levels of growth hormone. IGF-1 appears to have a negative feedback on growth hormone secretion by the pituitary.

References and recommended reading

Papers of particular interest, published within the annual period of review, have been highlighted as:

- • Of special interest
- •• Of outstanding interest

1. •• The Veterans Affairs Total Parenteral Nutrition Cooperative Study Group: **Perioperative Total Parenteral Nutrition in Surgical Patients.** *N Engl J Med* 1991, **325**:525–532.

Malnourished patients ($n \leq 395$) requiring laparotomy or noncardiac thoracotomy were randomly assigned to receive either TPN for 7 to 15 days before surgery and 3 days afterwards or no perioperative TPN. Perioperative TPN was beneficial only in the most severely malnourished patients unless there were other specific indications.

2. Hwang T-L, Huang S-L, Chen M-F: **The Use of Indirect Calorimetry in Critically Ill Patients: The Relationship of Measured Energy Expenditure to Injury Severity Score, Septic Severity Score, and APACHE II Score.** *J Trauma* 1993, **34**:247–251.

3. •• Kudsk KA, Croce MA, Fabian TC, Minard G, Tolley EA, Poret HA, Kuhl MR, Brown RO: **Enteral Vs Parenteral Feeding: Effects on Septic Morbidity After Blunt and Penetrating Trauma.** *Ann Surg* 1992, **215**:503–512.

Ninety-eight severely injured trauma victims were randomly assigned to receive either enteral or parenteral feeding within 24 hours of surgery. Septic complications were reduced with enteral feeding, particularly in the most severely injured patient population.

4. Moore FA, Feliciano DAV, Andrassy RJ, McArdle AH, McL Booth FV, Morgenstein-Wagner TP, Kellum JM, Welling RE, Moore EE: **Early Enteral Feeding, Compared With Parenteral, Reduces Postoperative Septic Complications: The Results of a Meta-analysis.** *Ann Surg* 1992, **216**:172–183.

5. Bower RH: **Nutrition During Critical Illness and Sepsis.** *New Horizons* 1993, **1**:348–352.

6. Daly JM, Lieberman MD, Goldfine J, Shou J, Weintraub F, Rosato EF, Lavin P: **Enteral Nutrition With Supplemental Arginine, RNA, and Omega-3 Fatty Acids in Patients After Operation: Immunologic, Metabolic, and Clinical Outcome.** *Surgery* 1992, **112**:56–67.

7. Gottschlich MM, Jenkins M, Warden GD, Baumer T, Havens P, Snook JT, Alexander JW: **Differential Effects of Three Enteral Dietary Regimens on Selected Outcome Variables in Burn Patients.** *JPEN J Parenter Enteral Nutr* 1990, **14**:225–236.

8. •• Ziegler TR, Young LS; Benfell K, Scheltinga M, Hortos K, Bye R, Morrow FD, Jacobs DO, Smith RJ, Antin JH, Wilmore DW: **Clinical and Metabolic Efficacy of Glutamine-Supplemented Parenteral Nutrition After Bone Marrow Transplantation: A Randomized, Double-Blind, Controlled Study.** *Ann Intern Med* 1992, **16**:821–828.

Glutamine supplementation reduced microbial colonization and hospital stay in 45 allogenic bone marrow transplant patients randomly assigned to receive standard TPN or glutamine-supplemented TPN.

9. VAZQUES JA, DANIEL H, ADIBI SA: **Dipeptides in Parenteral Nutrition: From Basic Science to Clinical Applications**. *Nutr Clin Pract* 1993, **8**:95–105.

10. FÜRST P, STEHLE P: **The Potential Use of Parenteral Dipeptides in •• Clinical Nutrition**. *Nutr Clin Pract* 1993, **8**:106–114.

An excellent view of the practical aspects of using dipeptides in clinical nutrition.

11. VAN DER HULST RWJ, VAN KREEL BK, VON MEYENFELDT MF, BRUMMER R-JM, ARENDS J-W, DEUTZ NEP, SOETERS PB: **Glutamine in the Preservation of Gut Integrity**. *Lancet* 1993, **341**:1363–1365.

12. KIRK SJ, HURSON M, REGAN MC, HOLT DR, WASSERKRUG HL, BARBUL A: **Arginine Stimulates Wound Healing and Immune Function in Elderly Human Beings**. *Surgery* 1993, **114**:155–160.

13. VARA-THORBECK R, GUERRERO JA, RUIZ-REQUENA ME, CAPITAN J, RODRIQUEZ M, ROSELL J, MEKINASSI K, MALDONADO M, MARTIN R: **Effects of Growth Hormone in Patients Receiving Total Parenteral Nutrition Following Major Gastrointestinal Surgery**. *Hepatogastroenterology* 1992, 39:270–272.

14. KUDSK KA, MOWATT-LARSSEN C, BUKAR J, FABIAN T, OELLERICH S, DENT DL, BROWN R: **Effect of rhIGF-I and Early TPN on Immune Depression Following Severe Head Injury**. *Arch Surg*, in press.

15. STEVENS LE: **Gauging the Severity of Surgical Sepsis**. *Arch Surg* 1983, **118**:1190–1192.

Kenneth A. Kudsk, MD, and Gayle Minard, MD, Department of Surgery, The University of Tennessee, 956 Court Avenue, Suite E228, Memphis, TN 38163, USA.

Peripheral vascular injury

Timothy C. Flynn, MD

University of Florida College of Medicine, Gainesville, Florida, USA

Over the past 20 years, the predominant trend in the care of the civilian trauma patient has been toward less invasive therapy. Splenic injuries that are now being identified with computed tomography scan or ultrasound are managed without laparotomy. Similarly, in caring for the patient with potential vascular injury of the extremity, the trend has been toward less invasive means of diagnosis and therapy. Defining which patients need angiography and how to use duplex scanning and pressure indices are still evolving issues.

Current Opinion in General Surgery 1994:30–34

Penetrating injuries

Patients with so-called "hard" signs of vascular injury have valid indications to go directly to the operating room without preoperative arteriography (Table 1) [1••]. In patients without hard signs of injury, the real cruxes of the issue are which vascular injuries need repair and whether physical examination or noninvasive tests can identify those that do. Although exclusion angiography has become the standard of care, the yield for finding significant injuries in patients whose only indication for arteriography is proximity of the penetration to a vessel is only 2% to 12% [2–5]. In addition, angiography has its own complications and also identifies a number of lesions considered so trivial that operative intervention is not warranted.

Table 1. Signs of vascular injury

"Hard" signs*
Arterial hemorrhage
Pulsatile or expanding hematoma
Bruit and thrill
Pulse deficit
Ischemic extremity
"Soft" signs†
Hematoma
History of bleeding
Neurologic deficit
Proximity of penetration

*Valid indications to go directly to surgery without preoperative arteriography.
†Surgeon must determine which injuries need repair and whether examination and noninvasive tests can determine them.

Weaver *et al.* [6] described 157 patients who had proximity as the only indication for arteriography. In these patients, 17 injuries were identified, of which only one required operative repair. Kaufman *et al.* [7] described 85 patients, of whom twenty-four showed positive arteriographic findings; only five patients had lesions in major vessels, and none of these underwent operative procedures. Although it is dangerous to extrapolate the experience from the arteriography suite to a traumatic injury, many vascular surgeons note that most small pseudoaneurysms and arterial-venous fistulas created by arteriography spontaneously heal [8,9]. For the most part, the natural history of such lesions in the trauma patient is not well known.

Stain *et al.* [10] prospectively followed 24 injuries in major arteries with serial arteriography. Of these, 42% resolved, 29% improved, 17% were stable, and 12% progressed. The authors concluded that with appropriate follow-up and judgment the majority of nonocclusive injuries, small aneurysms, and small arterial-venous fistulas could be followed.

Frykberg *et al.* [11] prospectively followed 46 clinically occult injuries of major arteries seen on angiography for a mean period of 3 months; 39 injuries had repeat angiography. One patient required emergency repair of a pseudoaneurysm of the superficial femoral artery 2 weeks after injury, and five patients required elective repair of expanding pseudoaneurysms. The remaining lesions were either stable or improved. Since there were no serious sequelae of this practice, a prospective protocol was established wherein patients with hard signs of vascular injury were taken directly to the operating room, and patients with clinically occult proximity injuries were followed for 24 hours in the hospital and then released. Of the 286 patients with clinically occult proximity injuries who had no angiography, two required surgical intervention. The authors concluded that there was a 0.7% false negative rate for physical examination alone in patients with asymptomatic proximity injuries. This is close to the numbers of false negatives reported by angiography, 0.3% to 6% [12].

Others have questioned this policy of expectantly following penetrating injuries. Kerstein *et al.* [13•] re-

© 1994 Current Science ISBN 1-85922-671-X ISSN 1065–6243

ported 118 cases with soft signs of vascular injury. These patients all underwent arteriography, and 23 abnormalities were identified, 16 of which were explored. The remaining seven cases were followed up. These were all categorized as minor intimal flaps. Six of the seven patients returned with new symptoms that required surgical intervention between 9 and 39 months after injury. This represents a considerably longer follow-up than is reported in the previous papers recommending conservative management. Feliciano *et al.* [14] and Perry [15•] have both reported cases of delayed presentations of vascular injuries, many of them years remote from the injury. They concluded that nonoperative management can potentially result in serious injury to the patient and that before recommending that some vascular injuries can be treated expectantly, studies with a longer period of follow-up and a larger number of patients are necessary to define the natural history of these injuries.

Laboratory experience with these lesions is minimal because models that approximate the human injury are difficult to create. Hsiang [16] created intimal flaps with an endoscope in 37 canine arteries. These were observed for 4 weeks and only one of the 37 lesions (2.7%) progressed to hemodynamically significant stenosis. Light and electron microscopy showed that the arteries healed with return of endothelium. Hernandez-Maldonado *et al.* [17] created flaps by doing arteriotomy and then raising a 4-mm long intimal flap in dogs. In this model at 3 weeks, patency was only 67% in the untreated group. Although this model is considerably different from the patient with a gunshot wound, residual defects were common and healing did not continue to complete resolution.

Despite the low yield from exclusion arteriography in patients with proximity injury, many trauma surgeons are uncomfortable with the notion that these injuries should go totally uninvestigated. This has led several authors to study the use of duplex ultrasonography or arterial pressure indices as simple screening tests to identify those patients who may need further investigation. Bynoe *et al.* [18] described 198 patients, 23 of whom had injury diagnosed by duplex ultrasonography and whose injuries were confirmed by operation or arteriography. There were two false negative results, both shotgun wounds. Duplex scan was 99% accurate in excluding vascular injury and 98% accurate in the diagnosis of a vascular injury.

On the other hand, color-flow Doppler scanning was used by Schwartz *et al.* [19] to examine 12 patients with 12 arteriographically documented nonocclusive arterial injuries. Only seven of the 12 documented injuries were detected by color-flow Doppler scanning, although these were all major injuries. Five missed injuries included small intimal defects, a side branch occlusion of superficial femoral artery, and a l-mm pseudoaneurysm of the distal radial artery. There was clearly a learning curve, with the more experienced sonographers identifying a much higher percentage of all injuries. Bergstein *et al.* [20••] reported color-flow Doppler scanning on 67 patients with 75 penetrating injuries and compared it with arteriography. Color-flow Doppler scanning had a specificity of 99%, although a sensitivity of only 50%. Fry *et al.* [21••] reported 500 duplex scans obtained from scans of penetrating trauma to the neck and extremities (Table 2). There were 49 arterial or venous injuries identified; 28 of the arterial and seven of the venous injuries were confirmed by exploration or arteriography. The possibility of making a diagnosis of venous injuries was an added benefit of the use of duplex scans. In this series, there was one false positive and no false negatives, for an accuracy of 98.6%. Panetta *et al.* [22,23] described a canine model, finding ultrasonography to be 95% accurate when compared with histologic examination and even somewhat more sensitive than angiography.

Arterial pressure indices have been used to identify lesions that cause proximal stenosis or occlusion. Lynch and Johansen [24] reported 100 consecutive injured limbs in 93 trauma patients who had arterial pressure indices and arteriography. In this series, ankle pressure indices less than 0.9 were thought to be abnormal. Using clinical outcome as the gold standard, the overall accuracy was 97% compared with 98% with arteriography. A prospective study involving 100 extremity injuries in 96 patients was undertaken by Johansen *et al.* [25]. Patients with a pressure index of less than 0.9 had arteriography. Patients with an arterial pressure index greater than 0.9 underwent serial Doppler determinations and, in the majority of the cases, duplex sonogra-

Table 2. Diagnostic criteria of duplex scanning for vascular trauma*

	Thrombosis	Stenosis	Pseudoaneurysm	Arteriovenous fistula	Spasm
Ultrasonography	Complete luminal defect	Irregular luminal defect	Widened luminal diameter	Sonolucent connection between artery and vein	Smooth intima with luminal tapering
Color-flow Doppler scanning	Absent	Accelerated	Variable	Accelerated many velocities	Accelerated
Spectral analysis	Absent	Accelerated peak with spectral broadening	Variable	Accelerated with marked spectral broadening	Accelerated with mild spectral broadening

**From* Fry *et al.* [21••]; with permission.

phy. Seventeen limbs with arterial pressure indices of less than 0.9 underwent angiography. Of these, 16 had positive arteriographic findings and seven patients underwent operation for vascular repair. Four patients underwent angiography for proximity at the discretion of the treating physician despite a pressure index greater than 0.9, and all were normal. Of the remaining 79 limbs, all with arterial pressure index greater than 0.9, only one required a subsequent procedure. That one was repair of an arterial venous fistula between the profunda femoris artery and vein. Doppler pressure measurements can identify only occlusive injuries to major vessels and may miss injuries to the peroneal and profunda femoris arteries. Likewise, in the patient with multiextremity injuries and patients with hemorrhagic shock, pressure measurements may not be accurate. Lesions that are not obstructive, such as small intimal flaps, small pseudoaneurysm, or arterial-venous fistula, will not be detected by measuring pressure distal to the injury. Others have investigated whether the threshold for declaring an ankle pressure index abnormal should be 0.9 or 1.0. Schwartz *et al.* [26] combined pressure indices with physical examination to define patients as having low, medium, or high risk. By regression curves, they concluded that declaring a pressure index below 1.0 as abnormal yields the highest sensitivity but at some sacrifice to specificity.

One can expect that a new modality used for the diagnosis and treatment of atherosclerotic disease will be used for trauma as well. Although it has not been reported, intravascular ultrasound could be used to examine arterial injuries and may help in identifying lesions seen on angiography that may be managed nonoperatively. Angioscopy has been used to resect small intimal defects as a result of trauma [27,28]. Magnetic resonance imaging has been used to investigate extremity injuries [29]. Arteriographic embolization has been reported as therapeutic for small pseudoaneurysms and the obliteration of arterial-venous fistulas [30]. In addition, although not reported, one might consider the use of stents to repair intimal flaps and the deployment of intraluminal grafts for more extensive injuries.

Blunt injury

Treiman *et al.* [31••] has questioned the widely held policy of routine arteriography in all patients with knee dislocations. Of 220 patients with knee dislocation from blunt trauma whom the authors studied, 105 presented with severe ischemia and underwent immediate operations and 115 were clinically stable and underwent angiography. In the 86 stable patients with normal pulses on serial examination, none required surgery, whereas 76% of patients with abnormal pulses required operation (Table 3). The authors concluded that patients with obvious injuries should undergo repair and that patients with an abnormal pulse should undergo arteriography. For patients with normal pulses, they recommend that serial examinations be performed while observing the patient in the hospital. Patients with a deterioration of the pulse should undergo angiography or exploration. In the discussion of this paper, there were several who suggested that ankle brachial indices or duplex scanning may be useful as a more objective way to define a normal pulse. At the very least, it would appear that the dogma that requires all knee dislocations have an angiogram may be under some questioning.

Table 3. Accuracy of pulse examination in detecting a popliteal artery injury requiring operation*†

	Patients, *n*	
	No injury	Injury
Pulse intact	86	0
Pulse deficit	7	22

**From* Treiman *et al.* [31••]; with permission.
†The sensitivity in predicting an injury requiring arterial repair was 1.000; specificity, 0.924; positive predictive value, 0.758; negative predictive value, 1.000; and accuracy, 0.939.

It is difficult to salvage extremities with bone, soft-tissue, and vascular injuries. Katzman and Dickson [32] reviewed 19 patients with open tibial fractures and associated arterial injuries. All limbs were thought to be initially salvagable; however, 58% of the patients ultimately underwent amputation. Isolated anterior tibial or peroneal artery injuries had a good prognosis, whereas poor outcome was predicted in those patients with posterior tibial and popliteal artery injuries or injuries involving all three tibia vessels. Predictive indices have not been widely accepted, and as has been repeatedly emphasized, nerve injuries portend a poor outcome [33]. Padberg *et al.* [34••] reported a 41% amputation rate after infrapopliteal blunt injury. This series also observed that single-vessel injury could be safely treated with ligation and that only one tibial vessel was necessary for viability. Ballard *et al.* [35•] reviewed 99 injuries distal to the brachial bifurcation or popliteal trifurcation and concluded that only one functional artery distal to the elbow or knee is necessary for limb viability.

Venous injury

Cargile *et al.* [36•] reviewed injuries to the femoral artery and vein at Parkland Hospital in Dallas, Texas. Of interest in this paper are the 131 venous injuries, of which 91% were repaired. Eighteen of the venous repairs were noted to be occluded in the initial hospitalization, and four of these patients suffered pulmonary emboli, none of which were fatal. Although these numbers are small, they do represent a 22% incidence, whereas the overall incidence of pulmonary embolism in the remaining patients who did not have a venous repair was only 2.5%. As in most of these series, the long-term outcome of venous repairs could not be determined. Nypaver *et al.* [37], however, did collect a series of 32 cases with venous repair who had a follow-up of 49 months, with a range of 6 to 108 months. Of these patients, 56% underwent simple repair, 22% had a graft, 12% had a patch repair, and 9.5% had an end-to-end repair. Seventeen of these patients underwent venography, and thrombosis occurred in nine patients (54%) in the early postoperative period. Interestingly, follow-up color-flow Doppler scanning found 90% of the venous repairs to be patent, including eight of the nine repairs with early evidence of occlusion by venography. Only two of the patients in this series had significant edema. Sharma *et al.* [38] reported 38 venous repairs; 17 of these patients had meticulous reconstruction and intraoperative venography. The rate of patency within 2 weeks of surgery was 100%. A group of 20 patients who did not have confirmatory venography after reconstruction had a 38% occlusion rate in the early postoperative period. The authors conclude that meticulous attention to detail will result in improvement in vein patency. Alternatively, Yelon and Scalea [39] compared patients who had ligation of venous injuries with those whose injuries were repaired and found no difference in the incidence of edema in early follow-up.

Thoracic outlet and carotid injuries

The Jacksonville group, which has so aggressively questioned the use of angiography in extremity injuries, now brings into the question the use of routine angiography in penetrating zone II neck injuries [40•]. In 110 cases, there was only one lesion that required surgical intervention without evidence of hard signs of vascular injury. The authors elected to follow several patients with small intimal defects of the carotid or asymptomatic vertebral occlusions. In short-term follow-up, these had no negative consequences. Once again, the group questions whether or not routine angiography in the absence of hard signs is valid. Richardson *et al.* [41•] authored a multi-institutional review of 133 patients with penetrating carotid injuries to determine whether or not repair or ligation is appropriate. The limited numbers precluded significant statistical analysis and leave open the issue of whether or not the patient with a severe deficit should undergo repair or ligation. Of interest, even with the small numbers, when repair was attempted whenever possible, roughly half of these patients improved. Actually, I think that if technically feasible, all patients should have carotid repair regardless of preoperative status since there seems little to lose by repair.

Conclusions

The current trend in the care of penetrating injuries to the extremities is that fewer and fewer angiograms are being done in patients without signs of injury. Even those patients with knee dislocations may not need angiography but, at the very least, pressure indices should be done and, where available, duplex scan should also be considered. The mangled extremity with multiple vessel injuries should probably be considered for primary amputation as the results in this group are very poor. Venous repairs, even though they may clot initially, may provide long-term patency with recanalization, and therefore the policy continues to be that venous injuries should be repaired if at all possible. The risk of pulmonary embolism seems to be slightly increased should the venous repairs occlude and those patients should be treated with anticoagulation when venous occlusion is recognized. Angioscopy, intravascular ultrasound, and the varied techniques of interventional radiologists will probably play a greater role in the nonoperative therapy of vascular injuries. I still think that in institutions without these sophisticated techniques and when dealing with unreliable patients who will not be available for follow-up, a policy of thorough diagnostic studies and early repair of all but the most minor of injuries is most prudent.

References and recommended reading

Papers of particular interest, published within the annual period of review, have been highlighted as:

- • Of special interest
- •• Of outstanding interest

1. •• Martin RR, Mattox KL, Burch JM, Richardson RJ: **Advances in Treatment of Vascular Injuries From Blunt and Penetrating Limb Trauma.** *World J Surg* 1992, **16**:930–937.

This review from the Baylor group reflects the current practice at that busy trauma center.

2. Menzolan JO, Doyle JE, LoGerfo FW, Cantelmo N, Weitzman AF, Sequiera JC: **Evaluation and Management of Vascular Injuries of the Extremities.** *Arch Surg* 1983, **118**:93–95.
3. King TA, Perse JA, Marmen C, Darvin HI: **Utility of Arteriography in Penetrating Extremity Injuries.** *Am J Surg* 1991, **162**:163–165.
4. Francis H III, Thal ER, Weigelt JA, Redman HC: **Vascular Proximity: Is It a Valid Indication for Arteriography in Asymptomatic Patients?** *J Trauma* 1991, **31**:512–514.
5. Dennis JW, Frykberg ER, Crump JM, Vines FS, Alexander RH: **New Perspectives on the Management of Penetrating Trauma in Proximity to Major Limb Arteries.** *J Vasc Surg* 1990, **11**:84–93.
6. Weaver FA, Yellin AE, Bauer M, Oberg J, Ghalambor N, Emmanuel RP, Applebaum RM, Pentecost MJ, Shorr RM: **Is Arterial Proximity a Valid Indication for Arteriography in Penetrating Extremity Trauma?** *Arch Surg* 1990, **125**:1256–1260.
7. Kaufman JA, Parker JE, Gillespie DL, Greenfield AJ, Woodson J, Menzoian JO: **Arteriography for Proximity of Injury in Penetrating Extremity Trauma.** *J Vasc Interv Radiol* 1992, **3**:719–727.
8. Allen BT, Munn JS, Stevens SL, Sicard GA, Anderson CB, Droste ML, Ludbrook PA: **Selective Non-operative Management of Pseudoaneurysms and Arteriovenous Fistulae Complicating Femoral Artery Catheterization.** *J Cardiovasc Surg (Torino)* 1992, **33**:440–447.
9. Rivers SP, Lee ES, Lyon RT, Monrad S, Hoffman T, Veith FJ: **Successful Conservative Management of Iatrogenic Femoral Arterial Trauma.** *Ann Vasc Surg* 1992, **6**:45–49.
10. Stain SC, Yellin AE, Weaver FA, Pentecost MJ: **Selective Management of Nonocclusive Arterial Injuries.** *Arch Surg* 1989, **124**:1136–1141.
11. Frykberg ER, Crump JM, Dennis JW, Vines FS, Alexander RH: **Nonoperative Observation of Clinically Occult Arterial Injuries: A Prospective Evaluation.** *Surgery* 1991, **109**:85–96.
12. Frykberg ER, Dennis JW, Bishop K, Laneve L, Alexander RH: **The Reliability of Physical Examination in the Evaluation of Penetrating Extremity Trauma for Vascular Injury: Results at One Year.** *J Trauma* 1991, **31**:502–511.
13. • Kerstein M, Field CK, Arnold T, Matsomoto T: **The Adverse Outcome of Nonoperative Management of Intimal Injury Secondary to Penetrating Trauma [Abstract].** *J Vasc Surg* 1993, **17**:1118.

This abstract cautions against the widespread acceptance of observation alone as standard treatment for intimal injuries.

14. FELICAINO DV, CRUSE PA, BURCH JM, BITONDO CG: **Delayed Diagnosis of Arterial Injuries.** *Am J Surg* 1987, **154**:579–584.

15. PERRY MO: **Complications of Missed Arterial Injuries.** *J Vasc Surg*
• 1993, **17**:399–407.
This is a report of several cases treated by the author over several years and clearly states the bias against nonoperative management of vascular injuries.

16. HSIANG YN, FRAGOSO M, LUNDKIST A, WEIS M: **The Natural History of Intimal Flaps Caused by Angioscopy.** *Ann Vasc Surg* 1992, 6:38–44.

17. HERNANDEZ-MALDONADO JJ, PADBERG FT, TEEHAN E, NEVILLE R, DEFOUW D, DURAN WN, HOBSON RW II: **Arterial Intimal Flaps: A Comparison of Primary Repair, Aspirin, and Endovascular Excision in an Experimental Model.** *J Trauma* 1993, **34**:565–570.

18. BYNOE RP, MILES WS, BELL RM, GREENWOLD DR, SESSIONS G, HAYNES JL, RUSH DS: **Noninvasive Diagnosis of Vascular Trauma by Duplex Ultrasonography.** *J Vasc Surg* 1991, **14**:346–352.

19. SCHWARTZ M, WEAVER F, YELLIN A, RALLS P: **The Utility of Color Flow Doppler Examination in Penetrating Extremity Arterial Trauma.** *Am Surg* 1993, **59**:375–378.

20. BERGSTEIN JM, BLAIR JF, EDWARDS J, TOWNE JB, WITTMANN DH,
•• APRAHAMIAN C, QUEBBEMAN EJ: **Pitfalls in the Use of Color-Flow Duplex Ultrasound for Screening of Suspected Arterial Injuries in Penetrated Extremities.** *J Trauma* 1992, **33**:395–402.
This study provides a reasonable approach to the evolving use of ultrasound in vascular trauma.

21. FRY WR, SMITH RS, SAYERS DV, HENDERSON VJ, MORBITO DJ: **Duplex**
•• **Scanning: Diagnostic Criteria for Vascular Trauma.** *J Vasc Surg* 1993, **17**:1125–1126.
This is the largest reported series of duplex scans in trauma and gives criteria for the ultrasonographic diagnosis of vascular injuries.

22. PANETTA TF, SALES CM, MARIN ML, SCHWARTZ ML, JONES AM, BERDEJO GL, WENGERTER KR, VEITH FJ: **Natural History, Duplex Characteristics, and Histopathologic Correlation of Arterial Injuries in a Canine Model.** *J Vasc Surg* 1992, **16**:867–876.

23. PANETTA TF, HUNT JP, BUECHTER KJ, POTTMEYER A, BATTI JS: **Duplex Ultrasonography Versus Arteriography in the Diagnosis of Arterial Injury: An Experimental Study.** *J Trauma* 1992, **33**:627–635.

24. LYNCH K, JOHANSEN K: **Can Doppler Pressure Measurement Replace "Exclusion" Arteriography in the Diagnosis of Occult Extremity Arterial Trauma?** *Ann Surg* 1991, **214**:737–741.

25. JOHANSEN K, LYNCH K, PAUN M, COPASS M: **Non-invasive Vascular Tests Reliably Exclude Occult Arterial Trauma in Injured Extremities.** *J Trauma* 1991, **31**:515–522.

26. SCHWARTZ MR, WEAVER FA, BAUER M, SIEGEL A, YELLIN AE: **Refining the Indications for Arteriography in Penetrating Extremity Trauma: A Prospective Analysis.** *J Vasc Surg* 1993, **17**:116–124.

27. NEVILLE RF, YASUHARA H, WATANABE BI, CANADY J, DURAN W, HOBSON RW II: **Endovascular Management of Arterial Intimal Defects: An Experimental Comparison by Arteriography, Angioscopy, and Intravascular Ultrasonography.** *J Vasc Surg* 1991, **13**:496–502.

28. WHITE GH, WHITE RA, KOPCHOK GE, COLMAN PD, WILSON SE: **Endoscopic Intravascular Surgery Removes Intraluminal Flaps, Dissections, and Thrombus.** *J Vasc Surg* 1990, **11**:280–288.

29. YAQUINTO JJ, HARMS SE, SIEMERS PT, FLAMIG DP, GRIFFEY RH, FOREMAN ML: **Arterial Injury From Penetrating Trauma: Evaluation With Single-Acquisition Fat-Suppressed MR Imaging.** *AJR Am J Roentgenol* 1992, **158**:631–633.

30. PANETTA T, SCLAFANI SJ, GOLDSTEIN AS, PHILLIPS TF: **Percutaneous Transcatheter Embolization for Arterial Trauma.** *J Vasc Surg* 1985, 2:54–64.

31. TREIMAN GS, YELLIN AE, WEAVER FA, WANG S, GHALAMBOR N, BARLOW
•• W, SNYDER B, PENTECOST MJ: **Examination of the Patient With a Knee Dislocation: The Case for Selective Arteriography.** *Arch Surg* 1992, 127:1056–1063.
An iconoclastic suggestion that not all knee dislocations need an angiogram.

32. KATZMAN SS, DICKSON K: **Determining the Prognosis for Limb Salvage in Major Vascular Injuries With Associated Open Tibial Fractures.** *Orthop Rev* 1992, **21**:195–199.

33. SCHLICKEWEI W, KUNER EH, MULLAJI AB, GOTZE B: **Upper and Lower Limb Fractures With Concomitant Arterial Injury.** *J Bone Joint Surg Br* 1992, 74:181–188.

34. PADBERG FT JR, RUBELOWSKY JJ, HERNANDEZ-MALDONADO JJ, MILAZZO
•• V, SWAN KG, LEE BC, HOBSON RW II: **Infrapopliteal Arterial Injury: Prompt Revascularization Affords Optimal Limb Salvage.** *J Vasc Surg* 1992, **16**:877–886.
Despite successful arterial repair, the prognosis for limb salvage in combined blunt trauma injuries is dismal.

35. BALLARD JL, BLUNT TJ, MALONE JM: **Management of Small Artery Vas-**
• **cular Trauma.** *Am J Surg* 1992, **164**:316–319.
Confirms that only one patent artery is needed distal to the popliteal or brachial artery.

36. CARGILE JS III, HUNT JL, PURDUE GF: **Acute Trauma of the Femoral**
• **Artery and Vein.** *J Trauma* 1992, **32**:364–371.
This is a summary from Parkland in Dallas, Texas. Venous injuries were preferentially repaired, but those that clotted had a high incidence of pulmonary emboli.

37. NYPAVER TJ, SCHULER JJ, MCDONNELL P, ELLENBY MI, MONTALVO J, BARANIEWSKI H, PIANO G: **Long-Term Results of Venous Reconstruction After Vascular Trauma in Civilian Practice.** *J Vasc Surg* 1992, **16**:762–768.

38. SHARMA PVP, SHAH PM, VINZONS AT, PALLAN TM, CLAUSS RH, STAHL WM: **Meticulously Restored Lumina of Injured Veins Remain Patent.** *Surgery* 1992, **112**:928–932.

39. YELON JA, SCALEA TM: **Venous Injuries of the Lower Extremities and Pelvis: Repair Versus Ligation.** *J Trauma* 1992, **33**:532–538.

40. MENAWAT SS, DENNIS JW, LANEVE LM, FRYKBERG ER: **Are Arteriograms**
• **Necessary in Penetrating Zone II Neck Injuries?** *J Vasc Surg* 1992, **16**:397–401.
Significant arterial injuries all had hard signs of injury.

41. RICHARDSON R, OBEID FN, RICHARDSON JD, HOYT DB, WISNER DH,
• GOMEZ GA, JOHANSEN K, MCSWAIN NE, WEIGELT JA, BLAISDELL FW: **Neurologic Consequences of Cerebrovascular Injury.** *J Trauma* 1992, 32:755–760.
The issue of repair or ligation in the neurologically compromised patient remains in doubt.

Timothy C. Flynn, MD, Veterans Affairs Medical Center, Surgical Service (112), 1601 SW Archer Road, Gainesville, FL 32608-1197, USA.

New diagnostic techniques in trauma

David H. Livingston, MD

University of Medicine and Dentistry of New Jersey, Newark, New Jersey, USA

Advances in diagnostic and therapeutic interventions originally intended for use under elective circumstances have been applied to the trauma victim. This review examines the use of three of these techniques—transesophageal echocardiography (TEE), laparoscopy, and thoracoscopy—in the evaluation and treatment of the trauma patient. Initial experiences with TEE show it to be superior to transthoracic echocardiography in the evaluation of the heart. In limited studies, TEE appears to have the sensitivity to use as a screening tool for aortic disruption; however, it is severely limited by its ability to evaluate the distal aorta only. TEE cannot be used to visualize the ascending aorta or brachiocephalic vessels, which may account for 15% to 20% of injuries. Use of laparoscopy has been reported in more than 350 patients. Its primary use appears to be in decreasing negative and nontherapeutic laparotomies associated with penetrating trauma. The ability to operate through the scope continues to increase as additional improvements in instrumentation are introduced. Thoracoscopy has recently been shown to be able to evacuate retained hemothoraces and even drain empyemas and decorticate the pleural cavity.

Current Opinion in General Surgery 1994:35–40

New diagnostic and therapeutic modalities have advanced the treatment of many conditions. The use of laparoscopy has revolutionized the treatment of gallstones and has become the primary method of cholecystectomy. Though these technologic advancements were not originally designed for the trauma patient, investigators looking for improved diagnostic techniques have applied them in this setting. This is similar to what occurred with the adaptation of abdominal computed tomography (CT) for suspected abdominal injury. The use of abdominal CT has allowed injuries that were previously treated by operation to be successfully observed. This review assesses the use and impact of three new diagnostic and therapeutic procedures—transesophageal echocardiography (TEE), laparoscopy, and thoracoscopy—on the care of the trauma victim.

Transesophageal echocardiography

The use of two-dimensional echocardiography in the emergency department has been advocated by some authors as a useful means of detecting pericardial tamponade and ventricular dysfunction [1–4]. Fluid and air within the thoracic cavities can also be visualized. Jimenez *et al.* [5] compared transthoracic echocardiography and subxiphoid pericardial window in the diagnosis of occult cardiac injuries in 73 patients and found the results to be equivalent. Significant problems with transthoracic echocardiography occur with the presence of chest tubes or bandages and air in the subcutaneous tissue, and body habitus limits the windows available to image the heart. Furthermore, the technique does not allow imaging of the thoracic aorta.

TEE has become the initial imaging modality of choice for aortic pathology under elective or nontraumatic emergent circumstances. Its ability to provide better evaluation of cardiac and valvular function has also made TEE superior to transthoracic echocardiography in many cases. Brooks *et al.* [6••] found that TEE was significantly better than transthoracic echocardiography in diagnosing cardiac dysfunction following blunt chest trauma. For imaging of the acutely injured patient, TEE has been studied as a means to diagnose aortic rupture and to evaluate cardiac function [6••].

Angiography is the "gold standard" for the diagnosis of aortic and brachiocephalic vessel injuries and the technique which all other modalities must be prospectively compared. Because angiography is invasive, requires the patient to be transported to a specialized angiographic suite where resuscitation may not be able to proceed, and has positive rate of only 10%, investigators have continually searched for screening tools that could decrease the need for aortography. Although ad-

Abbreviations

CT—computed tomography; **DPL**—diagnostic peritoneal lavage; **TEE**—transesophageal echocardiography.

 ISBN 1-85922-671-X ISSN 1065–6243

vocated as an ideal screening test by some, routine CT of the chest has been found to be inconsistent in its ability to accurately predict which patients need angiography [7,8]. Miller *et al.* [8] found that thoracic CT had a sensitivity of 55% and a specificity of 65% for diagnosing aortic injury. By using CT as a screening modality, they would have missed two aortic and three great vessel injuries.

Advantages of TEE are that it is minimally invasive and can be performed quickly at the bedside. In June 1991, three groups simultaneously reported their experience with TEE for thoracic trauma [9–11]. Shapiro *et al.* [10] used TEE in 19 patients and found that the modality was very good for detecting cardiac pathology, but it missed two intimal tears in the descending aorta that were seen on angiography. Neither patient required operation. Sparks *et al.* [11] reported on 10 patients who underwent TEE and angiography for suspected injury. Results of TEE and aortography were positive in three patients. Aortography was considered positive in one where TEE was negative. This patient had no evidence of injury at exploration. TEE showed negative results in an additional two patients whose angiogram findings were initially thought to be positive, but which were considered as negative upon final interpretation. Both patients recovered uneventfully.

These initial studies have been followed by other case reports documenting the utility of TEE in the diagnosis of aortic and cardiac injury [12,13•,14,15]. Brooks *et al.* [6••] reported their experience with TEE and aortography in 21 patients with a mediastinal hematoma on chest radiography. They found that results of TEE and angiography were positive in three patients. The aorta was normal by TEE in 16 patients, which was confirmed by angiography in 14 and autopsy in 2. TEE detected three aortic lesions where the aorta was found to be normal by angiography. There were several limitations of this study that make interpretation of the utility of TEE difficult. Firstly, the investigators were using a single-plane TEE probe, which does not provide the resolution of the biplanar probe. The person performing the TEE was not blinded to the aortogram results and all three TEE studies with true positive results were performed knowing the injury was present. Furthermore, all three studies showing false positive results were performed before aortography, which may be attributable to the limitations of the instrumentation or inexperience of the examiner. There were no associated brachiocephalic vessel injuries present in this series.

The largest series to date was reported by Kearney *et al.* [16••]. They studied 69 patients with TEE and angiography after chest trauma. TEE was performed and interpreted by staff cardiologists or senior cardiology fellows using a two-dimensional echocardiograph. All of the TEE examinations occurred before angiography. Seven patients had aortic disruption seen on TEE. Four patients had positive aortography findings and one patient underwent repair based on the TEE alone. The remaining two patients had negative angiogram findings. One of these patients underwent exploratory surgery based on the TEE findings, and a 60% aortic disruption was repaired. The other patient died of other injuries and had an aortic intimal tear diagnosed at autopsy. All injuries occurred in the aorta distal to the left subclavian artery. The average time required for TEE was 27 minutes, which was significantly shorter than that for aortography (mean, 76 minutes) TEE was performed in the emergency department in 58%, and in the intensive care unit in 27%, of patients. Of concern in this series is the high false-negative rate of angiography results.

Although TEE appears to be a promising modality to diagnose distal aortic and cardiac injuries after chest trauma, several questions remain unanswered. First, who should be doing the procedure—the trauma surgeon, emergency department physician, or cardiologist? Although the latter group is undoubtedly better trained and more experienced, their unavailability at all hours of the day and night would significantly limit the applicability of TEE. Whether the technique can be learned by noncardiologists with the accuracy necessary is unclear. The study by Brooks *et al.* [6••], in which the examinations were done by trauma surgeons, is clouded by potential bias due to study design. The acquisition of other sonographic skills by surgeons and emergency department physicians has been reported to be possible and the results acceptable [1,17•].

TEE is also limited by its inability to evaluate the ascending aorta and the brachiocephalic vessels. These injuries comprise up to 20% of vascular injuries in blunt thoracic trauma. The ability of angiography to evaluate other blood vessels and body cavities as well as to perform therapeutic interventions is often not taken into account when comparing the two techniques. Lastly, it is unclear whether the surgeons involved in repairing these injured blood vessels would do so based on TEE findings alone. If not, the modality will merely place another layer of extraneous diagnostic testing between the patient and proper therapy.

Laparoscopy

The use of laparoscopy in the diagnosis and management of patients sustaining abdominal trauma had been proposed sporadically but failed to gain acceptance and widespread use [18–21]. Improvements in equipment and optics have resulted in general surgeons performing numerous laparoscopic surgical procedures, and laparoscopy is now part of the routine practice of the general surgeon. The incidence of nontherapeutic celiotomies has been reported to be 5% to 14% for blunt trauma and as high as 25% for stab wounds [22–24]. Negative celiotomies for tangential gunshot wounds and thoracoabdominal injuries are also frequent, and laparoscopy would appear to be an ideal way of decreasing the negative and nontherapeutic celiotomy rate.

Five recent studies evaluating the use of laparoscopy in abdominal trauma have been published since 1992 (Table 1) [25••,26••,27•,28,29]. All of them evaluated hemodynamically stable patients prior to planned celiotomy. The vast majority of the patients (91%) sustained penetrating injury, and most of the conclusions drawn from these studies pertain solely to penetrating trauma.

Laparoscopy was performed using a 0° laparoscope in all cases. The camera was positioned through a subumbilical port in most cases and additional ports were placed in about one half to three quarters of the patients. The instrumentation used was that which was available from late 1990 until early 1992 and consisted mainly of laparoscopic cholecystectomy instruments with some additions later in the series. Because laparoscopic surgery is very instrument-dependent, the published success or failure of this technique depends on what equipment was available. Fabian *et al.* [26••] reported that one complication occurred when a cholecystectomy grasper was used on the small intestine. Livingston *et al.* [25••], using basic laparoscopic cholecystectomy instruments, found that examination of the small bowel was practically impossible and all three small bowel injuries in their series were undiagnosed. This problem with small bowel and colonic injuries was echoed by Ivatury *et al.* [27•], who reported an 18% missed injury rate. In the discussion of his paper, Fabian *et al.* [26••] reported that the small bowel could be visualized accurately using newer laparoscopic intestinal instruments (Fig. 1).

While the advantages of laparoscopy in penetrating trauma are obvious, the potential use of laparoscopy in blunt trauma remains more undefined and is probably more limited. Abdominal CT scanning provides more anatomic information regarding liver and splenic injuries, the retroperitoneum, pelvic hematomas, and pelvic fractures. It is possible that some of the patients in these series who underwent laparoscopy following blunt trauma might have been treated by observation alone.

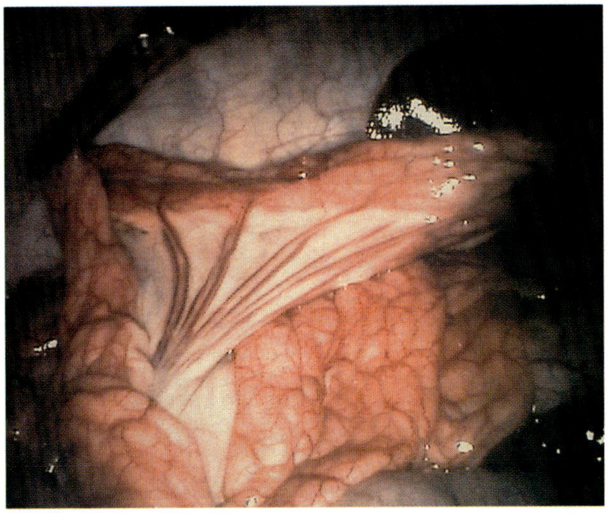

Fig. 1. Experimental study (porcine model) using advanced instruments to demonstrate the ability to view the small bowel. (*Courtesy* of G. Larsen, Louisville, KY.)

The use of a 0° laparoscope also limits the ability to explore the abdomen. We now routinely use a 30° laparoscope for trauma cases and find it more useful. The 30° scope allows for better visualization of the spleen, liver, diaphragm, and colonic gutters. In several cases, injuries not apparent on inspection with the 0° scope were obvious using the 30° instrument.

Table 1. Preliminary studies of laparoscopy for trauma

Study	Patients, *n*	Mechanism of injury, *n*		DL (−), no laparatomy, *n*		DL (+), no laparatomy, *n*		DL (+), nontherapeutic laparatomy, *n*	
Sosa *et al.* [29]	8	GSW	8	GSW	6		0		0
Livingston *et al.* [25••]	39	SW	16	SW	4		0	SW	2
		GSW	15	GSW	1			GSW	1
		Blunt	8	Blunt	2			Blunt	1
Ivatury *et al.* [27•]	100	SW	65	SW	22	SW	3	SW	12
		GSW	35	GSW	21	GSW	0	GSW	1
Fabian *et al.* [26••]	182	SW	99	SW	49	SW	2	SW	19
		GSW	66	GSW	41	GSW	0	GSW	6
		Blunt	17	Blunt	3	Blunt	4	Blunt	1
Smith *et al.* [28]	34	SW	13	SW	4	SW	0	SW	4
		GSW	15	GSW	6	GSW	0	GSW	0
		Blunt	6	Blunt	0	Blunt	5	Blunt	0
Totals	363	SW	193	SW	79	SW	5	SW	37
		GSW	139	GSW	73	GSW	0	GSW	8
		Blunt	31	Blunt	5	Blunt	9	Blunt	2

+, findings positive; –,findings negative.
DL—diagnostic laparoscopy; GSW—gunshot wound; SW—stab wound.

Laparoscopy was able to determine whether peritoneal penetration occurred, and 45% of patients listed in Table 1 were able to avoid laparotomy (Fig. 2). This benefit was most apparent for victims of gunshot wounds. Several patients who underwent nontherapeutic laparotomies during these studies would now probably not be operated upon, further increasing the number of patients not requiring laparotomy. Laparoscopy missed a significant number of small bowel and colonic injuries, as mentioned previously [27•]. Another difficulty is the evaluation of the abdomen that contains a significant hemoperitoneum. Improvements in instrumentation and technique may decrease these problems. Complications of laparoscopy were few and included two tension pneumothoraces, one small bowel perforation, and one missed splenic injury [25••,26••].

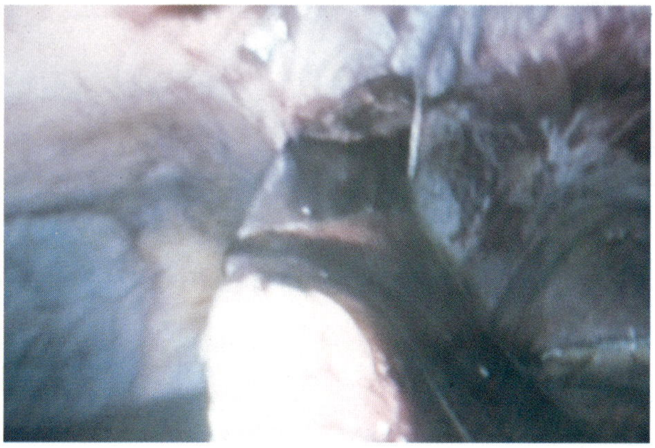

Fig. 2. Laparoscopic view of a knife entering the peritoneal cavity. The shaft of the blade is exposed and reflective. The tip of the knife was embedded in and elevated the anterior surface of the stomach. Adherent hematoma is seen on the right. The knife had broken off below the skin and was not present on physical examination or on chest radiograph.

Still debated in the use of laparoscopy in trauma are whether to perform the procedure in the operating room or the emergency department, and under what type of anesthesia, local or general. Another issue is the place of laparoscopy in the diagnostic work-up of the trauma patient. All of the studies reported in Table 1 were performed in the operating room, with most patients under general anesthesia. In their original description of laparoscopy for trauma, Berci *et al.* [19] used local anesthesia in the emergency department. Cuschieri *et al.* [30] reported a small series comparing laparoscopy done in the emergency department to diagnostic peritoneal lavage (DPL) in patients sustaining blunt trauma. Recently Salvino *et al.* [31•] compared DPL to laparoscopy in the emergency department setting. Of these procedures, 41% were performed using local anesthesia. In 59 patients who sustained blunt trauma, the use of laparoscopy offered no advantage over DPL as a primary screening tool. Using laparoscopy, they found four diaphragmatic injuries in patients with stab wounds (Fig. 3) who had DPL with fewer than 10,000 erythrocytes/mL. It is unknown whether these four studies were performed with patients under local or general anesthesia. The advantage to performing the procedure in the operating room under general anesthesia is the improved ability to evaluate the viscera, place additional ports, and potentially perform therapeutic procedures such as repair of the diaphragm. It remains to be seen whether emergency department laparoscopy is advantageous.

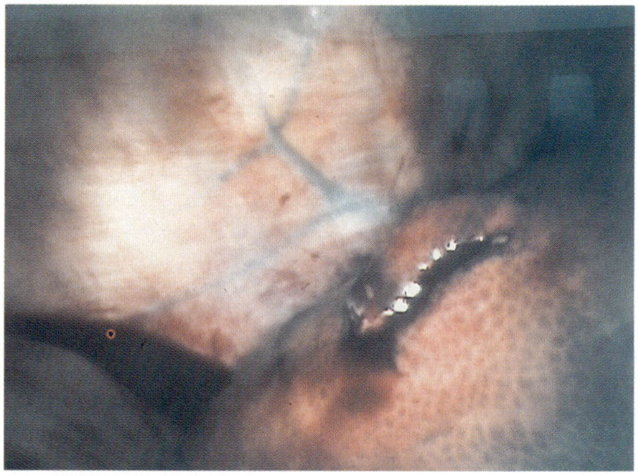

Fig. 3. Stab wound to the liver, not bleeding at the time of laparoscopy. Blood is seen in the right gutter, and the diaphragm is visible behind the liver.

Thoracoscopy

Thoracoscopy, like laparoscopy, is a technique that has been around for a number of years and now is seeing a resurgence due to improved video and optics. Jones *et al.* [32] in 1981, prior to the introduction of the newer instruments, reported their experience with thoracoscopy in chest trauma. The procedure was performed in the operating room under local anesthesia. They found the procedure to be useful. They believe that it altered the management in 44% of cases, and they were able to avoid thoracotomy in 16 patients. Once again, as with the experience with laparoscopy, this was the last report of the technique in trauma until the recent advances in video equipment.

Thoracoscopy following chest trauma has been used to visualize the diaphragm and remove clotted blood or empyemas. Ochsner *et al.* [33] believed that the evaluation of the diaphragm was best made through the chest rather than by laparoscopy. In their series of penetrating injuries ($n = 14$), 9 patients, had diaphragmatic injuries. In that group, seven sustained liver injuries and one had a retroperitoneal hematoma. One patient began bleeding from the lung following a negative thoracoscopy and required lower lobectomy. The problem with viewing the diaphragm from the chest is that it is not the diaphragmatic injury *per se* that is the problem but rather the injury to the liver or stomach that is important. Also, the diaphragm can be readily inspected in its entirety from the abdomen using a 30° scope.

The more likely application of thoracoscopy for trauma is in the evacuation of blood and pus from the thoracic cavity [34,35•]. While several studies have demonstrated the benefit of the early evacuation of retained hemothoraces in the trauma patient, there was great reluctance among many surgeons to subject patients to early operation in the hopes that the clot would resolve or cause no long-term problems [36,37]. Also differentiating pleural collections from parenchymal pathology, *eg*, atelectasis or pneumonia, was not always easy on plain chest radiography. Another unanswered question was how much blood in the pleural space following chest trauma could be reabsorbed. Thoracoscopy provides an ideal modality to evacuate the clot without the morbidity of a thoracotomy. Mancini *et al.* [34] recently reported on two patients whose clots were evacuated on day two and day four following injury. Thoracoscopy was attempted on day 7 after injury in a third patient, but the procedure failed due to dense adhesions.

We have successfully performed thoracoscopy in 12 patients for retained hemothorax. In one instance the patient had an empyema, which was successfully evacuated and the chest cavity debrided. In our experience several technical problems and solutions became obvious. The procedure required a functioning double lumen tube to allow the appropriate lung to be collapsed. Often the lung will not fully deflate and retract from the chest wall secondary to adhesions and the clotted blood. The scope should be initially placed away from the area of pathology in order to visualize a free area of chest wall. Two additional incisions are made for the retraction of the lung and the irrigation and evacuation of the clot. We have found the high-pressure pulsatile irrigation devices indispensable in loosening the clot.

The ability to evacuate empyemas requires more patience and skill that does evacuating early clotted blood. Before the general use of video thoracoscopy, Ridley and Bainbridge [38] reported their results in the debridement and irrigation of empyemas in 18 patients. They were successful in 12 patients. Recently O'Brien *et al.* [35•] reported the successful drainage and decortication in 6 patients with posttraumatic empyemas. No patient required a second procedure.

Conclusions

As new diagnostic modalities and refinements in older procedures continue to be introduced into clinical medicine, the work-up and evaluation of the trauma victim will continue to evolve, just as the era of mandatory exploratory surgery for many conditions was replaced by previous diagnostic advances such as angiography and CT scanning. It remains the responsibility of the trauma surgeon to carefully evaluate each new "advance" to determine if the technique adds important diagnostic information and can potentially reduce nontherapeutic procedures. Otherwise, these modalities merely waste resources and dollars and keep patients from prompt and appropriate treatment.

References and recommended reading

Papers of particular interest, published within the annual period of review, have been highlighted as:

• Of special interest
•• Of outstanding interest

1. Mayron R, Gaudio F, Plummer D, Asinger R, Elsperger J: **Echocardiography, Performed by Emergency Physicians: Impact on Diagnosis and Therapy**. *Ann Emerg Med* 1988, **17**:150–154.

2. Turturo M: **Emergency Echocardiography**. *Emerg Med Clin North Am* 1992, **10**:47–57.

3. Plummer D, Brunette D, Asinger R, Ruiz E: **Emergency Department Echocardiography Improves Outcome in Penetrating Cardiac Injury**. *Ann Emerg Med* 1992, **21**:709–712.

4. Kuwagata Y, Sugimoto H, Yoshioka T, Sugimoto T: **Left Ventricular Performance in Patients With Thermal Injury Or Multiple Trauma: A Clinical Study With Echocardiography**. *J Trauma* 1992, **32**:158–165.

5. Jimenez E, Martin M, Krukenkamp I, Barrett J: **Subxiphoid Pericardiotomy Versus Echocardiography: A Prospective Evaluation of the Diagnosis of Occult Penetrating Cardiac Injury**. *Surgery* 1990, **108**:676–680.

6. •• Brooks S, Young J, Cmolik B, Schina M, Dianzumba S, Townsend R, Diamond D: **The Use of Transesophageal Echocardiography in the Evaluation of Chest Trauma**. *J Trauma* 1992, **32**:761–768.

Follow-up series of authors' initial case report. Demonstrates the superiority of TEE over transthoracic echocardiography but fails to make a convincing case for TEE in the diagnosis of aortic injury.

7. Mirvis S, Kostrubiak I, Whitley N, Goldstein L, Rodriguez A: **Role of CT in Excluding Major Arterial Injury After Blunt Thoracic Trauma**. *AJR Am J Roentgenol* 1987, **149**:601–605.

8. Miller F, Richardson J, Thomas H, Cryer H, Willing S: **Role of CT in Diagnosis of Major Arterial Injury After Blunt Thoracic Trauma**. *Surgery* 1989, **106**:596–603.

9. Brooks S, Cmolik B, Young J, Towsend R, Diamond D: **Transesophageal Echocardiographic Examination of a Patient With Traumatic Aortic Transection From Blunt Chest Trauma: A Case Report**. *J Trauma* 1991, **31**:841–845.

10. Shapiro M, Yanofsky S, Trapp J, Durham R, Labovitz A, Sear J, Barth C, Pearson A: **Cardiovascular Evaluation in Blunt Thoracic Trauma Using Transesophageal Echocardiography (TEE)**. *J Trauma* 1991, **31**:835–840.

11. Sparks M, Burchard K, Marrin C, Bean C, Nugent W, Plehn J: **Transesophageal Echocardiography: Preliminary Results in Patients With Traumatic Aortic Rupture**. *Arch Surg* 1991, **126**:711–714.

12. Brathwaite C, Weiss R, Baldino W, Hoganson N, Ross S: **Multichamber Gunshot Wounds of the Heart: The Utility of Transesophageal Echocardiography**. *Chest* 1992, **101**:287–288.

13. • Goarin J, LeBret F, Riou B, Jacquens Y, Viars P: **Early Diagnosis of Traumatic Thoracic Aortic Rupture by Transesophageal Echocardiography**. *Chest* 1993, **103**:618–619.

Case reports of two patients who underwent TEE in an emergency department.

14. Goldberg S, Karalis D, Ross J, Chandrasekaran K: **Severe Right Ventricular Contusion Mimicking Cardiac Tamponade: The Value of Transesophageal Echocardiography in Blunt Chest Trauma**. *Ann Emerg Med* 1993, **22**:745–747.

15. Mitchell M: **Detection of Occult Hemopericardium Using Intraoperative Transesophageal Echocardiography**. *Anesthesiology* 1992, **76**:145–147.

16. •• Kearny P, Smith D, Johnson S, Barker D, Smith M, Sapin P: **Use of Transesophageal Echocardiography in the Evaluation of Traumatic Aortic Injury**. *J Trauma* 1993, **34**:696–703.

Largest prospective series of TEE in the diagnosis of aortic injury. High false-negative rate of angiography and the lack of brachiocephalic injuries clouds paper's conclusions.

17. • Tso P, Rodriguez A, Cooper C, Militello P, Mirvis S, Badellino M, Boulanger B, Foss F Jr, Hinson D, Mighty H, Nasrallah D, Raimonde A, Yates W, Yuschak J: **Sonography in Blunt Abdominal Trauma: A Preliminary Report**. *J Trauma* 1992, **33**:39–44.

Paper demonstrates that trauma surgeons can be trained to perform ultrasonography with a good deal of accuracy.

18. Adamthwaite DN: **Traumatic Diaphragmatic Hernia: A New Indication for Laparoscopy**. *Br J Surg* 1984, **71**:315.

19. Berci G, Dunkelman D, Michel SL, Sanders G, Wahlstrom E, Morgenstern L: **Emergency Minilaparoscopy in Abdominal Trauma: An Update**. *Am J Surg* 1983, **146**:261–265.

20. Carnevale N, Baron N, Delany HM: **Peritoneoscopy as an Aid in the Diagnosis of Abdominal Trauma: A Preliminary Report.** *J Trauma* 1976, **17**:634–641.

21. Gazzaniga AB, Stanton WW, Bartlett RH: **Laparoscopy in the Diagnosis of Blunt and Penetrating Injuries to the Abdomen.** *Am J Surg* 1976, **131**:315–318.

22. Henneman PL, Marx JA, Moore EE, Cantrill SV, Ammons LA: **Diagnostic Peritoneal Lavage: Accuracy in Predicting Necessary Laparotomy Following Blunt and Penetrating Trauma.** *J Trauma* 1990, **30**:1345–1355.

23. Miller FB, Cryer HM, Chilikuri S, Creech P, Richardson JD: **Negative Findings on Laparotomy for Trauma.** *South Med J* 1989, **82**:1231–1234.

24. Sorkey AJ, Farnell MB, Williams HJ Jr, Mucha P Jr, Ilstrup DM: **The Complementary Roles of Diagnostic Peritoneal Lavage and Computed Tomography in the Evaluation of Blunt Abdominal Trauma.** *Surgery* 1989, **106**:794–801.

25. Livingston DH, Tortella BJ, Blackwood J, Machiedo GW, Rush BF
•• Jr: **The Role of Laparoscopy in Abdominal Trauma.** *J Trauma* 1992, **33**:471–475.

Report on the authors' initial experience with laparoscopy in cases of abdominal trauma. Clearly defines the limitations (evaluation of the spleen) and small bowel and the strength (determination of peritoneal penetration) of the procedure.

26. Fabian T, Croce M, Stewart R, Pritchard F, Minard G, Kudsk K:
•• **A Prospective Analysis of Diagnostic Laparoscopy in Trauma.** *Ann Surg* 1993, **217**:557–565.

Largest series (182 patients) of laparoscopy for trauma in the literature. Reviews the pitfalls and capabilities of the technique. Presents a good discussion of the future of diagnostic and interventional laparoscopy for trauma.

27. Ivatury R, Simon R, Stahl W: **A Critical Evaluation of Laparoscopy**
• **in Penetrating Abdominal Trauma.** *J Trauma* 1993, **34**:822–828.

Describes use of laparoscopy in penetrating trauma. Includes the first 40 patients reported by authors using a nonvideo system.

28. Smith R, Tsoi E, Fry W, Henderson V, Kohler R, Bohman H, Morabito D, Organ C: **Laparoscopic Evaluation of Abdominal Trauma: A Preliminary Report.** *Contemp Surg* 1993, **42**:13–18.

29. Sosa JL, Sims D, Martin L, Zeppa R: **Laparoscopic Evaluation of Tangential Abdominal Gunshot Wounds.** *Arch Surg* 1992, **127**:109–110.

30. Cuschieri A, Hennessey TPJ, Stephens RB, Berci G: **Diagnosis of Significant Abdominal Trauma After Road Accidents: Preliminary Results of a Multicentre Clinical Trial Comparing Minilaparoscopy With Peritoneal Lavage.** *Ann R Coll Surg Engl* 1988, **70**:153–155.

31. Salvino C, Esposito T, Marshall W, Dries D, Morris R, Gamelli R:
• **The Role of Diagnostic Laparoscopy in Trauma Patients: A Preliminary Assessment [Abstract].** *J Trauma* 1992, **33**:162.

The most extensive use of laparoscopy in the emergency department setting for abdominal trauma.

32. Jones J, Kitahama A, Webb W, McSwain N: **Emergency Thoracoscopy: A Logical Approach to Chest Trauma Management.** *J Trauma* 1981, **21**:280–284.

33. Ochsner M, Rozycki G, Lucente F, Wherry D, Champion H: **Prospective Evaluation of Thoracoscopy for Diagnosing Diaphragmatic Injury in Thoracoabdominal Trauma: A Preliminary Report.** *J Trauma* 1993, **34**:704–710.

34. Mancini M, Smith L, Nein A, Buechter K: **Early Evacuation of Clotted Blood in Hemothorax Using Thoracoscopy: Case Reports.** *J Trauma* 1993, **34**:144–147.

35. O'Brien J, Cohen M, Solit R, Solit R, Lindenbaum G, Finnegan J,
• Vernick J: **Thoracoscopic Drainage and Decortication as Definitive Treatment for Empyema Thoracis Following Penetrating Chest Injury [Abstract].** *J Trauma* 1993, **35**:167.

Abstract of paper presented at the 1993 meeting of the American Association for the Surgery of Trauma, New Orleans, LA. Procedure is reported to be 100% successful at evacuating pus and decorticating thoracic cavity.

36. Milfeld D, Mattox K, Beall A Jr: **Early Evacuation of Clotted Hemothorax.** *Am J Surg* 1978, **136**:686–692.

37. Coselli J, Mattox K, Beall A: **Reevaluation of Early Evacuation of Clotted Hemothorax.** *Am Surg* 1984, **50**:21–24.

38. Ridley P, Braimbridge M: **Thoracoscopic Debridement and Pleural Irrigation in the Management of Empyema Thoracis.** *Ann Thorac Surg* 1991, **51**:461–464.

David H. Livingston, MD, University Hospital C-384, 150 Bergen Street, Newark, NJ 07103, USA.

Advances in the treatment of pediatric trauma

Matthew L. Moront, MD, and Martin R. Eichelberger, MD

Children's National Medical Center, Washington, DC, USA

Injury is the leading cause of death among US children over 1 year of age. The financial burden of acute care is over $15 billion annually. The unique anatomic and physiologic differences of children predispose them to certain types of injuries and require a specialized approach to pediatric trauma care. This article reviews the common etiologies of injuries to children and identifies injury subgroups at increased risk of mortality. Resuscitation and assessment are discussed, emphasizing fluid management, rapid intravenous access, and the physiologic evaluation of the child in shock. Protocols for evaluating head, thoracic, abdominal, and pelvic injuries are presented in light of recent advances in the diagnosis, treatment, and rehabilitation of children sustaining these injuries.

Current Opinion in General Surgery 1994:41–49

The children of the United States face a frightening challenge. They must learn to survive in a society where childhood injury is the number one threat to life and accounts for more deaths than all other causes combined [1]. Over 20,000 children died in 1992 as a result of injury. Recent statistics indicate an even greater number will die in 1993 [1,2••]. As sobering as these figures are, they only suggest the magnitude of this tragedy.

For every child in this country who dies of injury, 40 more will require hospitalization, and over 1100 will be examined in emergency departments. It is estimated that 50,000 children will suffer permanent disability due to brain injury, and that one child in four will seek some type of medical treatment [3]. The financial burden is immense. The Institute of Medicine in Washington, DC, estimates that in 1985, injuries to children less than 15 years of age cost almost $16 billion. In the 15- to 24-year-old age group, the total was over $39 billion with less than $9 million going toward direct hospital care [1,3].

Unique aspects of pediatric anatomy and physiology

Children's anatomic and physiologic differences require a distinct clinical approach from that used with the adult patient. Evaluation of a child must bear in mind these differences. Children's larger ratio of body surface area to mass makes them much more susceptible to hypothermia and dehydration [4]. This is especially true in infants whose immature shivering mechanism and lack of subcutaneous fat make hypothermia-induced vasoconstriction, pulmonary hypertension, and subsequent metabolic acidosis very real possibilities [5]. The disproportionately large head size and poorly developed neck musculature of young children raise the center of gravity and increase the risk of head and upper cervical spine injury [6]. The increased compliance of a child's skeletal system and the lack of protection afforded by the rib cage increase the potential of injury to the lung, liver, and spleen without associated rib fracture [7,8].

The child's airway deserves special mention because it is unlike the adult airway in several important ways. A child's tongue is proportionately larger, the larynx shorter and more anterior, and the epiglottis softer, making intubation difficult [9,10]. The most narrow point in a child's airway is distal to the focal cords, at the cricoid cartilage, making endotracheal tube selection challenging and necessitating the use of uncuffed endotracheal tubes in children under 8 years of age to prevent tracheal stenosis [11••].

Components of care

Comprehensive care for the injured child includes injury prevention, short-term treatment, and rehabilitation and community reintegration. Providing the best trauma care possible for children starts with sound injury prevention principles. This is possible through organizations such as the SAFE KIDS Campaign, the first nonprofit nationwide effort to reduce preventable childhood injury. The campaign strategy works through community coalitions and local organizations to promote child safety through modification of public policy, media education, and improved product engineering [12].

Abbreviation

CT—computed tomography.

 ISBN 1-85922-671-X ISSN 1065–6243

Remarkable advances have been made in the area of prevention. A most notable example involves the use of bicycle helmets by children. Bicycle-related injury constitutes a significant portion of blunt trauma; over 50% of these children sustain some type of head injury [13]. In an attempt to combat this problem, a cooperative study was undertaken in Seattle, Washington [14]. By increasing public awareness, reducing helmet costs, and creating usage incentives, the percentage of children wearing helmets in Seattle tripled, and the number of children sustaining head injuries decreased; the risk of head injury was reduced by 85%. Other areas where extensive progress continues include limiting the maximum temperature on hot water heaters in the home to reduce the incidence and severity of scald burns from tap water, institution of passive restraint systems in automobiles, use of children's car seats, and finally, installation of window guards on the elevated windows of homes where children live, thereby reducing the number of falls.

The recognition that children constitute a distinct and physiologically different subset of patients has stimulated the evolution of specialized emergency medical services for children [2••]. To provide for their needs, specialized educational courses such as Pediatric Advanced Life Support and Advanced Pediatric Life Support for prehospital care providers, nurses, and physicians have been developed [15,16].

The final component of care essential to the injured child is rehabilitation. This process begins at admission, continues throughout the acute care of the child, and ends only when complete reintegration into the community is achieved. A multidisciplinary team of health professionals assesses the degree of functional impairment, offers treatment options, and guides the family through the rehabilitation process [13].

Etiology of injury

Blunt force accounts for more than 60% of the trauma admissions of children less than 14 years of age, with over half of these children presenting with head injury [17••,18]. The most common mechanism of injury is motor-vehicle related (pedestrians, bicyclists, or vehicle occupants), accounting for 30% of the trauma admissions to a level I pediatric trauma center. Many of these children sustain multisystem injury [17••]. Falls comprise the next most common mechanism of injury (24%) and usually occur in younger children. Fortunately, severe injury or death due to a fall is uncommon [18]. Child abuse, both underrecognized and underreported, occurs with alarming frequency in the younger age group and accounts for 25% of the mortality for children under 1 year of age [19,20]. Penetrating injury in the pediatric population (0 to 19 years of age) has increased dramatically in the last decade; nearly 12% of the pediatric deaths reported in 1989 were due to gunshot wounds. Firearm homicides are the leading cause of death among urban black teenagers 15 to 19 years of age [21•,22]. Burn injury constitutes approximately 20% of all trauma admissions nationally, and although not usually fatal, it is a tremendous drain on resources. Statistics show that 50% of all children with burn injuries will require at least 1 month of hospitalization and some type of reconstructive surgery. An additional 25% will need up to 2 months of hospitalization [11••,23].

Resuscitation and assessment

Restorative care begins soon after admission and continues through discharge and rehabilitation to ensure maximum recovery and integration for the injured child and his family [24,25]. Although all phases of the continuum of care are equally important, this review focuses on the emergency care component. In the emergency department, the resuscitation of the injured child begins with activation of the specially designated trauma team accustomed to the systematic guidelines of Advanced Trauma Life Support and the Pediatric Advanced Life Support protocol [16,26]. Assessment and stabilization of the airway are the highest priority, followed be ventilation and evaluation for signs of inadequate tissue perfusion. Immobilization of the cervical spine is essential until evaluation reveals no injury [16,26–28].

In children with inadequate tissue perfusion, reliable indicators of shock are tachycardia, tachypnea, and physical signs such as cool mottled skin, delayed capillary refill, or altered mental status. Surprisingly, systolic blood pressure will remain within the normal range despite significant blood loss. Also, intravenous access in children presents a formidable challenge. This is especially true in an infant, whose fat accumulation is at its peak around 9 months of age, or in an older child with vascular collapse. An intraosseous infusion device placed in the anterior tibial plateau in children under 3 years of age and in the medial malleolus in older children permits infusion of both volume and medications when peripheral venous access is unavailable [29•,30]. Alternative sites for intraosseous infusion of fluids include the iliac crest and the distal femur (Fig. 1). After establishment of intravenous access, a rapid infusion of lactated Ringer's solution at 20 mL/kg is administered (Fig. 2); persistent inadequate tissue perfusion signifies the need for a repeat bolus of crystalloid infusion to a level of 40 mL/kg. If further volume expansion is needed, administration of 10 mL/kg of the most type-specific packed erythrocytes is begun. Persistent fluid and blood requirements indicate ongoing hemorrhage and compel prompt surgical hemostasis.

Pneumatic antishock trousers are used for prehospital treatment of hypotension in adults [31]. Use of pneumatic trouser is contraindicated in children since a compromise of ventilation occurs and trouser inflation may promote pulmonary edema during fluid infusion. An exception to this is a child with an unstable pelvic fracture, where inflation of the pelvic portion helps stabilize the fracture and reduce bleeding at the fracture site until external fixation is possible. Recently, clinical trials using 7.5% sodium chloride for crystalloid

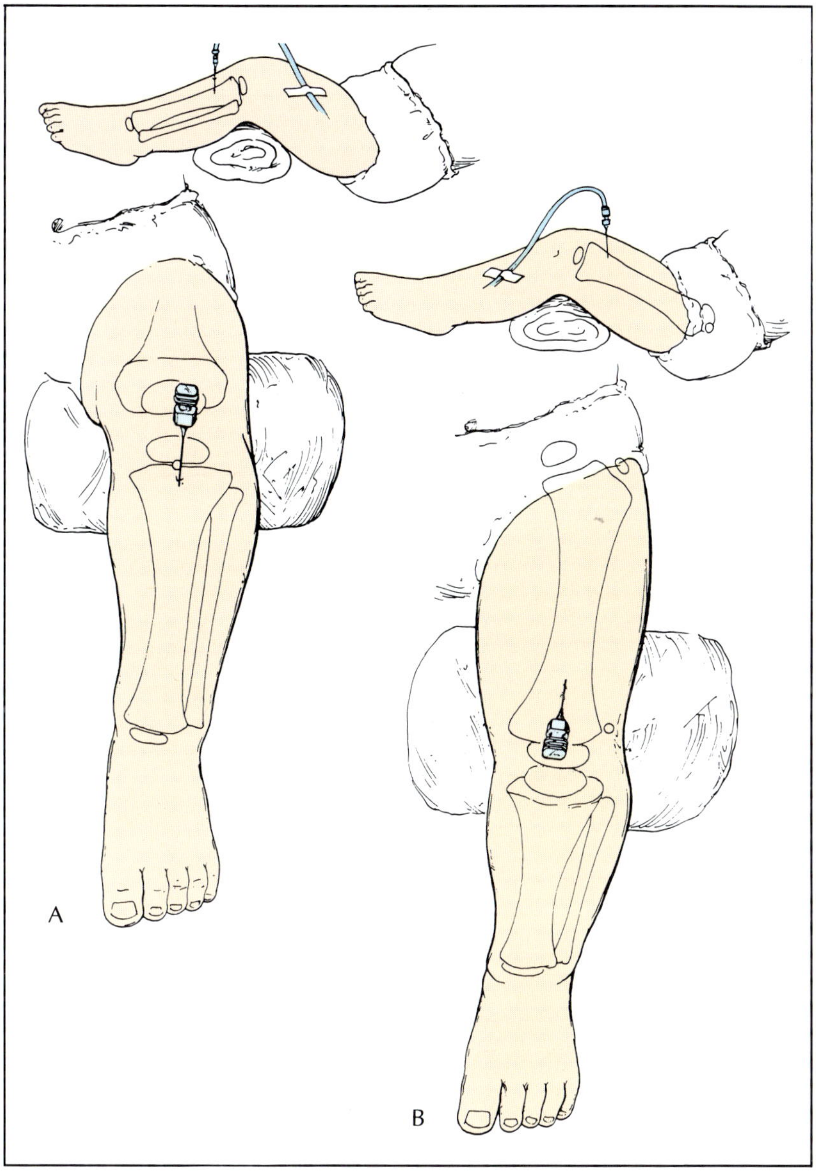

Fig. 1. Intraosseous line placement in the proximal tibia (*A*) and distal femur (*B*). (*From* Fleisher and Ludwig [69]; with permission.)

fluid infusion show a survival advantage in hypotensive adult trauma victims [32]. While this technology is promising, its usefulness in the pediatric population remains unproven.

After the initial assessment and resuscitation, all severely injured children require portable radiographs of the cervical spine, chest, and pelvis [8,11••,33]. Computed tomography (CT) is currently the study of choice for the hemodynamically stable child in whom serious abdominal injury exists or in whom multisystem trauma occurs [34,35]. The presence of concomitant head injury or of gross hematuria with associated abdominal findings are also indications for obtaining a CT scan [34,36,37].

The technique of diagnostic peritoneal lavage, commonly used in adult trauma victims, is less useful in the pediatric population, where the successful nonoperative management of the majority of solid organ injuries has minimized the usefulness of this invasive procedure [38••,39,40]. If CT scan is not available or if a high suspicion of gastrointestinal perforation exists, diagnostic peritoneal lavage is a sensitive and useful diagnostic adjunct to the clinician's armamentarium [38••,41,42].

The use of ultrasonography in the initial evaluation of blunt trauma in the pediatric population is currently undergoing study [43–47]. A recent Canadian trial evaluated the clinical usefulness of ultrasonography as a first-line imaging modality and found it to be both sensitive (89%) and specific (96%) when compared with CT [18,42–44]. Another new application of a well-known diagnostic technique is the evaluation of the abdomen using laparoscopy, which could allow surgeons to assess suspected injury under direct vision in the emergency department and treat bleeding through the laparoscopic cannula [48,49].

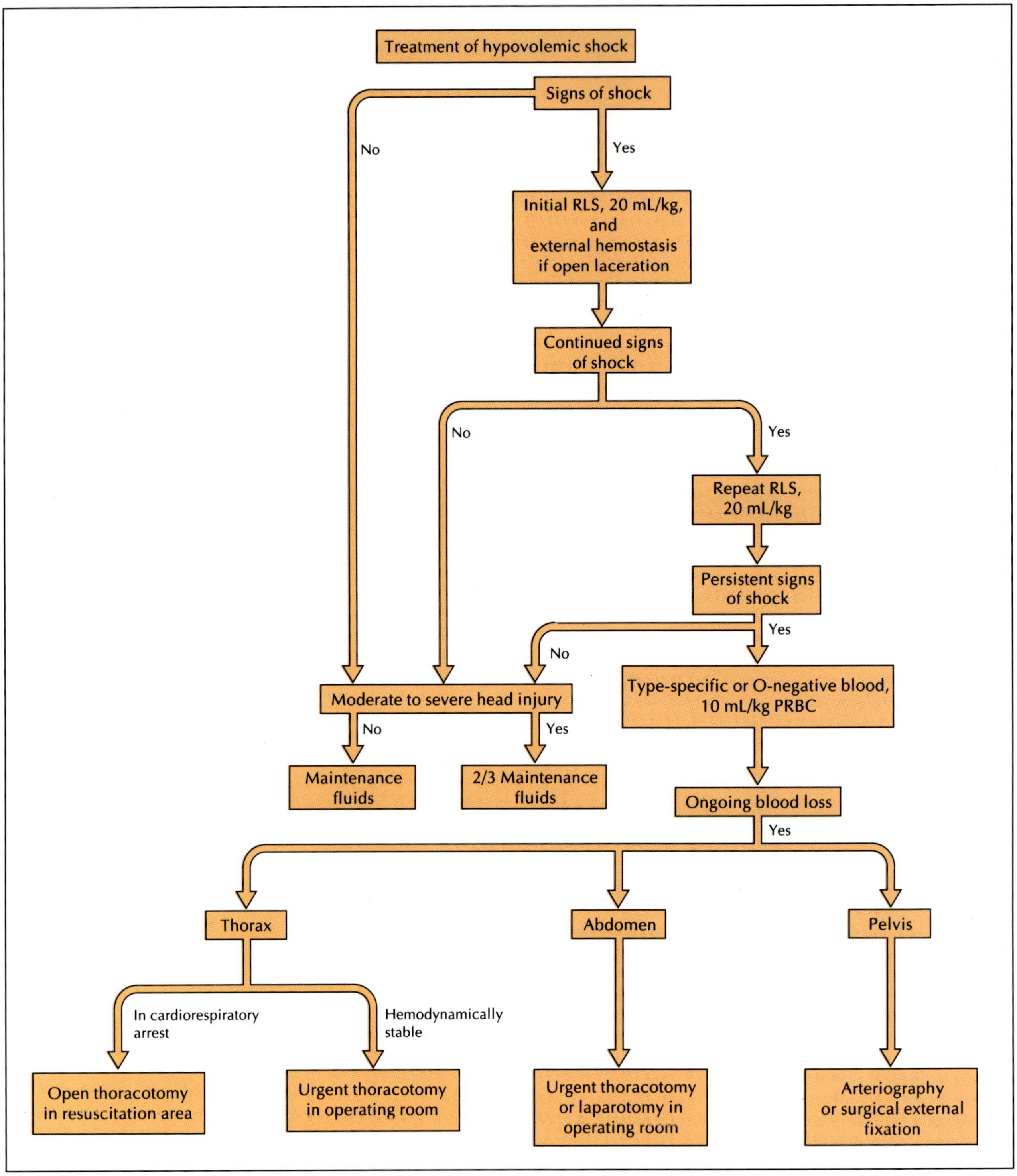

Fig. 2. An algorithm for treating hypovolemic shock in the injured child. PRBC—packed red blood cells; RLS—Ringer's lactated solution. (*From* Young and Eichelberger [70]; with permission.)

Head injury

Injury to the central nervous system ranks as the number one cause of death among children. Families are forced to endure pain and anguish, not only from the loss of a child, but from the tremendous emotional and financial drain of long-term rehabilitation necessary for children who survive head injury. The mechanism of pediatric head injury changes with increasing age; homicide is the predominant cause of head injury deaths in infants [19]. In the adolescent years, motor vehicle involvement (passengers, bicyclists, pedestrians) signals the start of a trend of increasing mortality with increasing age [11••].

Initial treatment of the child with a head injury begins with a thorough assessment of airway, ventilation, and circulation. Early neurosurgical examination, prior to sedation or intubation, is helpful in determining the extent of injury and in predicting prognosis. Children who arrive with a Glasgow score of 8 or less undergo intubation of the airway and hyperventilation [11••]. An urgent CT scan is necessary prior to operative intervention or placement of intracranial monitoring devices to determine the presence of a mass effect, a significant intracranial hematoma, or cerebral edema. Abnormal coagulation profile is associated with precipitous rise in the incidence of secondary brain injury and increases the necessity for early CT scan follow-up [50•]. Factors most predictive of survival include severity of extracranial injuries as assessed by the Abbreviated Injury Scale and pupillary response in the resuscitation area [51].

Monitoring arterial pressure and documenting cerebral perfusion pressure are essential for the prevention of the deleterious effects of hypotension [52]. In an attempt to measure changes in the cerebral circulation more accurately, transcranial Doppler ultrasonography has been successfully used to correlate the relationship between blood flow velocity, neurologic deficit, and clinical outcome [53••]. Finally, although mannitol has long been used to reduce intracranial pressure by promoting an osmotic diuresis, preliminary data on the use of tromethamine for this purpose has been very encouraging and warrants further study [54].

Before a child leaves the intensive care unit, preparations for appropriate rehabilitation are continued. Comprehensive follow-up of children with head injuries is essential to meet the needs of the family and child. Factors most accurate in the prediction of disability after severe head injury include level of oxygenation in the emergency department and Glasgow Motor Score at 72 hours [51]. Combining these disability predictors with constant clinical assessment facilitates successful identification of the child who requires intensive rehabilitation.

Thoracic injury

Injury to the thoracic cavity of a child is usually accompanied by a large transfer of energy and is asso-

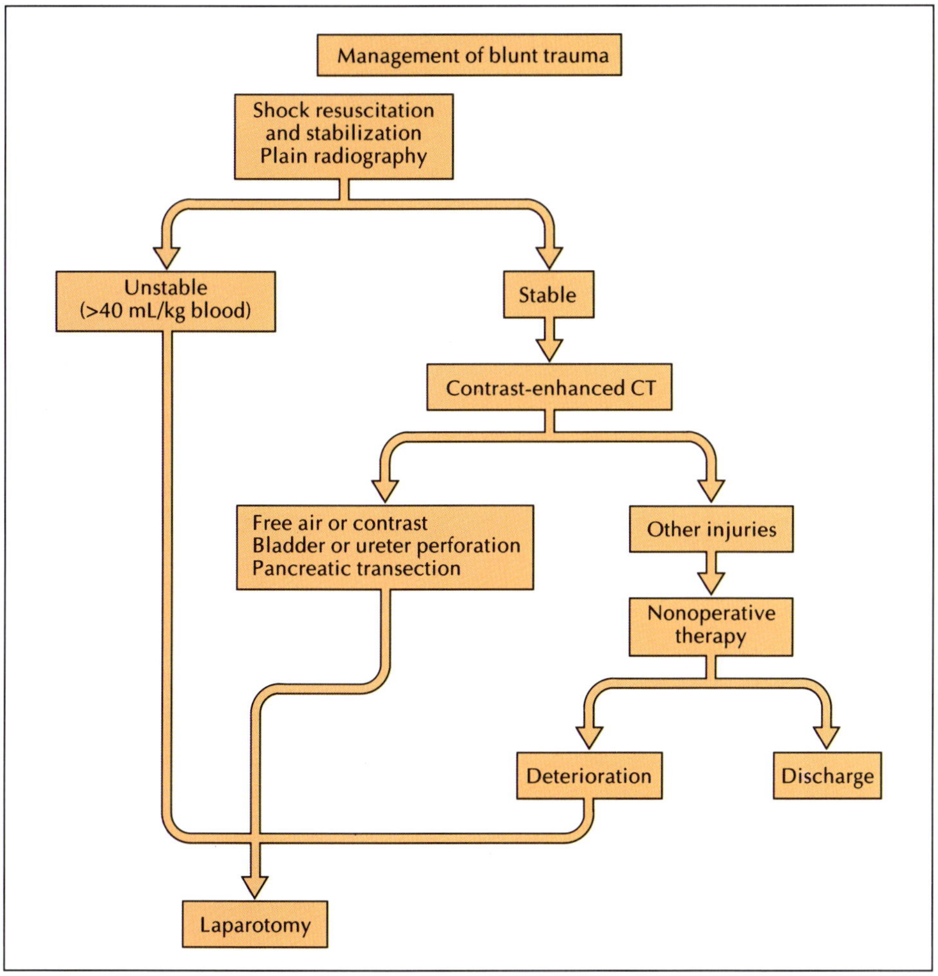

Fig. 3. Algorithm for management of blunt abdominal trauma. CT—computed tomography. (*From* Eichelberger [11••]; with permission.)

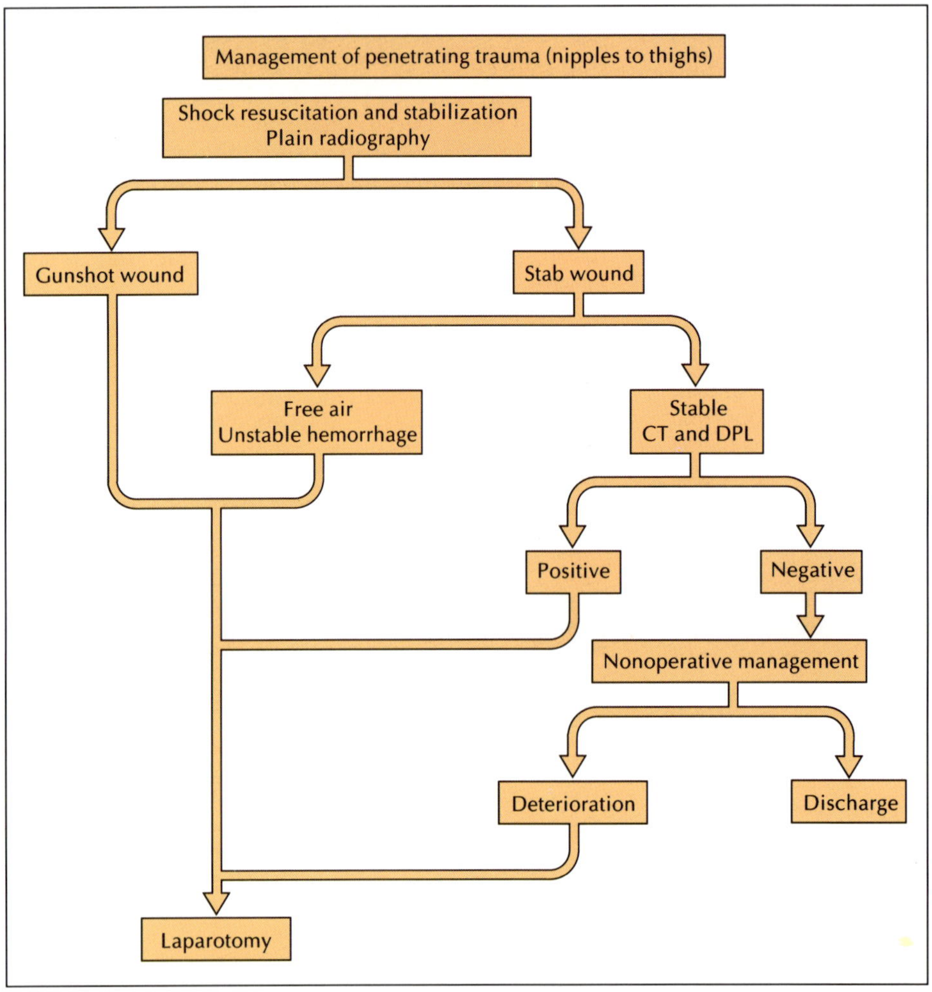

Fig. 4. Algorithm for management of penetrating abdominal trauma. CT—computed tomography; DPL—diagnostic peritoneal lavage. (*From* Eichelberger [11••]; with permission.)

ciated with an overall mortality rate of approximately 26% [55]; in contrast, less than 2% mortality occurs in children without concomitant thoracic injury [28]. Multisystem trauma is the rule with thoracic injuries, occurring in more than 80% of the cases. Head injuries are frequently involved (58%), and they raise the mortality rate to 36%. Another injury that significantly increases mortality is multiple rib fracture, which further increases mortality to 42% [7,18]. Nevertheless, an isolated single rib fracture is rarely associated with death or severe injury. The most ominous finding consists of multiple rib fractures and head injury, which raise the mortality to a staggering 71% [17••,56]. Despite these dismal statistics, most children with thoracic injury only require tube thoracostomy.

The most common thoracic injury in children is pulmonary contusion, which often occurs in the absence of rib fractures and that misleads the examiner as to the severity of the underlying pathology. Initial radiographic assessment of the chest by plain film will miss or underestimate this injury in approximately 40% of cases [18]. The possibility of pneumothorax is always considered when thoracic trauma occurs; needle decompression of the thorax in the midclavicular line in the second intercostal space and insertion of a thoracostomy tube are effective treatments. For hemothorax, thoracostomy is the initial treatment of choice. Children with ongoing hourly blood loss greater than 1 to 2 mL/kg require thoracotomy for assessment and control of hemorrhage. Decompression of the tension pneumothorax is essential, because the mediastinal structures in children are more mobile than in adults, making great vessel injury unusual, but resulting in significant vessel angulation, which causes circulatory compromise. Cardiac contusion is rare in the pediatric population and only infrequently causes detectable dysrhythmia [57,58]. Children with suspected cardiac contusion are treated conservatively without difficulty [58,59].

The indications for performing an emergency-room thoracotomy during resuscitation are subject to debate [60,61••,62]. Children with either blunt or penetrating trauma who have no obtainable pulse or blood pressure on arrival do not derive any benefit from emergency-department thoracotomy. Emergency thoracotomy is useful for children with penetrating thoracoabdominal trauma who have an obtainable pulse and refractory hypotension on arrival [60,61••].

Abdominal trauma

The evaluation of abdominal trauma in the injured child is a challenging task; mortality in these children is approximately 14% [17••]. The approach to treatment is divided into two distinct algorithms (Figs. 3 and 4). Stab wounds, missile injuries, and gunshot wounds are responsible for most penetrating trauma and require rapid fluid resuscitation and urgent exploratory laparotomy. The exception to this is stab wounds in children who are hemodynamically stable. These children undergo additional diagnostic evaluation of the solid organs and the gastrointestinal system; this assessment incudes plain radiographs, CT scanning, and if the diagnosis is still unclear, diagnostic peritoneal lavage [37,40,41].

Exploratory laparotomy is indicated for suspected ongoing hemorrhage after adequate crystalloid infusion (40 mL/kg) and packed erythrocyte transfusion of up to 50% of the total blood volume (40 mg/kg), obvious peritoneal signs, or a rapidly expanding abdomen. If the child is hemodynamically stable, additional diagnostic evaluation begins with an abdominal CT scan [38••]. Children with neurologic impairment following blunt trauma undergo assessment based on physical examination and do not routinely require CT scan [35]. Children with head injury following an assault or a bicycle crash were found to have an increased incidence of abdominal trauma, more than other injury subgroups [33]. In a recent study, 50% of children with confirmed blunt abdominal injury manifested hemoperitoneum on CT scanning [8]. The treatment strategy for hemodynamically stable children with specific types of solid organ injury has gradually shifted towards nonoperative management. This concept was initially suggested for blunt splenic injury in children but has now been extended to many grades of hepatic and renal injuries [63,64•]. A new strategy of early operative intervention using autotransfusion, combined with selective nonoperative management, resulted in a splenic salvage rate of 85% in moderate and severe (grades 3–5) blunt trauma [64•].

The increased use of seat belts has greatly reduced the number of fatalities from motor vehicle crashes, but a new pattern of injury is evident. Children presenting with lap belt ecchymoses have a significant number of lumbar spine and hollow viscus injuries. An examination of 61 children with abdominal wall ecchymosis revealed that 21% suffered lumbar spine injuries and 23% injured a hollow viscus [65]. Early exploratory laparotomy is useful in this group of children with the "lap belt complex" [65].

Pelvic injury

Pelvic fractures are uncommon in children, occurring in less than 3% of all blunt trauma admissions [66–68]. Motor vehicles cause 89% of these cases, with an overall mortality rate of 11.1% [66]. Head injury is the predominant cause of death in these children (77%), while mortality due to severe hemorrhage is rare (1.3%). The presence of multiple fracture sites within the pelvic circle is a strong indicator of visceral injury, with 80% of children with multiple fractures having concomitant intra-abdominal or genitourinary injury [66,67]. The probability of abdominal injury is reduced to 6% for an isolated pubic ramus fracture.

Conclusions

The tragedy of childhood injury continues unabated. It is clear that prevention is the cornerstone of reducing the childhood epidemic of injury. Accurate intervention by physicians and by nurses will have the greatest impact on the outcome of injured children. Analysis of the patterns of childhood injury and of the current methods of treatment is essential for the improvement of pediatric trauma care in America.

References and recommended reading

Papers of particular interest, published within the annual period of review, have been highlighted as:

- • Of special interest
- •• Of outstanding interest

1. Buckly J: **The Shame of Emergency Medicine: Kids at Risk.** *US News World Rep*, January 27, 1992.

2. Durch JS, Lohr KW, eds: **Emergency Medical Service for Children.**
•• Washington, DC: National Academy Press: 1993.
This report was created by a distinguished panel of pediatricians, surgeons, and emergency medicine specialists to examine the problem of emergency medical services for children in the United States. The report comprehensively details the current status of prehospital provider training and education, communication systems, integration of emergency medical service agencies, and issues concerning funding, evaluation, and research. The committee makes specific recommendations for improvement and emphasizes the need for increasing public awareness concerning emergency services for children.

3. Guyers B, Elers B: **The Causes, Impact, and Preventability of Childhood Injuries in the United States: The Magnitude of the Problem: An Overview.** *Am J Dis Child* 1990, **144**:627–646.

4. De Bruin WJ, Greenwald BM, Notterman DA: **Fluid Resuscitation in Pediatrics.** *Crit Care Clin* 1992, **8**:423–438.

5. Kissoon ND, Dreyer J, Walia M: **Pediatric Trauma: Differences in Pathophysiology, Injury Patterns and Treatment Compared With Adult Trauma.** *Can Med Assoc J* 1990, **14**:27–34.

6. Dickman CA, Rekate HL, Sonntag VK, *et al.*: **Pediatric Spinal Trauma: Vertebral Column and Spinal Cord Injuries in Children.** *Pediatr Neurosci* 1989, **15**:237–256.

7. Garcia V, Gotschall CS, Eichelberger MR, *et al.*: **Rib Fractures in Children: A Marker of Severe Injury.** *J Trauma* 1990, **30**:695–700.

8. Rouse T, Eichelberger M: **Trends in Pediatric Management.** *Surg Clin North Am* 1992, **72**:1347–1364.

9. Aijian P, Tsai A, Knopp R: **Endotracheal Intubation of Pediatric Patients by Paramedics.** *Ann Emerg Med* 1989, **18**:489–494.

10. Nakayama DK, Gardner MJ, Rowe MI: **Emergency Endotracheal Intubation in Pediatric Population.** *Ann Surg* 1990, **211**:218–223.

11. Eichelberger M: *Pediatric Trauma-Prevention, Acute Care, Rehabil-*
•• *itation,* edn 1. Philadelphia: Mosby; 1993.
A comprehensive reference that examines a broad range of pediatric trauma topics. The book begins with an examination of the disease process of childhood injury and goes on to describe the unique features of children. What follows is a series of detailed chapters by noted authors on the specific issues involved in the prevention, acute care, and rehabilitation on the injured child.

12. *National SAFE KIDS CAMPAIGN.* Washington, DC: Children's National Medical Center, 1987.

13. Seidel JS, Henderson DP, eds: **Emergency Medical Services for Children: A Report to the Nation.** Washington, DC: National Center for Education in Maternal and Child Health; 1991.

14. Thompson RS, Rivea FP, Thompson DC: **A Case-Control Study of the Effectiveness of Bicycle Safety Helmets**. *New Engl J Med* 1989, **320**:1361–1367.

15. Silverman B, *et al.*: **Advanced Pediatric Life Support**. Elk Grove Village, IL: American Academy of Pediatrics; 1993.

16. American Heart Association: **Pediatric Advanced Life Support**. Dallas: American Heart Association; 1988.

17. Allshouse MJ, Rouse T, Eichelberger M: **Childhood Injury: A Current •• Perspective**. *Pediatr Emerg Care* 1993, 9:159–164.
This is a well-written, concise review describing the impact and patterns of childhood injury. The authors discuss the treatment of specific injuries by anatomic region and review the most current strategies for fluid management, radiographic evaluation, and therapeutic decision making for blunt abdominal trauma.

18. Sivit CJ, Taylor GA, Newman KD, *et al.*: **Chest Injury in Children With Blunt Abdominal Trauma: Evaluation With CT**. *Radiology* 1989, **8**:815–819.

19. Peclet MH, Newman KD, Eichelberger MR, *et al.*: **Patterns of Injury in Children**. *J Pediatr Surg* 1990, **25**:85–91.

20. Sivit CJ, Taylor GA, Eichelberger MR: **Visceral Injury in Battered Children: A Changing Perspective**. *Radiology* 1989, **173**:658–661.

21. Committee on Injury and Poison Prevention: **Firearm Injuries Af- • fecting the Pediatric Population**. *Pediatrics* 1992, **89**:788–790.
This article reveals the shocking trends and statistics involved in pediatric death and injury by firearms. Details outlining the increased use of firearms in teenage suicides and homicides are provided as well as recommendations on how to reduce this tragic loss of life.

22. Fingerhut LA, Ingram DD, Feldman JJ: **Firearm Homicide Among Black Teenage Males in Metropolitan Counties: Comparison of Death Rates in Two Periods, 1983 Through 1985 and 1987 Through 1989**. *JAMA* 1992, **267**:3054–3058.

23. Finkelstein JL, Schwartz SB, Madden MR, *et al.*: **Pediatric Burns: An Overview**. *Pediatr Clin North Am* 1992, **39**:1145-1163.

24. Alexander MA, Demasco PW, Gilbert M, *et al.*: **Rehabilitation Technology for Disabled Children**. *Arch Phys Med Rehabil* 1991,15:

25. Savage RC: **Identification, Classification, and Placement Issues for Students With Traumatic Brain Injuries**. *J Head Trauma Rehabil* 1991, 6:1–9.

26. American College of Surgeons, The Committee on Trauma: **Advanced Trauma Life Support Course**. Chicago: American College of Surgeons; 1993.

27. Davis JW, Phreaner DL, Hoyt DB, *et al.*: **The Etiology of Missed Cervical Spine Injuries**. *J Trauma* 1993, **34**:342–346.

28. Gerretts BD, Peterson EU, Mabry J, *et al.*: **Delayed Diagnosis of Cervical Spine Injuries**. *J Trauma* 1991, **31**:16–22.

29. Guy J, Haley K, Zuspan S: **Use of Intraosseous Infusion in the Pe- • diatric Trauma Patient**. *J Pediatr Surg* 1993, **28**:158–161.
This study evaluated the indications, complications, and insertion sites of intraosseous line placement in 27 children. The results confirm that intraosseous line placement is a simple, safe, and effective method for obtaining rapid short-term access with minimal complications.

30. Neufeld JD, Marx JA, Moore EE, *et al.*: **Comparison of Intraosseous, Central, and Peripheral Routes of Crystalloid Infusion for Resuscitation of Hemorrhagic Shock in a Swine Model**. *J Trauma* 1993, 34:422–428.

31. Cayton GC, Berendt BM, *et al.*: **A Study of Pneumatic Antishock Garments in Severely Hypotensive Trauma Patients**. *J Trauma* 1993, 34:728–735.

32. Vasser MJ, Perry CA, Holcroft JW: **Prehospital Resuscitation of Hypotensive Trauma Patients With 7.5% NaCl With Added Dextran: A Controlled Trial**. *J Trauma* 1993, 34:622–633.

33. Koury HI, Peschiera JL, Welling RE: **Selective Use of Pelvic Roentgenograms in Blunt Trauma Patients**. *J Trauma* 1993, 34:236–238.

34. Taylor GA, Eichelberger MR, O'Donnell R, *et al.*: **Indications for Computed Tomography in Children After Blunt Trauma**. *Ann Surg* 1991, **213**:121–126.

35. Freshman SP, Wisner D, *et al.*: **Secondary Survey Following Blunt Trauma: A New Role for Abdominal CT**. *J Trauma* 1993, 34:337–341.

36. Taylor GA, Eichelberger MR: **Abdominal CT in Children With Neurologic Impairment Following Blunt Trauma**. *Ann Surg* 1989, **210**:229–233.

37. Taylor GA, Eichelberger MR, Potter BM: **Hematuria: A Marker of Abdominal Injury in Children After Blunt Trauma**. *Ann Surg* 1988, **208**:688–693.

38. Yurt RW: **Triage, Initial Assessment, and Early Treatment of the •• Pediatric Trauma Patient**. *Pediatr Clin North Am* 1992, **39**:1083–1091.
This is a thoughtful, step-by-step introduction to the principles necessary to care for the pediatric trauma victim. A description of different trauma scoring systems is provided, as well as an outline of the management priorities necessary in the assessment, resuscitation, and acute care of the injured child.

39. Perry JF, Strate RG: **Diagnostic Peritoneal Lavage in Blunt Abdominal Trauma: Indications and Results**. *Surgery* 1972, **71**:898–901.

40. Davis JW, Hoyt DB, Macckerkie RC: **Complications in Evaluating Abdominal Trauma: Diagnostic Peritoneal Lavage Versus Computed Axial Tomography**. *J Trauma* 1990, **30**:1506–1509.

41. Drew R, Perry JF, Fischer RP: **The Expediency of Peritoneal Lavage for Blunt Trauma in Children**. *Surg Gynecol Obstet* 1977, **145**:885–888.

42. Jaffin JH, Ochsner MG, *et al.*: **Alkaline Phosphatase Levels in Diagnostic Peritoneal Lavage Fluid as a Predictor of Hollow Viscus Injury**. *J Trauma* 1993, 34:829–833.

43. Bode PJ, Niezen A, *et al.*: **Abdominal Ultrasound as a Reliable Indicator for Conclusive Laparotomy in Blunt Abdominal Trauma**. *J Trauma* 1993, 3:27–31.

44. Luks FI, Lemire A, Dickens SV, *et al.*: **Blunt Abdominal Trauma in Children: The Practical Value of Ultrasonography**. *J Trauma* 1993, 34:607–611.

45. Forster R, Pillasch J, Zielke A, *et al.*: **Ultrasonography in Blunt Abdominal Trauma: Influence of the Investigators' Experience**. *J Trauma* 1993, 34:264–269.

46. Rozycki GS, Ochsner MG, Jaffin JH: **Prospective Evaluation of Surgeons' Use of Ultrasound in the Evaluation of Trauma Patients**. *J Trauma* 1993, 34:516–527.

47. Rothlin MA, Naf R, Amgwerd M, *et al.*: **Ultrasound in Blunt and Thoracic Trauma**. *J Trauma* 1993, 34:488–495.

48. Rogers DA, Lobe TE, Schropp KP: **Evolving Uses of Laparoscopy in Children**. *Surg Clin North Am* 1992, 72:1299–1313.

49. Salvino CK, Esposito TJ, Marshall WJ, *et al.*: **The Role of Diagnostic Laparoscopy in the Management of Trauma Patients: A Preliminary Assessment**. *J Trauma* 1993, 34:488–495.

50. Stein SC, Young GS, *et al.*: **Delayed Brain Injury After Head Trauma: • Significance of Coagulopathy**. *Neurosurgery* 1992, **30**:160–165.
A revealing retrospective study of patients with head injury who manifested an abnormality in prothrombin time, partial thromboplastin time, or platelet count. Evidence of delayed or progressive brain injury was present in 55% of the patients with abnormal clotting studies and only 9% of those with normal clotting studies. Careful monitoring and an early repeat CT scan is necessary in this group of patients.

51. Michaud LJ, Rivara FP, Grady MS, Reay DT: **Predictors of Survival and Severity of Disability After Severe Brain Injury in Children**. *Neurosurgery* 1992, **31**:254–264.

52. Chesnut RM, Marshall LF, *et al.*: **The Role of Secondary Brain Injury in Determining Outcome From Severe Head Injury**. *J Trauma* 1993, 34:216–222.

53. Chan HK, Miller JD, Dearden NM: **Intracranial Blood Flow Velocity •• After Head Injury: Relationship to Severity of Injury, Time, Neurological Status and Outcome**. *J Neurol Neurosurg Psychiatry* 1992, **55**:787–791.
Middle cerebral artery blood-flow velocity was measured by transcranial Doppler ultrasonography in patients with mild, moderate, and severe head injuries and compared with matched controls. The initial mean flow velocity was significantly lower in the severe head injury group, and at discharge, than the control group. Patients with persistently low Doppler flow velocities consistently had a worse prognosis, while those whose flow velocity returned to near normal had significantly better outcomes.

54. Wolf AL, Levi L, *et al.*: **Effect of THAM Upon Outcome in Severe Head Injury: A Randomized Prospective Clinical Trial**. *J Neurosurg* 1993, 78:54–59.

55. Reilly JP, Brant ML, Mattox KL: **Thoracic Trauma in Children**. *J Trauma* 1993, 34:329–331.

56. Peclet MH, Newman KD, Eichelberger MR, *et al.*: **Thoracic Trauma in Children: An Indicator of Increased Mortality**. *J Pediatr Surg* 1990, 25:961–966.

57. Beaver BL, Laschinger JC: **Pediatric Thoracic Trauma**. *Semin Thorac Cardiovasc Surg* 1992, 4:255–262.

58. Ildstad ST, Tollerud DJ, Weiss RG, *et al.*: **Cardiac Contusion in Pediatric Patients With Blunt Thoracic Trauma**. *J Pediatr Surg* 1990, 25:287–289.

59. Langer JC, Winthrop AL, Wesson DE, *et al.*: **Diagnosis and Incidence of Cardiac Injury in Children With Blunt Thoracic Trauma**. *J Pediatr Surg* 1989, 24:1091–1094.

60. Millham FR, Grindlinger GA: **Survival Determinants in Patients Undergoing Emergency Room Thoracotomy for Penetrating Chest Injury.** *J Trauma* 1993, 34:332–336.

61. Sheikh AA, Culbertson CB: **Emergency Department Thoracotomy in Children: Rationale for Selective Application.** *J Trauma* 1993, 34:323–328.
•• A retrospective review of 23 children who underwent emergency-department thoracotomy at a level one trauma center after sustaining blunt and penetrating trauma. This data confirm the futility of emergency-department thoracotomy for trauma patients who arrive with no cardiac rhythm after sustaining blunt or penetrating trauma. The authors note that only children with penetrating thoracic trauma who arrive in the emergency department with vital signs that then deteriorate are potentially salvageable.

62. Rothenberg SS, Moore EE, Moore FA, *et al.*: **Emergency Department Thoracotomy in Children: A Critical Analysis.** *J Trauma* 1989, 29:1322–1325.

63. Witte CL, Esser MJ, Rappaport WD: **Updating the Management in Salvageable Splenic Injury.** *Ann Surg* 1992, **215**:261–265.

64. Smith EM, Elder JS, Spirnak JP: **Major Blunt Renal Trauma in the Pediatric Population: Is a Nonoperative Approach Indicated?** *J Urol* 1993, **149**:546–549.
• Conservative management for liver and spleen injuries in children sustaining blunt trauma is successful in the majority of cases. This study describes the results of nonoperative management for major renal lacerations (grades 3 to 5) and shows that this approach is also acceptable for renal injuries.

65. Sivit CJ, Taylor GA, Newman KD, *et al.*: **Safety-Belt Injuries in Children With Lap Belt Ecchymosis: CT Findings in 61 Patients.** *AJR Am J Roentgol* 1991, **157**:111–114.

66. Bond SJ, Gotschall CS, Eichelberger MR: **Predictors of Abdominal Injury in Children With Pelvic Fracture.** *J Trauma* 1991, **31**:1169–1173.

67. Musemeche CA, Fischer RP, *et al.*: **Selective Management of Pediatric Pelvic Fractures: A Conservative Approach.** *J Pediatr Surg* 1987, **22**:538–540.

68. Torode I, Zieg D: **Pelvic Fractures in Children.** *J Pediatr Orthop* 1985, **5**:76–84.

69. Fleisher G, Ludwig S, eds: *Textbook of Pediatric Emergency Medicine.* Baltimore: Williams & Wilkins; 1988.

70. Young G, Eichelberger MR: **Initial Resuscitation of the Child With Multiple Injuries.** In *Pediatric Emergency Medicine.* Edited by Grossman M, Dieckmann RA. Philadelphia: JB Lippencott; 1991.

Matthew L. Moront, MD, and Martin R. Eichelberger, MD, Trauma Center, Children's National Medical Center, 111 Michigan Avenue, NW, Washington, DC 20010-2970, USA.

Endocrine

Editorial overview

Norman W. Thompson, MD

University of Michigan Medical Center, Ann Arbor, Michigan, USA

Current Opinion in General Surgery 1994:51–52

The paper by Brian Stephenson, Malcolm Wheeler, and Orlo Clark (pp 53–59) represents the viewpoints of two highly experienced and sophisticated groups, one on each side of the Atlantic, managing large numbers of patients with thyroid carcinomas. They address the controversy surrounding the optimal extent of thyroidectomy in treating differentiated thyroid carcinoma. Specifically, they focus on the role of total thyroidectomy, a subject that remains controversial even among experienced thyroid surgeons. The authors conclude that there are several compelling reasons why total thyroidectomy, as an initial procedure, offers the best opportunity for eradication of the malignancy with the lowest risk of recurrence and ultimate mortality. While recognizing that prognostic scoring systems may be helpful and that the extent of operation may make a significant impact in only about 15% of all patients, they espouse total thyroidectomy as the treatment of choice for most patients with this disease. For minimal papillary carcinomas (< 1 cm) and minimally invasive follicular carcinomas, a thyroid lobectomy is usually sufficient. They emphasize that a total thyroidectomy is a safe procedure and that the high morbidity figures frequently quoted in the past are unacceptable today and do not occur in the hands of experienced surgeons.

The recent developments in application of molecular genetic techniques to the study of inherited endocrinopathies have important implications for surgeons involved with patients proven to have these syndromes. The paper by Kerstin Sandelin, Catharina Larsson, and Ruth Decker (pp 60–68) constitutes a state-of-the-art review of these recent advances. The group at the Karolinska Hospital has been at the forefront of attempts to localize and clone the *MEN1* gene, whereas Decker in Ann Arbor has done extensive genetic linkage studies in families affected by multiple endocrine neoplasia type 2A (MEN-2A) . They emphasize the important discoveries that are or soon will be applicable in the evaluation of family members at risk for developing either the MEN-1 or the MEN-2A syndrome. Because both syndromes are inherited as autosomal dominant gene defects, affected individuals transmit the disease to 50% of their offspring. Periodic biochemical testing of MEN-2A family members at risk will subsequently be limited to those with proven mutation-specific diagnosis obtained after the testing of a single blood sample. Currently, DNA-based methods can distinguish gene carriers in MEN-1 families, but this requires the indirect method of genetic linkage involving blood sampling from at least several other affected family members. When the *MEN1* gene has been identified, mutational analysis will simplify the study not only of family members at risk, but of individuals who may be probands with this syndrome. Considering the acceleration of developments in this field, it is likely that the *MEN1* gene will soon be isolated.

With the isolation of the *RET* protooncogene as the putative *MEN2A* gene, effective screening by DNA mutational analysis has already become a reality. As Decker states, "All this requires is a single blood sample with results that are objective and independent of the age of the person at risk." This is clearly a major breakthrough, for it now allows an early prophylactic total thyroidectomy in MEN-2A family members affected before they develop medullary carcinoma with metastases. Furthermore, all patients with apparent sporadic medullary thyroid carcinoma can be evaluated for possible *RET* protooncogene mutations. Hereditary disease can be excluded in these patients with a high degree of certainty. This will eliminate the need to study other family members. Furthermore, individuals with proven sporadic medullary carcinoma will not need to be studied for the presence or future development of pheochromocytomas.

Regardless of the developments in DNA based testing for MEN-1, the practical problem of how best to treat patients with that disease who develop gastrinomas and the Zollinger-Ellison Syndrome (ZES) remains to be resolved. More than a third of all patients with the ZES are found in MEN-1 family members, and until genetic therapy is developed, these patients will require both medical and surgical management. In their comprehensive and informative review, Romano Delcore and Stanley Friesen (pp 69–76) address the status of the surgical management of the ZES in both sporadic and familial cases. These authors have had a long and distinguished record in contributing to the man-

Abbreviations

MEN—multiple endocrine neoplasia; **ZES**—Zollinger-Ellison syndrome.

 ISBN 1-85922-671-X ISSN 1065–6243

agement of this disease, and their observations and opinions are based on an extensive experience during which treatment has evolved. They emphasize that many patients previously considered incurable can be successfully treated, provided the primary tumor and any involved lymph nodes are resected. Through the use of localization techniques and an awareness that gastrinomas not detected preoperatively are most likely to be found in the duodenal wall, surgeons have become more effective in the surgical treatment of this disease. In their opinion, all patients with ZES, including those with the MEN-1 syndrome, should be explored with intent to cure. In patients without liver metastases, regardless of lymph node involvement, it has been shown conclusively that cure can be achieved if the resection is adequate. Despite the evidence that the majority of even small duodenal tumors are malignant and have metastasized to lymph nodes, the biological behavior of these tumors does not preclude cure. Based on their own experience, excellent results reported in the literature, and the current low morbidity and mortality of this operation, Delcore and Friesen make a case for a pancreaticoduodenectomy in those patients with larger, locally invasive duodenal tumors or those with extensive lymph node metastases. They note that the most controversial aspect of ZES management lies in the surgical treatment of MEN-1 patients. They emphasize, however, that these patients develop metastases just as frequently as those without the syndrome and that treatment should be directed at the malignant potential of the neoplasm just as in patients with the sporadic form of the syndrome. An aggressive surgical approach in all ZES patients is emphasized because of the malignant potential of these tumors and the fact that it has now been shown that complete surgical resection of gastrinomas results in eugastrinemia with a 90% to 100% 10-year survival rate, even when lymph nodes have been involved. In contrast, patients with unresectable or incompletely resected gastrinomas have 5 - and 10 -year survival rates of 43% and 25%, respectively. This paper clearly and succinctly updates the dramatic changes that have occurred in the management of ZES patients during the past decade.

Norman W. Thompson, MD, University of Michigan Medical Center, Room 2920, Taubman Building, 1500 Medical Center Drive, Ann Arbor, MI 48109, USA.

The role of total thyroidectomy in the management of differentiated thyroid cancer

Brian M. Stephenson, MS, FRCS, Malcolm H. Wheeler, MD, FRCS, and Orlo H. Clark, MD

Cardiff Royal Infirmary, Cardiff, UK, and Mount Zion Medical Center, University of California at San Francisco, San Francisco, California, USA

The extent of surgical resection required in the optimal management of differentiated (papillary and follicular) thyroid carcinoma remains controversial. Arguments in favor of total thyroidectomy include the adequate treatment of tumor multifocality, reduction in local recurrence rates and anaplastic transformation, and creating a suitable environment for radioactive iodine scanning and treatment of metastases. The benefits of this procedure have to be weighed against the potential but minimal morbidity.

Current Opinion in General Surgery 1994:53–59

Although thyroid cancer is rare (the incidence is 3.7 to 4.7 per 100,000) [1] and accounts for only 0.5% of all cancer deaths [2], there is considerable interest in its diagnosis and surgical management. Palpable thyroid nodules are common, occurring in 4.2% of patients aged 30 to 59 [3]. Although the vast majority of such lesions are benign, accurate identification of the malignant nodule is of paramount importance because thyroid cancer is in most instances an eminently treatable condition. The main types of thyroid cancer, with their cell of origin and frequency, are shown in Table 1. Papillary and follicular carcinomas arising from the follicular cell are considered to be differentiated and usually maintain the ability to trap iodine, respond to thyroid-stimulating hormone, and thus synthesize thyroglobulin.

As a consequence of the infrequency and heterogeneity of the disease and, until recently, discrepancies in the histologic classification, there remains considerable controversy as to the best strategy for treating patients with differentiated thyroid cancer. Long-term follow-up of patients with differentiated thyroid cancer and randomized trials comparing the merits of various surgical and other therapies must be considered before the ideal treatment can be determined. This review focuses on the place of total thyroidectomy in the surgical treatment of such patients.

Papillary carcinoma

Papillary carcinoma is the commonest type of thyroid cancer; it frequently appears in late childhood or early adult life. These tumors are divided into three main categories depending primarily on the size and extent of the disease (Table 1). The term *minimal* (tumors ≤1 cm in size and not clinically obvious) is probably more appropriate than *occult* (tumors ≤1.5 cm in size, many of which are clinically apparent, often with cervical lymphadenopathy [lateral aberrant thyroid]). Although these tumors are rarely associated with distant metastatic disease, a study from the Mayo Clinic reported four deaths in 396 patients with tumors 1.5 cm or less in diameter [4]. Nevertheless, small microcarcinomas are common, being detected in 6% to 13% of thyroid glands of patients dying from causes other than thyroid disease [1,5,6]. This observation raises important issues relating to the natural history and possibly benign course of many papillary tumors.

Intrathyroid primary tumors are situated totally within the thyroid. Patients with these tumors have a significantly better prognosis than do patients with extra-thyroid tumors, which extend through the thyroid capsule and may involve adjacent structures such as the recurrent laryngeal nerve, trachea, and esophagus. Patients with invasive tumors also have a worse prognosis than do patients who have regional nodal involvement.

There is general agreement that thyroidectomy is the treatment of choice for patients with papillary carcinoma. However, the extent of the thyroidectomy, ranging from excisional biopsy to total thyroidectomy, remains controversial [7–16]. It is therefore important to consider known factors that influence the prognosis of patients with differentiated thyroid cancer and to define precise treatment objectives (Table 2). Sev-

 ISBN 1-85922-671-X ISSN 1065–6243

Table 1. Types of thyroid cancer

Type	Cell of origin	Description	Frequency, %
Papillary	Follicular	Occult or minimal Intrathyroidal Extrathyroidal	75
Follicular	Follicular	Minimally invasive Frankly invasive (Hürthle cell)	10
Anaplastic	Follicular		<5
Medullary	Parafollicular C cells		8
Lymphoma	Nonthyroid cells		2
Metastatic	From other sites		<1

eral prognostic scoring systems have been developed [17,18]. It is obviously necessary to accurately stage the disease to compare the merits of different surgical therapies. Multivariate analysis has demonstrated that patients with papillary carcinoma can be divided into high- and low-risk groups in terms of risk for recurrence and long-term survival, primarily on the basis of the age of the patient at the time of initial diagnosis. In the AGES (age of the patient, the microscopic histologic grade, extent, and size of the tumor) score system from the Mayo Clinic [18], over 85% of 860 patients fitted into the low-risk group in terms of risk of cancer-related mortality, which was 2% at 25 years. The higher risk groups, with AGES scores of 4 to 4.99, 5 to 5.99, and more than 6, had 25-year mortalities of 24%, 49%, and 93%, respectively. The most recent scoring system, MACIS (metastasis, age, complications of resection, invasion, size), also from the Mayo Clinic, similarly places emphasis on the age of the patient and size and extent of tumor, but also considers completeness of resection and distant metastases (Table 3). The use of these scoring systems helps to compare various modalities of therapy.

Table 2. Treatment objectives in differentiated thyroid cancer

Eradicate primary disease
Reduce incidence of local and distant recurrence
Facilitate treatment of metastases
Cure maximum number of patients
Achieve all of the above with minimal morbidity

The arguments for and against total thyroidectomy are shown in Table 4. The multifocal nature of papillary carcinoma has been well documented in a number of carefully performed histologic studies (Fig. 1). Although the disease may only be microscopic, the frequency with which multifocality is detected ranges from 30% to 87.5% [6,12,19••,20•,21•]. This observation suggests that procedures such as unilateral lobectomy, subtotal thyroidectomy, or even near-total thyroidectomy (total lobectomy, isthmusectomy, and subtotal lobectomy on the contralateral side) are likely to leave at least microscopic papillary carcinomas. The biologic behavior and full clinical significance of such microscopic foci are unknown, and most patients treated with less-than-total thyroidectomy do not develop recurrent tumor in the remaining thyroid tissue.

Table 3. Prognostic index system for papillary carcinoma*

Factors	Score†
Age <39	3.1
>40	0.08 × age
Diameter of primary tumor	0.3 × cm
Incomplete resection	1
Extrathyroidal invasion	1
Distant metastases	3

*The MACIS score from the Mayo clinic.
†Low risk<6; high risk>8.

Local recurrence after surgery for papillary carcinoma is undoubtedly a clinical disaster. The incidence of local recurrence in a number of studies of variable follow-up has ranged from 5% to 24% [1,9,22,23,24••]. Although there is no doubt that some patients do well after unilateral lobectomy, it is a disturbing fact that approximately 50% of patients who suffer a recurrence ultimately die of the disease. Such recurrences may not occur until 20 years after the primary surgery, but the fact remains that a local recurrence in the remaining thyroid lobe or remnant is as much a harbinger of death as it is in other types of cancer. In Cady *et al.*'s [9] series at the Lahey Clinic there was an 11% recurrence rate for patients categorized as low risk, and the subsequent mortality was 36%. Mazzaferri *et al.* [10–11] retrospectively analyzed the impact of treatment on recurrence and survival in 576 patients followed up for a median of 10 years. Among 310 patients treated by total thyroidectomy, there was an 11% recurrence rate compared with that of 19% in 261 patients treated by subtotal resection, a clinically and statistically significant difference.

More recently, a series of articles from the Mayo Clinic [18,25,26••] addressed the question of the extent of thyroidectomy. Local recurrence rates were examined in low- and high-risk patients (AGES score <3.99 vs ≥4, respectively). In patients at low risk (AGES score <3.99), the recurrence rate at 20-years' follow up was significantly higher for unilateral resection than for bilateral resection, 14% and 2%, respectively. Among high-risk patients who were followed up for 20 years, the recurrence rates were 45% and 20%, respectively, for the two surgical strategies. The authors found no benefit, however, in either high- or low-risk groups with respect to recurrence when bilateral resection or near-total thyroidectomy were compared with total thyroidectomy. However, it must be appreciated that total lobectomy on one side and contralateral subto-

Table 4. Advantages and disadvantages of total thyroidectomy in differentiated thyroid cancer

Advantages	Disadvantages
Tumor multifocality (30% to 80%)	Recurrent laryngeal nerve damage
Decreases local recurrence	Hypoparathyroidism
Decreases distant recurrence	
Reduces risk of anaplasia	
Facilitates treatment with ^{131}I	
Allows thyroglobulin measurement	

tal resection at the authors' institution usually involved leaving no more than 1 g of tissue [27], which might be considered virtually a total thyroidectomy by some surgeons. With this in mind it is interesting to note that although papillary microcarcinoma (minimal) has an excellent prognosis, both the 20-year cumulative local (thyroid bed) and nodal recurrence rates in a series of 535 patients with papillary microcarcinoma (median tumor size, 8 mm) was significantly higher among patients treated by lobectomy as compared with those treated by bilateral resection [26••].

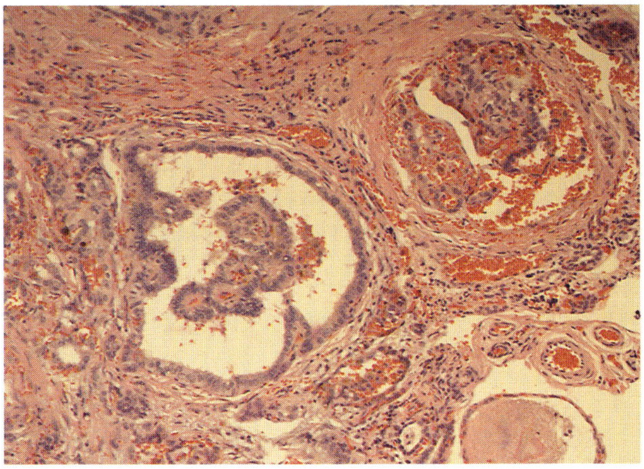

Fig. 1. Microscopic foci of papillary thyroid in a patient with multifocal thyroid cancer.

With the advent of these newer prognostic scoring systems, deaths from thyroid cancer have also been examined [18]. As expected, high-risk patients had a higher cumulative mortality at 25 years as compared with patients with low risk. Furthermore, there were more deaths in those patients treated by ipsilateral lobectomy rather than bilateral resection. However, total thyroidectomy did not offer any significant advantage compared with bilateral resection [18]. Lennquist (Personal communication), however, showed that in high-risk patients a strategy of total thyroidectomy as compared with subtotal resection has resulted in fewer recurrences and a prolonged survival. There is increasing clinical evidence that residual tumor foci may undergo anaplastic change in inadequately treated thyroid cancer [16,28]. The development of anaplasia inevitably leads to the rapid demise of the patient, and clearly this disaster can be averted by performance of total thyroidectomy.

A further and perhaps most important argument in favor of total thyroidectomy is that it permits radioactive iodine scanning to detect metastases and allows for their subsequent ablation by radioiodine [29,30,31••,32]. If there is competing residual normal thyroid tissue after less-than-total thyroidectomy, these important diagnostic and therapeutic options cannot be implemented. It has been argued that it is possible to ablate residual thyroid tissue by an initial dose of radioactive iodine, but this may require large doses of ^{131}I, exposing the patient to unnecessary risk and wasting radioactive iodine that might be subsequently required to treat recurrent or metastatic disease. Patients whose metastases are visible only on radioiodine scanning despite negative chest radiography or chest computed tomography scan [31••] have an excellent prognosis; indeed, Schlumberger *et al.* [30] reported that it is "much easier to cure micrometastases with radioiodine than it is to palliate macronodules." This approach can only be employed by using radioactive iodine after total thyroidectomy to identify functioning metastases and for subsequent ablation. About 75% of papillary thyroid cancers will take up radioiodine. Harness *et al.* [29] have shown that the treatment by total thyroidectomy and appropriate use of ^{131}I has reduced mortality in patients with differentiated thyroid carcinoma and distant metastases from a historical level of 75% within 5 years of diagnosis to a mortality from carcinoma of approximately 25%.

The final important benefit of total thyroidectomy is to facilitate the follow-up of thyroid cancer patients by measuring thyroglobulin levels [33]. The best time to determine the serum thyroglobulin level is when a patient is in a hypothyroid state and has a high endogenous serum thyroid-stimulating hormone level in preparation for a thyroid scan.

The minimum surgical procedure that should be performed for any patient with a unilateral nodule suspected of being cancer is total lobectomy on the side of the lesion with isthmusectomy. If papillary cancer is confirmed either by frozen section or definitive paraffin histology, total thyroidectomy is the most appropriate surgical treatment for intrathyroid and extrathyroid tumors. The small (< 1 cm) and rare encapsulated papillary cancers, which generally have an excellent prognosis, can be adequately treated by total lobectomy and isthmusectomy. If there is a previous history of head or neck irradiation, a total or near-total thyroidectomy is appropriate because of the multifocal nature of the neoplasms in these patients [1,34].

Follicular carcinoma

The incidence of follicular carcinoma has steadily decreased as a result of the increase in dietary iodine. In most series, this cancer accounts for about 10%

of cases of thyroid cancer. It usually presents later in life than papillary carcinoma, and unfortunately many patients have evidence of pulmonary or bony metastases at the time of diagnosis. Follicular carcinomas are classified according to their histopathologic features into two types: minimally invasive and frankly invasive [1,14,24••,35,36] (Fig. 2). The former is characterized by little or no invasion of the tumor capsule and adjacent veins and is rarely metastatic. Invasive follicular carcinomas have a marked propensity to metastasize to the bones and lungs. Patients with angioinvasion are more likely to have metastatic disease than those with capsular invasion. The diagnosis of follicular carcinoma cannot be made by cytologic assessment but about 20% of follicular neoplasms investigated by fine-needle aspiration biopsy cytology are found to be follicular carcinoma. Frozen section histology at the time of thyroidectomy is usually unhelpful, and the final diagnosis is only made on definitive paraffin section. Most would agree that the minimally invasive lesion can be adequately treated by a unilateral thyroid lobectomy including the isthmus and pyramidal lobe, because there is little indication for total thyroidectomy [14,16,24••]. However, patients with frankly invasive tumors have a poor prognosis, particularly those over the age of 40. There is general agreement that these patients benefit from total thyroidectomy [1,12,14,16,24••,35,36]. A decision to proceed to total thyroidectomy will often be made on the basis of the macroscopic appearances of the tumor at surgery and occasionally because of the involvement of lymph nodes. Frozen section histology is helpful if there are areas of definite invasion, and it can also sometimes diagnose follicular variants of papillary thyroid carcinoma. When the definitive paraffin histology reveals frankly invasive cancer completion, total thyroidectomy is indicated. In contrast, if the definitive histology is reported as minimal capsular invasion then no further surgery is usually necessary. A bone scan and serum thyroglobulin level may detect a rare patient with metastatic disease. Total thyroidectomy for patients with invasive follicular thyroid cancer allows for radioactive iodine scanning to detect and ablate functioning metastases.

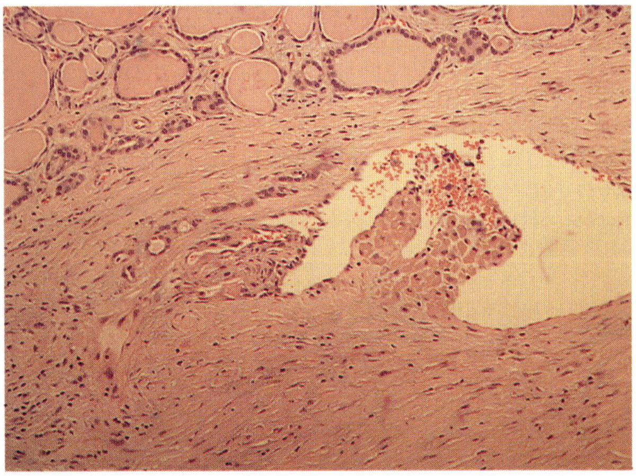

Fig. 2. Photomicrograph illustrates invasion of follicular cancer into veins (angioinvasion).

Hürthle cell carcinomas account for about 3% of all thyroid cancers. Although these tumors are often included with follicular cancer, they differ in that they are more likely than follicular cancers to be multifocal and metastasize to lymph nodes. Furthermore, they do not take up radioactive iodine but do synthesize thyroglobulin. Total thyroidectomy and central neck nodal dissection is therefore often advocated for this aggressive tumor. Lower recurrence rates and improved survival have been reported after total thyroidectomy when compared with patients treated by less extensive thyroidectomy [37].

Arguments against total thyroidectomy

Complications of total thyroidectomy are often quoted by clinicians who favor unilateral resection or near-total thyroidectomy as opposed to total removal of the thyroid gland. The earlier literature reported hypoparathyroidism rates of approximately 30% and a 10% incidence of recurrent laryngeal nerve palsy [1]; it is because of these complication rates that near-total rather than total thyroidectomy was popularized. However, it is clear that these unacceptable results can no longer be quoted in defense of a lesser surgical procedure, because in experienced hands total thyroidectomy can be performed with minimal morbidity. In current series, the incidence of permanent hypoparathyroidism and recurrent laryngeal nerve palsy is approximately 1% to 3% [1,12,14–16,20,24••,28,38–41,42••,43••]. Clark [12] reported an incidence of only 1% of permanent hypoparathyroidism and no permanent recurrent laryngeal nerve damage in 82 consecutive total thyroidectomies. Furthermore, these complications have usually occurred in patients undergoing surgery for extensive bilateral thyroid disease who also have metastatic lymphadenopathy. Nevertheless it is important to note that two recent reports documented the absence of recurrent laryngeal nerve palsy in children and adolescents undergoing total thyroidectomy for papillary carcinoma. Young patients with papillary thyroid cancer invariably have extensive cervical lymphadenopathy [39,44•]. If a comparison is to be made between the morbidity of total thyroidectomy and that of lesser procedures, then due consideration must be given to the higher risks, particularly those to the recurrent laryngeal nerve and parathyroid glands, when a technically difficult second operation is required for residual or recurrent disease after an inadequate initial procedure. Removal of the entire thyroid gland most importantly allows for early detection of metastatic disease, and radioactive therapy is much more effective for ablating micro- rather than macrometastases. In addition, the objective of performing one definitive operation aiming to achieve cure will certainly cause less emotional stress in these patients and their families.

Surgical technique

Several key points in the technique of total thyroidectomy are worthy of note. Identification of the recurrent laryngeal nerve, not only low in the neck but also at the level of the ligament of Berry and in its upper third before it enters the larynx, is essential to avoid damaging the nerve. An awareness of all the anomalies of the nerve, particularly that of nonrecurrence on the right, is equally important [45]. The external branch of the superior laryngeal nerve has received particular attention in the recent literature. This nerve usually runs on the midportion of the cricothyroid muscle. Injury to the nerve can be avoided by identifying it at this site and by ligating the individual branches of the superior thyroid artery close to the thyroid [46].

The main trunk of the inferior thyroid artery should not be ligated, but the individual branches should be tied close to the thyroid capsule, thereby preserving the small, delicate branches that supply the parathyroid glands. These glands must be identified and teased laterally on as broad a pedicle as possible from the thyroid gland to preserve their blood supply. Occasionally a parathyroid is situated well anteriorly on the thyroid and cannot be preserved in this manner. It is then appropriate to excise the gland and transplant it in several 1-mm pieces in separate pockets in the sternomastoid muscle. It is a wise precaution to carry out frozen section histology on this gland before transplantation to avoid transplanting thyroid cancer. One should remember that the inferior parathyroids are almost always situated anterior to the recurrent laryngeal nerves, whereas the superior parathyroid glands are usually situated within 1 cm of the intersection of the recurrent laryngeal nerve and the inferior thyroid artery.

Prophylactic lymph node clearance in papillary carcinoma has been controversial. This procedure is particularly relevant for the young; cervical lymph node metastases occur in 90% of patients 15 years of age or younger [24••]. In all patients with papillary carcinoma, it is important to remove visible lymph nodes in the paratracheal area. This can be done with preservation of the recurrent laryngeal nerve. A recurrent nerve that is functioning preoperatively should be functioning postoperatively. Occasionally it is necessary to use sharp dissection to remove tumor from the recurrent laryngeal nerve. When lateral neck nodes are palpable or there is extensive central neck nodal involvement, a modified neck dissection is performed to preserve the internal jugular vein, sternomastoid muscle, and spinal accessory nerve, unless they are directly involved with the tumor. There is no evidence that a more extensive formal block dissection confers any improved long-term benefit in these patients. Some patients will unfortunately develop lymph node recurrences in the lateral neck after the initial operation. Nodal involvement does not have an appreciable adverse effect on the prognosis of these patients. These nodes can be removed by a subsequent modified radical neck dissection or even be excised individually if few in number.

Conclusions

Differentiated thyroid carcinoma is an uncommon disease; although most patients have an excellent prognosis, some still die from it. The mainstay of management is surgical, and there are several compelling reasons why total thyroidectomy as an initial procedure offers the best opportunity to eradicate the malignancy with the lowest risk of recurrence and ultimate mortality. Retrospective series do not always fairy represent the virtues of totally thyroidectomy, because this procedure may have been employed for the more advanced and aggressive disease. It is likely that 80% of patients with differentiated thyroid cancer will do well, and 5% will die; but in the remaining 15%, the outcome can be significantly improved by total thyroidectomy, radioactive iodine scanning, and ablative therapy and thyroid-stimulating hormone–suppressive therapy. The AGES and MACIS prognostic index systems are helpful. Other predictors of tumor aggressiveness include 1) DNA ploidy [24,47,48•], 2) radioactive iodine uptake, 3) adenylate-cyclase response to thyroid-stimulating hormone [49], and 4) presence of various genetic changes, *ie*, *gsp* and *ras* oncogenes [50] or the *p53* tumor suppressor gene [51]. For the future, it may be reasonable to conclude that the wider acceptance of scoring and staging systems may facilitate a selective approach to therapy based on reliable parameters. More extensive treatment may then be reserved for tumors that are likely to display aggressive behavior. At present, total thyroidectomy is the treatment of choice for most patients with thyroid cancer. A near-total thyroidectomy is acceptable when there is concern about the viability of the parathyroid glands. A thyroid lobectomy is indicated for occult (< 1 cm) papillary thyroid cancers and minimally invasive follicular thyroid cancers. Thyroidectomy in experienced hands is a safe procedure, transfusions are almost never required, and almost all patients can be comfortably discharged within 2 to 3 days of surgery.

References and recommended reading

Papers of particular interest, published within the annual period of review, have been highlighted as:
- • Of special interest
- •• Of outstanding interest

1. THOMPSON NW, NISHIYAMA RH, HARNESS JK: **Thyroid Carcinoma: Current Controversies**. *Curr Probl Surg* 1978, 15:1–67.
2. REEVE TS: **Operations for Non-Medullary Cancer of the Thyroid Gland**. In *Surgery of the Thyroid and Parathyroid Glands*. Edited by Kaplan EL. London: Churchill Livingstone; 1983:62–74.
3. VANDER JB, GASTON EA, DAWBER DR: **Significance of Non Toxic Thyroid Nodules: Final Report of a 15 Year Study of the Incidence of Thyroid Malignancy**. *Ann Intern Med* 1968, 69:537–540.
4. MCCONAHEY WM, HAY ID, WOOLNER LB, VAN HEERDEN JA, TAYLOR WS: **Papillary Thyroid Cancer Treated at the Mayo Clinic, 1946 Through 1970: Initial Manifestations, Pathologic Findings, Therapy and Outcome**. *Mayo Clin Proc* 1986, 61:978–996.
5. NISHIYAMA RH, LUDWIG GK, THOMPSON NW: **The Prevalence of Papillary Small Papillary Thyroid Carcinomas in 100 Conservative Necropsies in an American Population:** In *Radiation-Associated Thyroid Carcinoma*. Edited by De Groot JL. New York: Grune and Strattan; 1977:123–135.

6. LANG W, BORRUSCH H, BAUER L: **Occult Carcinomas of the Thyroid: Evaluation of 1020 Sequential Autopsies.** *Am J Clin Pathol* 1988, **90**:72–76.

7. BLOCK MD: **Management of Carcinoma of the Thyroid.** *Ann Surg* 1977, **185**:133–144.

8. BUCKWALTER JA, THOMAS CG: **Selection of Surgical Treatment for Well Differentiated Thyroid Carcinoma.** *Ann Surg* 1972, **176**:565–578.

9. CADY B, SEDGEWICK C, MEISSNER WA, WOOL MS, SALTZMAN FA, WERBER J: **Risk Factor Analysis in Differentiated Thyroid Cancer.** *Cancer* 1979, **43**:810–820.

10. MAZZAFERRI EL, YOUNG RL, OERTEL JE, KEMMERER WT, PAGE CB: **Papillary Thyroid Carcinoma: The Impact of Therapy in 576 Patients.** *Medicine* 1977, **56**:171–196.

11. MAZZAFERRI EL, YOUNG RL: **Papillary Thyroid Carcinoma: A 10 Year Follow Up Report on the Impact of Therapy in 576 Patients.** *Am J Med* 1981, **70**:511–518.

12. CLARK OH: **Total Thyroidectomy: The Treatment of Choice for Patients With Differentiated Thyroid Cancer.** *Ann Surg* 1982, **196**:361–370.

13. THOMPSON NW, OLSEN WR, HOFFMAN GL: **The Continuing Development of the Technique of Thyroidectomy.** *Surgery* 1973, **73**:913–927.

14. REEVE TS, DELBRIDGE L: **Thyroid Cancers of Follicular Cell Origin: The Place of Radical or Limited Surgery.** *Prog Surg* 1988, **19**:113–132.

15. HARNESS JK, FUNG L, THOMPSON NW, BURNEY RE, MCLEOD MK: **Total Thyroidectomy: Complications and Technique.** *World J Surg* 1986, **10**:781.

16. FRIEDMAN M, PACELLA BL: **Total Versus Subtotal Thyroidectomy: Arguments, Approaches and Recommendations.** *Otolaryngol Clin North Am* 1990, **23**:413–427.

17. CADY B, ROSSI R: **An Expanded View of Risk Group Definition in Differentiated Thyroid Carcinoma.** *Surgery* 1988, **104**:947–953.

18. HAY ID, GRANT CS, TAYLOR WF, MCCONAHEY WM: **Ipsilateral Lobectomy Versus Bilateral Lobe Resection in Papillary Thyroid Carcinoma: A Retrospective Analysis of Surgical Outcome Using a Novel Prognostic Scoring System.** *Surgery* 1987, **102**:1088–1095.

19. •• PASIEKA JL, THOMPSON NW, MCLEOD MK, BURNEY RE, MACHA M: **The Incidence of Bilateral Well-Differentiated Thyroid Cancer Found at Completion Thyroidectomy.** *World J Surg* 1992, **16**:711–716.

Multifocal disease after lobectomy is associated with a high incidence of contralateral disease on completion thyroidectomy.

20. • DE-JONG SA, DEMETER JG, LAWRENCE AM, PALOYAN E: **Necessity and Safety of Completion Thyroidectomy for Differentiated Thyroid Carcinoma.** *Surgery* 1992, **112**:734–737.

Suggests that completion thyroidectomy be offered to patients with either papillary or follicular carcinoma.

21. • KATOH R, SASAKI J, KURIHARA H, SUZUKI K, IIDA Y, KAWAOI A: **Multiple Thyroid Involvement (Intraglandular Metastasis) in Papillary Thyroid Carcinoma: A Clinicopathologic Study of 105 Consecutive Patients.** *Cancer* 1992, **70**:1585–1590.

Foci of intrathyroidal papillary carcinoma were detected in 78% of patients.

22. ROSE RG, KELSEY MP, RUSSELL WO, IBANEZ ML, WHITE EC, CLARK RL: **Follow-Up Study of Thyroid Cancer Treated by Unilateral Lobectomy.** *Am J Surg* 1963, **106**:494–500.

23. TOLLEFSEN HR, SHAH JP, HUVOS AG: **Papillary Carcinoma of the Thyroid: Recurrence in the Thyroid Gland After Initial Surgical Treatment.** *Am J Surg* 1972, **124**:468–472.

24. •• THOMPSON NW: **Differentiated Thyroid Carcinoma.** In *Diseases of Thyroid: Pathophysiology and Management.* Edited by Wheeler MH, Lazarus JH: London: Chapman & Hall; in press.

A comprehensive review of the surgical management of differentiated thyroid carcinoma.

25. GRANT CS, HAY ID, GOUGH IR, BERGSTRALH EJ, GOELLNER JR, MCCONAHEY WM: **Local Recurrence in Papillary Carcinoma: Is Extent of Surgical Resection Important?** *Surgery* 1988, **104**:954–962.

26. •• HAY ID, GRANT CS, VAN HEERDEN JA, GOELLNER JR, EBERSOLD JR, BERGSTRALH EJ: **Papillary Thyroid Microcarcinoma: A Study of 535 Cases Observed in a 50 Year Period.** *Surgery* 1992, **102**:1139–1147.

An authoritative article on the outcome of patients in whom the median size of papillary tumor was only 8 mm.

27. HUBERT JP, KIERNAN PD, BEARHS OH, MCCONAHEY WM, WOOLNER LB: **Occult Papillary Carcinoma of the Thyroid Gland.** *Arch Surg* 1980, **115**:394–398.

28. GORETZKI PE, SIMON D, FRILLING A, WITTE J, REINERS C, GRUSSENDORF M, HORSTER FA, ROEHER H-D: **Surgical Reintervention for Differentiated Thyroid Cancer.** *Br J Surg* 1993, **80**:1009–1012.

29. HARNESS JK, THOMPSON NW, SISSON JC, BEIERWALTES WH: **Differentiated Thyroid Carcinoma: Treatment of Distant Metastases.** *Arch Surg* 1974, **108**:410–417.

30. SCHLUMBERGER M, TUBIANA M, DE VATHAIRE F, HILL C, GARDET P, TRAVAGLI JP, FRAGU P, LUMBROSO J, CAILLOU B, PARMENTIER C: **Long Term Results of Treatment of 283 Patients With Lung and Bone Metastases From Differentiated Thyroid Carcinomas.** *J Clin Endocrinol Metab* 1986, **63**:960–967.

31. •• VASSILOPOULOU-SELLIN R, KLEIN MJ, SMITH TH, SAMAAN NA, FRANKENTHALER RA, GOEPPERT H, CANGIR A, HAYNIE TP: **Pulmonary Metastases in Children and Young Adults With Differentiated Thyroid Cancer.** *Cancer* 1993, **71**:1348–1352.

Illustrates the importance of total thyroidectomy in allowing identification of pulmonary metastases in young patients whose chest radiographs are apparently normal.

32. BEIERWALTES WH, NISHIYAMA RH, THOMPSON NW: **Survival Time and Cure in Papillary and Follicular Thyroid Carcinoma With Distant Metastases.** *J Nucl Med* 1982, **23**:561–569.

33. VAN HERLE AJ, ULLER RP: **Elevated Serum Thyroglobulin: A Marker of Metastases in Differentiated Thyroid Carcinoma.** *J Clin Invest* 1975, **56**:270–277.

34. DE GROOT LJ, KAPLAN EL, MCCORMICK M, STRAUS FH: **Natural History, Treatment and Course of Papillary Thyroid Carcinoma.** *J Clin Endocrinol Metab* 1990, **71**:414.

35. YOUNG RL, MAZZAFERRI EL, RAHE AJ, DORFMAN SG: **Pure Follicular Thyroid Carcinoma: Impact of Therapy in 214 Patients.** *J Nucl Med* 1980, **21**:733–737.

36. YAMASHITA T, FUJIMOTO Y, KODAMA T, HIRAYAMA A, OBARA T, ITO Y, AIBA M, KUSAKABE K: **When is Total Thyroidectomy Indicated as a Treatment of "Follicular Carcinoma"?** *World J Surg* 1988, **12**:559–564.

37. THOMPSON NW: **Total Thyroidectomy in the Treatment of Thyroid Carcinoma.** In *Endocrine Surgical Update.* Edited by Thompson NW, Vinik AI. New York: Grune and Stratten; 1983:71–84.

38. ATTIE JN, KHAFIF RA: **The Preservation of Parathyroid Gland During Total Thyroidectomy.** *Am J Surg* 1975, **130**:399–403.

39. ZIMMERMAN D, HAY ID, GOUGH IR, GOELLNER JR, RYAN JJ, GRANT CS, MCCONAHEY WM: **Papillary Thyroid Carcinoma in Children and Adults: Long-Term Follow-Up of 1039 Patients Consecutively Treated at One Institution During Three Decades.** *Surgery* 1988, **104**:1157–1166.

40. CLARK OH, LEVIN K, ZENG Q-H, GREENSPAN FS, SIPERSTEIN A: **Thyroid Cancer: The Case for Total Thyroidectomy.** *Eur J Cancer Clin Oncol* 1988, **24**:305–313.

41. WAX MK, BRIANT TD: **Completion Thyroidectomy in the Management of Well-Differentiated Thyroid Carcinoma.** *Otolaryngol Head Neck Surg* 1992, **107**:63–68.

42. •• LEVIN KE, CLARK AH, DUH QY, SIPERSTEIN AE, CLARK OH: **Reoperative Thyroid Surgery.** *Surgery* 1992, **111**:604–609.

Completion thyroidectomy can be performed with minimal morbidity.

43. KHADRA M, DELBRIDGE L, REEVE TS, POOLE AG, CRUMMER P:
•• **Total Thyroidectomy: Its Role in the Management of Thyroid Disease**. *Aust N Z J Surg* 1992, **62**:91–95.
Total thyroidectomy can be safely performed in a variety of thyroid diseases.

44. HARNESS JK, THOMPSON NW, MCCLEOD MK, PASIEKA JL,
• FUKUUCHI A: **Differentiated Thyroid Carcinoma in Children and Adolescents**. *World J Surg* 1992, **16**:547–553.
Total thyroidectomy is the treatment of choice in children with papillary carcinoma of the thyroid.

45. WHEELER MH, RICHARDS SH: **Laryngeal Nerves**. In *Current Surgical Practice*, vol 5. Edited by Hadfield J, Hobsley M, Treasure T. London: Edward Arnold; 1990:237–250.

46. LENNQUIST C, CAHLIN C, SMEDS S: **The Superior Laryngeal Nerve in Thyroid Surgery**. *Surgery* 1987, **102**:999–1008.

47. COHN K, BACKDAHL M, FORSSLUND BM, AUER G, LUNDELL G, LOWHAGEN T, TALLROTH E, WILLEMS JS, ZETTERBERG A, GRANBERG PO: **Preoperative Value of Nuclear DNA Content in Papillary Thyroid Carcinoma**. *World J Surg* 1984, **12**:474–480.

48. PASIEKA JL, ZEDENIUS J, AUER G, GRIMELIUS L, HOOG A,
• LUNDELL G, WALLIN G, BACKDAHL M: **Addition of Nuclear DNA Content to the AMES Risk Group Classification for Papillary Thyroid Carcinoma**. *Surgery* 1992, **112**:1154–1159.
Suggests that preoperative DNA ploidy may allow individualization of surgical treatment in patients with papillary carcinoma.

49. SIPERSTEIN AE, ZENG QH, GUM ET, LEVIN KE, CLARK OH: **Adenylate-Cyclase Activity as a Predictor of Thyroid Tumour Aggressiveness**. *World J Surg* 1988, **12**:528–533.

50. GORETZKI PE, LYONS J, STACY-PHIPPS S, ROSENAU W, DEMEURE M, CLARK OH, MCCORMICK F, ROEHER H-D, BOURNE HR: **Mutational Activation of RAS and GSP Oncogenes in Differentiated Thyroid Cancer and Their Biological Implications**. *World J Surg* 1992, **16**:576–582.

51. ITO T, SEYAMA T, MIZUNO T, TSUYAMA N, HAYASHI T, HAYASHI Y, DOHI K, NAKAMURA N, AKIYAMA M: **Unique Association of *p53* Mutations With Undifferentiated But Not With Differentiated Carcinomas of the Thyroid Gland**. *Cancer Res* 1992, **52**:1369–1371.

Brian M. Stephenson, MS, FRCS, and Malcolm H. Wheeler, MD, FRCS, Department of Surgery, Cardiff Royal Infirmary, Newport Road, Cardiff CF2 1SZ, UK.

Orlo H. Clark, MD, Department of Surgery, Mount Zion Medical Center, University of California at San Francisco, 1600 Divisadero Street, San Francisco, CA 94120, USA.

Genetic aspects of multiple endocrine neoplasia types 1 and 2

Kerstin Sandelin, MD, PhD,* Catharina Larsson, MD, PhD,* and Ruth Anne Decker, MD†

*Karolinska Hospital, Stockholm, Sweden, and †University of Michigan Medical Center, Ann Arbor, Michigan, USA

Multiple endocrine neoplasia (MEN) type 1 is an autosomal, dominantly inherited predisposition to develop neoplastic lesions of the parathyroid glands, the neuroendocrine pancreas-duodenum, and the anterior pituitary. The genetic defect was mapped to the centromeric part of the long arm of chromosome 11 based on studies of somatic deletions in MEN-1–associated tumors and linkage analysis in families in whom the disease is segregated. Combined family and tumor analysis has shown that tumorigenesis in MEN-1 involves loss of the wild-type chromosome, indicating that the putative MEN-1 gene is a tumor suppressor gene. Similar deletions are also seen in a proportion of sporadic parathyroid and pancreatic tumors, suggesting that tumorigenesis involves related mechanisms in both sporadic and familial cases. Based on results from linkage analysis in more than 40 MEN-1 families, predictive testing for MEN-1 using DNA polymorphisms can now be performed with high accuracy. Hence, biochemical screening programs can focus on individuals at risk to identify early signs of tumor development. MEN-2, an autosomal dominant cancer syndrome of variable expressivity, has previously been localized to chromosome 10q11.2 by positional cloning tactics. The *RET* protooncogene mapping to the *MEN2* susceptibility locus has recently emerged as a candidate gene for MEN-2A. RET, a transmembrane receptor protein, has a large glycosylated extracellular domain containing clustered cysteine residues and calcium-binding motifs, a single hydrophobic transmembrane domain, and a cytoplasmic domain with tyrosine kinase catalytic activity. Several germline missense mutations in a codon specifying one of these highly conserved cysteine residues have been detected in patients affected with MEN-2A. The base substitution creates a nonconservative amino acid change at the boundary of the extracellular and transmembrane domains. A mutation in *RET* has not yet been disclosed in patients affected with the MEN-2B variant of the syndrome. Although the normal function of RET or its putative ligand is presently unknown, the receptor appears to have homology to the communicative cadherins.

Current Opinion in General Surgery 1994:60–68

Multiple endocrine neoplasia type 1

Multiple endocrine neoplasia (MEN) in its familial forms encompasses hyperfunctioning benign and malignant tumors. In MEN type 1, the parathyroid glands, the anterior pituitary, the duodenum, and the endocrine pancreas are most commonly affected. The thyroid, the thymus, and the adrenal glands are less common localizations. MEN-2A refers to malignancy of the thyroid (medullary thyroid carcinoma), hyperparathyroidism, and pheochromocytoma, whereas MEN-2B includes medullary thyroid carcinoma, pheochromocytoma, and neurogangliomatosis. Although both MEN-1 and MEN-2 are hereditary, their etiologic mechanisms are quite different.

Incidence

There are no true incidence figures for MEN-1 in the general population. Among patients with primary hyperparathyroidism, the overall incidence varies

Abbreviation

MEN—multiple endocrine neoplasia.

© 1994 Current Science ISBN 1-85922-671-X ISSN 1065–6243

from 1% to 18%. Approximately 50% of patients with Zollinger-Ellison syndrome and 4% of patients with insulinomas display the MEN-1 syndrome. The pituitary is associated with MEN-1 (in 30% of patients) [1].

The *MEN1* locus maps to the long arm of chromosome 11

The familial and genetic nature of MEN-1 was first pointed out in 1954 by Wermer, who suggested that an autosomal dominant gene with high penetrance controls the trait [2]. This means that an individual who is affected has a 50% chance of passing the disease to his or her offspring and that the trait is usually transmitted through a kindred from parent to child with no skipped generations. With the use of linkage analysis in MEN1 families, the chromosomal localization of the *MEN1* gene was determined. This method exploits the tendency for genes that lie close together on a chromosome (linked genes) to cosegregate during cell division in gonads (*ie*, meiosis).

DNA markers detecting restriction fragment length polymorphisms at the *PYGM* locus, located on 11q13, were found to cosegregate with the disease predisposition (Fig. 1) [3]. This chromosomal localization was then confirmed in several families, and despite extensive linkage analysis in more than 40 families, no meiotic recombinations between *MEN1* and *PYGM* have been detected so far [4,5•–7•]. This indicates that the *MEN1* gene is located close to the *PYGM* locus and that the disease is genetically homogenous. Isolation of additional polymorphic markers has allowed more precise localization of the *MEN1* gene to within a 1- to 2-Mb region, *ie*, approximately 1% of the entire chromosome 11 (Weber and Larsson, Unpublished data) [5•,8].

Because of the age-dependent penetrance, most individuals carrying the gene do not develop clinical manifestations until the third decade of life. Thus, DNA-based methods can distinguish gene carriers in MEN-1 families in order to avoid unnecessary biochemical screening of patients that are not at risk. When the disease gene has not been isolated or the disease-causing mutation cannot be identified, genetic linkage is used as an indirect method of diagnosis. In contrast to mutation-specific diagnosis, in which DNA from a single individual is tested, linkage requires samples (*eg*, peripheral leukocytes) from several family members. The disease-associated marker allele is the one shared by the affected family members; therefore, samples from at least two affected individuals in addition to those seeking presymptomatic diagnosis must be analyzed (Fig. 1). With the large number of markers closely linked to *MEN1*, nearly every member of an MEN-1 family can be diagnosed with a high degree of accuracy.

Tumor development

Studies of genetic alterations in MEN-1 tumors have given insight into the properties of the *MEN1* gene and its mode of involvement in tumor development in this syndrome. Through comparison of constitutional and tumor tissue genotypes from the same patient, loss of genetic material from chromosome 11 was detected in tumors from MEN-1 patients. This loss was seen in the majority of parathyroid and pancreatic tumors, as well as in a few of the pituitary and adrenocortical tumors analyzed [3,9–12]. Thus, gross chromosomal rearrangements are detected as allele losses for polymorphic DNA markers within the region. Restriction enzymes recognize specific base-pair combinations where they cleave the DNA. Individual variations in the DNA sequence occurring within restriction sites affect the cleavage pattern, which gives rise to restriction fragments of variable length. When the DNA fragments are size-separated and hybridized against complementary radiolabeled DNA markers, bands of dif-

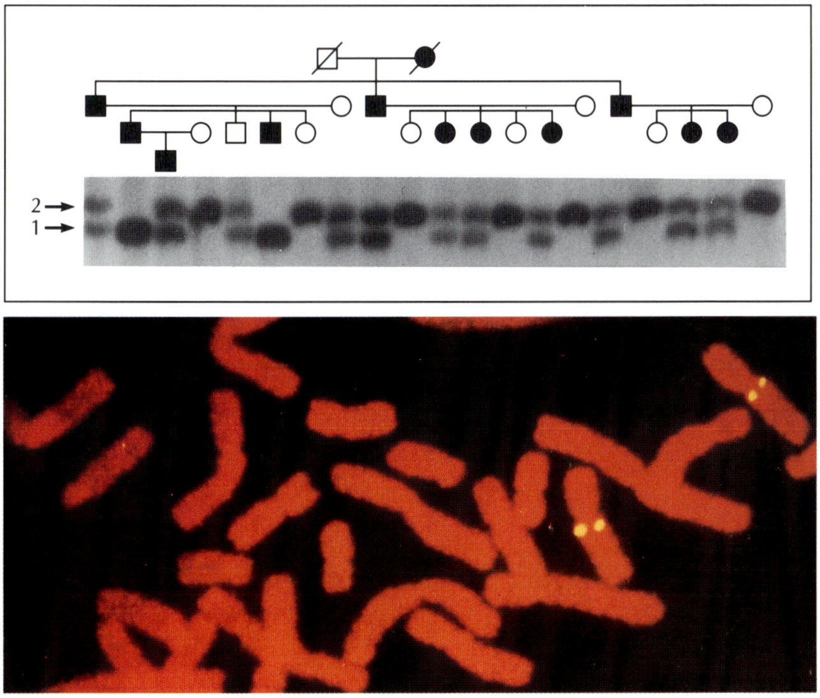

Fig. 1. Linkage of multiple endocrine neoplasia type 1 to the *PYGM* locus at 11q13. **Top**, *Solid squares* and *circles* in pedigree indicate affected members; *open squares* and *circles* in pedigree, unaffected members. Autoradiogram below shows the genotypes (*rows* [alleles] *1* and *2*) for the *PYGM* marker CL15. In this family the disease is inherited together with the 1-allele (lod = 3.46 at 0 cM). **Bottom**, Localization of the *PYGM* marker CL15 at the centromeric part of the long arm of chromosome 11, using fluorescent *in situ* hybridization to human chromosomes.

ferent sizes can be visualized on an autoradiogram. In cases of heterozygosity, one of the bands (fragments) represents the maternally derived chromosome, and the other, the paternally derived chromosome. Allele losses are then detected as loss of one of the alleles (bands) in the tumor tissue DNA as compared with the constitutional DNA (Fig. 2).

When the parental origin of the lost alleles was determined, it was evident that the chromosome derived from the unaffected parent was always lost, leaving only the mutated *MEN1* allele in the tumor. This pattern was seen in all pancreatic and parathyroid tumors and in the one pituitary and adrenocortical tumor analyzed, and it is generally believed to reflect inactivation of a tumor suppressor gene in this region [3,9,11–13]. Hence, tumorigenesis would require two subsequent inactivating mutations of the gene, the first of which would be heritable and would only predispose the patient to tumor development [14]. The tumors would develop when a second mutation leading to complete elimination of the gene or gene function occurred in one of the cells in the target tissue. Consequently, it should be possible to determine on which chromosome the gene for a heritable form of a neoplasia is situated simply by detecting chromosomal rearrangements in these tumors, and in fact this approach was used to localize the *MEN1* gene to chromosome 11.

In keeping with the two-mutation model in MEN-1, the finding that homozygosity for *MEN1* does not result in a more severe hyperparathyroidism or pancreatic disease indicates additional events in tumor development. This idea is supported by several different observations, as exemplified in the following discussion. Histopathologic examination of pancreatic tissue specimens from many MEN-1 patients reveals multiple microadenomas, often referred to as *microadenomatous islet cell hyperplasia*, in addition to hormone-secreting adenomas and carcinomas [15]. In one examined case, loss of chromosome 11 was present already in microadenomatous tissue [3]. Karyotyping of MEN-1 pancreatic tumors has demonstrated chromosome abnormalities such as tetraploidy and the presence of double-minute chromosomes [16]. Although the latter is a phenomenon normally associated with oncogene amplification in neoplastic cells, it has also been identified in cultures of Epstein-Barr virus–transformed lymphocytes from MEN-1 patients [17]. These cells also had a high rate of chromosomal instability, with numerical and structural abnormalities. Another observation is the presence of a factor in plasma from MEN-1 patients that is mitogenic on normal parathyroid cells. Even if illegitimate expression of an oncogene is unlikely to account for the inherited mutation in *MEN1*, it may still be operative in tumor development [18–20]. For example, the stimulatory G-protein shows a specific mutation called *gsp* in a subset of pituitary tumors with constitutive activation of adenylate cyclase and autonomous cyclic AMP synthesis [21].

Oncogenesis of sporadic tumors

Patients with MEN-1 characteristically develop multiple primary tumors, equally distributed between men and women, at 20 to 30 years of age, whereas patients with sporadic disease show mainly single tumors with a later onset. Morphologically, the lesions are indistinguishable, suggesting that tumorigenesis in female and sporadic cases involves related mechanisms [22,23]. Indeed, both sporadic parathyroid, pancreatic, and pituitary tumors and adrenocortical carcinomas show deletions of chromosome 11, but this finding has a tendency to be less frequent in sporadic forms than in the familial tumor forms. Sporadic primary hyperparathyroidism is a frequent disorder that mainly affects postmenopausal women, for reasons not yet known. Malignancy of the parathyroid glands has not been reported in classic MEN-1 families, but it occurs in both sporadic and familial forms of isolated primary hyperparathyroidism [24–27,28]. In two recent publications, familial isolated primary hyperparathyroidism was neither linked to the *MEN1* region nor associated with chromosome 11 deletions [29,30]. These findings further sup-

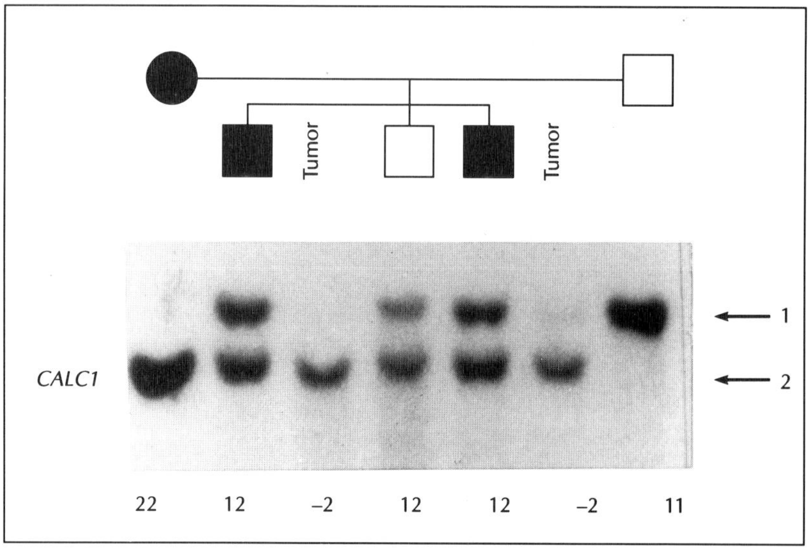

Fig. 2. Pedigree and autoradiogram showing hybridization to the calcitonin marker (*CALC*) from a family with three members affected by multiple endocrine neoplasia (*solid squares* and *circle*). Tumor tissue (insulinoma) from two brothers displayed loss of heterozygosity (*third and sixth lane from left*). The lost allele (*row 1*) derived from the unaffected father (*right lane*), whereas the retained allele (*row 2*) was transmitted from the affected mother (*left lane*).

port the hypothesis that primary hyperparathyroidism constitutes a genetically heterogenous entity.

Multiple endocrine neoplasia type 2

Multiple endocrine neoplasia type 2A is a rare familial cancer syndrome characterized by the expression of medullary thyroid carcinoma as the index lesion with the variable concurrence of additional neural crest abnormalities, including pheochromocytoma and congenital aganglionosis (Hirschsprung's disease) [31,32]. The less common subtype, MEN-2B, which is distinguished from MEN-2A by a ganglioneuromatosis of the intestine, Marfanoid habitus, and the presence of distinct dysmorphic facial features, has an earlier age of disease onset and an enhanced malignant course [33]. Genetically, segregation of the MEN-2 phenotype follows an autosomal dominant model, with complete but delayed, age-dependent biochemical and clinical penetrance [33]. Specifically, it is estimated that potentially 40% of *MEN2A* gene carriers will remain clinically silent into late adulthood [34]. Presymptomatic screening and earlier biochemical detection of the thyroid C-cell disease, medullary thyroid carcinoma or its premalignant precursor C-cell hyperplasia, can be accomplished by measuring an increase in the plasma calcitonin level after the intravenous injection of pentagastrin. This method will identify approximately 90% of asymptomatic gene carriers by the age of 25 years [35]. The majority of MEN-2A cases occur in a familial setting, with a spontaneous mutation rate of 0.0 and an estimated gene frequency of one in 50,000; this situation is in contrast to that of MEN-2B, in which a significant number of cases arise from novel germline mutations [36].

Strategy for isolating the *MEN2* gene

Linkage and physical mapping studies

Unfortunately, efforts to identify the *MEN2* gene were initially hampered by a lack of preexisting information and insight into the nature of the biochemical defect producing the disease phenotype. In addition, cytogenetic analyses of peripheral blood lymphocytes from patients affected with MEN-2 were unrevealing, with no visible gross alterations to reliably guide the search for the *MEN2* locus. As a result, the process of gene identification began with the more arduous but exciting approach of positional cloning. The chromosomal assignment of *MEN2* was supported by initial mapping information that emerged from genetic linkage analysis. In 1987, two independent groups mapped the genetic defect responsible for MEN-2A to the pericentromeric region of chromosome 10 between the flanking restriction fragment length polymorphism markers *RBP3* (10q11.2) and *FNRB* (10p11.2), the genes encoding the interstitial retinol-binding protein and the β-subunit of the fibronectin receptor, respectively [37,38]. Although this interval was subsequently narrowed proximally to encompass a sex-averaged genetic distance of 11.5 centiMorgans (cM), it remained unknown for several years thereafter whether *MEN2A* mapped to the long or the short arm of chromosome 10 [39]. The *MEN2B* gene localized to a region on the long arm of chromosome 10 between the centromeric probe *D10Z1* and *RBP3*, as determined by a single meiotic recombination in an unaffected individual [40]. Efforts to refine further the position of the *MEN2* gene by meiotic mapping were initially impeded by the paucity of identifiable critical crossovers detectable with existing restriction fragment length polymorphism markers, as well as by a repression of recombination noted in males in this region. However, all of the MEN-2 variants and families studied appeared to show linkage to a single region on chromosome 10 [41,42]. This finding suggested that each subtype might be due to a different allele at an identical locus, a pleiotropic effect of an identical, dominant mutation, or the presence of several contiguous genes all involved in neural crest cell differentiation. Subsequent to the localization studies, efforts were directed toward constructing a detailed and improved genetic map of the pericentromeric region of chromosome 10 using highly informative microsatellite polymorphisms (Fig. 3). This refined the *MEN2* region to a 0.55-cM interval on 10q11.2 between the flanking markers D10S141 and D10S94, encompassing the locus encoding the *RET* protooncogene [43••,44,45]. Interestingly, linkage studies in affected families had detected no meiotic recombinants between *MEN2A* and *RET*, suggesting close proximity between sites [46,47]. Previously, *RET* had been shown to be rearranged in human papillary thyroid cancers [48,49], and although papillary thyroid cancer is not a usual feature of MEN-2, a single MEN-2A kindred was identified in which expression of papillary thyroid cancer appeared to cosegregate with the *MEN2A* gene [50]. Detailed physical mapping of the region spanning the *MEN2* locus was then undertaken, with techniques such as pulsed-field gel electrophoresis and radiation-reduced hybrid panels confirming the results of the genetic linkage analysis. A yeast artificial chromosome contig was constructed that spanned more than 1 million consecutive base pairs from human chromosome band 10q11.2 and contained the markers D10S141, *RET*, and D10S94, all closely linked to the *MEN2A* gene [51••]. The three markers positioned on the yeast artificial chromosome contig assumed the relative order of cen-D10S141-*RET*-D10S94-qter and necessarily included the *MEN2A* disease locus, which fell between the flanking markers D10S141 and D10S94 and defined a region spanning a physical distance of 480 kb. The *RET* protooncogene known to lie within this region thus emerged as a serious candidate for the *MEN2A* gene.

Tumor analysis

Following localization of the putative *MEN2A* gene to chromosome 10, tumor allelotyping was undertaken to analyze tissues for possible loss of heterozygosity, which might lead to the unmasking of a mutant, inactive tumor suppressor gene allele. Surprisingly, constitutional heterozygosity for the linked *MEN2* locus could not be identified in medullary thyroid carcinomas or pheochromocytomas derived from these patients using several probes tightly linked to the *MEN2*

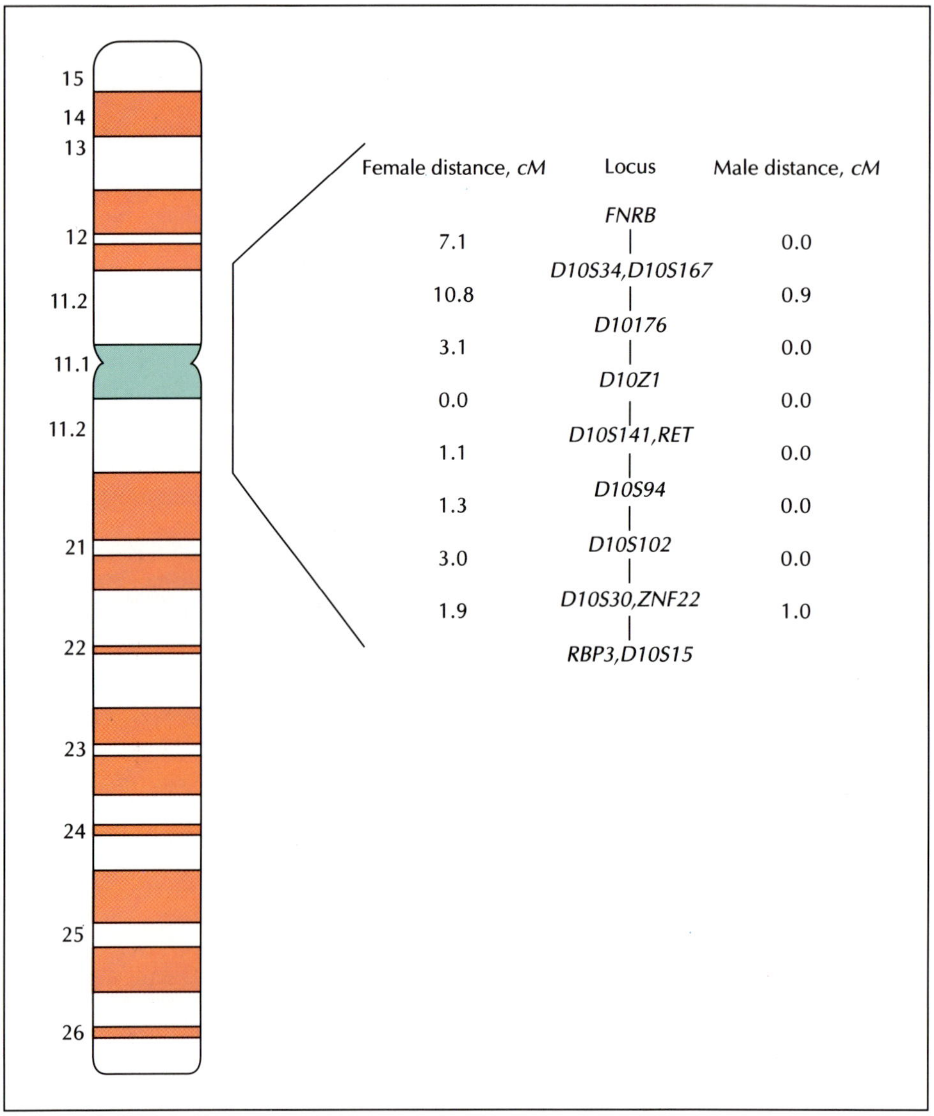

Fig. 3. Current genetic linkage map of the multiple endocrine neoplasia type 2 region on chromosome 10. Sex-specific distances are shown in centiMorgans (cM). (*From* Gardner *et al.* [43••]; with permission.)

locus [52••,53]. This finding suggested that perhaps the germline abnormality on chromosome 10 did not involve a tumor suppressor gene. Consequently, the quest for the *MEN2* gene was not amenable to such strategies as tumor deletion mapping. Although the predisposing event for expression of *MEN2* was believed to originate on chromosome 10, tumor allelic losses were observed on chromosomal arms 1p, 3q, 3p, 22q, 11p, 13q, and 17p (in order of decreasing frequency) [52••]. Furthermore, the regions deleted on chromosomes 11 (11pter-p13), 17 (17pter-p11.2), and 13 (13q) contained the known tumor suppressor loci *WT1, TP53,* and *RB1,* respectively, which could contribute to tumor progression in MEN-2.

The oncogenic potential of RET, a receptor tyrosine kinase, was previously recognized in human papillary thyroid cancers, in which it was shown to be structurally rearranged and activated [49]. The mutated oncogene was found to result from a somatic intrachromosomal rearrangement that produced a chimeric transforming sequence created by substituting the 5′ sequence of *RET* with a distant sequence designated D10S170 (H4). However, no constitutional or transcriptional abnormalities in *RET* were apparent in MEN-2 patients, at least at the Southern blot level or by pulsed-field gel electrophoresis analysis, although the gene appeared to be expressed in pheochromocytomas and medullary thyroid carcinomas [54••,55•].

Molecular cloning

Finally, early in 1993, researchers in Cambridge uncovered several germline mutations of the *RET* protooncogene in 20 of 23 distinct MEN-2A families [54••]. Mutational analysis of the *RET* coding sequence in these patients had been complicated by the fact that RET is not normally expressed in lymphocytes or the majority of adult tissues. In addition, although the *RET* complementary DNA sequence was available [56,57], knowledge of the intron and exon structure of the gene was initially absent, which precluded strategies employing direct amplification of genomic DNA with the polymerase chain reaction and simple sequencing of resultant products. Thus, screening of the *RET* transcripts was necessarily undertaken using RNA derived from the medullary thyroid carcinomas and pheochromo-

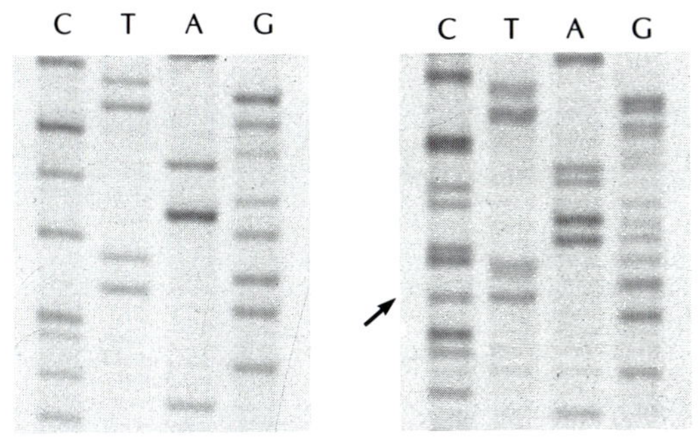

Fig. 4. Germ line sequence of a normal subject (*left panel*) and a patient affected with multiple endocrine neoplasia type 2A (*right panel*). Note T→C transition in affected individual (*arrow*) resulting in a nonconservative amino acid change (Cys →Arg).

cytomas of six MEN-2A patients, all of whom were known to express the gene. The search for sequence variations was accomplished using the chemical mismatch cleavage technique following polymerase chain reaction amplification of reversed transcribed tumor RNA. Direct sequencing of the detected variants identified altered sequences in codons 364, 378 to 380, and 380, respectively (Fig. 4). In each instance, a single base-pair substitution led to the replacement of a conserved cysteine residue with another amino acid. These changes were not observed in sporadic controls. In most cases, the tumor sample appeared to express both the normal and the mutant alleles. To determine whether the *RET* mutation was germline or somatic in origin, genomic DNA from the affected individuals was analyzed as well, and the identical sequence variation was observed. In addition, *RET* mutations of codon 380 were detected in 17 germline samples from 21 distinct MEN-2A families, and the codon 364 mutation was detected in another, demonstrating that the point mutation segregated with the disease phenotype. A normal *RET* sequence was present in all controls. Subsequently, other investigators reported mutations in *RET* of a similar nature, confirming the initial findings (Fig. 5) [58••]. Interestingly, a mutation in *RET* has not been found as of yet in patients affected with the more virulent MEN-2B subtype [54••,58••]. Expression studies will be necessary to verify that the observed mutations and dominant action of the oncogene indeed confer a predisposition to the MEN-2A disease.

Structural analysis and characteristics of the *RET* protooncogene

The *RET* protooncogene encodes a tyrosine kinase transmembrane receptor whose ligand is presently unknown [57]. The protein consists of a large glycosylated extracellular domain with a highly conserved cysteine-rich region of unknown function immediately proximal to a single transmembrane segment followed by an intracellular tyrosine kinase domain. In addition, the extracellular domain contains several related consensus sequences and seven putative calcium-binding motifs that show sequence similarity to the communicative cadherins [59•,60]. The cadherins are a superfamily of transmembrane proteins that mediate homophilic calcium-dependent cell-cell adhesion and are known

1759 * AAC-**TGC**-TTC-CCT-GAG-GAG-GAG-AAG-**TGC**-TTC-**TGC**-GAG-CCC-GAA
356 † Asn **Cys** Phe Pro Glu Glu Glu Lys **Cys** Phe **Cys** Glu Pro Glu

TG**G**
Trp

CGC
Arg
AGC
Ser
T**A**C
Tyr
GGC
Gly

CGC
Arg
T**A**C
Tyr

1816 CTG-**TGC**-GAC-GAG-CTG-**TGC**-CGC
375 Leu **Cys** Asp Glu Leu **Cys** Arg

CGC
Arg
GGC
Gly
T**A**C
Tyr
T**C**C
Ser
T**T**C
Phe

Fig. 5. *RET* mutations in multiple endocrine neoplasia type 2A. Amino acid (*dagger*) and codon (*asterisk*) sequences refer to the normal *RET* sequence. (*Data from* Takahashi *et al.* [57].) DNA sequence mutations (*bold type*) in the cysteine residues and predicted amino acid changes are indicated below the sequences. (*Data from* Mulligan *et al.* [54••] and Donis-Keller *et al.* [58••].)

to play a role in cell differentiation, morphogenesis, and tumor suppression [61]. The genetic structure of *RET* is comprised of no less than 21 exons spanning 30 kb of genomic DNA [62]. The protooncogene encodes several major messenger RNA species ranging in size from 3.9 to 7.0 kb as a result of alternative 3′ splicing and polyadenylation [63]. Expression of *RET* has been detected by Northern blot analysis in normal adrenal medulla and thyroid, and is transcribed in high amounts in various tumors or neuroectodermal origin, such as neuroblastoma, medullary thyroid carcinoma, and pheochromocytoma [55•,64,65]. Activation of the receptor results in its autophosphorylation on tyrosine residues; no other target protein has of yet been identified by Western blotting [66]. Long-term induction of RET expression by retinoic acid results in morphologic differentiation and extensive clustering of neuroblastoma cells, indicating that it may have a role in neuroendocrine cell growth [67]. In addition, elevated levels of RET transcripts have been detected in the embryonic rat, suggesting it may be expressed in fetal development [68].

Conclusions

A putative MEN-2A gene, the *RET* protooncogene mapping to chromosome 10q11.2, has been isolated. The normal function of the RET receptor-type tyrosine kinase or its ligand is presently unknown. It is unclear how the cysteine mutations in *RET* predispose to tumor formation in MEN-2; however, the changes appear to result in constitutive activation of the oncogene. The mutation responsible for the MEN-2B subtype has not been declared.

With characterization of the MEN-2A mutation in the kindreds under study, effective screening by DNA analysis is now a reality. The availability of genetic testing introduces the possibility of early, curative surgical treatment in those identified to be affected. Other advantages of a DNA approach to diagnosis are that it requires a single blood sample and that the results are objective in nature and independent of age. Furthermore, negative test results will obviate the need for the unpleasant and costly biochemical pentagastrin testing presently employed, which often extends into adulthood given the delayed penetrance of the disease.

Further characterization of *RET* and understanding of its function should provide insight into the molecular dynamics of tumor onset in general and medullary thyroid carcinoma onset in particular, as well as into the function of the normal gene in controlling the growth of neural crest–derived tissues. In addition to early surgical intervention, isolation of the molecular defect could provide the opportunity for preimplantation prevention of the disease.

Acknowledgments

The portion of this article on MEN-1 was supported by the Swedish Medical Research Council, the Swedish Cancer Foundation, and the Magnus Bergwall Foundation.

The portion of this article on MEN-2 was supported by National Institutes of Health grant 1K08DK02176-01, the American Cancer Society (VM-71281), and the John and Suzanne Munn Endowed Research Fund of the University of Michigan Comprehensive Cancer Center.

References and recommended reading

Papers of particular interest, published within the annual period of review, have been highlighted as:
• Of special interest
•• Of outstanding interest

1. Metz D, Jensen RT, Bale A, Skarulis MC, Eastman R, Nieman L, Norton J, Friedman E, Larsson C, Amorosi A, Brandi ML, Marx SJ: **Multiple Endocrine Neoplasia Type 1: Clinical Features and Management**. In *The Parathyroids*. Edited by Bileziken JP. New York: Raven Press; 1993.

2. Wermer P: **Genetic Aspects of Adenomatosis of Endocrine Glands**. *Am J Med* 1954, **16**:363–371.

3. Larsson C, Skogseid B, Öberg K, Nakamura K, Nordenskjöld M: **Multiple Endocrine Neoplasia Type 1 Maps to Chromosome 11 and Is Lost in Insulinoma**. *Nature* 1988, **332**:85–87.

4. Iwasaki H, Stewart PW, Dilley WG, Holt MS, Steinbreuk TD, Wells JR, Donis-Keller H: **A Minisatellite and a Microsatellite Polymorphism Within 1.5 kb at the Human Muscle Glycogen Phosphorylase (PYGM) Locus Can Be Amplified by PCR and Have Combined Informativeness of PIC 0.95**. *Genomics* 1992, **13**:7–15.

5. • Fujimori M, Wells SA Jr, Nakamura Y: **Fine Scale Mapping of the Gene Responsible for Multiple Endocrine Neoplasia Type I (MENI)**. *Am J Hum Genet* 1993, **50**:399–403.
A genetic map of newly isolated polymorphic markers was established by linkage analysis in reference families, and the location of the *MEN1* locus within this map was determined.

6. • Thakker RV, Wooding C, Pang JT, Farren B, Harding B, Anderson DC, Besser GM, Bouloux P, Brenton DP, Buchanan KD, Edwards CR, Heath DA, Jackson CE, Jansen S, Lips K, Norum R, Sampson J, Shalet SM, Taggart RT, Tailor D, Wheeler MH, Wollard PM, Yates J: **Linkage Analysis of 7 Polymorphic Markers at Chromosome 11p11.2-11q13 in 27 Multiple Endocrine Neoplasia Type 1 Families**. *Ann Hum Genet* 1993, **57**:17–25.
Linkage analysis in large panel of MEN-1 syndrome families established genetic homogeneity of the disease as well as a more precise location of the disease locus.

7. • Larsson C, Shepherd J, Nakamura Y, Blomberg C, Weber G, Werelius B, Hayward N, Teh B, Tokino T, Seizinger B, Skpgseid GB, Öberg K, Nordenskjöld M: **Predictive Testing for Multiple Endocrine Neoplasia Type 1 Using DNA Polymorphisms**. *J Clin Invest* 1992, **89**:1344–1349.
The authors describe accurate presymptomatic testing in MEN-1 using a large panel of polymorphic DNA markers.

8. Larsson C, Weber G, Kvanta E, Lewis K, Janson M, Jones C, Glaser T, Evans G, Nordenskjöld M: **Isolation and Mapping of Polymorphic Cosmid Clones for Sublocalization of the Multiple Endocrine Neoplasia Type 1 (MEN1) Locus**. *Hum Genet* 1992, **89**:187–193.

9. Byström C, Larsson C, Blomberg C, Sandelin K, Falkmer U, Skogseid B, Öberg K, Werner S, Nordenskjöld M: **Localization of the MEN1 Gene to a Small Region Within Chromosome 11 q13 by Deletion Mapping in Tumors**. *Proc Natl Acad Sci U S A* 1990, **87**:1968–1972.

10. Friedman E, Sakaguchi K, Bale AE, Falchetti A, Streeten E, Zimering M, Weinstein LS, McBride WO, Nakamura Y, Brandi ML, Norton JA, Aurbach GD, Spiegel AM, Marx SJ: **Clonality of Parathyroid Tumors in Familial Multiple Endocrine Neoplasia Type 1**. *N Engl J Med* 1989, **321**:213–218.

11. Skogseid B, Larson B, Lindgren P, Kvanta E, Rastad J, Theodorson E, Wide L, Wilander W, Öberg K: **Clinical and Genetic Features of Adrenocortical Lesions in Multiple Endocrine Neoplasia Type 1**. *J Clin Endocrinol Metab* 1992, **75**:142–148.

12. Thakker RV, Bouloux P, Wooding C, Chotai K, Broad PM, Spurr NK, Besser GM, O'Riordan JLH: **Association of Parathyroid Tumors in Multiple Endocrine Neoplasia Type 1 With Loss of Alleles on Chromosome 11**. *N Engl J Med* 1989, **321**:218–224.

13. Yoshimoto K, Iwahana H, Kobo K, Saito S, Itakura M: **Allele Loss on Chromosome 11 in a Pituitary Tumor From a Patient With Multiple Endocrine Neoplasia Type 1**. *Cancer Res* 1991, **82**:886–889.

14. Knudson AG: **Retinoblastoma: A Prototypic Hereditary Neoplasm**. *Semin Oncol* 1978, **5**:57–60.

15. Klöppel G, Heitz PU: **Pancreatic Endocrine Tumors**. *Pathol Res Pract* 1988, **183**:155–168.

16. Scappaticci S, Brandi ML, Capra E, Cortinovis M, Maraschio P: **Cytogenetics of Multiple Endocrine Neoplasia Syndrome: II. Chromosome Abnormalities in an Insulinoma and a Glucagonoma From a Subject With MEN1.** *Cancer Genet Cytogenet* 1992, **63**:17–21.

17. Scappaticci S, Maraschio P, Del Ciotto N, Fossati GS, Zonta A, Fraccarp M: **Chromosome Abnormalities in Lymphocytes and Fibroblasts of Subjects With Multiple Endocrine Neoplasia Type 1.** *Cancer Genet Cytogenet* 1991, **52**:85–92.

18. Brandi ML, Marx SJ, Aurbach GD, Fitzpatrick LA: **A New Look at Pathophysiology.** *Endocr Rev* 1987, **8**:391–405.

19. Brandi ML: **A Novel Endothelial Cell Growth Factor Circulates in Familial Endocrine Neoplasia Type 1.** *Nucl Med Biol* 1990, **17**:639–643.

20. Zimering MB, Katsumatu N, Sato Y, Brandi ML, Aurbach GD, Marx SJ, Friesen HG: **Increased Fibroblast Growth Factor in Plasma From Multiple Endocrine Neoplasia Type 1: Relation to Pituitary Tumors.** *J Clin Endocrinol Metab* 1993, **73**:1182–1187.

21. Hosoi E, Yokoguchi Y, Hosoi E, Yokoi K, Sano T, Saito S: **A Pituitary Specific Point Mutation of Codon 201 of the G Alpha Gene in a Pituitary Adenoma of a Patient With Multiple Endocrine Neoplasia (MEN) Type 1.** *Endocrinol Jpn* 1992, **39**:319–324.

22. Sandelin K, Larsson C, Falkmer UG, Farnebo L, Grimelius L, Nordenskjöld M: **Morphology, DNA Ploidy, and Allele Losses on Chromosome 11 in Sporadic Hyperparathyroidism and That Associated With Multiple Endocrine Neoplasia Type 1.** *Eur J Surg* 1992, **158**:199–206.

23. Harach HR, Jasane B: **Parathyroid Hyperplasia in Multiple Endocrine Neoplasia Type 1: A Pathological and Immunohistochemical Reappraisal.** *Histopathology* 1992, **20**:305–313.

24. Dinnen JS, Greenwood RH, Jones JH, Walker DA, Williams ED: **Parathyroid Carcinoma in Familial Hyperparathyroidism.** *J Clin Pathol* 1977, **30**:966–975.

25. Frayah RA, Nasar VH, Dagher F, Salti IS: **Familial Parathyroid Carcinoma.** *Lebanese Med J* 1972, **25**:299–309.

26. Lee C-H, Lee C, P'eng FK, Lui W-Y, Ho L-T, Lin H-D, Chhing K-N, Yeh PH-H: **Surgical Treatment of Primary Hyperparathyroidism.** *Endocr Surg* 1988, **5**:441–450.

27. Malette LE, Bilezikian JP, Ketcham AS, Aurbach GD: **Parathyroid Carcinoma in Familial Hyperparathyroidism.** *Am J Med* 1974, **57**:642–648.

28. Sandelin K, Auer G, Bondeson L, Grimelius L, Farnebo LO: **Prognostic Factors in Parathyroid Cancer: A Review of 95 Cases.** *World J Surg* 1992, **16**:724–731.

29. Streeten E, Weinstein LS, Norton JA, Mullvihill JJ, White BJ, Friedman E, Jaffe G, Brandi ML, Stewart K, Zimering MB, Spiegel AM, Aurbach GD, Marx SJ: **Studies in a Kindred With Parathyroid Carcinoma.** *J Clin Endocrinol Metab* 1992, **75**:362–366.

30. Wassif WS, Moniz CF, Friedman E, Wong S, Weber G, Nordenskjöld M, Peters TJ, Larsson C: **Familial Isolated Hyperparathyroidism: A Distinct Genetic Entity With Increased Risk of Parathyroid Cancer.** *J Clin Endocrinol Metab*, in press.

31. Decker RA, Wells SA: **Multiple Endocrine Neoplasia.** *Jpn J Surg* 1989, **19**:645–657.

32. Decker RA: **Long-Term Follow-Up of a Large North American Kindred With Multiple Endocrine Neoplasia Type 2A.** *Surgery* 1992, **112**:1066–1073.

33. Decker RA, Toyama WM, O'Neal LW, Telander RL, Wells SA: **Evaluation of Children With Multiple Endocrine Neoplasia Type IIb Following Thyroidectomy.** *J Pediatr Surg* 1990, **25**:939–943.

34. Easton DF, Ponder MA, Cummings T, Gagel RF, Hansen HH, Reichlin S, Tashjian AH, Telenius-Berg M, Ponder BA, and the Cancer Research Campaign Medullary Thyroid Group: **The Clinical and Screening Age-at-Onset Distribution for the MEN-2 Syndrome.** *Am J Hum Genet* 1989, **44**:208–215.

35. Ponder BA, Coffey R, Gagel RF, Semple P, Ponder MA, Pembrey ME, Telenius-Berg M, Easton DF, and the Cancer Research Campaign Medullary Thyroid Group: **Risk Estimation and Screening in Families of Patients With Medullary Thyroid Carcinoma.** *Lancet* 1988, **i**:397–401.

36. Carter C, Easton DF, Mathew CGP, Welander G, Telenius H, Telenius-Berg M, Ponder BAJ: **Exclusion of Linkage of Loci on Chromosome 19 With Multiple Endocrine Neoplasia Type 2.** *Cytogenet Cell Genet* 1987, **45**:33–37.

37. Mathew CG, Chin KS, Easton DF, Thorpe E, Carter C, Liou GI, Fong SL, Bridges CD, Haak H, Nieuwenhuijzen Kruseman AC, Schifter S, Hansen HH, Telenius H, Telenius-Berg M, Ponder BA: **A Linked Genetic Marker for Multiple Endocrine Neoplasia Type 2A on Chromosome 10.** *Nature* 1987, **328**:527–528.

38. Simpson NE, Kidd KK, Goodfellow PJ, McDermid H, Myers S, Kidd JR, Jackson CE, Duncan AM, Farrer LA, Brasch K, Castiglione C, Genel M, Gertner J, Greenberg CR, Gusella JF, Holden JJ, White BN: **Assignment of Multiple Endocrine Neoplasia Type 2A to Chromosome 10 by Linkage.** *Nature* 1987, **328**:528–530.

39. Gardner E, Easton D, Mole SE, Mulligan LM, Telenius H, Papi L, Ponder BA: **Extending the Genetic Map of the Pericentromeric Region of Chromosome 10.** *Cytogenet Cell Genet* 1991, **58**:1949.

40. Jackson CE, Norum RA: **Genetics of the Multiple Endocrine Neoplasia Type 2B Syndrome.** *Henry Ford Hosp Med J* 1992, **40**:232–235.

41. Narod SA, Morgan LM, Calmettes C, Sobol H, Goodfellow PJ, Lenior GM: **Genetic Analysis of 24 French Families With Multiple Endocrine Neoplasia Type 2A.** *Am J Hum Genet* 1992, **51**:469–477.

42. Lairmore TC, Howe JR, Korte HA, Dilley WG, Aine L, Aine E, Wells SA, Donis-Keller H: **Familial Medullary Thyroid Carcinoma and Multiple Endocrine Neoplasia Type 2B Map to the Same Region of Chromosome 10 as Multiple Endocrine Neoplasia Type 2A.** *Genomics* 1992, **9**:181–192.

43. •• Gardner E, Papi L, Easton DF, Cummings T, Jackson CE, Kaplan M, Love DR, Mole SE, Moore JK, Mulligan LM, Norum RA, Ponder MA, Reichlin S, Stall G, Telenius H, Telenius-Berg M, Tunnacliffe A, Ponder BA: **Genetic Linkage Studies Map the Multiple Endocrine Neoplasia Type 2 Loci to a Small Interval on Chromosome 10q11.2.** *Hum Mol Genet* 1993, **2**:241–246.

With the use of several newly isolated highly polymorphic DNA markers to uncover previously unrecognized meiotic recombinant events, the genetic interval encompassing the *MEN2A* gene was narrowed to less than 1 cM on 10q11.2.

44. Howe JR, Lairmore TC, Mishra SK, Dou S, Veile R, Wells SA, Donis-Keller H: **Improved Predictive Testing for MEN2 Using Flanking Dinucleotide Repeats and RFLPs.** *Am J Hum Genet* 1992, **51**:1430–1442.

45. Decker RA, Collins FS: **Dinucleotide Repeat Polymorphism at the D10S469 Locus.** *Hum Mol Genet* 1993, **2**:1330.

46. Lairmore TC, Dou S, Howe JR, Chi D, Carlson K, Veile R, Mishra SK, Wells SA, Donis-Keller H: **A 1.5-Megabase Yeast Artificial Chromosome Contig From Human Chromosome 10q11.2 Connecting Three Genetic Loci (RET, D10S94, and D10S102) Closely Linked to the MEN2A Locus.** *Proc Natl Acad Sci U S A* 1993, **90**:492–496.

47. Yamamoto M, Miki T, Tanaka N, Miya A, Shin E, Karakawa K, Kobayashi T, Tahira T, Ishizaka Y, Iton F, Nagao M, Mori T, Takai S: **Tight Linkage of the *ret* Proto-oncogene With the Multiple Endocrine Neoplasia Type 2A Locus.** *Jpn J Clin Oncol* 1991, **21**:149–152.

48. Ishizaka Y, Itoh F, Tahira T, Ikeda I, Ogura T, Sugimura T, Nagao M: **Presence of Aberrant Transcripts of *ret* Proto-oncogene in a Human Papillary Thyroid Carcinoma Cell Line.** *Jpn J Cancer Res* 1989, **80**:1149–1152.

49. Grieco M, Santoro M, Berlingieri MT, Melillo RM, Donghi R, Bongarzone I, Pierotti MA, Della Porta G, Fusco A, Vecchio G: **PTC Is a Novel Rearranged Form of the *ret* Proto-oncogene and Is Frequently Detected In Vivo in Human Thyroid Papillary Carcinomas.** *Cell* 1990, **60**:557–563.

50. Decker RA: **Expression of Papillary Thyroid Carcinoma in Multiple Endocrine Neoplasia Type 2A.** *Surgery* 1993, **114**:1059–1063.

51. •• Mole SE, Mulligan LM, Healey CS, Ponder BA, Tunnacliffe A: **Localisation of the Gene for Multiple Endocrine Neoplasia Type 2A to a 480 kb Region in Chromosome Band 10q11.2.** *Hum Mol Genet* 1993, **2**:247–252.

This physical mapping study describes a 480-kb yeast artificial chromosome contig spanning the *MEN2A* region.

52. •• Mulligan LM, Gardner E, Smith BA, Mathew CG, Ponder BA: **Genetic Events in Tumour Initiation and Progression in Multiple Endocrine Neoplasia Type 2.** *Genes Chromosom Cancer* 1993, **6**:166–177.

Highlights chromosomal regions involved in the loss of tumor heterozygosity.

53. Nelkin BD, Nakamura Y, White RW, De Bustros AC, Herman J, Wells SA, Baylin SB: **Low Incidence of Loss of Chromosome 10 in Sporadic and Hereditary Human Medullary Thyroid Carcinoma.** *Cancer Res* 1989, **49**:4114–4119.

54. •• Mulligan LM, Kwok JB, Healey CS, Elsdon MJ, Eng C, Gardner E, Love DR, Mole SE, Moore JK, Papi L, Ponder MA, Telenius H, Tunnacliffe A, Ponder BA: **Germ-Line Mutations of the *ret* Proto-oncogene in Multiple Endocrine Neoplasia Type 2A.** *Nature* 1993, **363**:458.

First publication describing a germline mutation in the *RET* protooncogene in 20 of 23 patients with MEN-2A.

55. • Miya A, Yamamoto M, Morimoto H, Tanaka N, Shin E, Karakawa K, Toyoshima K, Ishizaka Y, Mori T, Takai S: **Expression of the *ret* Proto-oncogene in Human Medullary Thyroid Carcinomas and Pheochromocytomas of MEN 2A.** *Henry Ford Hosp Med J* 1992, **40**:215–219.

Study analyzing the expression of the *RET* protooncogene in human medullary thyroid carcinomas and pheochromocytomas in patients with MEN-2A by Northern blot analysis.

56. Takahashi M, Buma Y, Hiai H: **Isolation of *ret* Proto-oncogene cDNA With an Amino-Terminal Signal Sequence.** *Oncogene* 1989, 4:805–806.

57. Takahashi M, Buma Y, Iwanmoto T, Inaguma Y, Ikeda H, Hiai H: **Cloning and Expression of the *ret* Proto-oncogene Encoding a Tyrosine Kinase With Two Potential Transmembrane Domains.** *Oncogene* 1988, **3**:571–578.

58. Donis-Keller H, Dou S, Chi D, Carlson KM, Toshima K, Lairmore TC,
•• Howe JR, Moley JF, Goodfellow P, Wells SA: **Mutations in the *ret* Proto-oncogene Are Associated With MEN 2A and FMTC.** *Hum Mol Genet* 1993, 7:851–856.

Mutational analysis study confirming the germline missense changes of *RET* in patients with MEN-2A and describing several new cysteine mutations.

59. Iwamoto T, Taniguchi M, Asai N, Ohkusu K, Nakashima I, Takahashi
• M: **cDNA Cloning of Mouse *ret* Proto-oncogene and Its Sequence Similarity to the Cadherin Superfamily.** *Oncogene* 1993, **8**:1087–1091.

The authors outline a DNA sequence analogy between *RET* and the communicative cadherins. This suggests that *RET* may play a role in cell-cell adhesion and morphogenesis.

60. Schneider R: **The Human Protooncogene *ret*: A Communicative Cadherin? [Abstract]** *Trends Biochem Sci* 1992, **17**:468–469.

61. Takeichi M: **Cadherin Cell Adhesion Receptors as a Morphogenetic Regulator.** *Science* 1991, **251**:1451–1455.

62. Kwok JB, Gardner E, Warner JP, Ponder BA, Mulligan LM: **Structural Analysis of the Human *ret* Proto-oncogene Using Exon Trapping.** *Oncogene* 1993, **8**:2575–2582.

63. Tahira T, Ishizaka Y, Itoh F, Sugimura T, Nagao M: **Characterization of *ret* Proto-oncogene mRNAs Encoding Two Isoforms of the Protein Product in a Human Neuroblastoma Cell Line.** *Oncogene* 1990, **5**:97–102.

64. Ikeda I, Ishizaka Y, Tahira T, Suzuki T, Onda M, Sugimura T, Nagao M: **Specific Expression of the *ret* Proto-oncogene in Human Neuroblastoma Lines.** *Oncogene* 1990, **5**:1291–1296.

65. Santoro M, Rosati R, Grieco M, Berlingieri MT, Lucacolucci G, Amato D, De Franciscis V, Fusco A: **The *ret* Proto-oncogene Is Consistently Expressed in Human Pheochromocytomas and Thyroid Medullary Carcinomas.** *Oncogene* 1990, **5**:1595–1598.

66. Taniguchi M, Iwamoto T, Hamaguchi M, Matsuyama M, Takahashi M: **The *ret* Oncogene Products Are Membrane-Bound Glycoproteins Phosphorylated on Tyrosine Residue In Vivo.** *Biochem Biophys Res Commun* 1991, **181**:416–422.

67. Tahira T, Ishizaka Y, Itoh F, Nakayasu M, Sugimura T, Nagao M: **Expression of the *ret* Proto-oncogene in Human Neuroblastoma Cell Lines and Its Increase During Neuronal Differentiation Induced by Retinoic Acid.** *Oncogene* 1991, **6**:2333–2338.

68. Tahira T, Ishizaka Y, Sugimura T, Nagao M: **Expression of Proto-*ret* mRNA in Embryonic and Adult Rat Tissues.** *Biochem Biophys Res Commun* 1988, **153**:1290–1295.

Kerstin Sandelin, MD, PhD, Department of Surgery, and Catharina Larsson, MD, PhD, Department of Clinical Genetics, Karolinska Hospital, S-104 01 Stockholm, Sweden.

Ruth Anne Decker, MD, Department of Surgery, University of Michigan Medical Center, 2920 Taubman Center, Ann Arbor, MI 48109–0331, USA.

The place for curative surgical procedures in the treatment of sporadic and familial Zollinger-Ellison syndrome

Romano Delcore, MD, and Stanley R. Friesen, MD, PhD

University of Kansas Medical Center, Kansas City, Kansas, USA

The surgical treatment of patients with the Zollinger-Ellison syndrome has undergone a dramatic evolution since the syndrome was originally described. It is now recognized that an aggressive surgical approach is mandatory because of the malignant potential of gastrinomas in both the sporadic and the familial forms of the syndrome. Although initially regarded as an incurable neoplasm, it is now known that complete surgical resection of gastrinomas can result in eugastrinemia even in the presence of lymph node metastases. It is now recognized that extrapancreatic gastrinomas are more common than pancreatic gastrinomas, and the most common location for an extrapancreatic gastrinoma is the duodenal wall. Major improvements in preoperative imaging and intraoperative localization techniques combined with an increased awareness of the anatomic distribution of gastrinomas have markedly increased the surgeon's ability to care for and cure patients with the Zollinger-Ellison syndrome.

Current Opinion in General Surgery 1994:69–76

A progressive evolution in the surgical management the Zollinger-Ellison syndrome (ZES) from surgical attempts to control gastric acid hypersecretion by removal of the end organ to the current emphasis on early tumor eradication has occurred since the original description of the syndrome [1]. Prior to the availability of effective pharmacologic control of acid hypersecretion, patients presented with severe, often fatal complications of acid peptic ulceration and required multiple gastric operations, including total gastrectomy. Recently, successful medical control of acid hypersecretion has led to fewer patients requiring total gastrectomy [2]. Patients with the ZES are now less likely to succumb to the complications of acid peptic ulceration and, instead, if not operated on, they may suffer the consequences of the malignant behavior of gastrinomas [3]. At least 60% of gastrinomas are malignant, and surgical resection remains the only potentially curative treatment. Most, if not all, patients with the ZES should therefore undergo surgical exploration to assess resectability and attempt removal of all neoplastic tissue [3–6,7•,8•,9••]. Nevertheless, several aspects of the surgical management of the ZES remain controversial [4,10–12].

Gastrinomas

Gastrinomas are neoplasms arising from gastrin-secreting cells located in pancreatic and extrapancreatic sites. Early studies reported almost exclusively pancreatic gastrinomas, but recent series have demonstrated that up to two thirds of gastrinomas are found in extrapancreatic sites [11,13–15]. The most common extrapancreatic location is in the duodenal wall, but extraintestinal gastrinomas have been reported occasionally [16–26,27•–29•].

Sporadic gastrinomas are characteristically single, but patients with multiple endocrine neoplasia type 1 (MEN-1) almost invariably have multiple gastrinomas. Approximately 25% of patients with gastrinomas have MEN-1 and, conversely, 50% of patients with MEN-1 have gastrinomas [30,31]. Ninety percent of gastrinomas are found in a specific anatomic area, designated the "gastrinoma triangle" [11,32]. A recent report has also emphasized that even remote extrapancreatic gastrinomas have an unexplained right-sided preponderance, with nine of 11 ovarian and renal gastrinomas being located to the right of the superior mesenteric artery [33]. There appears to be a significant difference

Abbreviations

MEN-1—multiple endocrine neoplasia type 1; **ZES**—Zollinger-Ellison syndrome.

 ISBN 1-85922-671-X ISSN 1065–6243

in the biologic behavior of gastrinomas located to the right and left of the superior mesenteric artery [34••].

Neither size nor histologic appearance accurately reflect the biologic behavior of gastrinomas [3]. Malignancy was assumed when gastrinomas were found in metastatic sites, such as a lymph node or the liver, and initially it was reported that either lymph node [35–37] or liver [16,38–41] metastases resulted in a decreased survival. However, Stabile and Passaro [42] called attention to the fact that lymph node metastases in the absence of hepatic involvement were not associated with a poor outcome. They further reported that liver metastases developed in only one of 15 patients with lymph node involvement, and this occurred late in the course of a disease spanning 26 years. They concluded that two distinct groups of patients with gastrinomas exist: those with "clinically benign disease" and those whose disease is "clinically malignant." These two groups cannot be differentiated by histologic criteria, they reported, but rather only by the distribution of gastrinoma within the abdomen. Their findings have since been confirmed by another study in which only one of 11 patients with lymph node involvement developed liver metastases after a mean follow-up of 10 years [19]. Others have reported similar findings [43,44].

The presence of hepatic metastases generally indicates the poorest prognosis. with mean survivals of only 1 to 5 years [4,10,38,41]. An occasional patient, however, will survive for 10 or even 20 years with intrahepatic metastatic gastrinoma [37–39,45,46], and prolonged eugastrinemia has been reported following resection of hepatic metastases [47–49].

Gastric surgery

Surgical exploration should be the initial treatment of choice in patients with the ZES because resection remains the only chance for cure [7•]. Because of the success of medical therapy [50–58,59•–61•], total gastrectomy is now rarely indicated [2] and is recommended only for those patients whose medical therapy has failed, who are noncompliant, or who do not have access to routine medical therapy and follow-up [3,4,6,12,15,30,39,45,62,63]. Medical therapy and total gastrectomy are comparable in the control of acid peptic ulceration in patients with the ZES but side effects of lifelong medical therapy and the requirement of long-term patient compliance must nevertheless be weighed against the proven efficacy and safety of total gastrectomy [30]. Proximal gastric vagotomy combined with H_2-receptor antagonists was at one time proposed as an alternative to either total gastrectomy or medical therapy alone for the treatment of patients with unresectable gastrinomas or those in whom no tumor was found at laparotomy [64–66]. While medication dosage requirements are decreased by vagotomy, the need for lifelong compliance and follow-up remain. Furthermore, it is still unknown whether vagotomy results in a permanent or even a long-term reduction in medication dosage. Some authors have stated that there is no indication for parietal cell vagotomy in the treatment of the ZES [8•] and others have recommended against its routine use [6].

Exploratory laparotomy

Operative technique

The operative technique for exploration of patients with the ZES has been described in detail [13,46,62]. It should be carried out through a midline incision and must include a thorough examination of the entire abdominal cavity for suspicious nodules in the pancreas, duodenum, liver, lesser omentum, greater omentum, small bowel mesentery, small intestine, stomach, and pelvis (including the ovaries). All suspicious lymph nodes and nodules must be removed for histologic examination.

The search for nodules and abnormal lymph nodes should be particularly exhaustive in the area of the gastrinoma triangle [3,67,68]. The lesser sac should be opened by widely dividing the gastrocolic ligament. The entire pancreas must then be completely mobilized by an extended Kocher maneuver and incision of the peritoneum along the inferior margin of the pancreas. Only then can the entire gland be carefully inspected and bimanually palpated. The splenic hilum must also be carefully inspected.

The techniques of duodenal transillumination [69], duodenotomy with meticulous bimanual palpation [5,19,70], intraoperative ultrasonography [71,72], secretin stimulation with rapid gastrin radioimmunoassay [73], and selective intra-arterial methylene blue injection [74•] should be used at this point to ensure identification and complete removal of all gastrinomas. With experience, careful attention to detail, and liberal utilization of all available intraoperative localization techniques, a gastrinoma was found in 95% of the last 37 patients explored at the National Institutes of Health [75•].

Occasionally, exploration reveals only a gastrinoma that appears confined to a lymph node. This raises the question of whether the neoplasm represents a primary lymph node gastrinoma or simply a metastatic lesion from an occult primary lesion (Fig. 1) [76]. Several authors have reported groups of patients in whom extirpation of such nodal gastrinomas resulted in eugastrinemia and cure [17,18,22,32,77–79]. These reports support the notion that isolated lymph node gastrinomas may represent primary lesions. In most of these cases, however, a total gastrectomy was performed, and it is possible that occult duodenal gastrinomas, which may be no larger than 2 to 3 mm in size or even microscopic (Fig. 2) were serendipitously removed as part of the gastrectomy specimens [5]. When the only finding at exploration is lymph node involvement with no evidence of hepatic metastases, the search for a primary tumor should be directed to the duodenum. The duodenum should not only be completely mobilized (Kocher maneuver) for meticulous palpation, but also opened via a generous pyloroduodenotomy so that careful bimanual palpation and a more complete search for possible submucosal lesions may be conducted [9••,19,62,70,80••]. Duodenal wall lesions should then be excised with a full thickness margin of normal duodenum.

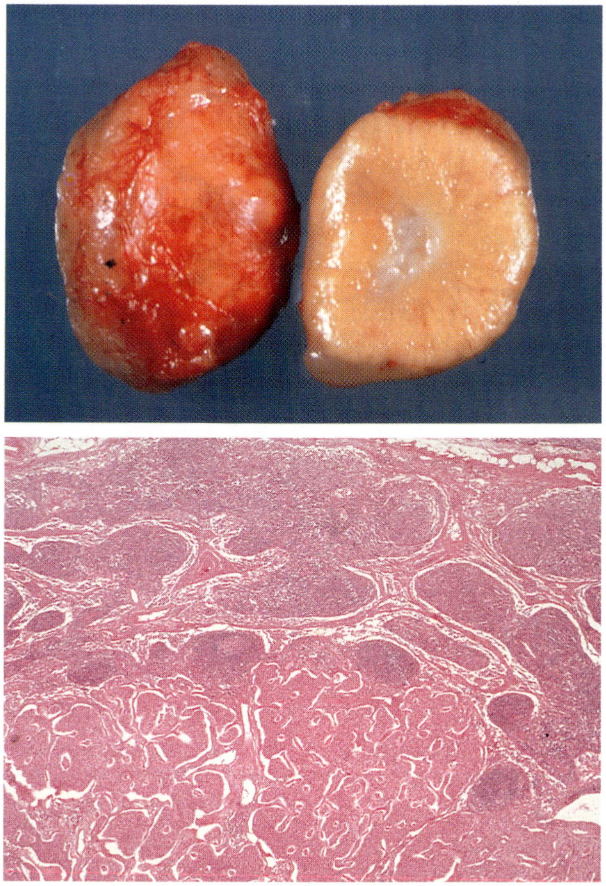

Fig. 1. Gross (*top panel*) and microscopic (*bottom panel*) appearance of a lymph node with gastrinoma. This was the only finding at laparotomy in a patient with the Zollinger-Ellison syndrome. (*From* Delcore *et al.* [19]; with permission.)

Results

In as many as 50% of patients with the ZES who do not have metastases, no gross tumor is found at exploration [65,81–83]. Failure to find tumor at operation or in the resected specimen may mean that the duodenum was not thoroughly examined. A recent report points out that occult gastrinomas are most often duodenal microgastrinomas [70] and these lesions are often missed not only by the surgeon despite a careful search but also by the pathologist (Fig. 3) [5]. Thus, it now appears that duodenal gastrinomas are more than likely the site of occult primaries in most, if not all, patients with isolated lymph node gastrinomas as well as in patients in whom the tumor is not found at operation. This may explain the excellent prognosis previously reported for patients with the ZES in whom no tumor was found at laparotomy [3,37,40,84]. Similarly, it is now recognized that serendipitous excision of occult duodenal microgastrinomas provides the most plausible explanation for the apparent "regressions" and eugastrinemia formerly believed to represent disappearance of retained primary or metastatic gastrinomas after total gastrectomy [85].

Pancreatoduodenectomy

Duodenal gastrinomas were originally considered to be a rare cause of the ZES and represented only 13% of all gastrinomas in a tumor registry review of 800 cases [86]. Duodenal gastrinomas are now recognized with increased frequency and account for 33% to 38% of gastrinomas [11,45,87,88]. Early on, duodenal gastrinomas were thought to be a more benign and more often curable cause of the ZES [3,86,89••]. A prospective study of 73 patients over a 10-year period recently demonstrated that duodenal gastrinomas have a significantly greater incidence of metastases (55% vs 22%) than pancreatic gastrinomas and a significantly shorter disease-free interval (12 vs 84 mo) following resection, "suggesting that duodenal gastrinomas may be more malignant and not more frequently curable than pancreatic gastrinomas" [9••]. The increased ability to locate and simply excise or enucleate more duodenal gastrinomas in this prospective study did not improve the observed short disease-free interval and may indicate that some occult duodenal gastrinomas were still overlooked. This possibility, coupled with the higher incidence of metastatic disease found in these patients, suggests that perhaps a more radical resection such as pancreatoduodenectomy, which includes areas of lymphatic drainage as well as surrounding tissues, should be carefully considered in the treatment of some patients with duodenal gastrinomas [90••].

Pancreatoduodenectomy was recommended for the treatment of duodenal gastrinomas as early as 1960 [91]. It failed to gain widespread acceptance because of the high morbidity and mortality rates associated with the operation, the apparent rarity of duodenal gastrinomas, and the initial low curative potential of gastrinoma resection in patients with the ZES. Even now, many authors consider this operation as too radical and dangerous and therefore advise against its use [4,6,9••,46,65,92]. Nevertheless, 19 patients treated by pancreatoduodenectomy for duodenal gastrinomas have been reported in the literature since 1960 [90••]. These patients were all biochemically "cured," with normal serum gastrin concentrations and negative secretin stimulation tests at 1 month to 11 years following resection [14,73,81,87,93–97]. Only one operative death, that of a patient who underwent operation in 1959, occurred in these 19 reported cases [98]. In the 1950s and 1960s, operative mortality of pancreatoduodenectomy was as high as 40% [99]. This high risk, which remained at 20% or greater throughout the 1970s [99], prevented more widespread application of this operation for the treatment of duodenal gastrinomas. A marked decline in the morbidity and mortality of pancreatoduodenectomy has occurred in the last decade, however, and operative mortality rates of 2% or less are now consistently reported from specialized centers [100–102].

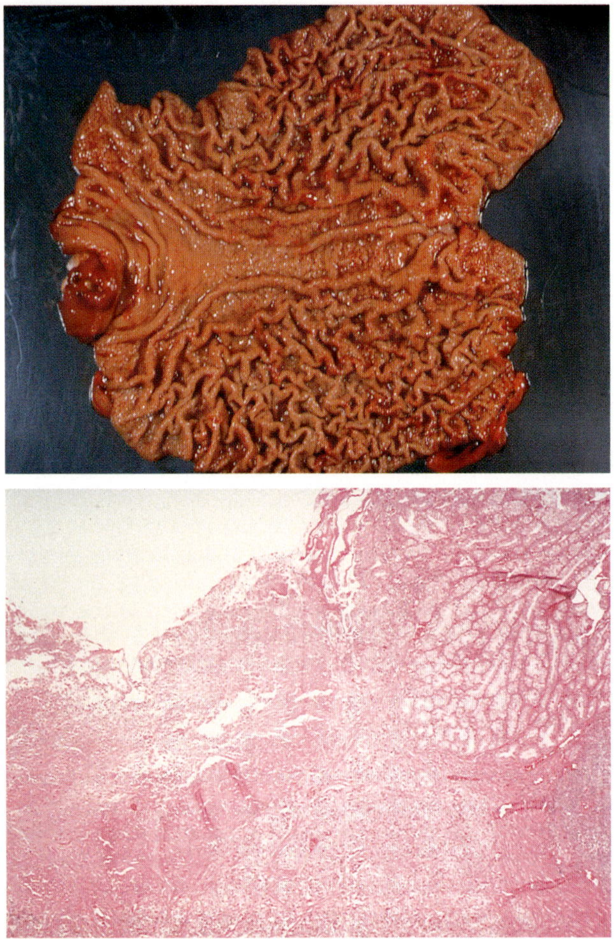

Fig. 2. Top, Total gastrectomy specimen with proximal duodenal ulcer from a patient with the Zollinger-Ellison syndrome in whom no tumor was identified at laparotomy. **Bottom**, Microscopic appearance of the ulcer shown in *top panel* demonstrates the base of the ulcer, duodenal Brunner's glands, and an occult submucosal duodenal gastrinoma.

Pancreatoduodenectomy should be considered indicated for the treatment of patients with invasive duodenal gastrinomas or with multiple pancreatoduodenal lymph node metastases from duodenal primaries that cannot be completely resected by lesser procedures. Pancreatoduodenectomy also provides a safe alternative to the need for numerous excisions of lymph node metastases and multiple submucosal duodenal lesions, some of which may otherwise be easily overlooked and lead to decreased cure rates and early recurrences. Curative pancreatoduodenectomy has also been performed with excellent long-term results in patients with otherwise unresectable gastrinomas located in the head of the pancreas [7•,73,93,103]. "Blind" pancreatoduodenectomy has recently been advocated for the treatment of patients with preoperative localization studies that unequivocally identify the pancreatoduodenal area as the source of the hypergastrinemia [14,73,81,95,96]. Although experience with blind pancreatoduodenectomy remains extremely limited, continued advances in preoperative localization and the present safety of pancreatoduodenectomy in experienced hands suggest that this operation may merit careful prospective evaluation in selected patients with the ZES. Pancreatoduodenectomy should no longer be considered contraindicated in the treatment of gastrinomas if a lesser procedure proves inadequate to accomplish a curative resection [7,90••].

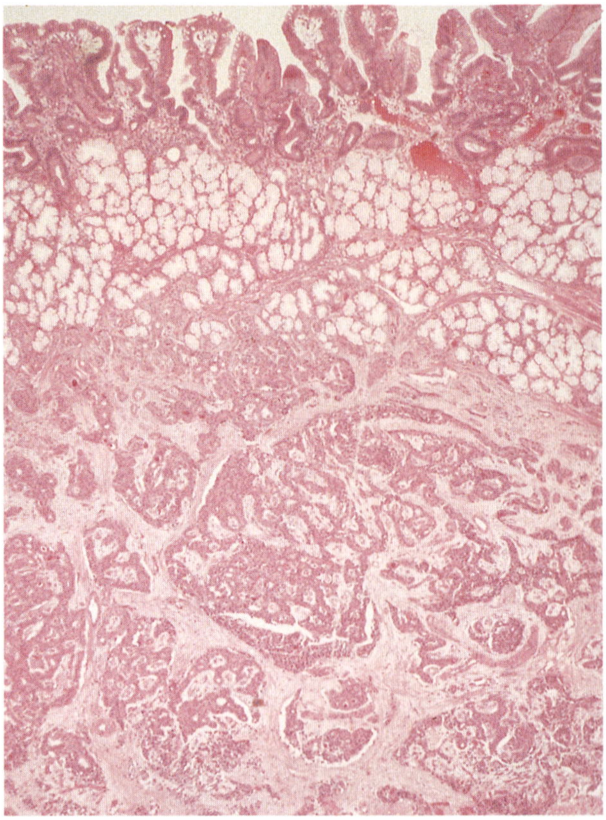

Fig. 3. Microscopic appearance of an occult submucosal duodenal microgastrinoma. This was found only after complete microscopic examination of the entire resected gastrectomy specimen in a patient in whom no tumor had been identified at laparotomy or during routine histologic examination.

Surgery in patients with familial gastrinomas and the multiple endocrine neoplasia type 1 syndrome

The role of surgery in the treatment of the ZES is perhaps most controversial in patients with the MEN-1 syndrome [8•,12,84]. These patients have multiple gastrinomas not only in the pancreas [104] but also at extrapancreatic sites [31]. This multicentricity has lead to low cure rates following resection, prompting some authors to recommend against routine surgical exploration in these patients [15,40,41,105]. Early reports also suggested that gastrinomas in patients with the MEN-1 syndrome were less malignant, less likely to metastasize, and thus had a better prognosis [16,38,40,105]. Others, however, failed to demonstrate a survival advantage for patients with MEN-1 [7•,37,42] and it is now recognized that these patients develop metastases as frequently as patients without the MEN-1 syndrome [45,106,107••].

Treatment of familial gastrinomas in patients with MEN-1 should therefore be directed at the malignant potential of the neoplasm just as in patients with the sporadic form of the syndrome. For this reason, several authors now recommend exploration and curative resection for patients with MEN-1 in whom preoperative studies directly image [3,106] or specifically localize [84,107••,108] gastrinomas.

In spite of the good results obtained by these and other investigators, a long-term cure by an aggressive surgical approach in the setting of MEN-1 was only recently achieved [107••], and total pancreatectomy has therefore been recommended as the only curative procedure for these patients [109]. However, it has been recently discovered [12,31] that although all patients with MEN-1 have multicentric pancreatic neuroendocrine tumors, these tumors may not all be gastrinomas. In fact, immunocytochemical examination of all resected pancreatic tumors in patients with MEN-1 has often demonstrated the absence of gastrin [31,110–113]. This suggests that the gastrinomas responsible for the ZES in patients with MEN-1 may be extrapancreatic, and recent studies have demonstrated duodenal gastrinomas to be much more common in MEN-1 patients than was previously assumed [31,87,106]. An aggressive surgical approach to patients with MEN-1 is thus justified and can result in cure even in the presence of hepatic metastases [107,114••]. The duodenum should be the first site examined for gastrinomas in patients with MEN-1 [31] and pancreatoduodenectomy may become necessary for curative resection of multiple lesions in these patients [108].

Surgery in patients with metastatic gastrinomas

Curative resection for gastrinomas was previously considered possible in only 20% of patients with the ZES [115] and early studies reported curative resection in only 5% of patients [3,39]. It is now estimated that gastrinomas should be curable in up to 42% of cases [78]; several selected series have achieved 30% to 40% cure rates [30], and a cure rate of 82% was recently reported [11]. In addition, it is now known that lymph node metastases do not preclude curative resection [19,42]. When simple excision or enucleation of the gastrinoma is not possible, more extensive resection should be performed to adequately excise large invasive tumors, tumors with multiple lymph nodes metastases, or multiple tumors [39,73]. In cases where curative resection is not feasible, removal of as much resectable tumor as possible (debulking) is indicated to prolong survival [39,48] and facilitate control of acid hypersecretion.

In general, orthotopic liver transplantation for metastatic neoplasms to the liver has been associated with poor results, but it has been suggested that this modality may have a place in the treatment of neoplasms with unusually indolent clinical courses such as pancreatic islet cell tumors [116]. A few patients with hepatic metastases have undergone successful orthotopic liver transplantation following complete resection of the primary gastrinoma [117–119]. Orthotopic liver transplantation may thus broaden the Halsteadian principle of radical resection of tumor and, in the future, may become a potential therapeutic approach for occasional, highly selected cases with otherwise unresectable hepatic metastases arising from gastrinomas [117]. At present, however, this therapeutic modality must be regarded as still experimental.

Conclusions

The treatment of patients with the ZES has undergone a dramatic evolution since the syndrome was originally described [1]. It is now recognized that an aggressive surgical approach is mandatory because of the malignant potential of gastrinomas. Although they were initially regarded as an incurable neoplasms, it is now known that complete surgical resection of gastrinomas results in eugastrinemia with 90% to 100% 10-year survival rates [92]. Even when lymph node metastases are present, aggressive and complete surgical resection results in eugastrinemia with 85% 10- and 20-year survivals [19]. In comparison, patients with unresectable or incompletely resected gastrinomas have 5- and 10-year survival rates of 43% and 25% respectively [92], emphasizing the importance of aggressive surgical resection in all patients with the ZES.

References and recommended reading

Papers of particular interest, published within the annual period of review, have been highlighted as:

- • Of special interest
- •• Of outstanding interest

1. Zollinger RM, Ellison EH: **Primary Peptic Ulcerations of the Jejunum Associated With Islet Cell Tumors of the Pancreas.** *Ann Surg* 1955, **142**:709–728.

2. McCarthy DM: **The Place of Surgery in the Zollinger-Ellison Syndrome.** *N Engl J Med* 1980, **302**:1344–1347.

3. Wolfe MM, Jensen RT: **Zollinger-Ellison Syndrome: Current Concepts in Diagnosis and Management.** *N Engl J Med* 1987, **317**:1200–1209.

4. Bonfils S, Landor JH, Mignon M, Hervoir P: **Results of Surgical Management in 92 Consecutive Patients With Zollinger-Ellison Syndrome.** *Ann Surg* 1981, **194**:692–697.

5. Delcore R, Hermreck AS, Friesen SR: **Selective Surgical Management of Correctable Hypergastrinemia.** *Surgery* 1989, **106**:1094–1102.

6. Berg CL, Wolfe MM: **Zollinger-Ellison Syndrome.** *Med Clin North Am* 1991, **75**:903–921.

7. • Farley DR, van Heerden JA, Grant CS, Miller LJ, Ilstrup DM: **The Zollinger-Ellison Syndrome: A Collective Surgical Experience.** *Ann Surg* 1992, **215**:561–570.

Study of 90 surgically treated patients with the ZES. Demonstrates that exploratory laparotomy provides the only chance for cure and identifies the significant prognostic factors associated with long-term patient survival.

8. • Jaffe BM: **Current Issues in the Management of Zollinger-Ellison Syndrome.** *Surgery* 1992, **111**:241–243.

Timely and complete review of current controversial issues in the management of the ZES.

9. NORTON JA, DOPPMAN JL, JENSEN RT: **Curative Resection in Zollinger-Ellison Syndrome: Results of a 10-Year Prospective Study.** *Ann Surg* 1992, **215**:8–18.
•• This prospective study of 73 patients suggests that all patients with localized sporadic ZES can have the gastric acid hypersecretion managed medically. Overall survival of these patients is excellent: most (78%) can have all gastrinoma found and resected, and some (30%) will be cured.

10. FRIESEN SR: **Treatment of the Zollinger-Ellison Syndrome: A 25-Year Assessment.** *Am J Surg* 1982, **143**:331–338.

11. HOWARD TJ, ZINNER MJ, STABILE BE, PASSARO E: **Gastrinoma Excision for Cure: A Prospective Analysis.** *Ann Surg* 1990, **211**:9–14.

12. NORTON JA, JENSEN RT: **Unresolved Surgical Issues in the Management of Patients With Zollinger-Ellison Syndrome.** *World J Surg* 1991, **15**:151–159.

13. NORTON JA, DOPPMAN JL, COLLEN MJ, HARMON MN, MATON PN, GARDNER JD, JENSEN RT: **Prospective Study of Gastrinoma Localization and Resection in Patients With Zollinger-Ellison Syndrome.** *Ann Surg* 1986, **204**:468–479.

14. VOGEL SB, WOLFE MM, MCGUIGAN JE, HAWKINS IF JR, HOWARD RJ, WOODWARD ER: **Localization and Resection of Gastrinomas in Zollinger-Ellison Syndrome.** *Ann Surg* 1987, **205**:550–556.

15. WISE SR, JOHNSTON J, SPARKS J, CAREY LC, ELLISON EC: **Gastrinoma: The Predictive Value of Preoperative Localization.** *Surgery* 1989, **106**:1087–1093.

16. THOMPSON JC, LEWIS BG, WIENER I, TOWNSEND CM: **The Role of Surgery in the Zollinger-Ellison Syndrome.** *Ann Surg* 1983, **197**:594–607.

17. WOLFE MM, ALEXANDER RW, MCGUIGAN JE: **Extrapancreatic, Extraintestinal Gastrinoma: Effective Treatment by Surgery.** *N Engl J Med* 1982, **306**:1533–1536.

18. BHAGAVAN BS, SLAVIN RE, GOLDBERG J, RAO RN: **Ectopic Gastrinoma and Zollinger-Ellison Syndrome.** *Hum Pathol* 1986, **17**:584–592.

19. DELCORE R, CHEUNG LY, FRIESEN SR: **Outcome of Lymph Node Involvement in Patients With the Zollinger-Ellison Syndrome.** *Ann Surg* 1988, **208**:291–298.

20. MACGILLIVRAY DC, RUSHIN JM, ZEIGER MA, SHAKIR KMM: **The Significance of Gastrinomas Found in Peripancreatic Lymph Nodes.** *Surgery* 199, 558–562.

21. ANTONIOLI DA, DAYAL Y, DVORAK AM, BANKS PA: **Zollinger-Ellison Syndrome: Cure by Surgical Resection of a Jejunal Gastrinoma Containing Growth Hormone Releasing Factor.** *Gastroenterology* 1987, **92**:814–823.

22. THOMPSON NW, VINIK AI, ECKHAUSER FE, STRODEL WE: **Extrapancreatic Gastrinomas.** *Surgery* 1985, **98**:1113–1119.

23. COCCO AE, CONWAY SJ: **Zollinger-Ellison Syndrome Associated With Ovarian Mucinous Cystadenocarcinoma.** *N Engl J Med* 1975, **293**:485–486.

24. LONG TT, BARTON TK, DRAFFIN R, REEVES WJ, MCCARTY KS JR: **Conservative Management of the Zollinger-Ellison Syndrome: Ectopic Gastrin Production by an Ovarian Cystadenoma.** *JAMA* 1980, **243**:1837–1839.

25. BOLLEN ECM, LAMERS CBHW, JANSEN JBMJ, LARSSON LI, JOOSTEN HJM: **Zollinger-Ellison Syndrome Due to a Gastrin-Producing Ovarian Cystadenocarcinoma.** *Br J Surg* 1981, **68**:776–777.

26. NORD KS, JOSHI V, HANNA M, KHADEMI M, SAAD S, MARQUIS J, PELZMAN H, VERNER E: **Zollinger-Ellison Syndrome Associated With a Renal Gastrinoma in a Child.** *J Pediatr Gastroenterol Nutr* 1986, **5**:980–986.

27. GOLETTI O, CHIARUGI M, BUCCIANTI P, TORTORA A, CASTAGNA M, DEL GUERRA P, VIACAVA P, CAVINA E : **Resection of Liver Gastrinoma Leading to Persistent Eugastrinemia: Case Report.** *Eur J Surg* 1992, **158**:55–57.
• In a 30-year-old man with the ZES, the only detectable gastrinoma was in the right lobe of the liver. Right hepatic lobectomy, without additional gastric surgery, resulted in eugastrinemia confirmed by 5 years' follow-up.

28. LARRIVA-SAHD J, ANGELES-ANGELES A, HERNANDEZ-PANDO R, FERNANDEZ LM, RONDAN A, ESTEVEZ O: **Ultrastructural and Immunocytochemical Study of a Primary Gastrinoma of the Liver.** *Ultrastruct Path* 1992, **16**:667–672.
• A primary hepatic gastrinoma found in a 13-year-old boy was studied by light microscopy, immunohistochemistry, electron microscopy, and immunoelectron microscopy. The patient, who had the ZES, was treated by surgical resection of the tumor and remained eugastrinemic after 24 months.

29. KAHN H, WAXMAN J: **Peripancreatic Lymph Node Gastrinoma in a Patient With Zollinger-Ellison Syndrome.** *Mt Sinai J Med* 1992, **59**:425–428.
• Case report of a patient with the ZES caused by a primary peripancreatic lymph node gastrinoma.

30. ANDERSEN DK: **Current Diagnosis and Management of Zollinger-Ellison Syndrome.** *Ann Surg* 1989, **210**:685–703.

31. PIPELEERS-MARICHAL M, SOMERS G, WILLEMS G, FOULIS A, IMRIE C, BISHOP AE, POLAK JM, HAICKI WH, STAMM B, HEITZ PU, KLOPPEL G: **Gastrinomas in the Duodenums of Patients With Multiple Endocrine Neoplasia Type 1 and the Zollinger-Ellison Syndrome.** *N Engl J Med* 1990, **322**:723–727.

32. STABILE BE, MORROW DJ, PASSARO E JR.: **The Gastrinoma Triangle: Operative Implications.** *Am J Surg* 1984, **147**:25–31.

33. SAWICKI MP, HOWARD TJ, DALTON M, STABILE BE, PASSARO E JR: **The Dichotomous Distribution of Gastrinomas.** *Arch Surg* 1990, **125**:1584–1587.

34. HOWARD TJ, SAWICKI MP, STABILE BE, WATT PC, PASSARO E JR: **Biologic Behavior of Sporadic Gastrinoma Located to the Right and Left of the Superior Mesenteric Artery.** *Am J Surg* 1993, **165**:101–106.
•• The findings of this study suggest two distinct populations of sporadic gastrinomas, one to the right (gastrinoma triangle) and the other to the left (outside triangle) of the superior mesenteric artery, which appear to have different biologic behaviors. These differences may reflect divergent etiologies for these two groups of tumors.

35. DEVENEY CW, DEVENEY KE: **Zollinger-Ellison Syndrome (Gastrinoma): Current Diagnosis and Treatment.** *Surg Clin North Am* 1987, **67**:411–422.

36. BRENNAN MF, JENSEN RT, WESLEY RA, DOPPMAN JL, MCCARTHY DM: **The Role of Surgery in Patients With Zollinger-Ellison Syndrome (ZES) Managed Medically.** *Ann Surg* 1982, **196**:239–245.

37. ELLISON EC, CAREY LC, SPARKS J, O'DORISIO TM, MEKHJIAN HS, FROMKES JJ, CALDWELL JH, THOMAS FB: **Early Surgical Treatment of Gastrinoma.** *Am J Med* 1987, **82(suppl 5B)**:17–24.

38. ZOLLINGER RM: **Gastrinoma: Factors Influencing Prognosis.** *Surgery* 1985, **97**:49–54.

39. ZOLLINGER RM, ELLISON EC, FABRI PJ, JOHNSON J, SPARKS J, CAREY LC: **Primary Peptic Ulcerations of the Jejunum Associated With Islet Cell Tumors: Twenty-five Year Appraisal.** *Ann Surg* 1980, **192**:422–430.

40. MALAGELADA J-R, EDIS AJ, ADSON MA, VAN HEERDEN JA, GO VLW: **Medical and Surgical Options in the Management of Patients With Gastrinoma.** *Gastroenterology* 1983, **84**:1524–1532.

41. MIGNON M, RUSZNIEWSKI P, HAFFAR S, RIGAUD D, RENE E, BONFILS S: **Current Approach to the Management of Tumoral Process in Patients With Gastrinoma.** *World J Surg* 1986, **10**:703–710.

42. STABILE BE, PASSARO E JR.: **Benign and Malignant Gastrinoma.** *Am J Surg* 1985, **149**:144–150.

43. LANDOR JH: **Control of the Zollinger-Ellison Syndrome by Excision of Primary and Metastatic Tumor.** *Am J Surg* 1984, **147**:406–409.

44. BORNMAN PC, MARKS IN, MEE AS, PRICE S: **Favourable Response to Conservative Surgery for Extrapancreatic Gastrinoma With Lymph Node Metastases.** *Br J Surg* 1987, **74**:198–201.

45. KAPLAN EL, HORVATH K, UDEKWU A, STRAUSS F II, SCHARK C, FERGUSON DJ, SKINNER DB: **Gastrinomas: A 42-Year Experience.** *World J Surg* 1990, **14**:365–376.

46. TOWNSEND CM, THOMPSON JC: **Gastrinoma.** *Semin Surg Oncol* 1990, **6**:91–97.

47. THOMPSON JC, REEDER DD, VILLAR HV, FENDER HR: **Natural History and Experience With Diagnosis and Treatment of the Zollinger-Ellison Syndrome.** *Surg Gynecol Obstet* 1975, **140**:721–739.

48. NORTON JA, SUGARBAKER PH, DOPPMAN, JL, WESLEY RA, MATON PN, GARDNER JD, JENSEN RT: **Aggressive Resection of Metastatic Disease in Selected Patients With Malignant Gastrinoma.** *Ann Surg* 1986, **203**:352–359.

49. WILSON SD, HERMRECK AS, FRIESEN SR: **Metastatic Duodenal Gastrinomas: Cure by Minimal and Maximal Operations.** *Postgrad Gen Surg* 1992, **4**:217–221.

50. MCCARTHY DM: **Report on the United States Experience With Cimetidine in Zollinger-Ellison Syndrome and Other Hypersecretory States.** *Gastroenterology* 1978, **74**:453–458.

51. BONFILS S, MIGNON M, GRATTON J: **Cimetidine Treatment of Acute and Chronic Zollinger-Ellison Syndrome.** *World J Surg* 1979, **3**:597–604.

52. COLLEN MJ, HOWARD JM, MCARTHUR KE, RAUFMAN JP, CIARLEGLIO CA, GARDER JD, JENSEN RT: **Comparison of Ranitidine and Cimetidine in the Treatment of Gastric Hypersecretion.** *Ann Intern Med* 1984, **100**:52–58.

53. HOWARD JM, CHREMOS AN, COLLEN MJ, MCARTHUR KE, CHERNER JA, MATON PN, CIARLEGLIO CA, CORNELIUS MJ, GARDNER JD, JENSEN RT: **Famotidine, A New Potent, Long-Acting Histamine H_2 Receptor Antagonist: Comparison With Cimetidine and Ranitidine in**

the Treatment of Zollinger-Ellison Syndrome. *Gastroenterology* 1985, **88**:1026–1033.

54. Vinayek R, Howard, JM, Maton PN, Wank SA, Slaff JI, Gardner JD, Jensen RT: **Famotidine in the Therapy of Gastric Hypersecretory States.** *Am J Med* 1986, **81**(suppl 4b):49–59.

55. Lamers CB, Lind T, Moberg S, Jansen JBMJ, Olbe L: **Omeprazole in Zollinger-Ellison Syndrome: Effects of a Single Dose and of Long-Term Treatment in Patients Resistant to Histamine H_2-Receptor Antagonists.** *N Engl J Med* 1984, **310**:758–761.

56. McArthur KE, Collen MJ, Maton PN, Cherner JA, Howard JM, Ciarleglio CA, Cornelius MJ, Jensen RT, Gardner JD: **Omeprazole: Effective, Convenient Therapy for Zollinger-Ellison Syndrome.** *Gastroenterology* 1985, **88**:939–944.

57. Maton PN, Vinayek R, Frucht H, McArthur KA, Miller LS, Saeed ZA, Gardner JD, Jensen RT: **Long Term Efficacy and Safety of Omeprazole in Patients With Zollinger-Ellison Syndrome: A Prospective Study.** *Gastroenterology* 1989, **97**:827–836.

58. Frucht H, Maton P, Jensen RT: **The Use of Omeprazole in Patients With Zollinger-Ellison Syndrome.** *Dig Dis Sci* 1991, **36**:394–404.

59. Mozell EJ, Cramer JA, O'Dorisio TM, Woltering EA: **Long-Term**
• **Efficacy of Octreotide in the Treatment of Zollinger-Ellison Syndrome.** *Arch Surg* 1992, **127**:1019–1026.

Octreotide acetate provides efficacious long-term suppression of elevated gastrin levels and excellent symptomatic relief in patients with the ZES.

60. Metz DC, Pisegna JR, Ringham GL, Feigenbaum K, Koviack PD,
• Maton PN, Gardner JD, Jensen RT: **Prospective Study of Efficacy and Safety of Lansoprazole in Zollinger-Ellison Syndrome.** *Dig Dis Sci* 1993, **38**:245–256.

The results demonstrate that lansoprazole is a safe and effective inhibitor of gastric acid hypersecretion in patients with the ZES.

61. Metz DC, Pisegna JR, Fishbeyn VA, Benya RV: **Currently Used Doses**
• **of Omeprazole in Zollinger-Ellison Syndrome Are too High.** *Gastroenterology* 1992, **103**:1498–1508.

While the efficacy of omeprazole increases during the first few days of administration, the authors suggest that long-term maintenance dosage requirements in patients with the ZES may be lower than dosages initially established by upward titration.

62. Howard TJ, Passaro E Jr.: **The Current Status of the Surgical and Medical Treatment of the Zollinger-Ellison Syndrome.** *Surg Annu* 1990, **22**:93–106.

63. Vellar D, Henderson M, Vellar ID, Desmond P: **The Zollinger-Ellison Syndrome: A Review of the St. Vincent's Hospital, Melbourne Experience.** *Aust N Z J Surg* 1985, **55**:455–462.

64. Richardson CT, Feldman M, McClelland RN, Dickermaan RM, Kumpuris D, Fordtran JS: **Effect of Vagotomy in Zollinger-Ellison Syndrome.** *Gastroenterology* 1979, **77**:682–686.

65. Richardson CT, Peters, MN, Feldman M, McClelland RN, Walsh JH, Cooper KA, Willeford G, Dickerman RM, Fordtran JS: **Treatment of Zollinger-Ellison Syndrome With Exploratory Laparotomy, Proximal Gastric Vagotomy, and H_2 Receptor Antagonists: A Prospective Study.** *Gastroenterology* 1985, **89**:357–367.

66. Malagelada JR: **Vagotomy in the Management of Patients With Zollinger-Ellison Syndrome: Pros and Cons.** *Gastroenterology* 1985, **89**:435–437.

67. Barton JC, Hirschowitz BI, Maton PN, Jensen RT: **Bone Metastases in Malignant Gastrinoma.** *Gastroenterology* 1986, **91**:915–925.

68. Howard TJ, Passaro E Jr: **Gastrinoma: New Medical and Surgical Approaches.** *Surg Clin North Am* 1989, **69**:667–681.

69. Frucht H, Norton JA, London JF, Vinayek R, Doppman JL, Gardner JD, Jensen RT, Maton PN: **Detection of Duodenal Gastrinomas by Operative Endoscopic Transillumination.** *Gastroenterology* 1990, **99**:1622–1627.

70. Thompson NW, Vinik AI, Eckhauser FE: **Microgastrinoma of the Duodenum: A Cause of Failed Operations for the Zollinger-Ellison Syndrome.** *Ann Surg* 1989, **209**:396–404.

71. Cromack DT, Norton JA, Sigel B, Shawker TH, Doppman JL, Maton PN, Jensen RT: **The Use of High-Resolution Intraoperative Ultrasound to Localize Gastrinomas: An Initial Report of a Prospective Study.** *World J Surg* 1987, **11**:648–653.

72. Norton JA, Cromack DT, Shawker TH, Doppman JL, Comi R, Goreden P, Maton PN, Gardner JD, Jensen RT: **Intraoperative Ultrasonographic Localization of Islet Cell Tumors: A Prospective Comparison to Palpation.** *Ann Surg* 1988, **207**:160–168.

73. Imamura M, Takahashi K, Isobe Y, Hattori H, Satomura K, Tobe T: **Curative Resection of Multiple Gastrinomas Aided by Selective Arterial Secretin Injection Test and Intraoperative Secretin Test.** *Ann Surg* 1989, **210**:710–718.

74. Ko TC, Flisak M, Prinz R: **Selective Intra-arterial Methylene Blue In-**
• **jection: A Novel Method of Localizing Gastrinoma.** *Gastroenterology* 1992, **102**:1062–1064.

Selective intra-arterial methylene blue injection can enhance intraoperative detection of small gastrinomas and may improve the rate of curative resection in the ZES. Further evaluation of this novel localizing technique is warranted.

75. Pisegna JR, Norton JA, Slimak GG, Metz DC, Maton PN, Gardner
• JD, Jensen RT: **Effects of Curative Gastrinoma Resection on Gastric Secretory Function and Antisecretory Drug Requirement in the Zollinger-Ellison Syndrome.** *Gastroenterology* 1992, **102**:767–778.

Chronic hypergastrinemia has trophic effects on the gastric mucosa, causing increased parietal cell mass. Careful monitoring of acid secretion is required after reversal of the chronic hypergastrinemia in diseases such as the ZES, because 55% of patients at 3 to 6 months and up to 67% at 4 years remain mild acid hypersecretors and require low doses of antisecretory drugs.

76. Friesen SR: **Are "Aberrant Nodal Gastrinomas" Pathogenetically Similar to "Lateral Aberrant Thyroid" Nodules?** *Surgery* 1990, **107**:236–238.

77. Wilson SD: **The Role of Surgery in Children With Zollinger-Ellison Syndrome.** *Surgery* 1982, **92**:682–692.

78. Harmon JW, Norton JA, Collin MJ, Krudy AG, Shawker TH, Doppman JL, D'Avis J, Jensen RT: **Removal of Gastrinomas for Control of Zollinger-Ellison Syndrome.** *Ann Surg* 1984, **200**:396–404.

79. Rawson AB, England MT, Gillam GG, French JN, Stammers FAR: **Zollinger-Ellison Syndrome With Diarrhea and Malabsorption: Observations on a Patient Before and After Pancreatic Islet-Cell Tumor Removal Without Resort to Gastric Surgery.** *Lancet* 1960, **2**:131–134.

80. Sugg SL, Norton JA, Fraker DL, Metz DC, Pisegna JR, Fishbeyn
•• V, Benya RV, Shawker TH, Doppman JL, Jensen RT: **A Prospective Study of Intraoperative Methods to Diagnose and Resect Duodenal Gastrinomas.** *Ann Surg* 1993, **218**:138–144.

This prospective study demonstrates that the duodenum is the most common location for gastrinoma in patients with the ZES (77%) and that duodenotomy to detect and remove duodenal gastrinomas should be routinely performed in all explorations for patients with the ZES.

81. Roche A, Raisonnier A, Gillon-Savouret MC: **Pancreatic Venous Sampling and Arteriography in Localizing Insulinomas and Gastrinomas: Procedure and Results in 55 Cases.** *Radiology* 1982, **145**:621–627.

82. Jensen RT, Gardner JD, Raufman JP, Pandol SJ, Doppman JL, Collen MJ: **Zollinger-Ellison Syndrome: Current Concepts and Management.** *Ann Intern Med* 1983, **98**:59–75.

83. Deveney CW, Deveney KE, Stark D, Moss A, Stein S, Way LW: **Resection of Gastrinomas.** *Ann Surg* 1983, **198**:546–553.

84. Vinik AI, Thompson NW: **Controversies in the Management of Zollinger-Ellison Syndrome.** *Ann Intern Med* 1986, **105**:956–959.

85. Delcore R, Friesen SR: **Zollinger-Ellison Syndrome: A New Look at Regression of Gastrinomas.** *Arch Surg* 1991, **126**:556–558.

86. Hofmann JW, Fox PS, Wilson SD: **Duodenal Wall Tumors and the Zollinger-Ellison Syndrome: Surgical Management.** *Arch Surg* 1973, **107**:334–339.

87. Delcore R, Cheung LY, Friesen SR: **Characteristics of Duodenal Wall Gastrinomas.** *Am J Surg* 1990, **160**:621–624.

88. Thom AK, Norton JA, Axiotix CA, Jensen RT: **Location, Incidence, and Malignant Potential of Duodenal Gastrinomas.** *Surgery* 1991, **110**:1086–1093.

89. Imamura M, Kanda M, Takahashi K, Shimada Y, Miyahara T, Wagata
•• T, Hashimoto M, Tobe T, Soga J: **Clinicopathological Characteristics of Duodenal Microgastrinomas.** *World J Surg* 1992, **16**:703–710.

This study demonstrates a difference in the cellular composition of duodenal and pancreatic gastrinomas, suggesting that the process of development and differentiation of gastrinoma cells is different and that there is an essential biological difference between duodenal and pancreatic gastrinomas.

90. Delcore R, Friesen SR: **The Role of Pancreatoduodenectomy in the**
•• **Management of Primary Duodenal Wall Gastrinomas in Patients With the Zollinger-Ellison Syndrome.** *Surgery* 1992, **112**:1–8.

Demonstrates that in patients with duodenal gastrinomas and the ZES, pancreatoduodenectomy should be considered the treatment of choice whenever complete tumor excision is not possible by a lesser procedure.

91. Oberhelman HA, Nelsen TS, Johnson AN, Dragstedt LR: **Ulcerogenic Tumors of the Duodenum.** *Ann Surg* 1961, **153**:214–227.

92. Vinayek R, Frucht H, Chiang HCV, Maton PN, Gardner JD, Jensen RT: **Zollinger-Ellison Syndrome: Recent Advances in the Management of the Gastrinoma.** *Gastroenterol Clin North Am* 1990, **19**:197–217.

93. Waddell WR, Coppinger WR, Loughry RW: **Pancreatoduodenectomy for Zollinger-Ellison Syndrome.** *Ann Surg* 1968, **168**:641–654.

94. Stamm B, Hedinger CE, Saremaslani P: **Duodenal and Ampullary Carcinoid Tumors: A Report of 12 Cases With Pathological Characteris-**

tics, Polypeptide Content and Relation to the MEN 1 Syndrome and von Recklinghausen's Disease (Neurofibromatosis). *Virchows Arch A Pathol Anat Histopathol* 1986, **408**:475–489.

95. Cavina E, Pagliai EF, Goletti O, Chiarugi M, Chirico A: **Pylorus Preserving Pancreatoduodenectomy for Gastrinoma: A Case Report.** *Ital J Surg Sci* 1986, **16**:291–295.

96. Rosato FE, Bonn J, Shapiro M, BarBot DJ, Furnary AM, Gardiner JA: **Selective Arterial Stimulation of Secretin in Localization of Gastrinomas.** *Surg Gynecol Obstet* 1990, **171**:196–200.

97. Oberhelman HA: **Excisional Therapy for Ulcerogenic Tumors of the Duodenum: Long Term Results.** *Arch Surg* 1972, **104**:447–453.

98. Oberhelman HA Jr, Nelsen TS: **Surgical Consideration in the Management of Ulcerogenic Tumors of the Pancreas and Duodenum.** *Am J Surg* 1964, **108**:132–141.

99. Gudjonsson B: **Cancer of the Pancreas: 50 Years of Surgery.** *Cancer* 1987, **60**:2284–2303.

100. Crist DW, Sitzmann JV, Cameron JL: **Improved Hospital Morbidity, Mortality, and Survival After the Whipple Procedure.** *Ann Surg* 1987, **206**:358–365.

101. Trede M, Schwall G, Saeger HD: **Survival After Pancreatoduodenectomy: 118 Consecutive Resections Without an Operative Mortality.** *Ann Surg* 1990, **211**:447–458.

102. Delcore R, Thomas JG, Pierce GE, Hermreck AS: **Pancreatogastrostomy: A Safe Drainage Procedure After Pancreatoduodenectomy.** *Surgery* 1990, **108**:641–647.

103. Stadil F: **Gastrinomas: Clinical Syndromes.** *Acta Oncol* 1989, **28**:379–381.

104. Thompson NW, Lloyd RV, Nishiyama RH, Vinik AI, Strodel WE, Allo MD, Eckhauser FE, Talpos G, Mervak T: **MEN-1 Pancreas: a Histological and Immuno-histochemical Study.** *World J Surg* 1984, **8**:561–574.

105. van Heerden JA, Smith SL, Miller LJ: **Management of the Zollinger-Ellison Syndrome in Patients With Multiple Endocrine Neoplasia Type I.** *Surgery* 1986, **100**:971–976.

106. Sheppard BC, Norton JA, Doppman JL, Maton PN, Gardner JD, Jensen RT: **Management of Islet Cell Tumors in Patients With Multiple Endocrine Neoplasia: A Prospective Study.** *Surgery* 1989, **106**:1108–1118.

107. •• Cherner JA, Sawyers JL: **Benefit of Resection of Metastatic Gastrinoma in Multiple Endocrine Neoplasia Type I.** *Gastroenterology* 1992, **102**:1049–1053.

By achieving a 16-month cure of gastrinoma, this case report demonstrates that an aggressive surgical approach can benefit certain patients with gastrinoma who have MEN-1 even in the presence of hepatic metastases.

108. Akerstrom G, Johansson H, Grama D: **Surgical Treatment of Endocrine Pancreatic Lesions in MEN-1.** *Acta Oncol* 1991, **30**:541–545.

109. Tisell LE, Ahlman H, Jansson S, Grimelius L: **Total Pancreatectomy in the MEN-1 Syndrome.** *Br J Surg* 1988, **75**:154–157.

110. Johnston CF, O'Hare MMT, Sloan JM, Buchanan KD: **MEN Type 1: Gastrinomas Are Extrapancreatic.** *Regul Pept* 1984, **8**:335.

111. Kloppel G, Willemer S, Stamm B, Hacki WH, Heitz PU: **Pancreatic Lesions and Hormonal Profile of Pancreatic Tumors in Multiple Endocrine Neoplasia Type 1: An Immunocytochemical Study of Nine Patients.** *Cancer* 1986, **57**:1824–1932.

112. Bordi C, De Vita O, Pilato FP, Carfagna G, D'Adda T, Missale G, Peracchia A: **Multiple Islet Cell Tumors With Predominance of Glucagon-Producing Cells and Ulcer Disease.** *Am J Clin Pathol* 1987, **88**:153–161.

113. Pilato FP, D'Adda T, Banchini E, Bordi C: **Nonrandom Expression of Polypeptide Hormones in Pancreatic Endocrine Tumors: An Immunohistochemical Study in a Case of Multiple Islet Cell Neoplasia.** *Cancer* 1988, **61**:1815–1820.

114. •• Thompson NW: **Surgical Treatment of the Endocrine Pancreas and Zollinger-Ellison Syndrome in the MEN-1 Syndrome.** *Henry Ford Hosp Med J* 1992, **40**:195–198.

This study demonstrates that duodenal gastrinomas are common in MEN-1 and can be managed successfully by appropriate operative intervention.

115. Deveney CW, Deveney KS, Way LW: **The Zollinger-Ellison Syndrome 23 Years Later.** *Ann Surg* 1978, **188**:384–393.

116. Lim SML, Pollard SG: **Liver Transplantation in Cancer: A Review.** *Ann Acad Med* 1990, **19**:275–280.

117. Makowka L, Tzakis A, Mazzaferro V, Teperman L, Demetris AJ, Iwatsuki S, Starzl TE: **Transplantation of the Liver for Metastatic Endocrine Tumors of the Intestine and Pancreas.** *Surg Gynecol Obstet* 1989, **168**:107–111.

118. Arnold JC, O'Grady JG, Bird GL, Calne RY, Williams R: **Liver Transplantation for Primary and Secondary Hepatic Apudomas.** *Br J Surg* 1989, **76**:248–249.

119. Alsina AE, Bartus S, Hull D, Rosson R, Schweizer RT: **Liver Transplant for Metastatic Neuroendocrine Tumor.** *J Clin Gastroenterol* 1990, **12**:533–537.

Romano Delcore, MD, and Stanley R. Friesen, MD, PhD, Department of Surgery, University of Kansas Medical Center, 4945 Murphy Building, 3901 Rainbow Boulevard, Kansas City, KS 66160-7309, USA.

Colorectal

Editorial overview

Richard L. Nelson, MD

University of Illinois College of Medicine, Chicago, Illinois, USA

Current Opinion in General Surgery 1994: 77–78

Cancer

In the past 18 months, a great deal of attention has been focused by the news media on colon and rectal disease because of the significant advances made in this period, particularly those related to cancer. The first general area of advance is the screening of asymptomatic individuals for colorectal cancer. In 1989, a group called the United States Preventive Services Task Force attempted as objectively as they could to assess the health advantages of screening for a number of diseases including colon and rectal cancer. They stated at that time that there was no statistical proof that screening was beneficial. There were certainly those who disagreed with that viewpoint. They could point to the rapid decline in mortality from colon and rectal cancer over the previous 15 years concomitant with the rapid rise in the incidence of the disease. However, this argument constituted only circumstantial evidence and not direct proof obtained from clinical studies or intervention trials that mortality was reduced by screening. Since that time, two major studies have been published: one relating to fiberoptic sigmoidoscopy and the other relating to fecal occult blood testing. Both showed large decreases in mortality in screened populations when compared either with individuals randomly allocated to control groups or retrospectively with those not screened in a cohort of individuals treated in a single health plan. The evidence is now compelling that colorectal cancer screening, although it is expensive and associated with some risks, can significantly diminish mortality from colorectal cancer [1,2].

The genetic events leading to the formation and spread of colon and rectal cancer have been elucidated with great rapidity over the past 3 to 4 years. Most recently, a gene has been identified on chromosome 2 that correlates with subsequent cancer risk. The major criticisms of current screening methods are that fecal occult blood testing lacks sensitivity and specificity, and sigmoidoscopy lacks sensitivity. Certainly, genetic data imply that quite specific markers of risks can now be identified before disease onset, and the genetic approach may indeed be the screening technique of the future [3].

Once a patients is diagnosed with colon cancer, a number of steps are taken in preparation for treatment, including the recommendation that the patient donate his or her own blood for surgery. This has not been shown to increase the risk of spreading cancer. In fact, there are data that imply that cancer-specific mortality is diminished by autologous blood donation. There are, of course, other major advantages to autologous blood donation, *ie*, the avoidance of allergic reaction or spread of infectious disease. These may be the only reasons to recommend autologous donation, since a well-conducted prospective randomized study has shown that when other clinical factors are controlled for, there is no survival advantage compared with homologous transfusion [4].

Following therapy, there is wide variation in the frequency of selection of tests performed to determine if cancer has recurred. Among the oldest of these tests is the carcinoembryonic antigen (CEA); the newest is the anti-CEA radio-labeled monoclonal antibody. It has recently been estimated that the laboratory costs alone of following up colorectal cancer patients in the United States exceed $1 billion per year. Yet surprisingly, none of these testing modalities was critically evaluated for its ability to diminish overall cancer mortality until very recently. CEA has just been subjected to such an evaluation and has been found wanting. No survival advantage could be attached to CEA screening [5]. No such study has been done regarding radio-labeled monoclonal antibodies, and it is therefore not possible to say if this very sensitive and apparently quite specific test will be able to pay for itself.

In the field of prevention, the National Polyp Study has recently demonstrated that polyp removal may prevent formation of some cancers. This was assumed for years to be the case, but surprisingly, it was never proven. In the field of primary prevention, the most active dietary item under discussion is aspirin, and despite at least five studies being published on this topic within the past 18 months, it is still uncertain whether aspirin itself is capable of diminishing colorectal cancer mortality or whether the diseases for which the aspirin is taken, such as rheumatoid disorders, might be associated with diminished risk of incidence. More studies

Abbreviation

CEA—carcinoembryonic antigen.

© 1994 Current Science ISBN 1-85922-671-X ISSN 1065-6243

have been published in the past 18 months on the dietary risk factors associated with adenoma than had been published in the previous 70 years. The purpose of such studies is of course related to the hope that dietary items that prevent adenoma formation might similarly prevent carcinomas.

Lastly, reports of more objective means of evaluating constipation as a risk factor for cancer were recently published. Patients found to have melanosis coli, a disorder caused by chronic herbal laxative abuse, had an increased risk of colorectal cancer when compared with those found not to have this abnormal pigmentation of the colon [6].

Inflammatory bowel disease

Regarding diagnostic techniques for inflammatory bowel disease, interest in radio-labeled white-cell scanning has been growing in the past decade. The isotope most commonly used is indium. In the past year, three studies have directly compared indium with technetium. Technetium has been shown to be the more useful isotope for identifying specific mucosal disease. A recent study has also demonstrated that intestinal inflammation can be detected with some sensitivity simply by performing a quantitative assay for the five-carbon alkane pentane in exhaled breath. Such a test may monitor effects of medical therapy and determine whether therapy should be diminished or withdrawn [7].

There is little news in the field of medical or surgical therapy for inflammatory bowel disease. Regarding etiology, there is the gradual and progressive accumulation of evidence that Crohn's disease probably has mycobacterial origin. This development has not led to any specific therapies, however.

Benign anorectal disease

The most prevalent colorectal diseases are of course the benign anorectal diseases: hemorrhoids, fissure-in-ano, and fistula in ano. Because of the very high prevalence of these disorders, their diagnosis and treatment will always be of great interest. It is astounding how little research is done regarding etiology, prevention, or appropriate choice of treatment regarding benign anorectal disease.

A great deal of research is being done in the area of pelvic floor muscular disorders: incontinence, constipation, and the varying combinations of the two. A physician now has a dizzying array of tools to choose from to evaluate a patient's ability to defecate. To the older modalities of digital examination, defecating proctography, electromyography, anorectal manometry, and motility testing has now been added endorectal ultrasonic evaluation of sphincter thickness. Studies have shown differing thickness of the internal anal sphincter in patients with various dysfunctional states when compared with eufunctional control subjects. It has also been demonstrated that external sphincter thickness diminishes and internal sphincter thickness increases with advancing age [8]. All of the tests listed are quite similar to those tests applied to postoperative colorectal cancer patients in one important way: the benefit to the patient has not been demonstrated by measuring relevant clinical outcomes.

Regarding surgical intervention for continence restoration, an old operation has been given new life through electrical pacing. That is the gracilis muscle wrap around the anal canal. What was once only a passive obstruction to defecation, the gracilis tendon, with electrical pacing of the muscle fibers can become apparently a controllable sphincter muscle. Perhaps the most important advance in this stems from a conference sponsored by the National Institutes of Health regarding urinary incontinence [9]. The study panel concluded that in spite of the apparent success of many operations in treating urinary incontinence, behavioral therapy (meaning biofeedback) should be the first choice before surgical intervention was undertaken. It seems very likely that similar recommendations will be made regarding pelvic floor dysfunction.

References

1. Mandel JS, Bond JH, Church TR, Snover DC, Bradley GM, Schuman LM, Ederer F: **Reducing Mortality From Colorectal Cancer by Screening for Fecal Occult Blood.** *New Engl J Med* 1993, **328**:1365–1371.
2. Selby JV, Friedman GD, Queensbury CP, Weiss NS: **A Case-Control Study of Screening Sigmoidoscopy and Mortality From Colorectal Cancer.** *New Engl J Med* 1992, **326**:653–657.
3. Marx J: **New Colon Cancer Gene Discovered.** *Science* 1993, **260**:751–752.
4. Hoynck van Papendrecht MAW, Marquet RL, Jeekel J: **Blood Transfusions and Prognosis in Colorectal Cancer.** *New Engl J Med* 1993, **328**:1372–1376.
5. Moertel CG, Fleming TR, MacDonald JS, Haller DG, Laurie JA, Tangen C: **An Evaluation of the Carcinoembryonic Antigen (CEA) Test for Monitoring Patients With Resected Colon Cancer.** *JAMA* 1993, **270**:943–947.
6. *Urinary Incontinence in Adults.* Washington DC: Department of Health and Human Services; 1992. [AHCPR publication no. 92-0038.]
7. Kokoszka J, Nelson RL, Swedler WI, Skosey J, Abcarian H: **Determination of Inflammatory Bowel Disease Activity by Breath Pentane Analysis.** *Dis Colon Rectum* 1993, **36**:597–601.
8. Papachrysostomou M, Pye SD, Wild SR, Smith AN: **Anal Endosonography in Asymptomatic Subjects.** *Scand J Gastroent* 1993, **28**:551–556.
9. Seigers CP, von Herzberg-Lotin E, Otte M, Schneider B: **Anthranoid Laxative Abuse: A Risk Factor for Colorectal Cancer.** *Gut* 1993, **34**:1099–1101.

Richard L. Nelson, MD, Department of Surgery, University of Illinois Hospital, 1740 West Taylor Street, Room 2204, Chicago, IL 60612-7238, USA.

Screening for colorectal cancer

Jack S. Mandel, PhD, MPH

University of Minnesota, Minneapolis, Minnesota, USA

This paper reviews studies on fecal occult blood testing and sigmoidoscopy screening for colorectal cancer. Recently published data from a randomized controlled trial provides the first concrete evidence that annual screening for fecal occult blood can reduce colorectal cancer mortality by at least 33%. These results are corroborated by a nonrandomized but controlled study that showed a 43% colorectal cancer mortality reduction with early detection through fecal occult blood testing and sigmoidoscopy, and by a case-control study that showed a 31% colorectal cancer mortality reduction associated with fecal occult blood testing. Persuasive data to support screening recommendations for sigmoidoscopy are not yet available; however, results from observational studies are suggestive and should stimulate further research to assess the benefit of sigmoidoscopy screening.

Current Opinion in General Surgery 1994:79–84

It is generally believed that most colorectal cancers develop slowly in a stepwise fashion from normal mucosa to enlarging adenomatous polyps to a localized, surgically curable malignancy to disseminated incurable disease. Early detection through screening, if effective, should interrupt this process and result in a reduction in mortality and possibly morbidity (by removing polyps) from this disease.

In 1993 there will be 152,000 new cases and 57,000 deaths from colorectal cancer [1]. The cause of the disease is unknown; thus primary prevention is not possible. At this time, secondary prevention, or screening, appears to be most promising strategy for reducing mortality.

This paper reviews the studies of fecal occult blood tests (FOBTs) and sigmoidoscopy, the two most widely recommended and used screening tests for colorectal cancers. The studies are limited to randomized controlled trials, nonrandomized but controlled prospective studies, and case-control studies.

During the past two decades, screening for colorectal cancer has increased [2]. Annual FOBTs and digital rectal examination and periodic flexible sigmoidoscopy are recommended by some organizations such as the American Cancer Society; however, the various organizations that offer screening recommendations have not agreed on a protocol for colorectal cancer screening because of the absence of definitive data showing a mortality reduction associated with screening. Recommendations have been formulated based on data from incomplete randomized trials, from descriptive studies, and from mathematical models that rely on various assumptions. The most persuasive evidence of screening effectiveness are data showing a mortality reduction from a well-designed randomized controlled clinical trial in which individuals are randomly assigned to a screen or to a control group. This method of group assignment increases the likelihood that the study groups are comparable in all factors that could influence the outcome of the trial. Demonstrating a mortality reduction rather than just an increased survival or a stage shift obviates the concerns with lead-time and length bias. Four such trials of FOBT are being conducted in Minnesota, the United States; Göteborg, Sweden; Funen, Denmark; and Nottingham, England [3,4,5••,6–14]. Results from one have recently been published [5••].

Fecal occult blood testing

Testing for occult blood was developed by Van Deen in 1864 (*reviewed in* Simon [15•]). Interest in its application as a test for home use for colorectal cancer screening was stimulated by Greegor [16] in 1967. Qualitative FOBTs using guaiac-impregnated slides are probably the most widely used screening test for colorectal cancer. Colorectal cancers bleed, and often blood is in such small quantities that it cannot be detected visually. Tests to detect occult blood in stool contain a reagent to hemoglobin. The peroxidase activity of hemoglobin acts as an oxidizing agent, which in the presence of the test reagent changes color, indicating a positive finding. The sensitivity of the test to colorectal cancers is diffi-

Abbreviation

FOBT—fecal occult blood test.

 ISBN 1-85922-671-X ISSN 1065–6243

cult to calculate precisely, but studies have shown that it could be as high as 92% [4].

Randomized controlled trials

The first trial was initiated in Minnesota in 1975. In this study, 46,551 participants aged 50 to 80 years were recruited between 1975 and 1977 and randomly assigned to annual screening, biennial screening, or a control group [5••].

Participants in the screened groups submitted six guaiac-impregnated paper slides, prepared by placing two smears from each of three consecutive stools on slides. Participants were instructed to abstain from red meat, poultry and fish, certain vegetables and fruits, and to discontinue the use of vitamin C tablets and aspirin for at least 24 hours before and during the collection of the samples. Slide processing was modified early in the trial to incorporate rehydration with a drop of deionized water to enhance test sensitivity, which was reduced because of drying. Participants with one or more positive test findings in the set of six slides underwent a colonoscopy examination (Fig. 1).

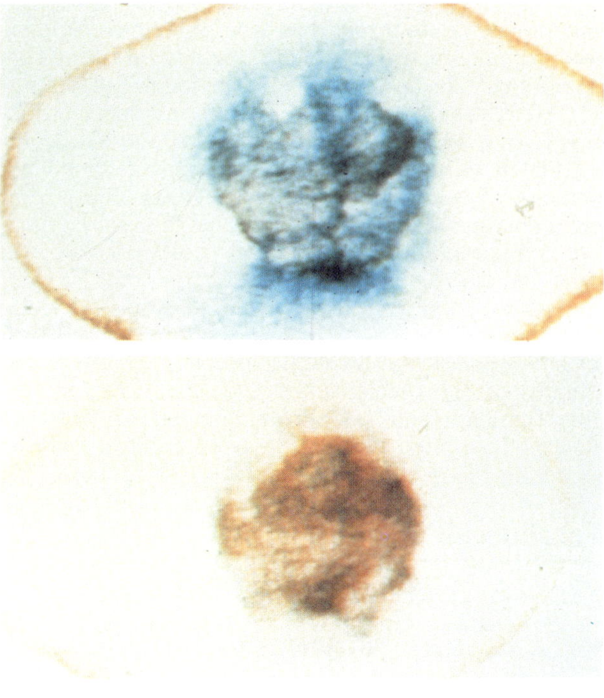

Fig. 1. Fecal occult blood screening. **Top,** Positive result. **Bottom,** Negative result.

All participants received a mailed questionnaire annually to ascertain vital status, the occurrence of colorectal cancer and polyps in the control group, and colorectal lesions discovered in members of the screened groups either as a result of a diagnostic procedure unrelated to a positive screening finding or in persons who were unwilling or unable to submit the slides. Follow-up for vital status was 100%.

In the Swedish study, the entire population of Göteborg born between 1918 and 1927 was enrolled in two phases, in 1982 and 1987 [6,7]. Participants were randomly allocated to a control group (25,670 persons) or to a screening group (26,655 persons). In the 1982 cohort, 13,759 screening group participants were screened between 1982 and 1983, with rescreening 16 to 22 months later (mean, 20 months after the first screen). The 1987 cohort of 11,896 participants was screened between 1987 and 1988; rescreening was conducted 14 to 17 months after the first screen.

Three guaiac-impregnated paper tests were mailed to participants, who collected two samples from each of three consecutive stools and mailed them back immediately after the last test. Fresh fruit and vegetables, meat, food made of blood, and vitamin C tablets were to be avoided two days before and during the testing. One half of the slides from the first screening and all the slides from the second screening were rehydrated.

Individuals with positive results from one or more tests were invited to the hospital for a work-up that included a digital rectal examination, proctoscopy, rectosigmoidoscopy (60 cm), and a double-contrast enema examination.

The study in Nottingham, which started in 1984, enrolled a population of 142,554 asymptomatic men and women, aged 50 to 74 years, living in the Nottingham area, who were randomly allocated to a control or screening group [8,9]. Study participants were identified from general practitioner records.

Participants who complied with the initial screening were rescreened every 2 years with FOBT. The initial tests were carried out without dietary restrictions. Since 1985, participants with a positive test result were asked to repeat the test over a 6-day period while excluding red meats and vegetables high in peroxidase from their diet. Those with a second positive test result were investigated by colonoscopy and, if this was incomplete, a double-contrast barium enema. Subjects with a negative second test result after dietary restrictions were asked to repeat the test, again with dietary restrictions, after 3 months.

In Funen, three fourteenths of the 139,400 residents aged 45 to 75 years were selected for screening and three fourteenths were selected as controls [10–14]. The two groups were stratified by age, and married couples were assigned to the same group. The randomized groups were similarly distributed by gender and residency even though these variables were not prestratified.

The randomized groups were generated from two files: the Central Person Register and the Patient File of the county. The latter file was used to exclude from randomization patients with known colorectal cancer, adenoma, and distant spread from all types of cancer.

Guaiac-impregnated slides were mailed to screening group participants with instructions for dietary (no red meat or fresh fruit) and medicine (no iron preparation, vitamin C, aspirin, or other nonsteroidal antirheumatics) restrictions during the 3-day testing period. Two samples were to be taken from each of three consecutive stools.

Rescreenings were at 2-year intervals. Only those participants completing the previous screening were invited for the following screening. Persons with positive FOBT slide results were examined by colonoscopy. A double-contrast barium enema was done when colonoscopy was incomplete or the person refused colonoscopy.

The salient features of these four randomized controlled trials are shown in Table 1. All the trials used an FOBT with dietary restrictions. The Minnesota and Göteborg trials used rehydrated slides, which resulted in an increase in positivity, higher sensitivity, lower specificity, and a lower positive predictive value. However, as shown in Table 2, the largest reduction in the proportion of Dukes D cancers between screening and control groups occurred in the Minnesota and Göteborg trials (48% and 38%, respectively) In the Funen and Nottingham trials, where slides were not rehydrated, the reduction in Dukes' D cancers were 5% and 10%, respectively.

The Minnesota trial is the only study to date that has demonstrated a mortality reduction (Fig. 2). Through 13 years of follow-up, there was a statistically significant 33% reduction in colorectal cancer mortality in the annual group compared with the control group [5]. The biennial group mortality reduction was 6%. A somewhat higher than expected mortality in the early years of the study, consistent with chance, contributed to the

Table 1. Summary of randomized controlled trials

	Minnesota	Göteborg	Nottingham	Funen
Date started	1975	1982	1984	1985
Participants, *n*	46,551	51,325	142,554	61,938
Age, *y*	50–80	60–64	50–74	45–74
Screening test	Hemoccult*	Hemoccult II*	Hemoccult*	Hemoccult II*
Slides rehydrated, %	83	75	0	0
Dietary restrictions	Yes	Yes	Yes†	Yes
Study groups, *n*	3	2	2	2
Frequency of screening	Annual, biennial	14–22 mo	Biennial	Biennial
Compliance with first screen, %	85	66	54	67
Rescreening compliance, %	78	60	76	93
Slides positive, %				
Rehydrated	9.8	6	—	—
Not rehydrated	2.4	2	2.1	0.9
Sensitivity for colorectal cancer, %	92‡	78	68	48
Specificity for colorectal cancer, %	90‡	96	98	99
Positive predictive value, %	2.2‡	3.3	14.7	8.2

*SmithKline Diagnostics, San Jose, CA.
†On retesting after a positive test result.
‡Rehydrated slides.

Table 2. Dukes stage of colorectal cancer for screen and control groups in fecal occult blood test randomized controlled screening trials*

	Minnesota		Göteborg		Funen		Nottingham	
Dukes stage	S	C	S	C	S	C	S	C
A	30	22	30	12	23	9	30	13
B	29	30	23	24	29	34	28	33
C	23	21	31	38	19	29	22	30
D	9	17	16	26	24	23	20	22
Unstaged	9	10	—	—	5	6	—	2

*Data are shown as percentage of patients in screened (S) and control (C) groups.

relatively small cumulative 13-year mortality reduction in the biennial group. A larger reduction may be observed with additional follow-up based on the stage distribution, which showed a 35% reduction in Dukes D cancers, and a survival rate for screen-detected cancers that is more similar to that of the annual group than of the control group [5••].

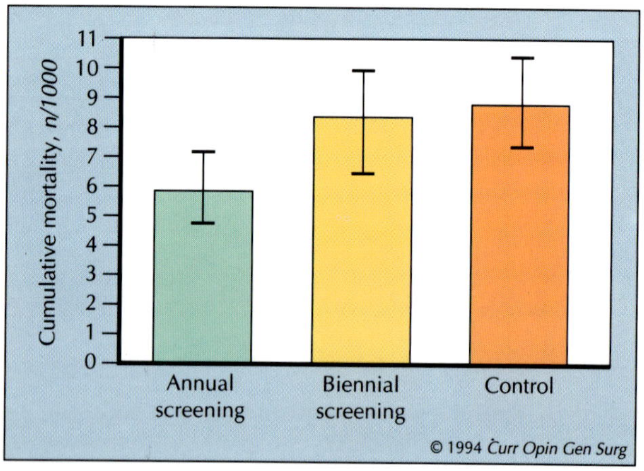

Fig. 2. Cumulative 13-year colorectal cancer mortality for participants in a randomized, controlled clinical trial demonstrating the relationship between mortality and fecal occult blood screening. *T bars* indicate SE.

Nonrandomized controlled studies

There are two prospective controlled, but nonrandomized studies of FOBT: one in the Burgundy area of France [17,18] and one in New York, the United States [19,20••]. The study in Burgundy, begun in 1988, involves 91,000 participants aged 45 to 74 years. All residents of certain towns and administrative districts of the department of Saone et Loire were invited to participate in the screening test. The control subjects are residents of areas of similar size and similar risk of colorectal cancer in the neighboring department of Côte d'Or.

The first screening with guaiac-impregnated paper slides was conducted in 1988 and 1989, the second in 1990. The third screening was scheduled to be conducted two years following the second.

Participants completed tests, using guaiac-impregnated paper slides, from three consecutive stools without adhering to any dietary restrictions. However, vitamin C and aspirin avoidance were suggested. Those with a positive screening test result have a colon examination, which is usually a colonoscopy. This study is still ongoing and results are not yet available.

The Colon Project, a controlled nonrandomized study conducted between 1975 and 1984 by the Memorial Sloan-Kettering Cancer Center in collaboration with the Preventive Medicine Institute–Strang Clinic in New York, was designed to evaluate the effectiveness of FOBT and rigid sigmoidoscopy.

From 1975 to 1979, 21,756 patients over the age of 40 years who presented at the clinic were enrolled. Those with a prior history of colon cancer or membership in group health insurance or corporate health plans were excluded.

There were two groups of patients coming to the clinic: one that responded regularly to reminders for annual check-ups and another that came for single visits, often because of specific health concerns. The former group were designated as *regulars* and the latter as *first timers.*

The regulars and first timers were separately allocated to study and control groups. Because it was decided that randomization was not feasible in the context of the operation of the clinic, allocation was based on enrollment date.

All participants underwent the standard Preventive Medicine Institute–Strang Clinic examination at enrollment, which included a 25-cm rigid proctosigmoidoscopy. Those assigned to a study group were sent three guaiac-impregnated slides and instructions for completing them before their clinic visit. They were asked to adhere to a meat-free, high-bulk diet for 1 day before and 3 three days during slide preparation. Slides were tested without hydration. Participants with a positive FOBT result were referred for double-contrast barium enema and full colonoscopy. In the screened group (first timers), there was a 43% reduction in colorectal cancer mortality, more early stage cancers, and an improved survival rate.

Case-control studies

Observational studies, such as case-control studies, provide suggestive, but inconclusive evidence of screening effectiveness. In a case-control study of FOBT screening among members of the Kaiser Permanente Medical Care Program of Northern California, potential cases were drawn from members over age 50 years who were diagnosed with colorectal adenocarcinoma between 1981 and 1987 and who subsequently died from the disease before December 1988 [21•]. One matched control was randomly selected for most cases from membership lists of the program; 96 of the cases had more than one control.

Outpatient medical records were reviewed for 10 years before the index date, which was defined as the date immediately before onset of symptoms or before the screening test that led to diagnosis. Only screening FOBTs, sigmoidoscopy, digital rectal examination, barium enema examination, and colonoscopy were analyzed.

An adjusted odds ratio (OR) of 0.69 (95% CI; range, 0.52 to 0.91) was observed for exposure to at least one screening FOBT during the 5-year interval. To address optimal screening intervals, odds ratios were calculated by number of years (0 through 5) since the most recent screening FOBT. The adjusted OR was 0.73 (95%

CI; range, 0.50 to 1.05) for the first year after the most recent screening FOBT and increased to 1.00 (95% CI; range, 0.47 to 2.11) 3 years after the last screening examination.

A population-based case-control study was conducted in Saarland, a southwestern state of Germany, to evaluate the effectiveness of colorectal cancer screening [22]. The FOBT was introduced as a component of the screening program under the statutory health insurance system in the Federal Republic of Germany in 1977 and was offered to all men and women aged 45 years or over.

Cases were histologically confirmed colorectal cancers in individuals 55 to 74 years of age who died between 1983 and 1986 and were identified by the pathology institutes serving the Saarland. Information about cause of death and screening history was obtained from physicians. Death certificates were not available because of privacy laws. Up to five age-matched controls were identified from the files of the physician of the corresponding case.

The use of screening FOBTs for cases were ascertained for the period 3 years before diagnosis for colorectal cancer and for a similar period for controls. The screening history for 429 cases (220 men, 209 women) and the control subjects (694 men and 2718 women) was obtained from gynecological and general practitioners' offices.

Six to 36 months prior to diagnosis, 13% of male cases and 14% of male control subjects had at least one asymptomatic FOBT result (OR = 0.92; 95% CI; range, 0.54 to 1.57). For the same prediagnostic period, 16% of female cases and 29% of female control subjects had at least one asymptomatic FOBT (OR = 0.43, 95% CI; range, 0.27 to 0.68). Thus, for men whose participation rates were generally low, there was no benefit, but for women, whose participation rates were higher, a benefit from screening was observed.

In a third case-control study, the medical records of 66 members of the Greater Marshfield Community Health Plan who died of large-bowel cancer from 1979 to 1988 and those of 196 members matched according to gender, age, and enrollment duration were reviewed for a history of screening for colorectal cancer [23]. Only screening tests done in the absence of symptoms were considered. FOBT screening was not associated with a lower colorectal cancer mortality (OR = 1.15; 95% CI = 0.93 to 1.44). The study was limited, however, since only 21% of the patients and 16% of the control subjects received multiple-slide evaluation of their stools. Most screening was completed on a single sample obtained during a digital rectal examination.

Screening with sigmoidoscopy

The American Cancer Society recommends screening with flexible sigmoidoscopy [24]. There are no data from randomized, controlled trials to support these recommendations, but the results of two recently published case-control studies of sigmoidoscopic screening conducted in health maintenance organizations provide some support for the recommendation.

At Kaiser Permanente Medical Care Program in Northern California, the cases studied were plan members 45 years of age or older diagnosed with adenocarcinoma of the colon or rectum between 1971 and 1987, who died of the cancer by the end of 1988 [25•]. There were 261 cases that could have been detected by rigid sigmoidoscopy (*ie*, cancers of the rectum or rectosigmoid and cancers of the sigmoid colon that were visualized by rigid sigmoidoscopy or described as within 20 cm of the anus in pathological or surgical reports) that were verified for inclusion in the primary analyses of the study. A random sample of 268 fatal cancers above 20 cm were selected from the remaining cases for separate analysis. Four matched controls per case were selected from membership lists. One control was selected for each of the 268 patients with cancer above 20 cm.

The analyses considered the 10-year period immediately before the onset of symptoms or the screening test that led to the diagnosis of fatal colorectal cancer. The same 10-year period was examined for the matched controls. A reviewer blinded to the subject's case-control status, reviewed outpatient medical records and abstracted all instances of screening tests with sigmoidoscopy, digital rectal examination, fecal occult blood testing, barium-enema examination, and colonoscopy.

Significantly fewer cases than controls had one or more screening rigid sigmoidoscopies during the 10-year period (adjusted OR = 0.41; 95% CI; range, 0.25 to 0.69). The optimum screening interval could not be determined because the small numbers of cases resulted in wide confidence intervals. Little evidence of the screening efficacy was found in the analysis of the 268 cases with cancer beyond the rigid sigmoidoscope (adjusted OR = 0.96; 95% CI; range, 0.61 to 1.50).

Newcomb *et al.* [23] conducted a study of 66 members of the Greater Marshfield Community Health Plan who died of cancer of the colon or rectum from 1979 to 1988 and for comparison, 196 plan members of the same gender, similar age, and enrollment duration.

Information was collected on dates, signs and symptoms, and results of only screening tests (FOBT, digital rectal examination, and sigmoidoscopy) done in the absence of symptoms. A total of 29.1% of control subjects had a screening sigmoidoscopy at least once compared with only 10.6% of cases. Both rigid and flexible sigmoidoscopy were used; however, a majority of the examinations were flexible sigmoidoscopies.

The risk for death from colorectal cancer was reduced among individuals having had a single screening sigmoidoscopy (OR = 0.21; 95% CI; range, 0.08 to 0.52). The reduction in cancer mortality risk appeared to be limited to cancer of the rectum and distal colon. The authors concluded that screening sigmoidoscopy can substantially reduce mortality from cancers of the rectum and distal colon.

Conclusions

Only one screening recommendation can be supported from the available literature: annual screening for fecal occult blood. The most compelling evidence comes from the Minnesota study, a randomized controlled trial, which showed a significant mortality reduction from annual screening with rehydrated tests using guaiac-impregnated slides [5••]. The other three studies with published results [20••,21•,22] support this recommendation, although slides were not rehydrated in these studies.

The literature does not support any argument for using other fecal occult blood tests including other qualitative tests, quantitative tests, or immunochemical tests. Some of the immunochemical tests show promising preliminary results, but it is premature to recommend them for mass screening [26].

Sigmoidoscopy screening has considerable appeal but insufficient evidence to recommend it for mass screening. Two observational studies [23,25•] suggest that sigmoidoscopy screening could reduce colorectal cancer mortality; however, these studies are not sufficient proof of effectiveness [27]. Further research is needed, preferably a randomized controlled trial to obtain definitive evidence of effectiveness.

References and recommended reading

Papers of particular interest, published within the annual period of review, have been highlighted as:

• Of special interest
•• Of outstanding interest

1. BORING CC, SQUIRES TS, TONG T: **Cancer Statistics, 1993**. *CA Cancer J Clin* 1993, **43**:7–26.

2. BROWN ML, POTOSKY AL, THOMPSON GB, KESSLER LG: **The Knowledge and Use of Screening Tests for Colorectal and Prostate Cancer: Data From the 1987 National Health Interview Survey**. *Prev Med* 1990, **19**:562–574.

3. GILBERTSON VA, CHURCH TR, GREIVE FJ, MANDEL, JS, MCHUGH RB, SCHUMAN LM, WILLIAMS SE: **The Design of a Study to Assess Occult Blood Screening for Colon Cancer**. *J Chronic Dis* 1980, **33**:107–114.

4. MANDEL JS, BOND JH, BRADLEY M, SNOVER DC, CHURCH TR, WILLIAMS S, WATT G, SCHUMAN LM, EDERER F, GILBERTSEN V: **Sensitivity, Specificity and Positive Predictivity of the Hemoccult® Test in Screening for Colorectal Cancers**. *Gastroenterology* 1989, **97**:597–600.

5. •• MANDEL JS, BOND JH, CHURCH TR, SNOVER DC, BRADLEY GM, SCHUMAN LM, EDERER F: **Reducing Mortality From Colorectal Cancer by Screening for Fecal Occult Blood**. *N Engl J Med* 1993, **328**:1365–1371.

This paper provides a description of the design, conduct, and analysis and presents the results of the first randomized controlled clinical trial to demonstrate a significant reduction in colorectal cancer mortality from annual screening for fecal occult blood.

6. KEWENTER J, BJÖRK S, HAGLIND E, SMITH L, SVANIK J, AHREN C: **Screening and Rescreening for Colorectal Cancer**. *Cancer* 1988, **62**:645–651.

7. KEWENTER J, ASZTELY M, ENGARAS B, HAGLUND E, SMITH L, SVANVIK J, AHERN C: **A Randomized Trial of Faecal Occult Blood Testing for Early Detection of Colorectal Cancer: Results of Screening and Rescreening of 51,325 Subjects.** In *Cancer Screening.* Edited by Miller AB, Chamberlain J, Day NE, Hakama M, Prorok PC. Cambridge: Cambridge University Press; 1991:117–125.

8. HARDCASTLE JD, FERRANDS PA, BALFOUR TW, CHAMBERLAIN J. AMAR SS, SHELDON MG: **Controlled Trial of Faecal Occult Blood Testing in the Detection of Colorectal Cancer**. *Lancet* 1983, **2**:1–4.

9. HARDCASTLE JD, THOMAS WM, CHAMBERLAIN J, *ET AL.*: **Randomised, Controlled Trial of Faecal Occult Blood Screening for Colorectal Cancer: Results for First 107,349 Subjects**. *Lancet* 1989, **1**:1160–1164.

10. KLAABORG K, MADSEN MS, SONDERGAARD O, KRONBORG O: **Participation in Mass Screening for Colorectal Cancer With Fecal Occult Blood Test**. *Scand J Gastroenterol* 1986, **21**:1180–1184.

11. KRONBORG O, FENGER C, SONDERGAARD O, PEDERSON KM, OLSEN J: **Initial Mass Screening for Colorectal Cancer With Fecal Occult Blood Test: A Prospective Randomized Study at Funen in Denmark**. *Scand J Gastroenterol* 1987, **22**:677–686.

12. KRONBORG O, FENGER C, OLSEN J, BECH K, SONDERGAARD O: **Repeated Screening for Colorectal Cancer With Fecal Occult Blood Test: A Prospective Randomized Study at Funen, Denmark**. *Scand J Gastroenterol* 1989, **24**:599–606.

13. KRONBORG O, FENGER C, WORM J, PEDERSEN SA, HEM J, BERTELSEN K, OLSEN K: **Causes of Death During the First 5 Years of a Randomized Trial of Mass Screening for Colorectal Cancer With Fecal Occult Blood Test**. *Scand J Gastroenterol* 1992, **27**:47–52.

14. JENSEN BM, KRONBORG O, FENGER C: **Interval Cancers in Screening With Fecal Occult Blood Test for Colorectal Cancer**. *Scand J Gastroenterol* 1992, **27**:779–782.

15. • SIMON JB: **Occult Blood Screening for Colorectal Carcinoma**. *Gastroenterology* 1985, **88**:820–837.

This is an excellent review paper on occult blood testing for colorectal cancer. It provides a historical overview of the development of the test and information on the test's characteristics and performance.

16. GREEGOR DH: **Diagnosis of Large-Bowel Cancer in the Asymptomatic Patient**. *JAMA* 1967, **201**:943–945.

17. FAIVRE J, ARVEAUX P, MILAN C, DURAND G, LAMOUR J, BEDENNE L: **Participation in Mass Screening for Colorectal Cancer: Results of Screening and Rescreening From the Burgundy Study**. *Eur J Cancer Prev* 1991, **1**:49–55.

18. ARVEUX P, DURAND G, MILAN C, BEDENNE L, LEVY D, DOAN BOH, FAIVRE J: **Views of a General Population on Mass Screening of Colorectal Cancer: The Burgundy Study**. *Prev Med* 1992, **21**:574–581.

19. WINAWER SJ, SCHOTTENFELD D, FLEHINGER BJ: **Colorectal Cancer Screening**. *J Natl Cancer Inst* 1991, **83**:243–253.

20. •• WINAWER SJ, FLEHINGER BJ, SCHOTTENFELD D, MILLER DG: **Screening for Colorectal Cancer With Fecal Occult Blood Testing and Sigmoidoscopy**. *J Natl Cancer Inst* 1993, **85**:1311–1318.

This prospective controlled but not randomized trial provides important information corroborating the effectiveness of occult blood testing.

21. • SELBY JV, FRIEDMAN GD, QUESENBERRY CP, WEISS NS: **Effects of Fecal Occult Blood Testing on Mortality From Colorectal Cancer: A Case-Control Study**. *Ann Intern Med* 1993, **118**:1–6.

Although this is an observational rather than experimental study, it is nevertheless a fairly well designed and conducted case-control study that presents evidence on screening effectiveness using fecal occult blood testing.

22. WAHRENDORF J, ROBRA BP, WIEBELT H, OBERHAUSEN R, WEILAND M, DHOM G: **Effectiveness of Colorectal Cancer Screening: Results From a Population-Based Case-Control Evaluation in Saarland, Germany**. *Eur J Cancer Prev* 1993, **2**:221–227.

23. NEWCOMB PA, NORFLEET RG, STORER BE, SURAWICZ TS, MARCUS PM: **Screening Sigmoidoscopy and Colorectal Cancer Mortality**. *J Natl Cancer Inst* 1992, **84**:1572–1575.

24. LEVIN B, MURPHY GP: **Revision in American Cancer Society Recommendations for the Early Detection of Colorectal Cancer**. *CA Cancer J Clin* 1992, **42**:296–299.

25. • SELBY JV, FRIEDMAN FD, QUESENBERRY CP, WEISS NS: **A Case-Control Study of Screening Sigmoidoscopy and Mortality From Colorectal Cancer**. *N Engl J Med* 1992, **326**:653–657.

This study provides the first convincing evidence that sigmoidoscopy screening may be effective in reducing mortality from colorectal cancer.

26. ST JOHN DBJB, YOUNG GP, ALEXEYEFF MA, DEACON MC, CUTHBERTSON AM, MACRAE FA, PENFOLD JCB: **Evaluation of New Occult Blood Tests for Detection of Colorectal Neoplasia**. *Gastroenterology* 1993, **104**:1661–1668.

27. SHAPIRO S: **Case-Control Studies of Colorectal Cancer Mortality: Is the Case Made for Screening Sigmoidoscopy?** *J Natl Cancer Inst* 1992, **84**:1546–1547.

Jack S. Mandel, PhD, MPH, School of Public Health, University of Minnesota, Box 807 UMHC, 420 Delaware Street SE, Minneapolis, MN 55455, USA.

Adjuvant radiation for rectal cancer: when and with what?

Bernard J. Cummings, MB, ChB, FRCPC, FRCR, FRACR

Faculty of Medicine, University of Toronto, Toronto, Ontario, Canada

This review outlines the progress made in recently reported trials to establish an effective adjuvant treatment for the surgical management of rectal cancer. Many of the trials of preoperative and postoperative radiation conducted over the past two decades are now mature. Moderate-to-high doses of radiation given prior to or following surgery reduce pelvic tumor recurrence rates but have little effect on survival. The coupling of radiation with cytotoxic chemotherapy, particularly 5-fluorouracil–based protocols, has been reported to improve survival as well as reduce the risk of recurrence in the pelvis and elsewhere. The status of ongoing trials is outlined.

Current Opinion in General Surgery 1994:85–93

The outlook for the patient newly diagnosed with adenocarcinoma of the rectum continues to improve as a result of the identification of more effective adjuvant therapy and advances in surgical technique. Recent information on the role of radiation alone or combined with chemotherapy as adjuvant therapy is surveyed here.

Improvements in surgical technique and reduction of the margin of normal rectal wall removed distal to the gross rectal tumor have reduced the number of patients who require a colostomy [1] and have increased the importance of maintaining anorectal function after adjuvant treatment. The margin of uninvolved tissue radial to the primary tumor and to any metastatic lymph nodes has become an important focus of attention as a likely source of local recurrence [2]. Opinion is still divided on whether surgical maneuvers, such as sharp dissection in the posterior and lateral pelvis, would consistently reduce the risk of local recurrence, and perhaps obviate adjuvant therapy in the pelvis [3,4]. The search for effective adjuvant therapy is based on the observation that despite changes in surgical technique, overall 5-year survival rates after apparently complete resection continue to average about 45% and range from 30% to 70%, with pelvic and extrapelvic recurrence rates each ranging from about 25% to 50%.

Improvements in survival and reductions in the risk of tumor recurrence are obvious measures of the effectiveness of adjuvant treatment. They must not, however, be offset by unacceptable increases in treatment-related complications. The studies reviewed do not always present all the data necessary for ready comparisons. Also, although the extent and technique of surgery may affect tumor recurrence patterns, the details of the surgery performed are discussed infrequently.

Conventional survival rate measurements are at 5 years, although this interval is arbitrary. A major trial reported by Krook *et al.* [5••] found that not all cancer-related events had occurred within 5 years, and this and previous studies [6] suggest that a 7-year follow-up may be more appropriate for evaluating the outcome of treatment for rectal cancer. Most authors think that truly effective treatment leads to improvements in overall survival rates, which encompass deaths from all causes. Disease-free rates, or cancer-related death rates, also provide useful information provided that all events due to the cancer and its treatment are identified. Data on patterns of failure and complications are often difficult to interpret. Actuarial rates are preferred because the risks of recurrence and complications can be assessed in the same way as survival rates. More frequently, these parameters are described in terms of incidence. The number of events recorded in patients followed up over different lengths of time is expressed as a proportion of the total number of patients entered on the study. This number tends to underestimate the risk. Some studies also report only the first sites of tumor recurrence, although this too can underestimate the risk of recurrence in a particular site, particularly if adjuvant therapy has delayed but not eradicated cancer growth.

Radiation alone

Adjuvant radiation, given preoperatively or postoperatively, has reduced the risk of pelvic recurrence in

Abbreviations

ECOG—Eastern Cooperative Oncology Group; **GITSG**—Gastrointestinal Tumour Study Group; **NCCTG**—North Central Cancer Treatment Group.

© 1994 Current Science ISBN 1-85922-671-X ISSN 1065–6243

many trials, but except in occasional studies has not had any significant influence on survival rates or on the risk of extrapelvic metastases. The results of recent randomized trials are shown in Tables 1 to 4, together with those of earlier studies selected for comparison.

Considerable controversy still exists over the most appropriate timing of adjuvant radiation relative to surgery, and the debate has not been resolved by recent publications. There are many reasons for favoring preoperative radiation. One is to reduce the risk of

Table 1. Survival after curative surgery with or without preoperative radiation in Dukes stages A to C of rectal carcinoma

Study	Patients, *n*	Radiation dose, *Gy/fractions/d*	5-Year overall survival rate, %		Cancer-related deaths, %	
			S	R and S	S	R and S
Norway (Dahl *et al.* [53])	259	31.5/18/24	58 (62*)	57 (68*)	NS	NS
EORTC (Gerard *et al.* [54])	341	34.5/15/19	59	69	NS	NS
Stockholm Rectal Cancer Study Group [7]	679	25/5/7	50	55	58†	68†

*5-Year disease-free survival rate.
†$P \leq 0.05$.
EORTC—European Organization for Research and Treatment of Cancer; NS—not stated; R—radiation; S—surgery.

Table 2. Failure after curative surgery with or without preoperative radiation in Dukes stages A to C of rectal carcinoma

Study	Radiation dose, *Gy/fractions/d*	Local recurrence incidence, % (5-year rate, %)		Extrapelvic recurrence incidence, % (5-year rate, %)		First or any failure
		S	S and R	S	S and R	
Norway (Dahl *et al.* [53])	31.5/18/24	23(NS)	15(NS)	18(NS)	18(NS)	First
EORTC (Gerard *et al.* [54])	34.5/15/19	28(30*)	15(15*)	22(NS)	23(NS)	First
Stockholm Rectal Cancer Study Group [7]	25/5/7	25(30*)	11(18*)	23(28)	17(25)	Any

*$P \leq 0.05$.
EORTC–European Organization for Research and Treatment of Cancer; NS—not stated; R—radiation; S—surgery.

Table 3. Survival after curative surgery with or without postoperative radiation in Dukes stages B and C of rectal carcinoma

Study	Patients, *n*	Radiation dose, *Gy/fractions/d*	5-Year overall survival, %		5-Year disease-free survival, %	
			S	S and R	S	S and R
Gastrointestinal Tumour Study Group [29]	108	40–48/20–26/32–39	46	52	45	53
National Surgical Adjuvant Breast and Bowel Project (Fisher *et al.* [31])	368	46–51/26–29/35–38	43	40	30	34
Denmark (Bentzen *et al.* [17•], Balslev *et al.* [20])	494	50/25/49 (split)	50	52	NS	NS
Netherlands (Treurniet-Donker *et al.* [18])	174	50/25/35	55	45	45	35

NS—not stated; R—radiation; S—surgery.

Table 4. Failure after curative surgery with or without postoperative radiation in Dukes stages B and C of rectal carcinoma

Study	Radiation dose, *Gy/fractions/d*	Local recurrence incidence, % (5-year rate, %)		Extrapelvic recurrence incidence, % (5-year rate, %)		First or any failure
		S	S and R	S	S and R	
Gastrointestinal Tumour Study Group [29]	40–48/20–26/32–39	24(NS)	20(NS)	34(NS)	30(NS)	First
National Surgical Adjuvant Breast and Bowel Project (Fisher *et al.* [31])	46–51/26–29/35–38	25(NS)	16(NS)	26(NS)	31(NS)	First
Denmark (Bentzen *et al.* [17•]; Balslev *et al.* [20])	50/25/49 (split)	18(27)	16(28)	24*(NS)	26*(NS)	Any
Netherlands (Treurniet-Donker *et al.* [18])	50/25/35	33(45)	24(35)	27(35)	39(48)	Any

*4-Year incidence.
NS—not stated; R—radiation; S—surgery.

both pelvic and extrapelvic recurrence, based on the assumption that some extrapelvic metastases arise from cancer cells released during intraoperative manipulation. Another is the lower likelihood of late-radiation enteritis because small bowel is less likely to be adherent in the pelvis prior to surgery. Another reason is the relatively greater radioresponsiveness of normally oxygenated cancer cells relative to that of cells and tissues hypoxic secondary to alterations in vascularity that result from pelvic surgery. Finally, if an interval of a few weeks is allowed between radiation and surgery, there may be some involution of the cancer, which could facilitate resection.

To allow more ready comparison with postoperative radiation, only patients who underwent curative resection after preoperative radiation are considered here. This selection highlights a criticism of preoperative treatment, which may be given inadvertently to patients who have a low risk of recurrence, or in whom complete resection of pelvic cancer proves impossible, or in whom extrapelvic metastases are found at laparotomy. Such patients are, of course, excluded from trials of postoperative adjuvant therapy. As imaging and other assessments improve, this objection to preoperative adjuvant treatment will become less important.

None of the randomized trials shown in Table 1 demonstrated a significant increase in 5-year overall survival rates. There was significant improvement ($P = 0.05$) in the Stockholm study when only cancer-related deaths were assessed [7]. The doses of radiation used in randomized trials of preoperative radiation have been relatively low. Trials with conventionally fractionated treatment, such as 45 Gy in 25 fractions in 5 weeks, may be more effective. Studies suggesting likely benefit with such doses either have not been randomized [8,9•] or have included too few patients to assess the merits of treatment adequately [10,11]. The significant improvement in patients in the Stockholm trial followed treatment with a short course of relatively intense fractionation of 25 Gy in five fractions in 1 week, an approach favored by several investigators in Sweden [7,12•]. This approach is not easily compared with more conventional fractionation (generally in the range of 1.7 to 2.5 Gy/d), but the Stockholm fractionation may be biologically equivalent to about 40 Gy in 20 fractions in 4 weeks. Examination of the failure patterns in the same studies shows that the higher radiation doses have led to significant reduction in local recurrence but have not affected the risk of extrapelvic metastases (Table 2). Preoperative radiation as given in the randomized trials has generally led to delays in perineal healing but not to any increased risk of breakdown of anastomoses. In nonrandomized series, doses of up to 45 Gy in 5 weeks have produced neither anastomotic leakage nor stricture, and diversionary colostomy is not required routinely after such doses [13]. Large-volume radiation (pelvis and para-aortic nodes) was associated with an increase in morbidity and mortality in the Stockholm trial, but further studies in which only the posterior pelvis was irradiated with the same dose proved safe [12•]. No late radiation enteritis has been reported, perhaps because the radiation doses used have been modest and well within small-bowel tolerance limits.

Several investigators reported that moderate-to-high doses of preoperative radiation facilitated resection with sphincter preservation and yielded good functional results [8,9•,14,15]. Comparing these results with the effects of postoperative radiation is difficult, although function may be relatively impaired by postoperative radiation following coloanal anastomosis [16].

Postoperative radiation therapy has been preferred by those who wish to select patients for adjuvant treatment by histopathologic features that have not been affected by prior radiation. Most randomized trials include patients in whom the cancer extended to pararectal tissues (Dukes stage B, American Joint Committee stage T3 or T4) or into regional lymph nodes (Dukes C, American Joint Committee N1 to 3). In randomized trials, no significant improvement in survival rates has been reported following doses as high as 50 Gy in 5 weeks (Table 3). Updates of the Danish and Netherlands trials were published in the past year [17•,18]. Although the incidence and rates of local recurrence were generally reduced following radiation treatment, the reductions did not reach conventional levels of statistical significance (Table 4). Similarly, no reduction occurred in the risk of extrapelvic recurrence (Table 4). In contrast to these disappointing results, a British Medical Research Council trial in which 40 Gy were given in 4 weeks has apparently led to both a decrease in pelvic recurrences and an improvement in survival [12,19••]. The full report of this study is awaited with interest. The incidence of small-bowel obstruction, radiation enteritis, or both, following postoperative radiation has varied widely, being significantly increased in the Danish study [20] but similar to the incidence of obstruction after pelvic surgery alone in other trials. The risks of radiation enteritis can be reduced by excluding small bowel from the pelvis surgically [21] and by careful attention to radiation therapy technique [22].

The first report of an unusual trial of postoperative radiation in which the para-aortic nodes and liver received 25 Gy in 20 fractions in 3 weeks, coupled with pelvic radiation of 50 Gy in 25 fractions in 5 weeks, showed no significant differences in survival rates at 5 years, or in local or extrapelvic recurrence rates, including liver metastases, when compared with irradiation of the pelvis only [23]. Wide-field radiation was less well tolerated during treatment, but there were no differences in late toxicity.

Some studies examined the merits of delivering radiation treatment both preoperatively and postoperatively (sandwich treatment). A nonrandomized study showed no advantage of dividing a dose of 45 Gy approximately equally preoperatively and postoperatively over postoperative treatment [24]. The preliminary report from a trial in which patients were randomly assigned to receive a single dose of 5 Gy or no radiation preoperatively, and in which those in whom the cancer had extended through the rectal wall or into regional nodes were treated with 45 Gy to 50 Gy in 5 weeks postoperatively, described no decrease in pelvic recurrence or increase in survival rates 3 years after surgery [25].

In studies in which preoperative and postoperative irradiation were compared, preoperative radiation was generally better tolerated than treatment given postoperatively [26]. Long-term results of a randomized trial performed in Sweden were presented. The trial compared preoperative radiation (25.5 Gy in five fractions in 1 week) with postoperative adjuvant treatment (60 Gy in 30 fractions in 8 weeks, split course after 40 Gy). The 5-year survival rates were similar, but there was a marked reduction of recurrence in the pelvis (incidence, 14% versus 27%, $P=0.02$) in patients receiving preoperative treatment. Perineal wound infections were more frequent after preoperative irradiation, but other perioperative morbidity was similar. The risk of later small-bowel obstruction was significantly greater after postoperative treatment (11% versus 5%; $P<0.01$) (Fig. 1) [27]. This trial has been criticized for its unconventional radiation schedules and its failure to compare identical radiation programs, but it provides further useful information on the merits of short-course intensive preoperative treatment.

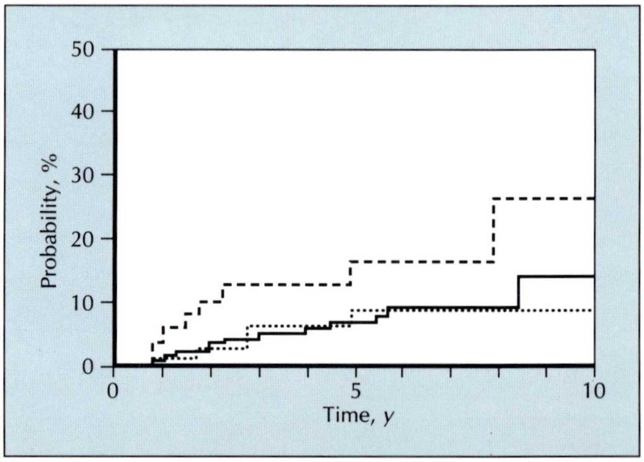

Fig. 1. Cumulative risk of developing a late bowel obstruction after surgery. *Solid line* indicates preoperative-irradiation group; *dashed line* indicates postoperative-irradiation group; *dotted line* indicates surgery-only group. (*From* Frykholm *et al.* [27]; with permission.)

Although the usual interpretation of the published trials of perioperative adjuvant radiation is that such treatment reduces the risk of local recurrence but does not influence mortality significantly, a recent meta-analysis suggests that radiotherapy as used in the published trials may have reduced mortality by about 10% [19••]. However, the authors also noted that the data are compatible either with radiation having no material effect on survival or with a reduction in the rate of cancer-related mortality of as much as 20%. It would be more convincing to see such a benefit demonstrated in a single trial, but this demonstration would require a much larger study than any conducted so far. In other meta-analyses discussed in the same paper, adjuvant systemic chemotherapy and portal vein infusion of 5-fluorouracil were each associated with reductions in mortality, although confidence limits ranged from almost no difference to about a 25% reduction in the odds of death. Meta-analyses do not identify the most effective regimens, although they may encourage further trials of a particular strategy.

Radiation and chemotherapy

The recognition that substantial numbers of patients experience both pelvic and extrapelvic recurrences after surgery and that single-modality adjuvant radiation or chemotherapy has proved relatively ineffective has led to increasing interest in trials combining radiation and chemotherapy. Several randomized trials of such combinations are in progress, but only a few have been completed (Tables 5 and 6).

Table 5. Survival after curative surgery for rectal carcinomas with or without perioperative radiation with or without chemotherapy

					5-Year overall survival, %			5-Year disease-free survival, %		
Study	Patients, *n*	Radiation dose, *Gy/fractions/d*	Concurrent 5-FU and R	Maintenance chemotherapy	S	S and R	S, R, and C	S	S and R	S, R, and C
Preoperative										
EORTC (Boulis-Wassif *et al.* [28])	247	34.5/15/19	Yes	None	—	59	46	—	60	65
Postoperative										
Gastrointestinal Tumour Study Group [29]	202	40–48/20–26/32–39	Yes	5-FU and semustine	46*	52	58*	45†	53	70†
Eastern Cooperative Oncology Group (Mansour *et al.* [30])	237	45–50.4/25–28/35–38	No	5-FU and semustine	—	46	50	—	40	46
North Central Cancer Treatment Group (Krook *et al.* [5••])	204	50.4/28/38	Yes	5-FU and semustine	—	47*	58*	—	38†	58†

*$P \leq 0.05$ after 7-year follow-up.
†$P \leq 0.05$.
C—chemotherapy; EORTC—European Organization for Research and Treatment of Cancer; 5-FU—5-fluorouracil; R—radiation; S—surgery.

The only trial of preoperative low-dose radiation and chemotherapy, in which a single 4-day course of bolus injections of 5-fluorouracil was given concurrently with low-dose radiation, disclosed no benefits [28]. The trials of postoperative combined modality therapy reported by the North Central Cancer Treatment Group (NCCTG) [5••] and by the Gastrointestinal Tumour Study Group (GITSG) [6,29] showed significant improvements in survival and in tumor recurrence patterns and stimulated interest in this strategy. In the GITSG study, there was an improvement in disease-free survival in combination therapy over surgery alone [29]. In the NCCTG trial, combined therapy was compared with radiation as adjuvant modalities [5••]. Overall survival rates were also improved by combined therapy in both trials when the patients were followed up for 7 years or longer [5••,6]. However, a trial of similar design conducted by the Eastern Cooperative Oncology Group (ECOG), and so far reported in abstract only, failed to demonstrate any advantage of the combination over one or other of the adjuvant modalities alone [30]. Only the GITSG, which studied combined radiation, chemotherapy, and surgery, included a surgery-only control arm [6,29]. Figure 2 from this trial shows how the benefit to combined modality treatment increased with time. The figure also shows that of the 202 patients entered in the trial (of whom, 58 were treated by surgery alone), only 46 distributed between all four treatment options were available for study at 8 years [6]. Although the results presented earlier suggest that the outcome of surgery and radiation are very similar to that of surgery alone, except the incidence of failure within the pelvis, unfortunately, most current trials do not include a surgical control arm. The influence of any changes in surgical management or in the natural history of rectal cancer is difficult to detect in trials lacking such controls. Local recurrence was reduced by combined radiation and chemotherapy in both the NCCTG [5••] and GITSG [29] trials when compared with radiation alone, although the difference was significant only in the larger, NCCTG study. There were fewer extrapelvic recurrences only in the NCCTG trial [5••].

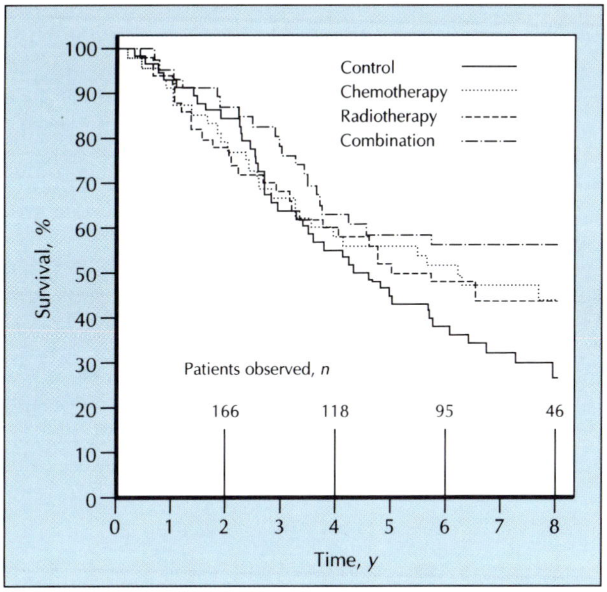

Fig. 2. Overall rates of survival after postoperative combination treatment for rectal cancer, by treatment type. (*From* Gastrointestinal Tumor Study Group [6]; with permission.)

The acute toxicity of combined-modality therapy is greater than that of adjuvant radiation alone. In the studies listed in Tables 5 and 6, acute morbidity was characterized by moderate-to-severe gastrointestinal and hematologic toxicity in about one third of patients. Late toxicity, particularly bowel obstruction or treatment-related enteritis, was not significantly increased by combining chemotherapy with radiation. As with trials of single-agent adjuvants, toxicity proved fatal in up to about 3% of the study group.

Table 6. Survival after curative surgery for rectal carcinomas with or without perioperative radiation with or without chemotherapy

Study	Radiation dose, *Gy/fractions/d*	Concurrent 5-FU and R	Maintenance chemotherapy	Local recurrence incidence, % (5-year rate, %)			Extrapelvic recurrence incidence, % (5-year rate, %)		
				S	S and R	S, R, and C	S	S and R	S, R, and C
Preoperative									
EORTC (Boulis-Wassif *et al.* [28])	34.5/15/19	Yes	None	—	NS(15)	NS(15)	—	No difference	
Postoperative									
Gastrointestinal Tumour Study Group [29]	40–48/20–26/32–39	Yes	5-FU and semustine	24(NS)	20(NS)	11(NS)	34(NS)	30(NS)	26(NS)
North Central Cancer Treatment Group (Krook *et al.* [5••])	50.4/28/38	Yes	5-FU and semustine	—	25*(NS)	14*(NS)	—	46*(NS)	29*(NS)

*$P \leq 0.05$.
C—chemotherapy; EORTC—European Organization for Research and Treatment of Cancer; 5-FU—5-fluorouracil; NS—not stated; R—radiation; S—surgery.

5-Fluorouracil remains the most effective drug in the treatment of advanced colorectal cancer and is the central agent in current trials of adjuvant therapy. Both trials of combined radiation and chemotherapy, which had positive outcomes [5••,6,29], and a National Surgical Adjuvant Breast and Bowel Project trial of adjuvant chemotherapy alone, which also showed survival benefit [31], included both semustine (methyl CCNU) and 5-fluorouracil. The ECOG study showed no advantage to combined therapy, although it, too, included semustine and 5-fluorouracil with radiation [30]. Semustine is a potentially toxic drug, associated in particular with nephrotoxicity and leukemia. Two randomized trials designed to compare the merits of 5-fluorouracil alone with those of 5-fluorouracil and semustine in combination with radiation suggested that semustine be omitted from rectal adjuvant protocols [32•,33]. Because both trials were designed to exclude survival differences of 20% or more, smaller advantages from the combination of semustine with 5-fluorouracil cannot be precluded. Pilot studies of other combinations presented during the survey period describe tumor responses but cannot be assessed adequately until they are compared with established regimens [34–36].

Considerable interest has arisen in evaluating different schedules of 5-fluorouracil in combination with radiation. Some studies of advanced colorectal cancer [37] or in the laboratory [38,39] suggested advantages due to possible interaction or sensitization from delivering 5-fluorouracil concomitantly with radiation. A detailed review of fluoropyrimidines as radiation sensitizers summarized the laboratory data [40•]. Despite such laboratory studies, interactions may not occur in clinical practice, and benefits attributed to concomitant therapy may simply result from additive cytotoxicity or from the reduction of delays in chemotherapy. Such delays can occur when radiation is integrated with chemotherapy schedules. Each of the studies surveyed in Tables 5 and 6 differed in the schedules and doses of radiation and chemotherapy delivered, as well as in whether radiation preceded or was intercalated during maintenance chemotherapy. The ideal schedule is not known. The failure of the ECOG trial [30] to reproduce the improvement in disease-free survival seen in the GITSG [29] and NCCTG [5••] trials of adjuvant 5-fluorouracil, semustine, and radiation may have resulted from the omission of the one or two short courses of 5-fluorouracil that were given concurrently with radiation in the other trials. The only trial in which the delivery of 5-fluorouracil concurrently with radiation was randomly compared with radiation alone without maintenance chemotherapy was the preoperative study conducted by the European Organization for Research and Treatment of Cancer, in which no significant differences were found [28]. A nonrandomized study of postoperative radiation with and without concurrent 5-fluorouracil and also without maintenance chemotherapy suggested improvements in local control and disease-free survival rates from combined radiation and 5-fluorouracil [41].

The merits of different schedules of administering 5-fluorouracil concurrently with radiation were evaluated in a randomized trial recently reported in abstract form [42]. Patients were randomly assigned to receive either 5-fluorouracil, 500 mg/m^2 intravenous bolus injection on 3 days in the 1st and 5th weeks of pelvic radiation, or 5-fluorouracil, 225 $mg/m^2/d$ continuous intravenous infusion throughout the 5- to 6-week course of pelvic radiation, 50.4 to 54 Gy at 1.8 Gy/d. Both groups received maintenance chemotherapy. There were significant advantages to the prolonged infusion for both 3-year, relapse-free survival (67% versus 56%; $P=0.01$) and overall survival (76% versus 68%; $P=0.02$). Prolonged infusion was associated with decreases in the incidence of both local and extrapelvic recurrences. No toxicity data were described. It will be important to confirm this result, both through longer follow-up and additional studies, in view of the resource implications of widespread use of continuous infusion chemotherapy.

5-Fluorouracil is usually combined with biochemical modifiers, such as folinic acid, when used to treat advanced colorectal cancer. The combinations of 5-fluorouracil and folinic acid [43], and of 5-fluorouracil and levamisole [44], improved survival as adjuvant treatments of colon cancer. Not surprisingly, these combinations and others that have shown benefits as systemic or portal vein–infusion adjuvants for colon cancer [19••,45] are now being evaluated for the treatment of rectal cancer, generally in combination with pelvic radiation. Preliminary studies of folinic acid and 5-fluorouracil given concurrently with radiation were reported [46,47] and the determination of the relative merits of such combinations compared with 5-fluorouracil alone will require randomized trials. Pilot studies have suggested that concurrent radiation, 5-fluorouracil, and folinic acid may be better tolerated, at least with respect to acute toxicity, when given preoperatively rather than postoperatively [47].

Conclusions

Review of the main reasons for favoring preoperative radiation shows that, although the risk of pelvic recurrence can be reduced, the incidence of extrapelvic metastases has not been reduced, and most metastases do not occur during surgical manipulation of the tumor. However, the delays in surgery that result from preoperative treatment have also not led to identifiable increases in the risk of metastases. There may well be less fixed small bowel within the pelvis prior to surgery, but the doses of radiation given have not been those that would be expected to cause enteritis, and methods are available to minimize the risk of enteritis whether radiation is given before or after surgery. Preoperative treatment can usually be given in a somewhat smaller volume than can postoperative radiation because the site of the primary tumor can be more readily localized, and the smaller volume may help to reduce late morbidity. The greater effectiveness of preoperative radiation in reducing local recurrence compared with even higher doses of postoperative treatment suggests some advantage for preoperative treatment. Whether this advantage results from postoperative hypoxic radioresistance remains moot. In postoperative radiation studies, patients have been selected according to histopathologic stages associated with greater risks of local recurrence, and patients unlikely to benefit from adjuvant treatment have been excluded. The impact of postoperative radiation on failure patterns and survival rates has been disappointing. Both preoperative and postoperative radiation continue to be advocated, but so far neither has been particularly effective apart from reducing the risk of local recurrence.

Combinations of chemotherapy and radiation therapy are intellectually attractive because they address the problems of pelvic and systemic recurrences. Much has been made of the two positive studies published, and correspondingly little has been written about the negative trials. Many other trials are in progress. The possibility of interaction between radiation and concurrent cytotoxic chemotherapy continues to be an area of very active clinical and laboratory studies, but with no firm conclusions. Efforts to refine the selection of patients for adjuvant trials and to predict outcome more accurately continue [48,49,50•], but none of the new methodologies can yet be recommended for general use.

Functional outcome other than serious morbidity was not addressed in the reports. As radiation doses are increased, and chemotherapy agents are combined with radiation, the risks of damage to all tissues irradiated, and particularly to the rectum and anal sphincter mechanisms, will need to be studied carefully. Possible advantages to delivering radiation prior to surgery so that the rectum can be reconstituted largely with unirradiated colon may then become apparent. Preoperative radiation is generally preferred for bulky and marginally resectable cancers, and regression of cancer after radiation has facilitated sphincter-sparing surgery even in very low rectal tumors.

European and North American commentators have tended to review the data differently. In Europe, the move to adopt combined chemotherapy and radiation therapy has been slower, and the inclusion of surgical controls in trials is still supported [51]. In North America, adjuvant radiation and 5-fluorouracil–based chemotherapy have been advocated more strongly [52]. All agree that the answers to whether radiation should be given prior to or after surgery, and to which chemotherapy should be coupled with radiation, will be answered most effectively through participation in appropriately designed clinical trials.

References and recommended reading

Papers of particular interest, published within the annual period of review, have been highlighted as:
- • Of special interest
- •• Of outstanding interest

1. WILLIAMS NS: **The Rationale for Preservation of the Anal Sphincter in Patients with Low Rectal Cancer.** *Br J Surg* 1984, 71:575–581.
2. QUIRKE P, DURDEY P, DIXON MF, WILLIAMS NS: **Local Recurrence of Rectal Adenocarcinoma Due to Inadequate Surgical Resection: Histopathological Study of Lateral Tumour Spread and Surgical Excision.** *Lancet* 1986, ii:996–999.
3. HEALD RJ, KARANJIA ND: **Results of Radical Surgery for Rectal Cancer.** *World J Surg* 1992, 16:848–857.
4. HOJO K, KAYAMA Y: **The Effectiveness of Wide Anatomical Resection and Radical Lymphadenectomy for Patients With Rectal Cancer.** *Jpn J Surg* 1982, 12:111–116.
5. •• KROOK JE, MOERTEL CG, GUNDERSON LL, WIEAND HS, COLLINS RT, BEART RW, KUBISTA TP, POON MA, MEYERS WC, MAILLIARD JA, TWITO DI, MORTON RF, VEEDER MH, WITZIG TE, CHA S, VIDYARTHI SC: **Effective Surgical Adjuvant Therapy for High-Risk Rectal Carcinoma.** *N Engl J Med* 1991, 324:709–715.

A well-designed and -reported trial of combined radiation and chemotherapy, which significantly decreased cancer recurrence and significantly increased survival rates. The basic design for several subsequent current trials.

6. Gastrointestinal Tumour Study Group: **Survival After Postoperative Combination Treatment of Rectal Cancer.** *N Engl J Med* 1986, **315**:1294.

7. Stockholm Rectal Cancer Study Group: **Preoperative Short-Term Radiation Therapy in Operable Rectal Carcinoma.** *Cancer* 1990, **66**:49–55.

8. Mohiuddin M, Marks G: **High Dose Preoperative Irradiation for Cancer of the Rectum, 1976-1988.** *Int J Radiat Oncol Biol Phys* 1991, **20**:37–43.

9. • Mendenhall WM, Bland KI, Copeland EM, Summers GE, Ptaff WW, Souba WW, Million RR: **Does Preoperative Radiation Therapy Enhance the Probability of Local Control and Survival in High-Risk Distal Rectal Cancer?** *Ann Surg* 1992, **215**:696–705.

A nonrandomized series that reviews the merits of different doses of preoperative radiation.

10. Kligerman M, Urdaneta N, Knowlton A, Vidone R, Hartman PR, Vera R: **Preoperative Irradiation of Rectosigmoid Carcinoma Including Its Regional Lymph Nodes.** *AJR Am J Roentgenol* 1972, **114**:498–503.

11. Reis Neto JA, Quilici FA, Reis JA Jr: **A Comparison of Nonoperative Versus Preoperative Radiotherapy in Rectal Carcinoma: A 10-Year Randomized Trial.** *Dis Colon Rectum* 1989, **32**:702–710.

12. • Pahlman L, Glimelius B: **Preoperative and Postoperative Radiotherapy and Rectal Cancer.** *World J Surg* 1992, **16**:858–865.

A detailed review of the merits of adjuvant radiation therapy including a discussion of various technical and biological aspects of radiation.

13. Kerman HD, Robertson SH, Bloom TS, Heron HC, Yaeger TE, Meese DL, Ritter AH, Tolland JT, Spangler AE: **Rectal Carcinoma: Long-Term Experience With Moderately High-Dose Preoperative Radiation and Low Anterior Resections.** *Cancer* 1992, **69**:2813–2819.

14. Berard P, Papillon J: **Role of Preoperative Irradiation for Anal Preservation in Cancer of the Low Rectum.** *World J Surg* 1992, **16**:502–509.

15. Minsky BD, Cohen AM, Enker WE, Sigurdson E: **Phase I/II Trial of Preoperative Radiation Therapy and Coloanal Anastomosis in Distal Invasive Resectable Rectal Cancer.** *Int J Radiat Oncol Biol Phys* 1992, **23**:387–392.

16. Berger A, Tiret E, Frileux P, Cugnenc PH, Nordlinger B, Hannoun L, Parc R: **Impact de la Radiothérapie Postoperatoire Sur le Résultat Fonctionnel de l'Anastomose Coloanale.** *Lyon Chirurgical* 1991, **87**:39–41.

17. • Bentzen SM, Balsev I, Pedersen M, Teglbjaerg PS, Hanberg-Sorenson F, Bone J, Jacobsen NO, Sell A, Overgaard J, Bertelsen K, Hage E, Fenger C, Kronborg O, Hansen L, Hoestrup H, Norgaard-Pedersen B: **Time to Loco-regional Recurrence After Resection of Dukes B and C Colorectal Cancer With or Without Adjuvant Postoperative Radiotherapy: A Multi-variate Regression Analysis.** *Br J Cancer* 1992, **65**:102–107.

One of several reports of a national study that has illustrated many of the problems encountered in multicenter trials.

18. Treurniet-Donker AD, Van Putten WL, Wereldsma JC, Bruggink ED, Hoogenraad WJ, Roukema JA, Snijders-Keilholz A, Meijer WS, Meerwaldt JH, Wijnmoolen AJ, Wiggers T: **Postoperative Radiation Therapy for Rectal Cancer: An Interim Analysis of a Prospective, Randomized Multicenter Trial in the Netherlands.** *Cancer* 1991, **67**:2042–2048.

19. •• Gray R, James R, Mossman J, Stenning S: **AXIS: A Suitable Case for Treatment.** *Br J Cancer* 1991, **634**:841–845.

Meta-analyses of adjuvant radiation therapy and chemotherapy. Also, a description of an unusual trial design intended to increase patient accrual.

20. Balslev I, Pederson M, Teglbjaeig PS, Hanberg-Soerensen F, Bone J, Jacobson NO, Overgaard J, Sell A, Bertelsen K, Hage E, Fenger C, Kronborg O, Hansen L, Hoestrip H, Noergaard-Pedersen B: **Postoperative Radiotherapy in Dukes B and C Carcinoma of the Rectum and Rectosigmoid.** *Cancer* 1986, **58**:22–28.

21. Thom A, Baumann J, Chandler JJ, Devereux DF: **Experience With High-Dose Radiation Therapy and the Intestinal Sling Procedure in Patients With Rectal Carcinoma.** *Cancer* 1992, **70**:581–584.

22. Herbert SH, Curran WJ, Solin LJ, Stafford PM, Lanciano RM, Hanks GE: **Decreasing Gastrointestinal Morbidity With the Use of Small Bowel Contrast During Treatment Planning for Pelvic Irradiation.** *Int J Radiat Oncol Biol Phys* 1991, **20**:835–842.

23. Horiot JC, Bosset JF, Hamers H, Cionini L, Bartelink H, Caspers R, Untereiner M, Ciambellotti E, Gonzalez DG, van den Weijngaert D, Milla Santos A, Arcangeli G, Le Floch O, van Glabbeke M, Pierart M: **Results of EORTC Trial 22831 in Resectable Rectal Cancer Using Postoperative Pelvic Radiation With and Without Irradiation of Paraaortic Nodes and Liver [Abstract].** *Radiother Oncol* 1992, **24(suppl)**:S102.

24. Cellini N, Valentini V, DeSantis M, Morganti AG, Trodella L, Coco C, Picciocchi A, Dobelbower RR Jr: **Radiosurgical Treatment Compared to Surgery Alone for Rectal Cancer.** *Int J Radiat Oncol Biol Phys* 1990, **19**:1159–1164.

25. Sause WT, Martz KL, Noyes D, Dobelbower RR, Fischbach AJ, Doggett S, Mohiuddin M: **RTOG 81-15 ECOG 83-23 Evaluation of Preoperative Radiation Therapy in Operable Rectal Carcinoma [Abstract].** *Int J Radiat Oncol Biol Phys* 1990, **19(suppl)**:179.

26. Pahlman L, Glimelius B: **Pre- or Postoperative Radiotherapy in Rectal and Rectosigmoid Carcinoma: Report From a Randomized Multicenter Trial.** *Ann Surg* 1990, **211**:187–195.

27. Frykholm GJ, Glimelius B, Pahlman L: **Preoperative or Postoperative Irradiation in Adenocarcinoma of the Rectum: Final Treatment Results of a Randomized Trial and an Evaluation of Late Secondary Effects.** *Dis Colon Rectum* 1993, **36**:564–572.

28. Boulis-Wassif S, Gerard A, Loygue J, Camelot D, Buyse M, Duez N: **Final Results of a Randomized Trial on the Treatment of Rectal Cancer With Preoperative Radiotherapy Alone or in Combination With 5-Fluorouracil, Followed by Radical Surgery.** *Cancer* 1984, **53**:1811–1818.

29. Gastrointestinal Tumour Study Group: **Prolongation of the Disease-Free Interval in Surgically Treated Rectal Carcinoma.** *N Engl J Med* 1985, **312**:1465–1472.

30. Mansour EG, Letkopoulou M, Johnson R, Douglass H Jr: **A Comparison of Postoperative Adjuvant Chemotherapy, Radiotherapy or Combination Therapy in Potentially Curable Rectal Carcinoma [Abstract].** *Proc Am Soc Clin Oncol* 1991, **10**:154.

31. Fisher B, Wolmark N, Rockette H, Redmond C, Deutsch M, Wickerham DL, Fisher ER, Caplan R, Jones J, Lerner H, Gordon P, Feldman M, Cruz A, Legault-Poisson S, Wexler M, Lawrence W, Robidoux A: **Postoperative Adjuvant Chemotherapy or Radiation Therapy for Rectal Cancer: Results From NSABP Protocol R-01.** *J Natl Cancer Inst* 1988, **80**:21–29.

32. • Gastrointestinal Tumour Study Group: **Radiation Therapy and Fluorouracil With or Without Semustine for the Treatment of Patients With Surgical Adjuvant Adenocarcinoma of the Rectum.** *J Clin Oncol* 1992, **10**:549–557.

Report of a randomized trial conducted to evaluate the need for semustine (methyl-CCNU) as a component of adjuvant cytotoxic chemotherapy in combination with radiation therapy.

33. O'Connell M, Wieand H, Krook J, Martenson J, Macdonald J, Rich T, Haller D, Mayer R, Gunderson L: **Lack of Value for Methyl-CCNU (MeCCNU) as a Component of Effective Rectal Cancer Surgical Adjuvant Therapy. Interim Analysis of Intergroup Protocol 86-47-51 [Abstract].** *Proc Am Soc Clin Oncol* 1991, **10**:134.

34. KIEL KD, STRYKER S, SHAW J, BENSON A, HARTZ W: **Concurrent 5-Fluorouracil, Mitomycin C and Radiation Followed by Low Anterior Resection for Carcinoma of the Distal Rectum [Abstract].** *Radiother Oncol* 1992, **24(suppl)**:S102.
35. SISCHY B, GRANEY MJ, HINSON EJ, QAZI R: **Preoperative Radiation Therapy With Sensitizers in the Management of Carcinoma of the Rectum.** *Dis Colon Rectum* 1985, **28**:56–57.
36. SARASHINA H, TODOROKI T, ORII K, OHARA K, OTSU H, IWASAKI Y: **Effects of Preoperative Radiotherapy on Rectal Cancer: Preliminary Report on Combining Radiation With Intratumour Injections of Peplomycin and Bromodeoxyuridine.** *Dis Colon Rectum* 1990, **33**:1017–1025.
37. MOERTEL CG, CHILDS DS, REITEMEIER RJ, COLBY MY, HOLBROOK MA: **Combined 5-Fluorouracil and Supervoltage Radiation Therapy of Locally Unresectable Gastrointestinal Cancer.** *Lancet* 1969, ii:865–867.
38. BYFIELD JE, CALABRO-JONES P, KLISAK I, KULHANIAN F: **Pharmacologic Requirements for Obtaining Sensitization of Human Cells In Vitro to Combined 5FU or Ftorafur and X-Rays.** *Int J Radiat Oncol Biol Phys* 1982, **8**:1923–1933.
39. STEEL GG: **The Search for Therapeutic Gain in the Combination of Radiotherapy and Chemotherapy.** *Radiother Oncol* 1988, **11**:31–53.
40. • LAWRENCE TS, MAYBAUM J: **Fluoropyrimidines as Radiation Sensitizers.** *Semin Radiat Oncol* 1993, **3**:20–28.

An up-to-date and comprehensive survey of the laboratory data concerning the interactions of one group of cytotoxic drugs, the fluoropyrimidines, with radiation.

41. WILLETT CG, TEPPER JE, KAUFMAN DS, SHELLITO PC, ELISEO R, CONVERY K, WOOD WC: **Adjuvant Postoperative Radiation Therapy for Rectal Adenocarcinoma.** *Am J Clin Oncol* 1992, **15**:371–375.
42. MARTENSON J, RICH T, WIEAND H, KROOK J, MACDONALD J, HALLER D, MAYER R, GUNDERSEN L: **Protracted Venous Infusion (PVI), 5 Fluorouracil (5FU) as a Component of Effective Combined Modality Postoperative Surgical Adjuvant Therapy for High-Risk Rectal Cancer [Abstract].** *Proc Am Soc Clin Oncol* 1993, **12**:193.
43. ZANIBONI A, ERLICHMAN C, SEITZ JF, SHEPHERD L, MILAN C, LABIANCA R, TORRI V, PIGNON JP, ZEE B, MARSONI S: **FUFA Increases Disease-Free Survival in Resected B2C Colon Cancer: Results of a Prospective Pooled Analysis of 3 Randomized Trials [Abstract].** *Proc Am Soc Clin Oncol* 1993, **12**:189.
44. MOERTEL CG, FLEMING TR, MACDONALD JS, HALLER DG, LAURIE JA, GOODMAN PJ, UNGERLEIDER JS, EMERSON WA, TORMEY DC, GLICK JH, VEEDER MH, MAILLIARD JA: **Effective Surgical Adjuvant Therapy of Colon Carcinoma: An Intergroup Study.** *N Engl J Med* 1990, **322**:352–358.
45. FUCHS CS, MAYER RJ: **Adjuvant Chemotherapy for Colon and Rectal Cancer.** *Semin Radiat Oncol* 1993, **3**:29–41.
46. MAILLIARD JA, MOERTEL CG, GUNDERSEN LL, MCKENNA PJ: **Early Evaluation of 5FU Plus Leucovorin (LV) As a Radiation Enhancer for Gastrointestinal Carcinoma [Abstract].** *Proc Am Soc Clin Oncol* 1991, **10**:151.
47. MINSKY BD, COHEN AM, KEMENY N, ENKER WE, KELSEN DP, REICHMAN B, SALTZ L, SIGURDSON ER, FRANKEL J: **Combined Modality Therapy of Rectal Cancer: Decreased Acute Toxicity With the Preoperative Approach.** *J Clin Oncol* 1992, **10**:1218–1224.
48. JONES DJ, ZALOUDIK J, JAMES RD, HABOUBI N, MOORE M, SCHOFIELD PF: **Predicting Local Recurrence of Carcinoma of the Rectum After Preoperative Radiotherapy and Surgery.** *Br J Surg* 1989, **76**:1172–1175.
49. REW DA, WILSON GD, TAYLOR I, WEAVER PC: **Proliferative Characteristics of Human Colorectal Carcinomas Measured In Vivo.** *Br J Surg* 1991, **78**:60–66.
50. • WITZIG TE, LOPRINZI CL, GONCHOROFF NJ, REIMAN HM, CHA SS, WEIAND HS, KATZMANN JA, PAULSEN JK, MOERTEL CG: **DNA Ploidy and Cell Kinetic Measurements or Predictors of Recurrence and Survival in Stages B2 and C Colorectal Adenocarcinoma.** *Cancer* 1991, **68**:879–888.

An illustration of some of the benefits of large trials and an indication of the potential merits of predictive assays to allow selection of patients for adjuvant therapy.

51. WILS J, WAGENER DJ: **Combined Modality Adjuvant Treatment of High-Risk Rectal Cancer: A Treatment of Choice or a Choice of Treatment?** *Ann Oncol* 1992, **3**:197–199.
52. NIH CONSENSUS CONFERENCE: **Adjuvant Therapy for Patients With Colon and Rectal Cancer.** *JAMA* 1990, **11**:1444–1450.
53. DAHL O, HORN A, MORILD I, HALVORSEN JF, ODLAND G, REINERTSEN S, REISAETER A, KAVLI H, THUNOLD J: **Low-Dose Preoperative Radiation Postpones Recurrences in Operable Rectal Cancer.** *Cancer* 1990, **66**:2286–2294.
54. GERARD A, BUYSE M, NORDLINGER B, LOYGUE J, PENE F, KEMPF P, BOSSET JF, GIGNOUX M, ARNARD JP, DESAIVE C, DUEZ N: **Preoperative Radiotherapy as Adjuvant Treatment in Rectal Cancer.** *Ann Surg* 1988, **208**:606–614.

Bernard Cummings, MB, ChB, FRCP, FRCR, FRACR, Department of Radiation Oncology, The Princess Margaret Hospital, 500 Sherbourne Street, Toronto, Ontario, M4X 1K9, Canada.

Sensitivity versus cost effectiveness in postoperative follow-up for colorectal cancer

Carina G. Biggs, MD, and Garth H. Ballantyne, MD

Yale University School of Medicine, New Haven, and
St. Mary's Hospital, Waterbury, Connecticut, USA

The incidence of colorectal cancer is increasing. Approximately 20% of patients present with untreatable, disseminated disease. The remaining 80% are generally treated by intended curative resection. Unfortunately, about 40% of the Dukes B_2 and C patients will develop recurrent disease. Of these patients, about one third will develop hepatic metastases, one fifth pulmonary metastases, one fifth intra-abdominal metastases, one tenth retroperitoneal metastases, and one twentieth anastomotic recurrences. Rectal cancer patients may have pelvic recurrence rates as high as one third. Unfortunately, only about one fifth of the Dukes B_2 and C patients will initially develop recurrences at only one site and are, thus, potentially curable. Indeed, when considering all colorectal cancer patients, resectable recurrences will be detected in the liver in only 2%, regional recurrences in about 10%, in the lungs in 2%, anastomotic recurrences in less than 1%, and in the ovaries in 1%. In general, long-term survival can be achieved in about 30% of these patients with salvage surgery. The goal of intensive follow-up programs has been to identify these sole site recurrences at an earlier, asymptomatic stage and thereby improve survival. Unfortunately this laudable goal has not been achieved. Intensive (and expensive) follow-up programs consistently achieve long-term survival in 0% to 4% of patients. Reliance on symptoms, however, achieves remarkably similar end results. Consequently, in this era of limited resources, we recommend two strategies for follow-up in the noninvestigational setting: 1) history and physical examination by a primary care physician every 3 months for 2 years and then annually (including rigid or flexible sigmoidoscopy for patients with colorectal anastomoses), or 2) instruction of the patient about the symptoms of recurrence. When patients develop symptoms, they return to their primary care physician for evaluation.

Current Opinion in General Surgery 1994:94–102

Colorectal cancer is the second most common malignancy in the United States. Unfortunately, the incidence of colorectal cancer continues to increase [1]. In 1992, 156,000 Americans developed new cases of colorectal cancer and 58,000 died from it [2]. Many of these patients succumbed to recurrence of their colorectal cancers. Consequently, considerable effort is expended by physicians in the postoperative follow-up of patients after curative resections for colorectal carcinoma. The purpose of these efforts is to identify these recurrences at an early and localized stage because surgical excision remains the only effective treatment. Five years ago, we questioned whether this laudable goal could be accomplished and concluded that postoperative follow-up for colorectal cancer patients had "failed to make any substantial impact on survival" [3].

We have now entered an era in which the resources of society can no longer meet the increasing expenses of health care in the United States. As a result, many issues in health care delivery are being reexamined. The best strategy for follow-up of patients after curative resections for colorectal carcinoma has entered a phase of vigorous debate [4]. Two different strategies have emerged based on two different goals. One strategy is to find all recurrences of colorectal cancers at the

Abbreviations

CEA—carcinoembryonic antigen; **CT**—computed tomography; **MRI**—magnetic resonance imaging; **SEER**—Surveillance, Epidemiology, and End Results.

ISBN 1-85922-671-X ISSN 1065–6243

earliest possible time. This is based on the unproven assumption that "newer techniques of postoperative monitoring after resection of primary lesion, more sensitive preoperative and intraoperative staging of recurrences, and the use of intraoperative radiation therapy may increase surgical salvage of recurrent colorectal cancer" [5]. In contrast, an alternative strategy is to identify treatable recurrences of colorectal carcinoma in the most cost-effective manner. This is based on the poor impact on end results achieved by follow-up efforts. Steele [6], for example, writes, "Is there any evidence that earlier diagnosis of asymptomatic or even symptomatic colon and rectum carcinoma recurrences will lead to any greater chance for cure? The answer is quite simply, no."

The purpose of this review is to clarify the scope of the problem, to detail the pattern of recurrences after curative resections for colorectal carcinomas, to review the end results for treatment of recurrences at specific sites, to examine the effectiveness of individual mechanisms used for the detection of recurrences, to focus on the end results of intensive prospective programs of follow-up for colorectal cancer patients, and finally to offer two strategies for the follow-up of colorectal cancer patients. We focus primarily on recent publications but also cite older literature to fill in areas not addressed by recent works.

The extent of colorectal cancer

Incidence

The incidence of colorectal cancer is increasing. Information on incidence is only available from a limited number of areas in the United States. The Connecticut Tumor Registry, founded in 1935, is the oldest state tumor registry in the United States and the second oldest in the world. Consequently, it provides excellent information regarding the incidence of colorectal cancer over the past 50 years. Between 1973 and 1985, 28,082 patients with colorectal cancer were reported to the Connecticut Tumor Registry [7]. During this period, the number of patients per year almost doubled. Part of the increased number of patients with colorectal cancer can be attributed to the advancing age of the population. However, the age-adjusted incidence of colorectal cancer is also increasing. Since 1935, the age-adjusted incidence of colorectal cancer has increased from 35.2 to 70.2 cases per 100,000 population per year for men, and from 32.1 to 49.2 cases per 100,000 population per year for women. Thus, the total number of colorectal cancer patients is rapidly increasing.

The incidence of colorectal cancer is increasing in other areas of the United States. The age-adjusted incidence of colorectal cancer was calculated in five states and four metropolitan areas by the Surveillance, Epidemiology, and End Results (SEER) Program of the National Cancer Institute. The SEER Program reported a 9.4% increase in age-adjusted incidence of colorectal cancer between 1973 and 1986. The age-adjusted incidence of colon and rectal cancer was 50.5 cases per 100,000 population per year for all age groups. For men, the age-adjusted incidence was 61 cases per 100,000 population per year; for women, 42.2 cases per 100,000 population per year [8]. These data from the SEER Program were recently updated; they indicate that blacks have suffered a particularly striking increase in incidence of colorectal cancer [1], and that notable increases of incidence have been reported since 1973 among all races and both sexes. Therefore it appears that colorectal cancer is becoming an increasing danger for all segments of the US population.

Stage at presentation

The stage of disease at the time of presentation is gradually changing. Stage at presentation according to Dukes classification have been reported by the SEER Program [9]. In 1977, 21.5% of patients presented with Dukes A carcinomas whereas in 1987 this rate increased to 26.8%. Concomitantly, the percentage of Dukes D lesions dropped from 22.9% to 18.4% during the same time period. This resulted in an improvement of relative 5-year survival from 49% to 56%. This slight improvement in stage at presentation is attributed to efforts at screening asymptomatic patients. These results indicate that one fifth of patients are already afflicted with incurable disease at the time of diagnosis. Additionally, this trend toward earlier diagnosis suggests that screening efforts can have an impact on stage of disease at the time of diagnosis and, more importantly, significantly improve end results.

Pattern of recurrence

General pattern

Approximately 80% of patients present with potentially curable colorectal cancer and undergo curative resections. Unfortunately, about two fifths of these patients will develop recurrent disease [10]. These recurrences are detected within 30 months of the first operation in 85% of patients [11]. Unfortunately, the overwhelming majority of these are unresectable and, thus, untreatable [12]. The pattern of recurrences differs somewhat for carcinomas of the colon and rectum [13].

Differences between colon and rectal cancer

The differences in sites of recurrence for colon and rectal cancer were studied in patients who were entered into three different adjuvant treatment protocols following curative resections [14•]. Among 818 patients with Dukes B_2 or C carcinomas, 353 (43%) suffered from recurrence of their disease: 52% of patients with rectal carcinoma and 40% of colon cancer patients. Median time to recurrence was 16.7 months. The most common sites of recurrence were hepatic (33%), pulmonary (22%), intra-abdominal (18%), retroperitoneal (10%), and in the peripheral lymph nodes (4%). Rectal lesions recurred locally or regionally more frequently than colon carcinomas. In contrast, colon carcinomas tended to involve more commonly the retroperitoneal or peripheral lymph nodes.

The rate of local recurrence for colon cancer patients is lower than for rectal cancer patients. At the Peter

Bent Brigham Hospital, local or regional recurrence was identified in 5.3% of patients with right colon lesions and 0% with transverse and left colon lesions [15••]. In contrast, regional recurrences were noted in 9.4% of patients with sigmoid lesions and 10.9% with rectal carcinomas. Distal sigmoid and rectal carcinomas account for most local or regional recurrences.

Treatable recurrences

Detection of treatable recurrences in the most important issue. In Galandiuk *et al.*'s [14•] study, initial recurrence was detected in only one site in 267 of 818 (33%) patients. These patients, however, had only Dukes B_2 and C disease. If one considers all patients after curative resections, this percentage decreases. At Memorial Sloan-Kettering Cancer Center, for example, 103 of 412 (25%) patients who had undergone curative resections for rectal cancer developed recurrences limited to one site [16]. This rate decreases to about 20% if one considers all patients with colorectal carcinomas, not only those who undergo curative resection. Thus, about one fifth of all colorectal cancer patients develop recurrences that are initially limited to one site. It is these sole site recurrences on which we must focus because these are the only resectable, and therefore treatable, recurrences.

Location of sole site recurrences

Liver

The liver is a common site of recurrence after primary excision of a colorectal carcinoma, but is the sole site of metastases in a very limited number of patients. At the Massachusetts General Hospital, 118 of 533 (22%) patients treated by curative resection for colonic carcinoma developed liver metastases [17]. Only 31% of these 118 patients (5.8% of the entire group), however, had the liver as the sole site of recurrence at the time of diagnosis.

Liver metastases are only treatable when limited to one lobe. Among 217 patients treated at Memorial Sloan-Kettering Cancer Center for liver metastases, lesions were limited to the right lobe in 48 (22%), the left lobe in 24 (11%) and both lobes in 145 (67%) [18]. The University of Alabama in Birmingham reported a similar rate of unilobar disease for patients with colorectal cancers [19]. Only one third of patients with liver metastases had lesions limited to one lobe. This finding suggests that only 2% of colorectal cancer patients will develop liver metastases that are potentially treatable.

Local or regional recurrence

Locoregional recurrence most commonly afflicts patients with sigmoid or rectal carcinomas. In a recent review, Turk and Wanebo [5] found local recurrence as the sole site of recurrence in 1% to 19% of colon cancer patients after curative resections and in 7% to 33% of rectal cancer patients. Only a fraction of these patients, however, were candidates for reresections.

Local or regional recurrence of carcinomas in the pelvis is often difficult to treat surgically. In Rome, 17 (14%) pelvic recurrences were identified in 120 patients following curative resections for rectal carcinoma [20]. Only eight (6.7%), however, were candidates for reexcision.

Pulmonary

The lungs are the most common site of extra-abdominal recurrence of colorectal cancer. Carcinomas of the rectum are associated with a significantly higher number of pulmonary recurrences than are carcinomas of the proximal colon [14•]. In one study, pulmonary metastases were diagnosed in 117 of 1013 (11.6%) patients with rectal cancers but in only 20 of 565 (3.5%) patients with colon cancers [21]. Nonetheless, overall only 2% to 4% of all colorectal cancer patients develop pulmonary metastases as the sole site of recurrence [22]. Furthermore, since the first resection of a solitary pulmonary metastasis from a colorectal cancer was reported in 1944, only 500 similar resections have been described in the literature [23]. The surgical treatment of a colorectal pulmonary metastasis would seem a fairly uncommon event.

Anastomotic

Isolated anastomotic recurrences are uncommon. Of the 818 patients reported by Galandiuk *et al.* [14•], only 5.6% suffered intraluminal recurrence. Anastomotic recurrences are found in rectal cancer patients more frequently than in colon cancer patients. Malcolm *et al.* [24•] followed up 259 patients for at least 5 years after curative resections for colorectal cancer. Overall, 20 (7.7%) patients developed suture line recurrences. Among patients with right colon lesions, these anatomic lesions were found in 3 of 93 (3.2%) transverse colon lesions in none of 10 (0%) sigmoid colon lesions in 13 of 88 (14.7%), and rectal cancers in 7 of 68 (10.2%).

These recurrences, however, are frequently associated with recurrent disease elsewhere [5]. At Roswell Park Cancer Institute, 50 patients with intraluminal anastomotic recurrences were identified among 3879 patients treated over a 17-year period [25]. Locoregional and disseminated recurrence was present in 90% of patients with anastomotic recurrences. Among the 259 patients described by Malcolm *et al.* [24•], only one recurrence (0.3%) was limited to the anastomosis. Similarly, among 1193 patients treated by curative resection at the Massachusetts General Hospital, resectable anastomotic recurrences were found in only six (0.5%) [26]. Most anastomotic recurrences form part of a pattern of disseminated recurrence. The chances of finding an anastomotic recurrence as the sole site of recurrence appear to be less than 1%.

Ovaries

Colorectal metastases spread to the ovaries in approximately 3% to 10% of women [5]. More than half (55.5%) of women with ovarian metastases also have developed recurrent disease at other sites [27]. Following curative resections for colorectal cancers, only 13 of

882 (1.4%) women underwent a second operation for ovarian recurrences [28]. The identification of ovarian metastases at a curable stage is difficult. As a result, some investigators advocate prophylactic oophorectomy at the time of the initial curative resection for colorectal cancer in women [29].

Survival after resection of recurrent cancers

Surgical excision is the only successful modality for the treatment of recurrent colorectal cancer. The end results of treatment of recurrent disease by resection is surprisingly consistent across various sites [30•]. The 5-year survival for a compiled series of 1387 patients who underwent resection for a solitary liver metastasis was 36% [7]. Survival after resections for multiple metastases varied from 0% to 50% depending on the criteria of patient selection. End results for patients after resections for nonhepatic recurrence is similar. Resection of locally or regional recurrent disease in 109 patients resulted in a 30% survival rate at 35 months [31]. Five-year survival rates for reresection of recurrent rectal cancer are somewhat worse, ranging from 9% to 14% [5]. Nonetheless, even pelvic exenteration or abdominal-sacral resections for pelvic recurrence can achieve cure rates of 30% to 50% in carefully selected patients [5]. Resection of isolated anastomotic recurrences is also often successful. Among 30 patients treated for anastomotic recurrences, 15 underwent successful complete reresection, and estimated 5-year survival was 49% [32]. Resection of pulmonary metastases from colorectal cancers results in a 5-year survival rate ranging from 30% to 40% [33,34]. These studies suggest that reresection of recurrent colorectal cancer will yield a 5-year survival rate of about one third for carefully selected patients.

Specific follow-up techniques

The goal of follow-up programs in patients who have undergone curative resections for colorectal cancers is "the detection of recurrent tumor at a stage when it is still curable" [35]. Consequently, follow-up efforts center on detection of recurrences in the liver, pelvis, lung, and anastomosis. These are pursued with a variety of methods. Some are aimed at detection of any recurrence, and others are site-specific. The yield for these modalities varies widely.

History and physical examination

A thorough history and physical examination often first reveals a recurrence. Camunas *et al.* [36] reported an initial suspicion of recurrences in 49% of patients based on history and physical examination in whom further evaluation demonstrated recurrent disease. This was also noted by Ovaska *et al.* [37], who detected clinical recurrence in 83% of patients prior to confirmation by standard diagnostic modalities.

Guaiac test

Testing stool for occult blood is a simple and inexpensive method of low sensitivity for the identification of intraluminal recurrences. Ahlquist [38] focused attention on the limitations of this study. Jahn *et al.* [39] found it to be positive in only three of nine patients who were shown to have local recurrence by colonoscopy. Crowson *et al.* [40] prospectively studied the efficacy of guaiac testing in 100 patients who had undergone surgical resection for colorectal cancer. Anastomotic recurrence was found in five of 14 patients who developed a positive guaiac test. Ahlquist *et al.* [41] evaluated 1217 patients who underwent annual surveillance after resection of a colorectal malignancy. Guaiac testing was found to be positive in only 21% of patients who were shown to have intraluminal recurrence by colonoscopy. These studies indicate that guaiac testing in the postoperative follow-up of patients after curative resections for colorectal cancers is a cheap but ineffective technique.

Colonoscopy

Colonoscopy is the most sensitive diagnostic modality for the detection of intraluminal malignancy and is usually included in the follow-up regimen after curative resection of a colorectal carcinoma. It provides direct visualization of an anastomotic recurrence and allows histologic confirmation [42]. Granquist and Karlsson [43] retrospectively evaluated 390 patients who had undergone surgical resection of a colorectal cancer. The first colonoscopy was performed 6 months postoperatively. The second examination was done 2 years later. The following examinations were performed every 4th year until the age of 70. Fourteen asymptomatic patients were found to have anastomotic recurrence (3.5%). Eleven recurrences were found within the first 6 months after surgery. Only eight (2%) patients, however, had disease that was amenable to surgery. The most striking finding of this study, however, was the identification of 12 (3%) new primary colorectal lesions. Periodic colonoscopy for the detection of suture line recurrence more than 1 year after surgical resection in asymptomatic patients may therefore be unwarranted. The disadvantages of colonoscopy also include patient discomfort, risk of perforation, bleeding, and expense [44]. Nonetheless, surveillance colonoscopy may be useful for the detection of metachronous lesions in patients who have been cured of their primary colorectal carcinoma.

Barium enema

The trend toward a "rightward shift" in primary colorectal cancers over the past 15 years has necessitated a more thorough postoperative investigation of the more proximal remaining large bowel [45]. A double-contrast study can identify 98% of the polyps greater than 1 cm in diameter found during colonoscopy [46]. Furthermore, barium enema has comparable accuracy to colonoscopy in the detection of colorectal carcinoma (Fig. 1). Its safety and cost-effectiveness may make it the preferred test in some patients [47].

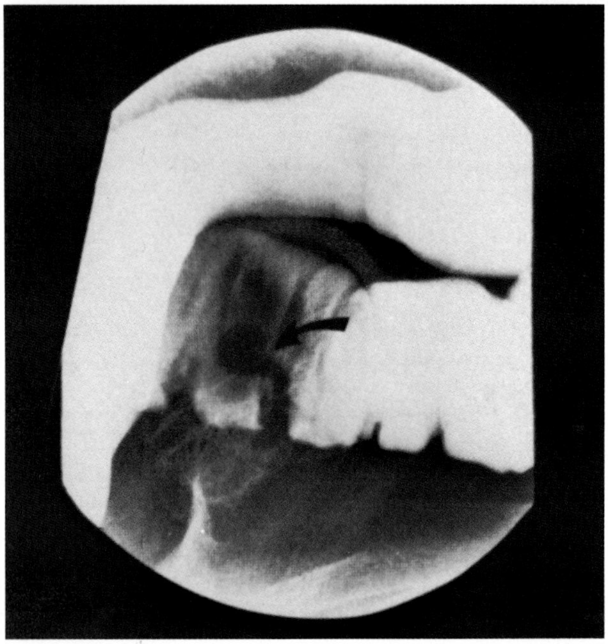

Fig. 1. Barium enema examination reveals a 1-cm pedunculated adenoma (*arrow*) in sigmoid colon. (*From* McCarty [47]; with permission.)

Endoscopic ultrasound

Endoscopic ultrasound has been of primary use in the staging of rectal cancer [48,49]. Endoscopic ultrasound is highly specific and sensitive in the detection of locally recurrent rectal carcinoma. Mascagni *et al.* [50] performed endoscopic ultrasound in 120 patients who underwent resection of a rectal carcinoma. It should be noted that in women who have undergone abdominal perineal resections, the pelvis can be assessed through the vagina. In the study by Mascagni *et al.*, local recurrence was detected in 17 (14%) patients; 5 (4%) were diagnosed by endovaginal ultrasonography, and 12 (10%) were diagnosed by endorectal sonography. Histologic confirmation was made by echo-guided biopsy. The authors reported 97% accuracy and 98% specificity.

In another study, 85 patients underwent surgical resection of a rectal carcinoma [51]. Twenty-two (26%) patients developed locally recurrent disease. Although local recurrence in 19 of the 22 (86%) patients was suspected by digital examination and sigmoidoscopy, endosonography was useful in making management decisions. Local recurrence was detected in three (3.5%) patients who had no other evidence of recurrent disease.

Hawes [52] has pointed out some of the limitations of endoscopic ultrasonography. The ultrasound characteristics of inflammation and malignancy are difficult to discern. The ability to assess microscopic involvement of tumor and lymph node recurrence is limited. The advantages of endorectal ultrasonography include high accuracy, low cost, absence of X-ray exposure, and minimal risks. Unfortunately, few individuals are trained in this technique at the present time.

Computed tomography

Computed tomography (CT) is useful in the detection of hepatic metastases of colorectal cancer. Abdominal CT scans with vascular contrast medium achieve greater sensitivity than magnetic resonance imaging (MRI) in the differentiation of metastatic liver lesions from benign processes. Assessment of extrahepatic colonic metastasis is more clearly made by CT than by MRI [53].

Computed tomography with arterial photography involves cannulation of the superior mesenteric artery via the femoral artery, and liver scanning done during delivery of contrast material [54]. In a study of over 100 patients, Karl *et al.* [55] found CT with arterial photography to be more sensitive than either conventional CT scan or CT scan 4 hours after administration of contrast material in the delineation of intrahepatic disease. Advances in the technique of abdominal CT scan continue to improve the sensitivity and specificity of this modality in the identification of recurrences of colorectal carcinoma.

Magnetic resonance imaging

Magnetic resonance contrast agents have added increased sensitivity and accuracy to conventional MRI in the detection of focal hepatic disease [56]. Mn-DPDP (manganese (II) N,N^{1}-dipyridoxylethylenediamine-N, N^{1}-diacetate $5,5^{1}$bis[phosphate]) is a hepatic-specific agent that is incorporated into normal hepatocytes, but not into tissue that lacks hepatocytes. Thus, tumors appear as negative defects and normal liver shows an increase in signal intensity [57]. In one multi-institutional study of Mn-DPDP, 96 patients with suspected or known focal hepatic tumors were evaluated with T1-weighted imaging parameters. More hepatic tumors were demonstrated by Mn-DPDP–enhanced T1-weighted imaging in 10 patients than were seen in both T1- and T2-weighted nonenhanced imaging [58].

In summary, nonenhanced MRI is inferior to Mn-DPDP–enhanced MRI in the detection of liver tumors [35]. Further studies may demonstrate comparable sensitivity and accuracy between CT with arterial photography and Mn-DPDP–enhanced MRI.

Immunoscintigraphy

Immunoscintigraphy is a promising new modality that permits the delineation of a malignancy through specific binding of radiolabeled monoclonal antibodies to tumor-associated antigens (Fig. 2). Its value in the preoperative stage and postoperative evaluation has been well described [59–61].

Collier *et al.* [62] evaluated 169 patients with colorectal cancer who underwent immunoscintigraphy, CT scan, and confirmatory laparotomy. Immunoscintigraphy was found to have greater sensitivity than CT scan in the detection of pelvic tumors (74% vs 57%; $P = 0.035$) and extrahepatic abdominal tumors (66% vs

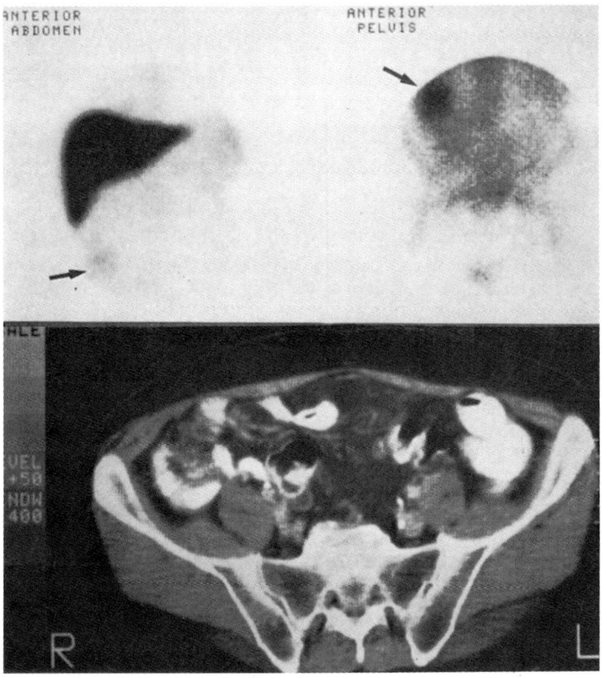

Fig. 2. Top, Demonstration of a monoclonal antibody–positive local recurrence (*arrows*) at the site of previous right hemicolectomy. (Patient had negative colonoscopy results.) **Bottom**, Computed tomographic scan fails to identify local recurrence. (*From* Doerr *et al.* [60]; with permission.)

34%; $P < 0.001$). Sensitivity of immunoscintigraphy was lower than that of CT scan in the detection of intrahepatic tumor recurrence. Griffin *et al.* [63] studied 23 patients who had undergone surgical resection of a colorectal carcinoma. All were suspected of having recurrent disease based on clinical evaluation or elevation of postoperative carcinoembryonic antigen (CEA) levels. Abdominal and pelvic CT showed no evidence of recurrence. Twenty patients were found to have abnormal antibody localization after injection of ^{111}In-labeled anti-CEA antibody. Accurate tumor localization was confirmed by biopsy in 19 patients. One author has suggested the use of immunoscintigraphy at regular intervals in the postoperative period in those patients who are at high risk for recurrence [64]. Further studies will be required to determine the clinical role of this technology.

Carcinoembryonic antigen

Carcinoembryonic antigen is an oncofetal antigen produced in several benign and malignant gastrointestinal conditions. CEA levels usually return to normal after curative resection. An elevated titer in the postoperative period may be associated with tumor recurrence and may warrant further evaluation [65]. Although this test has been a mainstay of postoperative follow-up for colorectal cancers, its effectiveness in the improvement of end results remains unproven.

Elevated preoperative CEA levels are associated with a higher risk of postoperative recurrence. Bohm *et al.* [66] identified recurrent disease in 56% of patients who had preoperative CEA levels greater than 5 ng/mL. Regression analysis showed an elevated preoperative CEA level to be an independent risk factor for recurrence.

A sustained postoperative elevation in CEA levels may have a particular significance in the detection of hepatic recurrence. Chu *et al.* [67] evaluated the distribution of colorectal cancer recurrences by site of recurrence in 132 patients. Of 45 patients who developed liver recurrence, 87% had postoperative CEA levels greater than 10 ng/mL. Locoregional recurrence was detected in 46 patients. Fifty-five percent of these patients had postoperative CEA levels over 10 ng/mL. Of those patients who developed pulmonary recurrence, postoperative CEA levels higher than 10 ng/mL were found in only 48%.

When directly compared, CEA identifies more recurrences than do liver function studies. Rocklin *et al.* [68] retrospectively analyzed CEA titers and liver function studies in 92 patients who developed liver recurrence after resection of a colorectal cancer. CEA was found to be elevated more often than any other liver function study.

Recently, the value of CEA in the detection of surgically curable recurrences of colorectal cancer was examined [69]. A total of 1017 patients who had undergone curative resections for Dukes B_2 and C colon cancers were followed up with CEA assays. These patients were all enrolled in national surgical adjuvant trials in which CEA monitoring was elective. Recurrent colon cancer developed in 417 (41%). The CEA was elevated in only 247 (59%) before symptoms developed and, thus, the rate of false-negative levels of CEA was 41%. Sixteen percent of 600 patients without recurrence of colorectal cancer developed false-positive elevations of CEA. Elevated levels of CEA led to the surgical exploration of 115 (11.3% of 1017) patients but curative resections, usually of hepatic metastases, were accomplished in only 47 (4.6%) patients. Eleven (1%) of these patients remained clinically free of further recurrence 1 year after the salvage operation. In contrast, 38 (3.7% of 1017) patients with normal CEA levels underwent surgical exploration and curative resections were accomplished in 23 (2.2%). Similarly, 23 of 199 (11.5%) patients not followed up with CEA also underwent curative resections for recurrent disease. In the patients with nonelevated levels of CEA, curative resections were usually performed for pulmonary or local recurrences. The rates of disease-free intervals for the CEA-normal patients and the patients not followed-up with CEA were similar to the rates for the patients followed up with CEA. The authors concluded that "cancer cures attributable to CEA monitoring are, at best, infrequent. It is questionable whether this small gain justifies the substantial cost in dollars and physical and emotional stress that this intervention may cause for patients."

Other tumor markers

Several other tumor-associated antigens may be helpful in the diagnosis of initial or recurrent disease [70,71].

Haglund *et al.* [72] compared the sensitivity of CA 19-9 and CA 50 for the detection of colorectal cancer recurrences in 24 patients. At the time of clinically recurrent disease, 46% of patients had elevated CA 19-9 levels, and 38% had elevated CA 50 levels. These tumor markers also are present in a variety of benign and malignant gastrointestinal conditions [72]. Plasma prolactin levels in recurrent disease have been shown to have a predictive value of 94% by Bhatavdekar *et al.* [73]. In another study, serum arginase levels were found to be significantly elevated in 31 patients with colorectal cancer in comparison with control subjects [74]. The clinical utility of these new tumor markers remains unproven.

Value of postoperative surveillance

The end results of intensive follow-up of patients following curative resections have been studied intensely. The investigators all shared the hope that they would improve 5-year survival for their patients by detecting recurrences at an early curable, *ie*, resectable, stage. Unfortunately, improvement of end results has proven to be an elusive Holy Grail.

Beart *et al.* [75] prospectively monitored 149 patients following curative resections for Dukes B_2 and C colorectal cancers at the Mayo Clinic. Patients were examined at least every 15 weeks. Patients were followed up from 1 to 3 years. Recurrences were detected in 34 (23%) patients. No resectable recurrences were detected. Outcome was not improved for a single patient.

Camunas *et al.* [36] in Madrid, Spain, prospectively evaluated the efficacy of postoperative monitoring in 151 (61%) patients who had undergone curative procedures for Dukes A, B, and C tumors of 246 patients treated for colorectal cancers. All patients were followed up for a minimum of 2 years. Evaluation took place every 2 to 3 months and included history, physical examination, blood tests, and CEA assay. Yearly chest radiographs and liver ultrasonography were performed. CT scans, colonoscopy, and barium enemas were also performed but not on a set protocol. Six resectable recurrences were identified: three of these patients were alive at 40, 43, and 69 months of follow-up. Despite this intensive follow-up, only three patients went on to have potentially curative second procedures. Thus, follow-up improved survival for 2% of the followed group but only 1% of the entire group of colorectal cancer patients.

Ovaska *et al.* [37] in Helsinki, Finland, retrospectively evaluated 402 patients from a group of 527 patients who had undergone curative surgery for colorectal cancer. A total of 709 patients had been treated for colorectal cancer during this time period. All patients were seen every 3 months for history, physical examination, blood test, CEA assay, stool guaiac test, and sigmoidoscopy. Chest radiographs and barium enemas were obtained every 6 months. Recurrent disease was found in 120 patients (30% of followed group). Twenty-six patients (6% of followed group) underwent reoperation with curative intent. They reported only 14 (3.5%) disease-free survivors. These efforts improved survival for 3.5% of the patients in the follow-up program but only 2% of the entire group of colorectal cancer patients.

Similar results were reported by Bohm *et al.* [66] who followed up 487 patients after curative surgery. All patients were seen every 3 months for a minimum of 2 years. Patients underwent histories and physicals, CEA assays, blood tests, and abdominal sonography every 3 months. Chest radiographs, rigid sigmoidoscopies, and colonoscopies, or barium enemas were obtained every 6 months. Recurrent cancer was discovered in 149 patients (31%). Only 36 patients (7%) underwent further curative surgery, nine (1.8%) of whom remained free of recurrent disease for more than 2 years.

Safi *et al.* [4] also noted the poor outcome of intensive postoperative surveillance. Over an 11-year period, 1050 patients underwent curative surgery for colorectal cancer. Recurrence was detected in 350 patients (33%) over a median time period of 9 to 14 months. A curative reoperation was performed in 56 (5%) patients. At the time of publication, 17 (1.6%) patients remained free of disease. Intensive postoperative surveillance permitted earlier detection of recurrent disease. However, few patients benefitted from such rigorous surveillance. These studies demonstrate that intensive and expensive efforts to detect early recurrence of colorectal cancer following curative resections will result in improved survival for at best 3% of the followed patients but for only about 1% to 2% of all colorectal cancer patients. In the vast majority of patients, these efforts serve to identify incurable disease.

Conclusions

The best strategy for the postoperative follow-up of patients after curative resection for colorectal cancers depends on the goals of the program. The greater the frequency of history and physical examinations, blood tests, CEA assays, imaging studies, and endoscopies, the earlier recurrences will be identified and the more that will be identified in asymptomatic patients. Unfortunately, few patients will benefit from this strategy. Moreover, there is little evidence to indicate that identification of the recurrent carcinoma at an asymptomatic stage makes any significant impact on outcome [76]. Indeed, survival of patients with symptomatic recurrences who can undergo reresection is similar to that of asymptomatic patients. Finally, the real outcome of intensive efforts of follow-up for the overwhelming majority of patients with recurrence of disease is the confirmation at an earlier time that they have developed untreatable disease. Consequently, although resection remains the only modality for the treatment of recurrent colorectal cancer, there is virtually no justification for intensive programs for follow-up. The only exception would be the investigational setting, in which new therapies for the identification or treatment of recurrent colorectal cancers are being studied.

Two methods of follow-up seem appropriate in non-investigational therapy. In the first, the patient undergoes a history and physical examination by his primary health care physician every 3 months for 2 years and then yearly. If the patient underwent a curative resection for sigmoid or rectal cancer with the construction of a colorectal anastomosis, a rigid or flexible sigmoidoscopy is included as part of the physical examination. When the patient develops symptoms or evidence of a recurrence is detected by physical examination, imaging techniques are used to determine whether the recurrence is resectable.

A second strategy eliminates routine follow-up all together. The patient is instructed about symptoms of recurrent disease. When symptoms develop, the patient returns to his or her primary care physician for evaluation.

Ideally, these two strategies should be compared in a randomized prospective study. Because of the expected low frequency of resectable recurrences and the even smaller chances of long-term survival, the number of patients required for entry into the two study groups would be extremely large. Consequently, it is unlikely that any feasible study will show a significant difference between these two strategies. Similarly, it is unlikely that any significant difference would be demonstrated if a third intensive follow-up arm was included in a proposed randomized trial.

This review does not address the issue of identification of metachronous colorectal cancers in patients who have previously undergone curative resections for colorectal cancers. This topic has been addressed by others [36,44].

References and recommended reading

Papers of particular interest, published within the annual period of review, have been highlighted as:

- • Of special interest
- •• Of outstanding interest

1. Greenwald P: **Colon Cancer Overview.** *Cancer* 1992, **70**(suppl 5):1206–1215.
2. Boring CC, Squire TS, Tong T: **Cancer Statistics.** *CA Cancer J Clin* 1992, **42**:19–38.
3. Ballantyne GH, Modlin IM: **Postoperative Follow-Up for Colorectal Cancer: Who Are We Kidding?** *J Clin Gastroenterol* 1988, **10**:359–364.
4. Safi F, Link KH, Beger HG: **Is Follow-Up of Colorectal Cancer Patients Worthwhile?** *Dis Colon Rectum* 1993, **36**:636–644.
5. Turk PS, Wanebo HJ: **Results of Surgical Treatment of Nonhepatic Recurrence of Colorectal Carcinoma.** *Cancer* 1993, **71**(suppl 12):4267–4277.
6. Steele G Jr: **Standard Postoperative Monitoring of Patients After Primary Resection of Colon and Rectum Cancer.** *Cancer* 1993, **71**(suppl 12):4225–4235.
7. Ballantyne GH, Quin J: **Surgical Treatment of Liver Metastasis in Patients With Colorectal Cancer.** *Cancer* 1993, **71**(suppl 12):4252–4266.
8. **Trends in Colorectal Cancer Incidence: United States.** *MMWR Morb Mortal Wkly Rep* 1989, **38**:728–731.
9. Shapiro S: **Goals of Screening.** *Cancer* 1992, **70**:1252–1258.
10. Cass AW, Million RR, Pfaff WW: **Pattern of Recurrence Following Surgery Alone for Adenocarcinoma of the Colon and Rectum.** *Cancer* 1976, **37**:2861–2865.
11. Sugarbaker PH, Gianola FJ, Dwyer A, Neuman N: **A Simplified Plan for Follow-Up of Patients With Colon and Rectal Cancer Supported by Prospective Studies of Laboratory and Radiologic Test Results.** *Surgery* 1987, **102**:79–87.
12. Bleday R, Wong WD: **Recent Advances in Surgery for Colon and Rectal Cancer.** *Curr Probl Cancer* 1993, **17**:1–68.
13. Niederhuber JE: **Colon and Rectum Cancer: Patterns of Spread and Implications for Workup.** *Cancer* 1993, **71**(suppl 12):4187–4192.
14. • Galandiuk S, Wieand HS, Moertel CG, Cha SS, Fitzgibbons RJ Jr, Pemberton JH, Wolff BG: **Patterns of Recurrence After Curative Resections of Carcinoma of the Colon and Rectum.** *Surg Gyncecol Obstet* 1992, **174**:27–32.

The authors present data on 818 patients who underwent curative resection for Dukes B_2 and Dukes C tumors. Patterns of recurrence are discussed.

15. •• Olson RM, Perencevich NP, Malcolm AW, Chaffey JT, Wilson RE: **Patterns of Recurrence Following Resection of Adenocarcinoma of the Colon and Rectum.** *Cancer* 1980, **45**:2969–2974.

The authors report the outcome of 818 patients who underwent resection for colorectal carcinoma. Data concerning sites of first recurrence and tumor stage are presented. Patterns and rates of recurrence are discussed.

16. Pilipshen SJ, Heilweil M, Quan SH, Sternberg SS, Enker WE: **Patterns of Pelvic Recurrence Following Definitive Resection of Rectal Cancer.** *Cancer* 1984, **53**:1354–1362.
17. Willett CG, Tepper JE, Cohen AM, Orlow E, Welch CE: **Failure Patterns Following Curative Resection of Colonic Carcinoma.** *Ann Surg* 1984, **200**:685–690.
18. Wanebo HJ, Semoglou C, Attiyeh F, Stearns MJ Jr: **Surgical Management of Patients With Primary Operable Colorectal Cancer and Synchronous Liver Metastases.** *Am J Surg* 1978, **135**:81–85.
19. Lahr CJ, Soong SJ, Cloud G, Smith JW, Urist MM, Balch CM: **A Multifactorial Analysis of Prognostic Factors in Patients With Liver Metastases From Colorectal Carcinoma.** *J Clin Oncol* 1983, **1**:720–725.
20. Mascagni D, Corbellini L, Di Matteo G: **Endoluminal Ultrasound for Early Detection of Local Recurrence of Rectal Cancer.** *Br J Surg* 1989, **76**:1176–1180.
21. Pihl E, Hughes ES, McDermott FT, Johnson WR, Katrrivessis H: **Lung Recurrence After Curative Surgery for Colorectal Cancer.** *Dis Colon Rectum* 1987, **30**:417–419.
22. Goya T, Miyasawa N, Kondo H, Tsuchiya R, Naruler T, Svemoser K: **Surgical Resection of Pulmonary Metastases From Colorectal Cancer.** *Cancer* 1989, **64**:1418–1421.
23. McAfee MK, Allen MS, Trastek VF, Ilstrup DM, Deschamps C, Pairolero PC: **Colorectal Lung Metastases: Results of Surgical Excision.** *Ann Thorac Surg* 1992, **53**:780–786.
24. • Malcolm AW, Perencevich NP, Olson RM, Hanley JA, Chaffey JT, Wilson RE: **Analysis of Recurrence Patterns Following Curative Resections for Carcinoma of the Colon and Rectum.** *Surg Gynecol Obstet* 1981, **152**:131–136.

Data regarding 139 patients who underwent resection of colorectal lung metastasis are presented. The authors discuss their indications for resection.

25. Rodriguez-Bigas MA, Stulc JP, Davidson B, Petrelli NJ: **Prognostic Significance of Anastomotic Recurrence From Colorectal Adenocarcinoma.** *Dis Colon Rectum* 1992, **35**:838–842.
26. Welch JP, Donaldson GA: **Detection and Treatment of Recurrent Cancer of the Colon and Rectum.** *Am J Surg* 1978, **135**:505–511.
27. MacKeigan J, Ferguson J: **Prophylactic Oophorectomy and Colorectal Cancer in Premenopausal Patients.** *Dis Colon Rectum* 1979, **22**:401–405.
28. Blamey SL, McDermott FT, Pihl E, Hughes ESR: **Resected Ovarian Recurrence From Colorectal Adenocarcinoma: A Study of 13 Cases.** *Dis Colon Rectum* 1981, **24**:272–275.
29. Ballantyne GH, Reigel M, Wolff B, Ilstrup DM: **Oophorectomy and Colon Cancer: Impact on Survival.** *Ann Surg* 1985, **202**:209–214.
30. • Austgen TR, Souba WW, Bland KI: **Reoperation for Colorectal Carcinoma.** *Surg Clin North Am* 1991, **71**:175–189.

The authors discuss diagnostic indicators and methods of detection for recurrent disease.

31. Schiessel R, Wunderlich M, Herbst F: **Local Recurrence of Colorectal Cancer: Effect of Early Detection and Aggressive Surgery.** *Br J Surg* 1986, **73**:342–344.
32. Vassilopoulos PP, Yoon JM, Ledesma EJ, Mittelman A: **Treatment of Recurrence of Adenocarcinoma of the Colon and Rectum at the Anastomotic Site.** *Surg Gynecol Obstet* 1981, **152**:777–780.
33. Tomoyuki G, Miyazawa N, Kondo H, Tsuchiya R, Naruke T, Seumasu K: **Surgical Resection of Pulmonary Metastases From Colorectal Cancer.** *Cancer* 1989, **64**:1418–1421.

34. McAfee MK, Allen MS, Trastek VF, Ilstrup DM, Deschamps C, Pairolero PC: Colorectal Lung Metastases: Results of Surgical Excision. *Ann Thorac Surg* 1992, 53:780–786.

35. Vignati PV, Roberts PL: Preoperative Evaluation and Postoperative Surveillance for Patients With Colorectal Carcinoma. *Surg Clin North Am* 1993, 73:67–84.

36. Camunas J, Enriquez JM, Devesa JM, Morales V, Millan I: Value of Follow-Up in the Management of Recurrent Colorectal Cancer. *Eur J Surg Oncol* 1991, 17:530–535.

37. Ovaska JT, Jarvinen HJ, Merklin JP: The Value of a Follow-Up Program After Radical Surgery for Colorectal Carcinoma. *Scand J Gastroenterol* 1989, 24:416–422.

38. Ahlquist DA: Occult Blood Screening. *Cancer* 1992, 70(suppl):1259–1265.

39. Jahn H, Joergensen OD, Kronborg O, Fenger C: Can Hemocult-II Replace Colonoscopy in Surveillance After Radical Surgery for Colorectal Cancer and After Polypectomy? *Dis Colon Rectum* 1992, 35:253–256.

40. Crowson MC, Jewkes AJ, Acheson N, Fielding J: Haemoccult Testing as an Indicator of Recurrent Colorectal Cancer: A Five-Year Prospective Study. *Eur J Surg Oncol* 1991, 17:281–284.

41. Ahlquist DA, Wieand HS, Moertel CG, McGill DB, Loprinzi CL, O'Connell MJ, Mailliard JA, Gerstner JB, Pandya K, Ellefson RD: Accuracy of Fecal Occult Blood Screening for Colorectal Neoplasia: A Prospective Study Using Hemocult and Hemo Quant Tests. *JAMA* 1993, 269:1262–1267.

42. Gowen GF: The Impact of Colonoscopy on Colorectal Carcinoma. *Am Surg* 1991, 57:254–257.

43. Granquist S, Karlsson T: Postoperative Follow-Up of Patients With Colorectal Carcinoma by Colonoscopy. *Eur J Surg* 1992, 158:307–312.

44. Stevenson GW: Radiology and Endoscopy in the Pretreatment Diagnostic Management of Colorectal Cancer. *Cancer* 1993, 71:4198–4206.

45. Sariego J, Burd ME, Kerstein M, Sano C, Matsumoto T: Changing Patterns in Colorectal Carcinoma: A 25-Year Experience. *Am Surg* 58:686–691.

46. Dodd GD: The Role of Barium Enema in the Detection of Colonic Neoplasms. *Cancer* 1992, 70(suppl 5):1272–1275.

47. MacCarty RL: Colorectal Cancer: The Case for the Barium Enema. *Mayo Clin Proc* 1992, 67:253–257.

48. Tio TL, Weijers O, Hulsman F, Jonkers L, Collins E, Sie LH, Tytgat GNJ: Endosonography of Colorectal Diseases. *Endoscopy* 1992, 24(suppl 1):309–314.

49. Cohen JL, Grotz RL, Welch JP, Deckers PJ: Intrarectal Sonography: A New Technique for the Assessment of Rectal Tumors. *Am Surg* 1991, 57:459–462.

50. Mascagni D, Corbellini L, Urciaoli P, DiMatteo G: Endoluminal Ultrasound for Early Detection of Local Recurrence of Rectal Cancer. *Br J Surg* 1989, 76:1176–1180.

51. Beynon J, Mortensen NJ McC, Foy DMA, Channer JL, Rigby H, Virgee J: The Detection and Evaluation of Locally Recurrent Rectal Cancer With Rectal Endosonography. *Dis Colon Rectum* 1989, 32:509–517.

52. Hawes RH: New Staging Techniques. *Cancer* 1993, 71(suppl 12):4207–4213.

53. Taylor AJ, Youker JE: Imaging in Colorectal Carcinoma. *Semin Oncol* 1991, 18:99–110.

54. Charnsangavej C: New Imaging Modalities for Follow-Up of Colorectal Carcinoma. *Cancer* 1993, 71:4236–4240.

55. Karl RC, Morse SS, Halpert RD, Clark RA: Preoperative Evaluation of Patients for Liver Research: Appropriate CT Imaging. *Ann Surg* 1993, 217:226–232.

56. Collier DB: New Radiographic Techniques for Colorectal Cancer. *Cancer* 1993, 71:4214–4216.

57. Bernardino ME, Young SW, Lee JKT, Weinred JC: Hepatic MR Imaging With Mn-DPDP: Safety, Image Quality, and Sensitivity. *Radiology* 1992, 183:53–58.

58. Hamm B, Vogl TJ, Branding G, Schnell B, Taupitz M, Wolf K, Lissner J: Focal Liver Lesions. MR Imaging With Mn-DPDP: Initial Clinical Results in 40 Patients. *Radiology* 1992, 182:167–174.

59. Patt YZ, Podoloff DA, Curley S, Smith R, Badkhamkar VA, Lamki L, Jessup MM, Hohn DC: Monoclonal Antibody Imaging in Patients With Colorectal Cancer and Increasing Levels of Serum Carcinoembryonic Antigen. *Cancer* 1993, 71:4293–4297.

60. Doerr RJ, Herrera L, Abdel-Nabi H: In-III CYT-103 Monoclonal Antibody Imaging in Patients With Suspected Recurrent Colorectal Cancer. *Cancer* 1993, 71:4241–4247.

61. Doerr RJ, Abdel-Nabi H, Krag D, Mitchel E: Radiolabeled Antibody Imaging in the Management of Colorectal Cancer. *Ann Surg* 1991, 314:118–124.

62. Collier DB, Abdel-Nabi H, Doerr R, Harwood SJ, Olsen J, Kaplan EH, Winzelberg GG, Grossman SJ, Krag DN, Mitchell EP: Immunoscintigraphy Performed With In-III-Labeled CYT-103 in the Management of Colorectal Cancer: Comparison With CT. *Radiology* 1993, 185:179–186.

63. Griffin TW, Brill AB, Stevens S, Collins JA, Bokhari F, Bushe H, Stochl MC, Gionet M, Rusckowski M, Stroupe SD, *et al.*: Initial Clinical Study of Indium-111-Labeled Clone 110 Anticarcinoembryonic Antigen Antibody in Patients With Colorectal Cancer. *J Clin Oncol* 1991, 9:631–640.

64. Galandiuk S: Immunoscintigraphy in the Surgical Management of Colorectal Cancer. *J Nucl Med* 1993, 34:541–544.

65. Hackford AW: Biochemical Markers for Colorectal Cancer: Diagnostic and Therapeutic Implications. *Surg Clin North Am* 1993, 73:85–102.

66. Bohm B, Schwenk W, Hucke HP, Stock W: Does Methodologic Long-Term Follow-Up Affect Survival After Curative Resection of Colorectal Carcinoma. *Dis Colon Rectum* 1993, 36:281–286.

67. Chu DZ, Erickson CA, Russell MP, Thompson C, Lang NP, Broadwater RJ, Westbrook KC: Prognostic Significance of Carcinoembryonic Antigen in Colorectal Carcinoma. *Arch Surg* 1991, 126:314–316.

68. Rocklin MS, Senagore AJ, Talbott TM: Role of Carcinoembryonic Antigen and Liver Function Tests in the Detection of Recurrent Colorectal Carcinoma. *Dis Colon Rectum* 1991, 34:794–797.

69. Moertel CG, Fleming TR, Macdonald JS, Haller DG, Laurie JA, Tangen C: An Evaluation of the Carcinoembryonic Antigen (CEA) Test for Monitoring Patients With Resected Colon Cancer. *JAMA* 1993, 270:943–947.

70. Angel CA, Pratt CB, Bhaskar NR, Schell MJ, Parham DM, Lobe TE, Fleming ID: Carcinoembryonic Antigen and Carbohydrate 19-9 Antigen as Markers for Colorectal Carcinoma in Children and Adolescents. *Cancer* 1992, 69:1487–1491.

71. van der Schow YT, Verbeek AL, Wobbes T, Segers MF, Thomas CM: Comparison of Four Serum Tumor Markers in the Diagnosis of Colorectal Carcinoma. *Br J Cancer* 1992, 66:148–154.

72. Haglund C, Roberts PJ, Jalanko H, Kuusela P: Tumor Markers CA 19-9 and CA 50 in Digestive Tract Malignancies. *Scand J Gastroenterol* 1992, 29:169–174.

73. Bhatavdekar JM, Partel DD, Giri DD, Karelia NH, Vora HH, Ghosh N, Shah NG, Trivedi SN, Balar DB: Comparison of Plasma Prolactin and CEA in Monitoring Patients With Adenocarcinoma of Colon and Rectum. *Br J Cancer* 1992, 66:977–980.

74. Leu SY, Wang SR: Clinical Significance of Arginase in Colorectal Cancer. *Cancer* 1992, 70:733–736.

75. Beart RW Jr, Metzger PP, O'Connell, Schutt AJ: Postoperative Screening of Patients With Carcinoma of the Colon. *Dis Colon Rectum* 1981, 24:585–588.

76. Lawrence W Jr: Summary of Workshop. *Cancer* 1993, 71(suppl 12):4314–4321.

Carina G. Biggs, MD, and Garth H. Ballantyne, MD, Department of Surgery, Yale University School of Medicine, 333 Cedar Street, PO Box 3333, New Haven, CT 06510, USA.

Rare anorectal pathologic conditions

J. Denis, MD, R. Ganansia, MD, and T. Puy-Montbrun, MD

Hôpital Leopold Bellan, Paris, France

Among the rare anorectal pathologic conditions published in the literature since 1992, except for malignant pathology, we have taken an interest in anal dermatology with Hailey-Hailey disease; infectious diseases, including tuberculosis, gangrene, actinomycosis, and cytomegalovirus ulcerations; vascular pathology with rectal varices and tumoral pathology with leiomyomas and lipomas; embryologic disorders, including gastric and salivary heterotopia; and a few exceptional lesions, such as spontaneous hematomas and certain traumatic lesions.

Current Opinion in General Surgery 1994:103–107

Hailey-Hailey disease

Described for the first time in 1939, Hailey-Hailey disease is an autosomal dominantly transmitted hereditary disease affecting the skin, and more rarely, the mucosa [1••,2•,3–5]. Histologically, the disease is characterized by a widespread suprabasal keratinocyte acantholysis. Ultrastructural study reveals a breakdown of desmosome-keratin filament complexes of uncertain pathogenesis, but possibly resulting from an anomaly in one of the constituents of the desmosomes. Hailey-Hailey disease usually makes its appearance during the third decade, with neither sex predominating. Diagnosis is frequently made late in the disease course. The lesions are found predominantly on the neck, in the armpits, and in the groin but more rarely may affect the anal region. Although the classic clinical presentation comprises a growth of bullae or vesicles, the atypical presentations occur very frequently, especially in the case of the anus, where verrucoid papules may be encountered. The verrucoid papules have frequently been misdiagnosed as anogenital warts. Their character is all the more deceptive in that the anal localization may be isolated, and the hereditary character is not always known.

In this context, it may assist diagnosis to examine the nails, which in 70% of cases exhibit asymptomatic white bands. These bands are different from those observed in patients with Darier's disease or with tumors of the nail matrix. Sometimes, the manifestation may be a candidiasis in the groove between the buttocks or other intertriginous sites, and the lesions are aggravated by heat, trauma, friction, and sweating.

Diagnosis is based on histologic examination, which reveals the characteristic intraepidermal acantholysis in all layers of the spinous zone. The existence of hyperkeratosis and acanthosis is correlated with the verrucoid clinical aspect. Histology can also exclude Darier's disease, which is not always easy to differentiate in the clinical diagnosis.

The treatment is essentially corticoid administration in the form of topical ointments applied continually or as required, often in association with topical antibiotics or oral antibiotics taken in prolonged, low doses.

In addition to these classic treatments, which are known to be effective, other treatments have been proposed: full-thickness excision of the lesions with grafting, dermabrasion, destruction of the lesions by carbon dioxide laser, and more recently, topically applied cyclosporine, which has not yet been used on a large enough sample to generalize the results.

Anal tuberculosis

Anal tuberculosis [6,7,8•] was very common prior to the introduction of antituberculous drugs. Sixteen percent of all fistulas in ano were tuberculous, and 80% of anal fistulas in tuberculosis patients resulted from anal tuberculosis involvement (Fig. 1). The incidence of tuberculosis decreased after 1950, but we now have a recrudescence in the immigrant population and, in our experience, in HIV-infected patients. Gastrointestinal tuberculosis comprises fewer than 1% of all cases of tuberculosis, and anal involvement is reported to occur in 10% of gastrointestinal tuberculosis. Usually, anal localization occurs in patients with tuberculosis in the lung; we have never seen primary anal location. Awareness is the prerequisite for correct diagnosis. The symptoms are not characteristic: anal and abdominal pain, blood or pus discharge, diarrhea, fever, and weight loss. Physical examination most frequently reveals ulcerations

(Fig. 2), multiple fistulas, and rarely, verrucous lesions and, in the rectum, a pseudotumoral aspect. Anorectal tuberculosis must be distinguished from other lesions (*eg*, mycoses, sarcoidosis, carcinoma, granuloma of foreign bodies, and Crohn's disease).

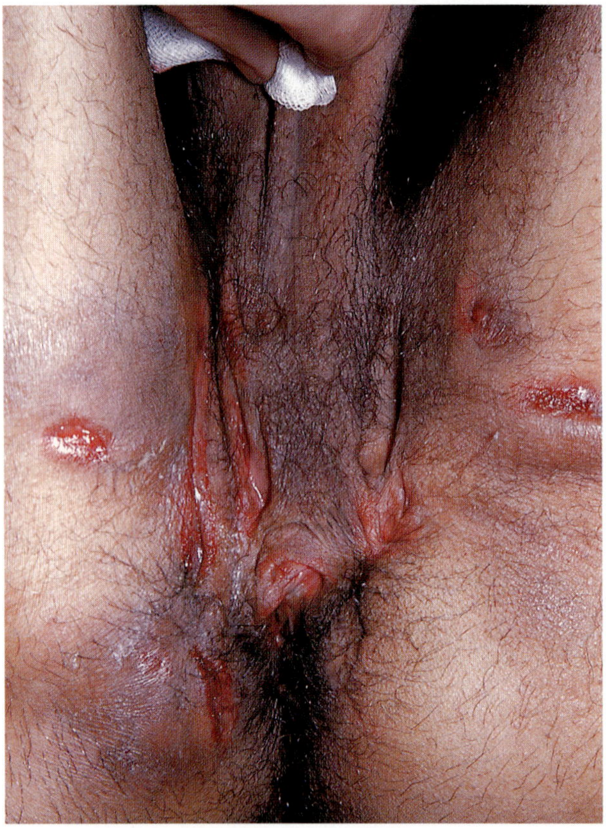

Fig. 1. Tubercular polyfistulous perineum.

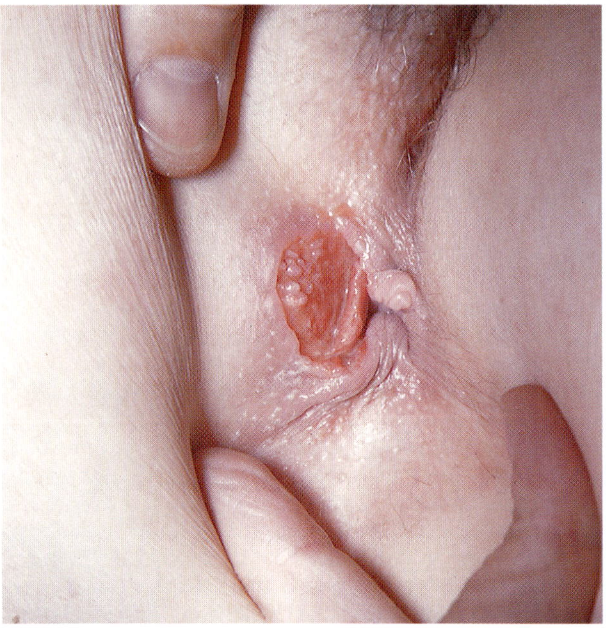

Fig. 2. Anal tuberculosis ulceration.

At histologic examination, the differential diagnosis from Crohn's disease is difficult: the presence of caseous necrosis and acid-fast bacilli establishes the correctness of the diagnosis. Pus should be cultured, and biopsies should be performed. The performance of chest radiography, tuberculin skin tests, sputum analysis, and colonoscopy is recommended. Treatment of anal tuberculosis consists of drainage of the abscess and administration of a multiple antituberculosis drugs.

Fournier's gangrene

Perineal necrotizing fasciitis, or Fournier's gangrene (Fig. 3) is a synergistic infection with toxicity that destroys soft tissues, initially in a single plane [9•,10••]. Since Fournier discovered this gangrene in 1883, only 500 cases have been reported. The most common predisposing factors are genitourinary infection and perianal abscess, preferentially in patients with diabetes mellitus, HIV, or cancer.

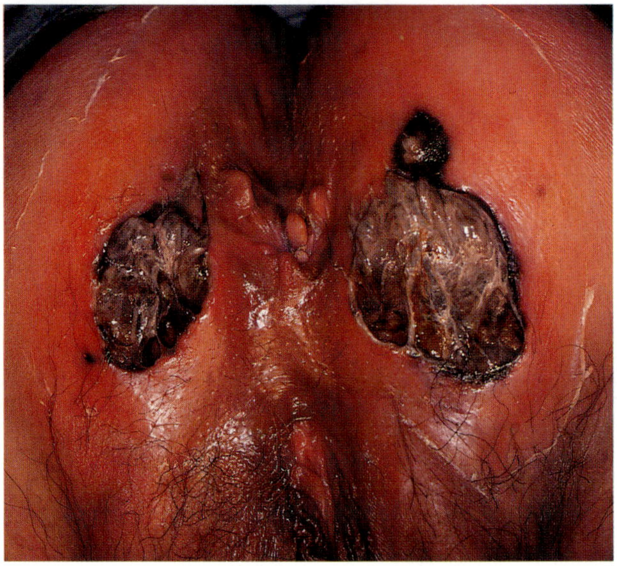

Fig. 3. Fournier's gangrene of the perineum. (*Courtesy of* P. Suduca, Toulouse, France.)

The first symptoms of Fournier's gangrene are pain or itching of rapid development, tenderness, swelling, necrotic skin, and enlarged scrotum. There is local crepitation in more than half the patients, and signs of systemic toxicity appear. The bacteriology is complex: anaerobic bacteria act in synergism with the aerobes; *Bacteroides fragilis* peptostreptococci, and *Escherichia coli* are the organisms most often cultured. *Clostridium perfringens* in Fournier's gangrene is rare, in contrast with gas gangrene, which involves all tissue.

The treatment for Fournier's gangrene includes surgery with excision of the clearly necrotic tissue and incisions in the area of compromised viability; antibiotic therapy must provide a broad spectrum of aerobic and anaerobic coverage. In addition, hyperbaric oxygen therapy at 2.5 atm for 120 minutes three times during the first 24 hours, then repeated twice daily has been described with good results.

Actinomycosis

Actinomyces species, gram-positive aerobic and anaerobic bacteria, have been misclassified in the past as a fungus. This species is a very unusual cause of anorectal suppuration as fistulas and chronic sinus tract even after appropriate surgical treatment. It presents as an indolent, hard, woody, nonfluent mass generally in patients with diabetes mellitus or in an immunocompromised state [11••].

Actinomycosis should be suspected when the suppuration contains small yellow particles in the purulent material: the sulfur granules consist of tiny bacterial colonies with a central core of intertwined branching filaments with club-shaped bodies at the periphery. These colonies are arranged spherically, creating a sunburst pattern.

Both surgical and antibiotic (penicillin or tetracycline) therapy are necessary to achieve complete eradication of actinomycotic infection.

Cytomegalovirus ulcerations

Cytomegalovirus ulceration (Fig. 4) constitutes another rare infection of the anus, occurring in immunodepressed patients infected with HIV [12•]. Invariably painful, the ulcerations may be single or multiple and may affect the anal margin, the anal canal, or both. Diagnosis is made from the histologic results rather than from culture. Treatment for cytomegalovirus ulcerations is by ganciclovir or foscarnet. However, relapse may occur when treatment ceases.

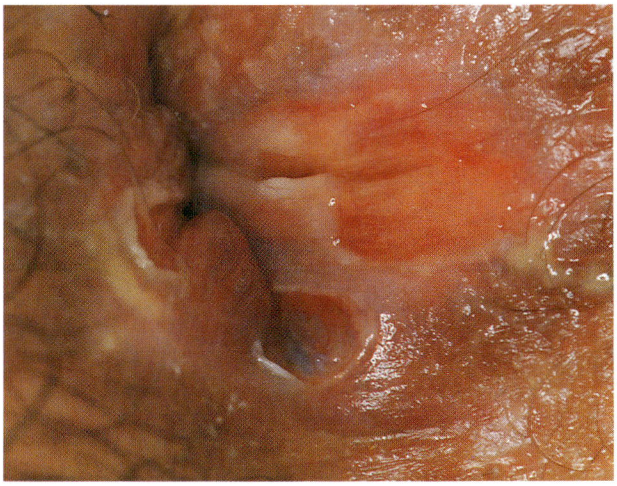

Fig. 4. Cytomegalovirus ulceration.

Anorectal varices

Anorectal varices are present in 44% to 99% of patients with portal hypertension. However, in this population, the frequency of hemorrhoids is the same as in the general population. The distinction between anorectal varices and hemorrhoids is clinically important because bleeding of anorectal varices can cause massive and fatal hemorrhage. Bleeding of the varices occurs in only 0.5% to 5.6% of cases, and its cause is unclear.

At endoscopic examination, the varices are blue-gray, 3 to 6 mm in diameter, and appear in the lower part of the rectum or in the anal canal; they do not prolapse, and they deflate with pressure. Transrectal ultrasonographic examination shows multiple, tortuous vascular structures. Magnetic resonance venography can also demonstrate prominent rectal varices, as distinct from hemorrhoids. These two noninvasive procedures allow follow-up after treatment for the condition.

The optimal therapy for anorectal varices has not yet been well defined. Cryosurgery and sclerotherapy can be dangerous. Suture of varices can be used to control bleeding, and recently, portal decompression with a transjugular intrahepatic shunt has been used with success [13,14,15•].

Rectal leiomyoma

Rectal myomatous tumors [16•,17] represent 0.1% to 0.6% of all benign and malignant rectal tumors. The symptoms are not characteristic: pain, the sensation of a foreign body in the rectum, and blood or mucus with the stools. The tumor is located in the lower part of the rectum; the size varies from 0.3 to 20 cm, usually around 5 cm (Fig. 5). At digital examination, leiomyoma has a dense, elastic consistency and is well limited. Biopsy is difficult to perform and is of little interest because the mucosa above the tumor is intact and mobile. Intrarectal ultrasound, radiography, and endoscopy show the tumor but fail to distinguish between leiomyoma and leiomyosarcoma. The probability of malignant transformation varies from 0 to 19.4%. The choice of surgical treatment depends on the size and localization of the tumor. Options are endoscopic electroexcision, transanal resection, and, for very large tumors, abdominorectal resection. Recurrence is possible.

Lipomas

Lipomas [18,19] are the most common tumors of the colon after adenomatous polyps, but location in the rectosigmoid is observed only in about 4% of cases. They are frequently asymptomatic and are accidental findings. The submucosal development of a lipoma can make a pedicle, and it can prolapse through the anal canal as a soft, rounded, yellow tumoral mass (Fig. 6). The treatment consists of endoscopic or surgical exci-

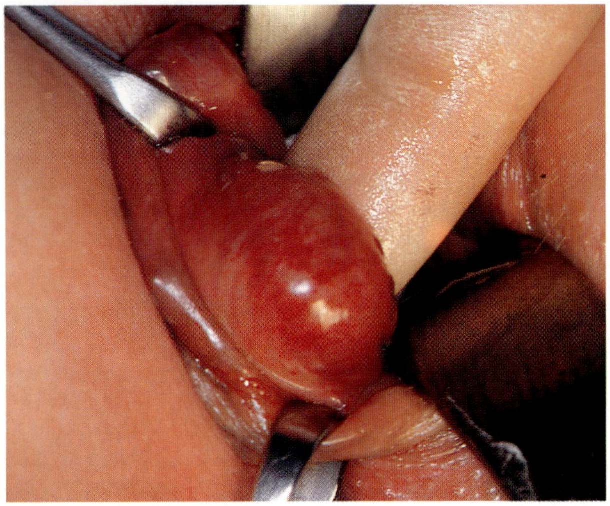

Fig. 5. Leiomyoma of the rectum.

sion of the tumor only if symptoms are present or when the histologic nature of the mass is uncertain.

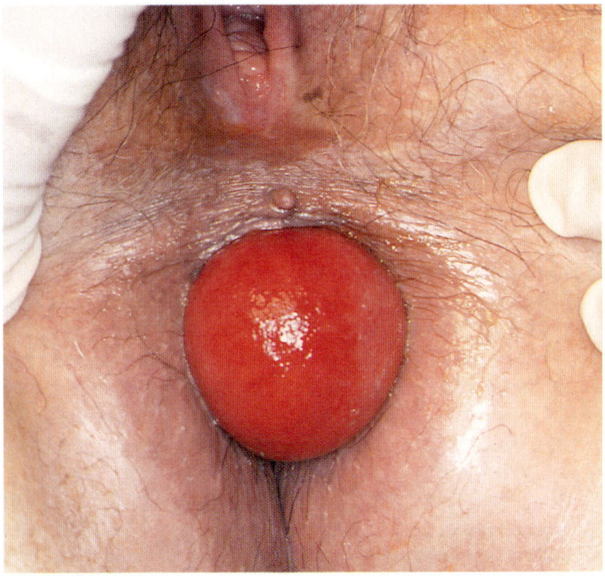

Fig. 6. Lipoma of the rectum prolapsed through the anal canal. (*Courtesy of* J. Faivre, Bourdeaux, France.)

Heterotopic tissue

Ectopic tissue in the rectum is a rare disease [20,21•]. More often, it is gastric mucosa (34 cases in the literature), and rarely, salivary gland tissue associated or not with gastric tissue (4 cases).

The etiology of ectopic epithelial tissue is still unknown. The usual presenting symptom is rectal bleeding with or without rectal ulceration, proctalgia, and tenesmus. Physical and endoscopic examination shows polypoid elevation or an irregular plaque of tissue with central umbilication. Biopsy results show gastric mucosa with fundic glands with or without *Helicobacter pylori.* The treatment consists of antisecretory drugs and transanal resection of the lesion.

Intramural hematomas

Intramural hematomas of the gastrointestinal tract occur commonly in the retroperitoneal duodenum secondary to blunt trauma; however, some intramural hematomas are spontaneous during hematologic disorders or therapeutic anticoagulation [22•]. These spontaneous hematomas can involve both the small and large bowel. The first reported case of spontaneous rectal hematoma occurred in a young man with chronic anticoagulation who presented an abdominal emergency with rectal bleeding; the rectal and endoscopic examination showed a large, boggy mass with edematous hemorrhagic mucosa. Computed tomographic scan revealed a large amount of intra-abdominal fluid, with marked soft tissue thickening in the region of the upper and midrectum. Enema confirmed a complete obstruction of the upper rectum. Surgical exploration showed the perforation of a large intramural hematoma of the rectum. A loop colostomy was fashioned, and 4 months later, continuity was established and the patient recovered.

Intrarectal tear from water skiing

Traumatic ruptures of the rectum can occur in exceptional conditions. One of these occurred in a young woman after a fall while water-skiing at high speed (60 mph) [23]. She was hospitalized when red-brown stools, and clots of blood appeared 2 hours after the fall.

Colonoscopy revealed a tear in the whole of the rectal wall, with pelvic and retroperitoneal hematoma. The treatment necessitated a procedure of diverting colostomy. The physical cause of the lesion was the violent entry of water, resulting in a high-pressure enema.

The same mechanism can give rise to vaginal lesions (laceration or rupture of the posterior cul-de-sac and lesions of the upper airway). The authors recommend avoidance of these rare lesions by the wearing of strengthened protection in the anoperineal region.

Atlas of rare diseases

Attention is drawn to the new *Atlas of Rare Diseases in Proctology* [24••], published in French. The Atlas illustrates 87 unusual lesions of the anorectum, including Darier's disease (autosomically transmitted dermatosis producing a vegetation of confluent keratosic papules forming a thick layer), molluscum contagiosum related to the poxvirus by way of enteropathic acrodermatitis due to a zinc deficiency of genetic origin, papilliferous hidradenoma, perianal amebiasis, Behçet's disease, larva migrans, cytomegalovirus ulceration, and X histiocytosis, to name only a few.

References and recommended reading

Papers of particular interest, published within the annual period of review, have been highlighted as:

- • Of special interest
- •• Of outstanding interest

1. BURGE SM: **Hailey-Hailey Disease: The Clinical Features Response to •• Treatment and Prognosis.** *Br J Dermatol* 1992, **126**:275–282.
Clinical study of 58 patients with biopsy results and special focus on manifestations in the nails.

2. LANGENBERG A, BERGER TG, CARDELLI M, RODMAN OG, ESTES S, BARRON • DR: **Genital Benign Chronic Pemphigus (Hailey-Hailey Disease) Presenting as Condylomas.** *J Am Acad Dermatol* 1992, **26**:951–955.
Description of clinical characteristics and histologic features of verrucous anogenital Hailey-Hailey disease in six patients, with review of literature.

3. KARTAMAA M, REITAMO S: **Familial Benign Chronic Pemphigus (Hailey-Hailey Disease).** *Arch Dermatol* 1992, **128**:646–648.

4. ZACHARIAE H: **Dermabrasion of Hailey-Hailey Disease and Darier's Disease.** *J Am Acad Dermatol* 1992, **128**:136.

5. JITSUKAWA K, RING J, WEYER U, KIMMING W, RADLOFF H: **Topical Cyclosporine in Chronic Benign Familial Pemphigus (Hailey-Hailey Disease).** *J Am Acad Dermatol* **128**:625–626.

6. ARCHIMANDRITIS A, KOLITSOPOULOS A, TZIVRAS M, FERTAKIS A, PALAMBROU E, KITTAS C: **Tuberculosis of the Anal Canal.** *J Clin Gastroenterol* 1993, **16**:89–90.

7. JAMIL D, TSMAIL R, MOUMEN A, EL MANSOURI A, BELLA-BAH A, CHERKAOUI A: **Tuberculose Pseudo-Tumorale du Rectum.** *Med Chir Dig* 1993, **22**:99–100.

8. HARLAND RW, VARKEY B: **Anal Tuberculosis: Report of Two Cases • and Literature Review.** *Am J Gastroenterol* 1992, **87**:1488–1490.
Two cases of anal tuberculosis are reported. The authors discuss the clinical features, and the difficulties of the diagnosis, especially in differentiating this condition from Crohn's disease, and they compare their data with those of the literature.

9. IORIANI P, OLIVER GC: **Synergistic Soft Tissue Infections of the Per- • ineum.** *Dis Colon Rectum* 1992, **35**:640–644.
Report on seven cases of necrotizing soft tissue infections of the perineum treated with radical debridement and antibiotic therapy. Includes review of the literature.

10. HIRN M: **Hyperbaric Oxygen in the Treatment of Gas Gangrene and •• Perineal Necrotizing Fasciitis.** *Eur J Surg* 1993, **suppl 570**:1–36.
Study of 32 patients with clostridial gas gangrene and 11 patients with Fournier's gangrene treated with surgery, antibiotic therapy, hyperbaric oxygen at 2.5 atm. Includes results of study of experimental models in rats.

11. FRY RD, BIRNBAUM EH, LACEY DL: **Actinomyces as a Cause of Recur- •• rent Perianal Fistula in the Immuno Compromised Patients.** *Surgery* 1992, **111**:591–594.
Report on two immunocompromised patients with recurrent perianal abscesses caused by *Actinomyces.* Macroscopic findings, histologic and bacteriologic diagnosis, and treatment are described.

12. PUY-MONTBRUN T, DENIS J, GANANSIA R, MATHONIERE F, LEMARCHAND • N, ARNOUS-DUBOIS N: **Anorectal Lesions in Human Immunodeficiency Virus Infected Patients.** *Int J Colorectal Dis* 1992, 7:26–30.
In a prospective study, the anorectal lesions observed in 148 HIV-infected patients are analyzed and compared with lesions described in the literature.

13. KILLI MR, OZTEMIZ O, SEVINC E: **Transrectal Ultrasonographic Demonstration of Anorectal Varices.** *Am J Gastroenterol* 1992, **87**:1685–1686.

14. SIPROUDHIS L, RENET C, BRETAGNE JF, RAOUL JL, HERESBACH D, FOSSELIN M: **Bleeding Anal Varix: Adverse Effects of Local Treatment With Histoacryl.** *Am J Gastroenterol* 1992, **87**:1886–1887.

15. KATZ JA, RUBIN R, COPE C, HOLLAND G, BRASS CA: **Recurrent Bleed- • ing From Anorectal Varices: Successful Treatment With a Trans jugular Intrahepatic Portosystemic Shunt.** *Am J Gastroenterol* 1993, **88**:1104–1107.
Report on a case with recurrent bleeding from anorectal varices successfully controlled by transjugular intrahepatic portosystemic shunt. Interesting for the description of diagnosis and follow-up of using magnetic resonance venography.

16. VOROBYOV GI, ODARYUK TS, KAPULLER LL, SHELYGIN YA, KORNYAK BS: • **Surgical Treatment of Benign, Myomatous Rectal Tumors.** *Dis Colon Rectum* 1992, **35**:328–331.
Retrospective study of 36 patients with leiomyomas operated on over an 18-year period, with clinical and surgical assessment.

17. VANDONI RE, GIVEL JC, ESSINGER AR: **Rectal Leiomyosarcoma: Acute Presentation After Local Injury.** *Eur J Surg* 1992, **158**:383–386.

18. ROIG JV, SOLANA A, HINOJOSA J, LLEDOS S: **Transanal Prolapse of Colorectal Lipomas.** *Colo-Proctology* 1993, **15**:88–90.

19. TAYLOR BA, WOLF BG: **Colonic Lipomas: Report of Two Unusual Cases and Review of the Mayo Clinic Experience, 1976-1985.** *Dis Colon Rectum* 1987, **30**:888–893.

20. GUADAGNI S, PISTOIA MA, CATARCI M, GOLAI P, CARDUCCI G, CARBONI J: **Salivary Gland Tissue in the Rectum.** *Colo-Proctology* 1992, **14**:371–373.

21. KESTEMBERG A, MARINO G, DE LIMA E, GARCIA FT, CARRASCAL E, • ARREDONDO JL: **Gastric Heterotopic Mucosa in the Rectum With *Helicobacter Pylori*-like Organisms: A Rare Cause of Rectal Bleeding.** *Int J Colorectal Dis* 1993, **8**:9–12.
A rare case of chronic rectal bleeding due to a gastric heterotopic mucosa in the rectum is described, as well as the diagnosis methods and treatment. Literature review of 30 cases of heterotopic mucosa in the rectum is included.

22. TERKONDA SP, NICHOLS FC III, SARR MG: **Spontaneous Perforating • Hematoma of the Rectum.** *Dis Colon Rectum* 1992, **35**:270–272.
The authors describe the first case of spontaneous perforating hematoma of the rectum in a young man with a history of chronic anticoagulation.

23. LEE RY, MILLER S, THORPE CH: **Intra-Rectal Tear From Water Skiing.** *Am J Gastroenterol* 1992, **87**:662–663.

24. DENIS J, ED: *Atlas des Maladies Rare en Proctologie.* Paris: Beaufour •• Pharmaceutical Group; 1993.
Comprehensive atlas illustrating 87 unusual lesions of the anorectum.

Professeur Jean Denis, MD, Department of Colo-proctologie, Hôpital Leopold Bellan, 19-21 rue Vercingetorix, 75674 Paris Cedex 14, France.

Esophageal, gastric, and small intestine*

Editorial overview

Robert J. Ginsberg, MD, Thomas A. Miller, MD, and Irvin M. Modlin, MD

Memorial Sloan-Kettering Cancer Center, New York, New York, University of Texas Medical School, Houston, Texas, and Yale University School of Medicine, New Haven, Connecticut, USA

*The articles on esophageal surgery in this section were edited by Dr. Ginsberg; those on gastric surgery, by Dr. Miller; and those on the small intestine, by Dr. Modlin.

Current Opinion in General Surgery 1994: 109–112

Esophageal

Surgical resection for cancer

The controversy over the optimum extent of resection for esophageal carcinoma continues. As Nasser Altorki (pp 113–116) rightly points out, there are "minimalists" who make no real attempt at wide excision or lymph node dissection, claiming that the ultimate 5-year survival from this type of resection (*eg*, transhiatal esophagectomy) is equal to that of radical en bloc resection with or without extensive lymphadenectomy. The extreme example of this latter approach is the current interest in Japan and elsewhere in three-field lymphadenectomy not only for esophageal carcinoma but also for treatment of bronchogenic carcinoma.

Proponents of these two extremes will offer statistics demonstrating the equality or superiority of their preferred technique. However, one must be very wary of comparing present-day surgical results with historical results. The advent of flexible endoscopy, computerized tomography, and endoscopic ultrasonography has allowed a better selection of patients, and with experience, surgeons almost certainly improve their selection of patients, not to mention their technical ability, both of which will result in better actuarial and crude survival rates.

To attribute improved results to an extended technique by comparing it with a previous decade's less extensive surgery results is fallacious. To compare one center's results utilizing one technique with another center's results utilizing a different technique is similarly fallacious, even if one matches patients stage for stage. Similarly, to attempt to compare the results of an extended technique with those of a standard technique in the same institution is just as fallacious as if there has been no randomization, resulting in a patient selection bias. This is certainly true in the DeMeester [1,2] series.

The fact that 20% of patients with supraclavicular disease identified in cervical lymphadenectomy specimens survived 5 years after three-field lymphadenectomy and esophagectomy is remarkable and warrants further study. Our Japanese colleagues are convinced of the validity of extending the lymphadenectomy and claim at least a 10% improvement in ultimate survival with this extended attempt at locoregional control [3].

The ultimate improvement in survival in esophageal cancer will result from earlier detection of early stage (stage I) disease, for which the survival rate following resection is extremely high, and the development of more effective systemic therapy used in an induction or adjuvant setting that has an effect on micrometastases. Most patients die from systemic disease following esophageal resection. On the whole, these metastases are believed to be present at the time of surgical resection. It appears that patients presenting with regional nodal and metastatic nodal disease have a higher proclivity for widespread systemic recurrence.

What can we learn from our colleagues who advocate radical en block resection and three-field lymphadenectomy? There is no doubt that a complete resection is required in dealing with esophageal carcinoma, because it is required in every solid tumor resection, no matter what the primary site. If a radical en bloc resection results in complete clearance of tumor, then the patient has a chance of having his primary tumor controlled. Similarly, if lymphadenectomy, even extended to three fields, results in locoregional tumor control, there may be a small chance to effect a cure even in patients with metastatic disease to nonregional

Abbreviation

NSAID—nonsteroidal anti-inflammatory drug.

lymph nodes (M1 disease). In treating patients with esophageal cancer, it seems reasonable to perform a complete resection, remove sufficient esophagus proximally to encompass any local lymphatic spread, and do a complete regional lymph node dissection, especially if the resultant perioperative morbidity and mortality are not increased. Whether further lymph node dissections in the neck and abdomen add a significant survival benefit is unknown. It is unlikely that a prospectively designed randomized trial comparing locoregional lymphadenectomy with three-field lymphadenectomy could ever be accomplished. We may have to extrapolate from the results of an ongoing European randomized trial regarding the value of extended lymphadenectomy in gastric carcinoma. When reporting results, however, it is important for authors not only to report survival, but to identify first and subsequent sites of recurrence, and especially, to report whether locoregional control was accomplished.

Minimally invasive therapeutic surgery

Spurred on by the remarkable success of laparoscopic cholecystectomy and thoracoscopic diagnostic procedures, surgeons have begun to explore the use of these minimally invasive techniques in managing benign and malignant diseases of the esophagus. Carlos Pellegrini (pp 117–119) reviews the early efforts of surgeons who have explored these new horizons.

The advantages of minimally invasive techniques to replace laparotomy include the potential for early return of gastrointestinal function, elimination of significant postoperative morbidity related to nausea and abdominal distension from ileus and decreased postoperative pain. The thoracoscopic approach, on the other hand, will eliminate morbidity related to pain but has few other advantages. Although both approaches could decrease hospital stay, this advantage has yet to be verified with video-assisted thoracoscopic surgery. The minimally invasive approaches, on the other hand, appear to lengthen the time of surgery even in the most experienced hands. It is also fair to say that esophageal surgery—even that utilizing open approaches—can be extremely demanding and involve significant postoperative complications in excisional surgery and late failures in benign reparative disease. For this reason, even experienced surgeons will have to approach minimally invasive techniques with extreme caution.

Despite these misgivings, it certainly appears that laparoscopic mobilization of the stomach for transposition and antireflux surgery are within the realm of possibility. The indications for antireflux surgery must remain strict, and the principles that have been developed over the past 30 years as well as fastidious attention to detail must be adhered to. Before surgeons embrace this approach, patients must be followed up closely for short-term and long-term failure. A good example of lack of adherence to these principles is the round ligament repair that was instituted as a "short cut" because of the laparoscopic approach. Short-cut approaches are doomed to failure.

Esophageal myotomy used in the treatment of specific motility disorders requires attention to detail to ensure that an adequate myotomy is performed both proximally and distally. The transthoracic thoracoscopic approach may fail to ensure adequate sphincter division, and the laparoscopic approach may provide an insufficient proximal length to the myotomy. It is likely that a laparoscopic approach will require an added antireflux procedure as part of the treatment. This may not be necessary when the esophagus is approached through the thorax, because the phrenoesophageal attachments do not necessarily have to be totally divided.

Mobilization of the esophagus in preparation for esophagectomy for carcinoma would be best handled thoracoscopically, allowing a wider excision and complete lymph node dissection vis-à-vis the endoscopic approach described by Buess, which limits lateral dissection.

There is no doubt that benign tumors can be easily enucleated and diverticula excised with minimal access techniques. One must remember the etiology of pulsion diverticulae and the necessity for accompanying myotomies in most patients.

All of these minimally invasive techniques must demonstrate an advantage over the open techniques that have been successfully developed over the years. All too frequently, the indications for and adherence to proper surgical technique are compromised for the sake of accomplishing a tour de force.

Gastric

In the present issue of *Current Opinion in General Surgery*, two articles appear that are worthy of serious consideration by all general surgeons, but particularly by those interested in diseases of the stomach and duodenum. The article by Mohammed Al-Assi and David Graham (pp 120–124) reviews the evidence for an infectious etiology of peptic ulcer disease and its implications for the surgical management of both gastric and duodenal ulcers. The paper by Martin Karpeh and Murray Brennan (pp 125–130) reviews recent developments in the preoperative staging of patients with gastric cancer and how these newer modalities may change the way in which malignancies of the stomach are managed in the future.

Al-Assi and Graham have provided compelling evidence for an infectious etiology of peptic ulcer disease. The organism responsible for this infection appears to be a gram-negative microaerophilic bacterium called *Helicobacter pylori*. The evidence implicating *H. pylori* is along three lines: First, with very few exceptions, patients who ultimately develop peptic ulcers can be shown to have *H. pylori* infection when cultures of gastric biopsy specimens are taken. This infection precedes the development of such ulcers, often by many years. In fact, current epidemiologic information suggests that many more patients are infected with *H. pylori* than actually have peptic ulcers, but over time, approximately 15% to 20% of these individuals will develop a true ulcer, in either the stomach or the duodenum. In those patients who develop ulcers without *H. pylori* infection, the most common causes are either nonsteroidal anti-inflammatory drugs (NSAIDs), or pathologic hypersecretory states such as Zollinger-Ellison syndrome. *H. pylori* infection and NSAID use appear to account for approximately 99% of ulcers. Second, although conventional medical treatment can certainly provide symptomatic relief and healing of ulcers, it does not in any way alter the natural history of the disease. If treatment is stopped, the ulcer commonly recurs, often within 6 to 12 months. In contrast, eradication of *H. pylori* infection not only provides symptom relief and ulcer healing, but , as demonstrated by multiple clinical trials, actually cures the ulcer. In fact, eradication has resulted in a recurrence rate of almost zero. In those cases in which ulcers do recur following therapy, either the ulcer is demonstrated to be related to incomplete eradication of infection or reinfection with *H. pylori* sometime later (although this appears to be a rare event), or the ulcer was actually caused by something else, most probably NSAID use. Third, eradication of *H. pylori* infection not only appears to cure ulcer disease, but also eliminates its complications. Intractability is virtually unheard of if *H. pylori* infection is eradicated, and patients with previous bleeding problems associated with ulceration have had this complication eliminated, as well as other complications such as perforation and obstruction. Whether individuals who present with perforation or obstruction from ulcer disease and are subsequently treated with agents to eradicate *H. pylori* infection will have these complications prevented from ever recurring remains to be demonstrated. If the *H. pylori* hypothesis is correct, one can presume that eradication of this organism will prevent these or any other complications from recurring.

The immediate response to these findings is logically something on the order of "This is too good to be true!" Although the data supporting the *H. pylori* hypothesis seem almost too neat, one must be careful not to write them off simply because they appear to be irrefutable. There is nothing wrong with skepticism, but one must not be so married to it that what appears to be truth is ignored. I am old enough to remember the skepticism that existed when the H_2-receptor blockers first became available for clinical use in 1977. Some thought these new agents would quickly demonstrate overriding toxic side effects, so that their clinical usefulness would be obviated. Others were willing to admit that these new antisecretory agents would play an adjunctive role in the management of peptic ulcer disease, but that surgical treatment would still be the mainstay of management for a significant number of patients. At that time, no one could have predicted the benefit that would ultimately be derived from the H_2 blockers and the tremendous change would take place in the management of gastric and duodenal ulcers. This change should be evident to everyone who trained in general surgery prior to the early 1980s, after which time these drugs became the mainstay of therapy for ulcer disease. The reality that all surgeons of the alimentary tract had to face was that peptic ulcer disease was no longer primarily a surgical-management disorder. The recent advances in knowledge concerning *H. pylori* and its link to peptic ulcer disease have the potential of changing treatment of gastric and duodenal ulcers even more radically, if elimination of this organism from the stomach does indeed result in permanent healing. One must therefore approach this new information with an open mind and be willing to accept the notion that peptic ulcer disease is an infectious disorder if the data ultimately demonstrate that to be the case, as accumulated findings to date strongly suggest.

In addition to the possible role that *H. pylori* seems to play in the pathogenesis of peptic ulcer disease, Al-Assi and Graham also indicate that this bacterium may play a role in the pathogenesis of gastric cancer. To date, however, the evidence is less compelling, and much more comprehensive epidemiologic study is required. Until the cause of gastric cancer can be identified, its prevention is obviously hampered. Thus, management of this disease focuses on issues that occur after its diagnosis and includes such concerns as the depth of tumor infiltration, the pattern and extent of lymph node involvement if present, and the absence or presence of metastatic disease. Until recently, most of these concerns could be dealt with adequately only by surgical exploration and visual inspection of the tumor and its presumed pathways of spread, and confirmation of such spread by frozen section, when appropriate. Careful follow-up of patients with gastric cancer, linking the stage of disease at diagnosis with ultimate survival, has done much to identify subpopulations of patients with disease that is clearly resectable, inoperable, unresectable, or at best palliatively resectable. Furthermore, new diagnostic modalities have provided important preoperative staging information that has helped greatly in surgical decision making with respect to individual patients. Both of these considerations are nicely summarized by Karpeh and Brennan.

With respect to surgery itself for carcinoma of the stomach, the extent of operation should be based on the likelihood of curative resection. Thus, in all patients, except those who have T3 tumors and/or are node positive, a resection margin of at least 5 cm should be effected after the stomach has been fully mobilized. Although total gastrectomy has been touted for many years as the procedure of choice for distal stomach cancers, no significant survival advantage over subtotal gastrectomy has been demonstrated in most series. Thus, as emphasized by Karpeh and Brennan, total gastrectomy is generally reserved only for those patients in whom a lesser procedure would severely compromise a safe margin. Furthermore, the likely benefits to be derived from an R2 node dissection have not been found to be uniform among all patients with potentially curable gastric cancer and appear to be influenced by the classification and histology of the tumor, its depth of penetration in the gastric wall, and its location and diameter.

Although preoperative staging of gastric cancer continues to pose a problem in the management of this disease, Karpeh and Brennan have nicely reviewed a number of technological advances that, with continuing experience, should result in the ability to distinguish those patients who would benefit from surgery from those who would not. While no one technique appears to be able to adequately determine tumor depth, nodal involvement, and metastatic disease, combined techniques could conceivably provide significant staging information to influence management decisions. For example, endoscopic ultrasonography has demonstrated considerable capability in determining tumor depth, particularly when T3 and T4 lesions are present. Although computed tomography is less discriminating in this regard, it is superior to endoscopic ultrasonography in determining the nodal and metastatic status of a patient and seems to be especially valuable when identifying liver metastases, unsuspected pelvic metastases (such as ovarian implants), and ascites. A particularly exciting preoperative diagnostic modality is laparoscopy. The role of laparoscopic approaches in removing gallbladders, appendices, and repairing hernias is already well known. The staging of gastric cancers seems a likely future application. Furthermore, the ability to perform intra-abdominal ultrasonography through the laparoscope may provide yet another means of identifying nodal and metastatic disease as well as of assessing tumor depth more accurately. With the use of these various techniques, it seems quite likely that in the years ahead patients with gastric cancer will be successfully screened preoperatively, and only those individuals with the greatest likelihood of cure subjected to operative management.

Small intestine

The paper by Gary Lawton and Irvin Modlin (pp 131–137) reviews the recent literature on the surgical management of duodenal gastrinomas. The paper by Marc Basson (pp 138–146) reviews the literature on mucosal repair in the small intestine.

References

1. DeMeester TR, Zaninotto G, Johansson KE: **Selective Approach to Cancer of the Lower Esophagus and Cardia**. *J Thorac Cardiovasc Surg* 1988, **95**:42–54.
2. DeMeester TR, Hagen JA, Peters JG: **Superiority of Extended En Bloc Esophagogastrectomy for Carcinoma of the Lower Esophagus and Cardia**. *J Thorac Cardiovasc Surg* 1993, in press.
3. Isono K, Sato H, Nakayama K: **Results of a Nationwide Study on the Three Field Lymph Node Dissection of Esophageal Cancer**. *Oncology* 1991, **48**:411–420.

Robert J. Ginsberg, MD, Memorial Sloan-Kettering Cancer Center, 1275 York Avenue, New York, NY 10021, USA.

Thomas A. Miller, MD, Department of Surgery, University of Texas Medical School, 6431 Fannin, Room 4264, Houston, TX 77030, USA.

Irvin M. Modlin, MD, Department of Surgery, FMB 109, Yale University School of Medicine, 333 Cedar Street, New Haven, CT 06510, USA.

Extended resections in the management of esophageal carcinoma

Nasser K. Altorki, MD

The New York Hospital, New York, New York, USA

The survival rate of patients with carcinoma of the esophagus is dismal. Improvement could be achieved only by earlier diagnosis and radical resection techniques to remove the esophagus and its draining lymphatic bed. En bloc esophagectomy and esophagectomy with three-field lymph node dissection are practiced in some centers in North America, Europe, and Japan. Survival rates with these techniques are better than those obtained with standard resection techniques.

Current Opinion in General Surgery 1994:113–116

Surgical resection, long considered the standard therapy for esophageal carcinoma, has become the subject of increasing scrutiny and controversy. An article published in 1980 by Earlam and Cunha-Melo [1] reviewed the world literature between 1953 and 1978. Over 83,000 patients were operated on for esophageal cancer. The operability, resectability, and mortality rates were 58%, 39%, and 29%, respectively, with a 5-year survival rate of 4%. These dismal results brought into question the role of surgical resection in the treatment of esophageal carcinoma. Some have suggested that the disease is nearly always systemic once the diagnosis is made, prompting a flurry of studies evaluating the role of chemotherapy, radiotherapy, or both as alternative modalities. Such was the state of the art in the West, when reports from the East indicated survival rates far exceeding those seen in Europe and North America [2,3]. In a classic article published in 1981, Akiyama *et al.* [4] reported an operative mortality of 1.4% and overall survival of 34.6% in 210 patients who underwent resection. Because advances in surgical techniques and perioperative care over the past decade have contributed to a significant improvement in early surgical results in the West, Earlam's and Cunha-Melo's findings are no longer justified. Muller *et al.* [5] reported on 47,000 patients operated on between January 1980 and December 1988, with an overall hospital mortality of 13%—less than half that reported a decade earlier. The hospital mortality in many centers with experienced esophageal surgeons is approximately 5% to 10% [6,7]. Despite dramatic improvement in perioperative outcome, long-term survival remains poor, averaging 20% for those undergoing resection and 10% for all patients [5].

With the increased safety of surgical resection established, the central issue became the improvement of long-term survival. Some have suggested that the good survival rates from the East were the result of a biologically more favorable disease rather than specific resection techniques [8]. Clearly, the primary hurdle is a delay in diagnosis, because the majority of the patients have advanced-stage disease at presentation. Altorki and Skinner [9] reported an 80% survival rate for patients with stage I disease, results comparable to those reported by Shao *et al.* [2] from China. More recently, Lerut *et al.* [10••] reported a 90% survival rate for patients with stage I disease, whereas Moghissi [11•] reported on 60 patients with early stage (stage I) adenocarcinoma of the esophagus and cardia with an absolute 5-year survival of 70% following esophageal resection. These results clearly negate the notion of differences in biological behavior and focus the debate on two central questions: 1) Is there a cost-effective method for earlier diagnosis of esophageal cancer, and 2) does the method of resection play a role in improving survival?

The common methods of esophageal resection include transhiatal esophagectomy and transthoracic esophagectomy. Neither approach specifically includes a complete mediastinal or abdominal lymphadenectomy. The proponents of these approaches maintain that surgical resection is essentially a palliative procedure, and that cure is a chance phenomenon. Those who favor extended resections [12] including en bloc resection and, more recently, three-field lymph node dissection [13], believe that these operations offer the best chance for cure in a select subgroup of patients with limited locoregional disease, namely those with stage IIA or IIB disease, and patients with stage III disease with fewer than four positive nodes. The controversy regarding the procedure of choice continues and is unlikely to be resolved. This article reviews extended esophageal resections, primarily en bloc resections and resections with three-field lymphadenectomy.

En bloc esophagectomy

The main object of en bloc esophagectomy is to resect the tumor-bearing esophagus with a wide envelope of tissue including the posterior mesoesophagus, both pleural surfaces laterally, and the pericardium where they abut on the esophagus, thus providing excellent local tumor control. Whereas en bloc resection has been used for tumors in other areas of the gastrointestinal tract with modest improvements in survival rates, the location of the esophagus (deep within the narrow confines of the mediastinum) and the lack of a well-defined esophageal mesentery have precluded its application as treatment of esophageal cancer. In the embryo, however, the esophagus distal to the aortic arch has a mesoesophagus, the adult counterpart of which is the

 ISBN 1-85922-671-X ISSN 1065-6243

lymphovascular tissue between the esophagus and the spine. This tissue, which includes the azygous vein and the thoracic duct,

is the esophageal equivalent of a well-defined mesentery and is considered an important pathway of lymphatic drainage from that organ.

In 1961, Logan [14] reported on 250 patients with carcinoma of the lower esophagus resected by an en bloc technique, with a 5-year survival of 16%, the best reported to date. An operative mortality of 21% discouraged wider adoption of the technique. Skinner [15] reintroduced its use in 1969 and extended its application to carcinoma of the thoracic and cervical esophagus. The technique is practiced in only a few centers in North America and Europe. Collard *et al.* [16] reported a 2.4% hospital mortality in 65 patients with esophageal carcinoma resected by the en bloc technique. Long-term survival was determined by the extent of penetration of the primary tumor into the esophageal wall and by the presence or absence of extrathoracic nodal metastases. In his series, the differences between N1 and N2 disease was not the number of involved nodes, as originally proposed by Skinner [15], but rather by whether the nodes were intra- (N1) or extrathoracic (N2). Survival of patients without nodal metastases was 58% at 3 years. Patients with intrathoracic nodal spread had a 3-year survival rate of 32% regardless of the degree of mural penetration. In an earlier report, DeMeester [17] reported an operative mortality of 7% following en bloc resection of carcinoma of the lower esophagus and cardia. The actuarial survival rates were 76%, 66%, and 53% at 1, 2, and 5 years, respectively.

A more recent report from the same group compared long-term outcome following esophageal resection for carcinoma of the distal esophagus and cardia in three groups of patients defined by preoperative and intraoperative staging [18•]. Group 3 patients ($n = 23$) received a palliative operation because of the presence of extensive disease. Patients in groups 1 and 2 had apparently limited disease and underwent either en bloc resection (group 1, $n = 30$) or transhiatal resection (group 2, $n = 16$) based on their ability to withstand transthoracic resection. Overall survival was significantly better after en bloc resection (41%) than in the 39 patients (groups 2 and 3) undergoing transhiatal resection (14%) ($P < 0.001$). Specifically, patients undergoing the en bloc procedure had survival better than patients of comparable staging (41% vs 21%) who underwent transhiatal resection (group 2). Patients with early lesions, defined as intramural tumors (T1 and T2) associated with fever than five positive nodes, had a 75% survival rate following en bloc resection compared with 20% for transhiatal resections. Survival of patients with advanced lesions, composed of transmural tumors associated with five or more positive nodes, was significantly better following en bloc than transhiatal resections (27% vs 9%). Lerut *et al.* [10••] reported on their experience with 232 patients undergoing resections for carcinoma of the esophagus, excluding those in the cervical esophagus and those located at the gastroesophageal junction. One hundred twenty-nine patients received a curative resection defined as clearance of all gross tumor. Fifty-four patients in the curative resection group were treated with en bloc resection. Hospital mortality was 7.4% for the curative en bloc group and 10.6% for the curative non–en bloc group. No differences in survival were found between adenocarcinoma and squamous carcinoma or by the location of the tumor in the esophagus. Survival was significantly better in patients treated by curative en bloc resection compared with those receiving a curative non–en bloc resection (48.5% vs 41%; $P < 0.002$) (Fig. 1). This survival advantage was especially evident in patients with nodal metastases rather than those with negative nodes. The survival advantage was apparent even when only stage III and IV patients treated with curative intent were compared (Fig. 2). At 5 years, survival rates were 22% versus 13% in favor of en bloc resections ($P < 0.05$). Significantly, 5-year survival for patients with stage I disease was 90%, indicating that early lesions are as curable as any other early-stage cancer.

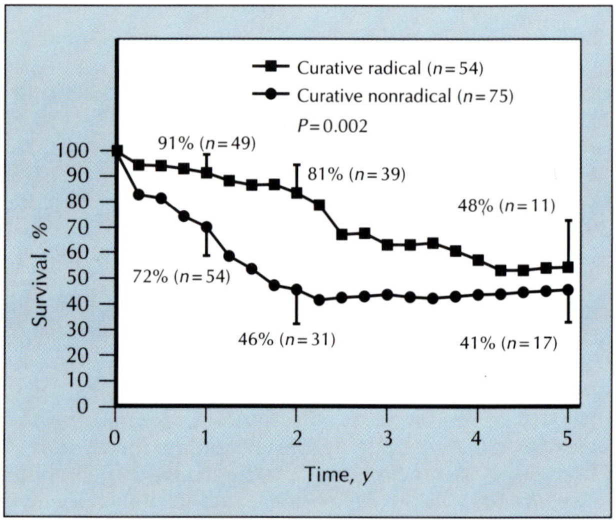

Fig. 1. Survival curves according to whether curative resection for thoracic esophageal carcinoma was radical. *T bars* indicate SD. (*From* Lerut *et al.* [10••]; with permission.)

Three-field lymphadenectomy

The concept of extended lymphadenectomy in carcinoma of the thoracic and abdominal esophagus stands in sharp contrast to the view generally held in the West with respect to nodal metastases. Prevailing philosophy in the West holds that nodal metastases, especially at distant sites, signify widespread disease. Treatment strategies based on less extensive surgical resections are generally favored, especially in breast cancer. In fact, even with en bloc resection, the presence of metastatic disease in lymph nodes at 10 cm on either side of the tumor signals incurability, and the procedure is converted to a standard resection. However, Japanese data, collected from a large number of patients undergoing resection for squamous carcinoma of the esophagus, clearly indicate that cervical nodal recurrence occurs in a significant number of cases [19]. A study of the patterns of recurrence following esophagectomy for cancer showed a 30% to 40% relapse rate in the cervical nodes following standard thoracic and abdominal lymphadenectomy

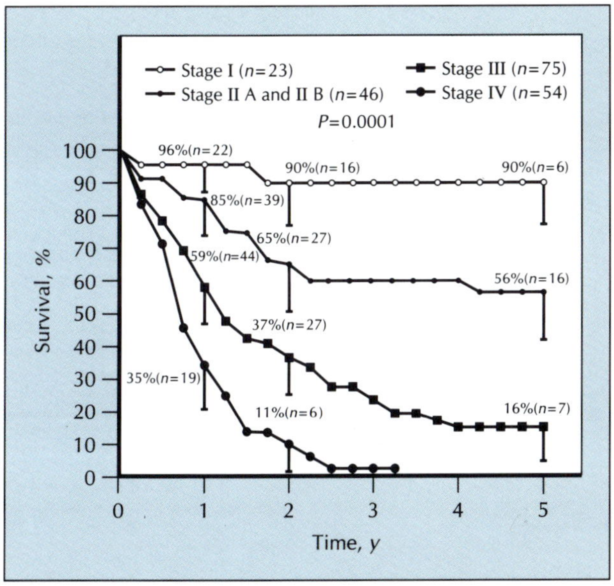

Fig. 2. Survival curves according to TNM stage after resection for thoracic esophageal carcinoma. *T bars* indicate SD. (*From* Lerut *et al.* [10••]; with permission.)

as proposed by Akiyama *et al.* [4]. An analysis of our own data showed that the cervical nodes were the site of first relapse in four of 20 patients who died of metastatic disease following en bloc esophagectomy for Barrett's adenocarcinoma [20]. A more recent analysis of 10 patients who underwent en bloc resection for squamous carcinoma of the thoracic esophagus demonstrated neck nodal recurrence in three patients [21•].

Japanese investigators have demonstrated the longitudinal lymphatic drainage of the esophagus along major intramural lymphatics [22]. With that rationale, Japanese surgeons employed three-field lymphadenectomy, defined as bilateral (not unilateral) cervical node dissection in addition to abdominal and mediastinal lymphadenectomy, for carcinoma of the thoracic esophagus. Isono *et al.* [23] reported on a large nationwide study analyzing the results obtained at 96 member institutions of the Japanese Society for Esophageal Disease. Thirty-five institutions performed three-field lymphadenectomy for carcinoma of the thoracic esophagus. The remaining institutions performed a two-field lymphadenectomy, *ie*, abdominal and mediastinal lymphadenectomy. The overall hospital mortality for 4590 patients was 3.9%, with a significantly lower mortality in the three-field lymphadenectomy group. Although the morbidity rate was essentially the same in both groups, the incidence of recurrent nerve paralysis was significantly higher following three-field (20%) compared with two-field dissection (14%). The rate of permanent recurrent nerve injury for en bloc resection in our experience is about 2%, but routine dissection of the intrathoracic portion of the right recurrent nodal chain is not routinely performed. Isono *et al.*'s report shows that among 1791 patients undergoing three-field lymphadenectomy, 27% had metastatic disease in the supraclavicular and deep cervical nodes without specific predilection for the left or right sides of the node. Although metastatic disease to the cervical nodes occurred regardless of tumor location, it was more common in carcinoma in the upper (41%) and middle (27%) thoracic esophagus than for tumors in the lower third (19%) or the intra-abdominal esophagus (11%). Survival rates were significantly better for patients undergoing three-field dissection (34% vs 26% 5-year survival). The salutary impact of three-field dissection was evident for all tumor locations except those in the intra-abdominal esophagus.

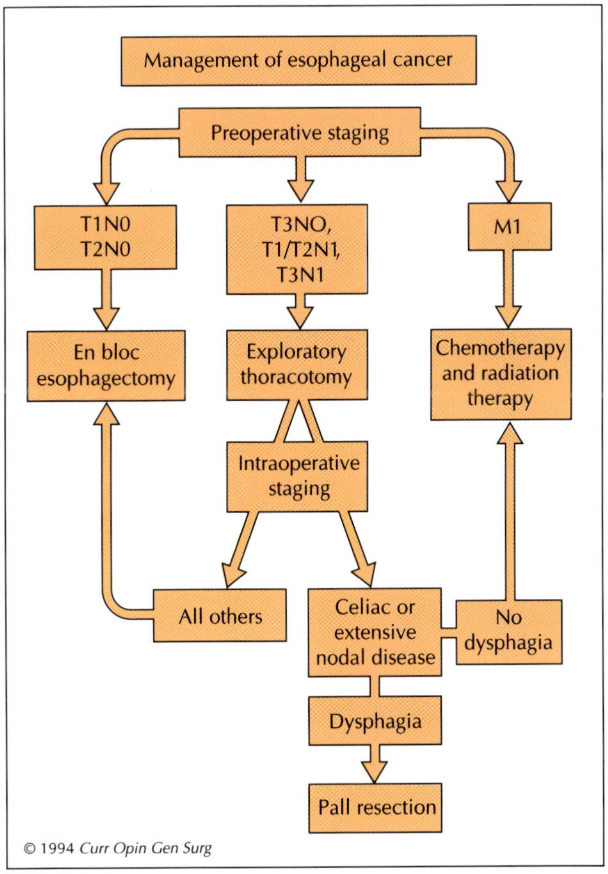

Fig. 3. Treatment of patients with esophageal cancer. Staging of carcinoma is shown according to American Joint Committee on Cancer TNM classification system.

In another report, Kato *et al.* [24] studied 150 patients operated on by two groups of surgeons with the same institution and time intervals. One surgeon performed a three-field dissection (group A) and the other a standard two-field lymphadenectomy (group B). The two groups of patients were matched with respect to tumor stages and patient characteristics, although patients receiving a two-field dissection were slightly older. The overall operative mortality was 7.3% (2.6% in group A and 12.3% in group B). There was no difference in postoperative morbidity between the two groups. There was no significant increase in the incidence of vocal cord paresis incurred by cervical node dissection. Twenty patients (26%) in group A had metastases in the neck nodes, and the 4-year survival rate in that group was 48%. Regardless of minor differences between the two patient groups, the 48% survival rate in patients with thoracic esophageal cancer and positive neck nodes is an important observation. There is no reported experience in the West about three-field dissection. The added impact of en bloc resection and three-field lymphadenectomy is unknown.

Isono *et al.* [23] state that a definite improvement in survival (about 10%) occurs after three-field lymph node dissection. These statements are along the same themes proposed by Lerut *et al.* [10••] in their report on radical resections. A conclusive statement on the therapeutic efficacy of three-field lymphadenectomy awaits further reports.

Conclusions

Our current approach to patients with esophageal carcinoma (Fig. 3) begins with a full preoperative staging work-up, which often includes barium esophagograms, endoscopy, and computed tomography of the chest and upper abdomen, endoscopic ultrasonography, and radionuclide bone scans. Bronchoscopy is done in patients with carcinoma of the middle and upper third of the thoracic esophagus. Patients with stage IV (distant visceral metastases) disease are treated nonoperatively. Patients with clinical T1N0 and T2N0 carcinoma are offered en bloc resections without neoadjuvant therapy. In the absence of a neoadjuvant protocol, all other patients (*ie,* those with T3N0, T1N1, T2N1, and T3N1 carcinoma) are explored. Careful intraoperative staging is performed to verify the absence of visceral metastases and exclude celiac nodal metastases or or nodal involvement 10 cm on either side of the tumor. Patients with extensive of celiac nodal metastases are subjected to to palliative resection only if significant dysphagia is present. All other patients undergo resection with the en bloc technique. The efficacy of cervical node dissection in the select group of patients with carcinoma of the thoracic esophagus is currently under investigation.

References and recommended reading

Papers of particular interest, published within the annual period of review, have been highlighted as:

- • Of special interest
- •• Of outstanding interest

1. EARLAM R, CUNHA-MELO JR: **Oesophageal Squamous Cell Carcinoma: A Critical Review of Surgery.** *Br J Surg* 1980, 67:381–390.

2. SHAO LF, HUANG GJ, ZHANG DW, *ET AL.*: **Detection and Surgical Treatment of Early Esophageal Carcinoma.** In *Proceedings of the Beijing Symposium on Cardiothoracic Surgery*. New York: John Wiley & Sons; 1981:168–171.

3. ORRINGER MB: **Palliative Procedures for Esophageal Cancer.** *Surg Clin North Am* 1983, **63**:941–950.

4. AKIYAMA H, TSURUMARU T, KAWAMURA T, ONO Y: **Principles of Surgical Treatment for Carcinoma of the Esophagus: Analysis of Lymph Node Involvement.** *Ann Surg* 1981, **194**:438–446.

5. MULLER JM, ERASMI H, STELZNER M, ZIEREN U, PICHLMAIER H: **Surgical Therapy of Oesophageal Carcinoma.** *Br J Surg* 1990, 77:845–857.

6. ELLIS FH JR, GIBB SP, WATKINS E JR: **Limited Esophogastrectomy for Carcinoma of the Cardia: Indication, Technique and Results.** *Ann Surg* 1988, **208**:354–361.

7. ORRINGER MB: **Transhiatal Esophagectomy Without Thoracotomy for Esophageal Carcinoma.** In *Debates in Clinical Surgery*. Edited by Simmons R. Chicago: Year Book Medical Publishers; 1990:177–188.

8. ORRINGER MB: **Ten-Year Survival After Esophagectomy for Carcinoma: Surgical Triumph or Biologic Variation?** *Chest* 1989:970–971.

9. ALTORKI NK, SKINNER DB: **Surgical Treatment of Esophageal Neoplasms.** In *Surgical Treatment of Digestive Disease*. Edited by Moody FG, Carey LC, Jones RS, Kelly KA, Nahrwold DL, Skinner DB. Chicago: Year Book Medical Publishers; 1989:109–120.

10. •• LERUT T, DELEYN P, COOSEMANS W, VAN RAEMDONCK D, SCHEYS I, LESAFFRE E: **Surgical Strategies in Esophageal Carcinoma With Emphasis on Radical Lymphadenectomy.** *Ann Surg* 1992, **216**:583–590.

A detailed article outlining a large experience with en bloc versus non–en bloc esophagectomy and clearly showing a survival advantage for extensive resections. The overall 5-year survival rate of 30% is impressive.

11. • MOGHISSI K: **Surgical Resection for Stage I Cancer of the Oesophagus and Cardia.** *Br J Surg* 1992, 79:935–937.

Analysis of survival for stage I cancer of the esophagus proves curability of early lesions.

12. SKINNER DB: **Esophageal Malignancies: Experience with 110 Cases.** *Surg Clin North Am* 1976, **56**:137–147.

13. TSURUMARU M, AKIYAMA H, UDAGAWA H, ONO Y, SUZUKI M, WATANABE G: **Cervical Thoracic Abdominal Lymph Node Dissection for Intrathoracic Esophageal Carcinoma.** In *Diseases of the Esophagus: Malignant Diseases*, vol 1. Edited by Ferguson MK, Little AG, Skinner DB. Mount Kisco: Futura; 1990:187–196.

14. LOGAN A: **The Surgical Treatment of Carcinoma of the Esophagus and Cardia.** *J Thorac Cardiovasc Surg* 1963, **46**:150–161.

15. SKINNER DB: **En Bloc Resection for Neoplasms of the Esophagus and Cardia.** *J Thorac Cardiovasc Surg* 1983, **85**:59–69.

16. COLLARD JM, OTTE JB, REYNAERT M, FIASSE R, KESTENS PJ: **Feasibility and Effectiveness of En Bloc Resection in the Esophagus for Esophageal Cancer: Results of a Prospective Study.** *Int Surg* 1991, 76:209–213.

17. DEMEESTER TR, ZANINOTTO G, JOHANSSON KE: **Selective Approach to Cancer of the Lower Esophagus and Cardia.** *J Thorac Cardiovasc Surg* 1988, **95**:42–54.

18. • DEMEESTER TR, HAGEN JA, PETERS JG: **Superiority of Extended En Bloc Esophagogastrectomy for Carcinoma of the Lower Esophagus and Cardia.** *J Thorac Cardiovasc Surg* 1993, in press.

An important comparative analysis of radical versus nonradical resections.

19. ISONO K, ONODA S, OKUYAMA K, SATO H: **Recurrence of Intrathoracic Esophageal Cancer.** *Jpn J Clin Oncol* 1985, **15**:49–60.

20. SKINNER DB: **Cervical Lymph Node Dissection for Thoracic Esophageal Cancer.** *Ann Thorac Surg* 1991, **51**:884–885.

21. • ALTORKI NK: **Squamous Carcinoma of the Esophagus in North America: A Therapeutic Dilemma.** *World J Surg*, in press.

Outlines the generally poor prognosis of squamous cell of the esophagus in North America, which is due primarily to extensive disease at presentation.

22. SAKATA K: **Über die Lymphgefässe des Oesophagus und Über seine regionären Lymphdrüsen mit Berücksichtigung der Verbreitung des Karcinoms.** *Mitt Grenzgeb Med Chir* 1983, **11**:634.

23. ISONO K, SATO H, NAKAYAMA K: **Results of a Nationwide Study on the Three Field Lymph Node Dissection of Esophageal Cancer.** *Oncology* 1991, **48**:411–420.

24. KATO H, WATANABE H, TACHIMORI Y, AND IIZUKA T: **Evaluation of Lymph Node Dissection for Thoracic Esophageal Carcinoma.** *Ann Thorac Surg* 1991, **51**:931–935.

Nasser K. Altorki, MD, The New York Hospital–Cornell Medical Center, 525 E. 68th Street, New York, NY 10021, USA.

The role of minimal-access surgery in esophageal disease

Carlos A. Pellegrini, MD

University of Washington, Seattle, Washington, USA

Modern advances in equipment and techniques have made it possible to treat many esophageal diseases with minimally invasive techniques. This chapter describes the impact of thoracoscopy and laparoscopy on esophageal surgery, with particular emphasis on the technique and results of esophageal myotomy, antireflux operations, and esophageal resection.

Current Opinion in General Surgery 1994:117–119

Advances in videoendoscopic equipment and techniques have opened new horizons in the treatment of diseases that affect intrathoracic organs. Mack *et al.* [1], for example, reported the initial experience with thoracoscopy in 70 patients who underwent various procedures previously accomplished with open techniques. These procedures included lung biopsies, wedge resections of pulmonary nodules, excision of the pericardium and drainage of the pericardial space, dorsal thoracic sympathectomy, apical blebectomy, and pleurodesis. These procedures, which previously required a thoracotomy with its attendant morbidity and discomfort, can now be performed with minimal hospital stay.

In a similar communication, Roviaro *et al.* [2] stressed the substantial decrease in pain, the expedient postoperative recovery, and the rapid return to work that is seen in patients undergoing thoracoscopic procedures. Cuschieri [3••] stressed some of the benefits of this approach and pointed out the need to obtain adequate data in order to assess the results of these newer techniques. He described in some detail the initial experience with the use of minimally invasive techniques in esophageal surgery. Considerable work has been done over the past 2 years in at least three areas: esophageal myotomy, antireflux surgery, and esophageal resection of benign and malignant tumors.

Esophageal myotomy

The use of minimally invasive techniques to perform esophageal myotomy has been applied to the treatment of patients with achalasia and those with other motility disorders. Achalasia is a disease characterized by a lack of peristalsis and inadequate relaxation of the lower esophageal sphincter. Current medical therapy is ineffective. The only recognized methods of treatment today are balloon dilatation and myotomy. Although myotomy has been proven to be more effective than balloon dilatation, previously there was a tendency to use the latter because it was quicker, was easier to perform, and required a minimal hospital stay.

Pellegrini *et al.* [4••] reported on an initial series of 17 patients treated with thoracoscopic or laparoscopic myotomy. They found that the use of an endoscope in the lumen of the esophagus greatly facilitated the identification of the organ and helped determine the extent to which the myotomy should be performed. They primarily used the thoracic approach and obtained good or excellent results in more than 80% of the patients. Follow-up was short, but because the technique used was similar to the original Heller myotomy, the authors believe the results will be comparable in the long term. Although this operation can be performed via a laparoscopic approach, it requires opening of the diaphragmatic hiatus to a greater extent and leads to reflux more often. When the myotomy is performed from the abdomen, an antireflux procedure should probably be done.

Shimi *et al.* [5] reported on the use of long esophageal myotomy to treat nutcracker esophagus causing odynophagia and chest pain. This disease is characterized by the presence of very high amplitude waves of esophageal peristalsis. The operation is performed through the left side of the chest, and the myotomy is carried out to the aortic arch. Good short-term relief of pain was achieved, and no complications were encountered. This operation can also be performed from the right side. Access to the esophagus is easier and the myotomy can be done over a longer area, but the lowest part of the esophagus is not easy to reach from the right side.

Antireflux surgery

The performance of antireflux surgery via minimally invasive techniques may have a major impact on a relatively common disease. Surgical therapy for abnormal reflux is very effective; however, the indications have been limited in the past because of the pain, discomfort, and relatively long recovery that are associated with traditional open techniques. With the reduction in postoperative pain and the rapid recovery associated with laparoscopy, laparoscopic repair of reflux may become the preferred form of therapy for this disease in the not-too-distant future.

The initial experience with antireflux surgery was reported by Shimi *et al.* [5] using the ligamentum teres. The technique involved mobilization of the round ligament from the falciform ligament, preserving its blood supply. The ligament was then rerouted around the previously dissected abnormal esophagus, creating a sling. Although preliminary results in a handful of patients

 ISBN 1-85922-671-X ISSN 1065–6243

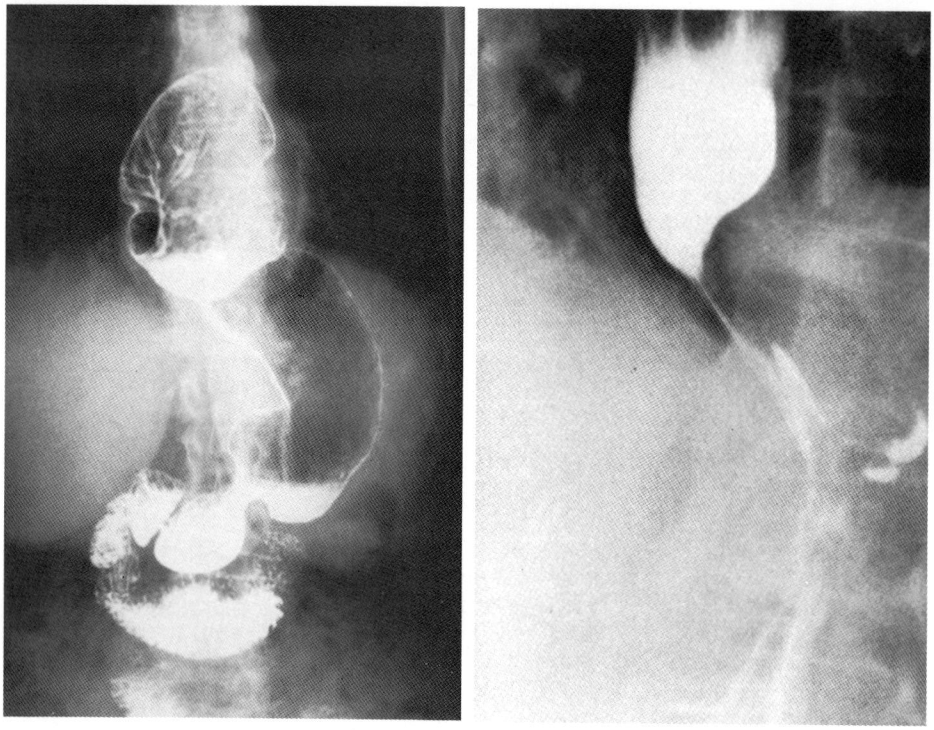

Fig. 1. Preoperative (*left panel*) and postoperative (*right panel*) results of barium swallows in a 72-year-old patient treated by laparoscopic repair of a mixed hiatal hernia. (*From* Cuschieri *et al.* [10]; with permission.)

showed that this procedure significantly raised the tone of the lower esophageal sphincter and relieved symptoms of chronic reflux, Shimi *et al.* abandoned its routine use in favor of a fundoplication.

Laparoscopic fundoplication was first reported on by Dallemagne *et al.* [6•] from Belgium. Falk *et al.* [7] in Australia and Cuschieri [8••] presented elaborate descriptions of the technique. The operation involves upward retraction of the left lobe of the liver, division of the peritoneum at the crura, dissection of the distal esophagus away from the right (first) and the left (later) crura, and eventually creation of the fundic wrap around the distal esophagus. In some cases, the short gastric vessels are divided to increase the size of the wrap and to allow a loose fundoplication, but the authors have not found that this is always needed. I believe that it is important to preserve the principles of antireflux surgery, so well described this year in a paper by Siewert *et al.* [9••]: *ie*, wide esophageal dissection and adequate wrapping with a loose fundoplication. As pointed out by Siewert *et al.*, the length of the wrap is probably not important, but the lack of tension is. Cuschieri [8••] stated that he prefers to use a partial fundoplication as advocated by Touppee for the majority of his patients, reserving the total fundoplication for those with large hiatal hernias.

In another interesting paper, Cuschieri *et al.* [10] described in detail the technique used to treat paraesophageal hernias with this approach (Fig. 1). The operation is similar to fundoplication performed in the absence of a hernia, but it is somewhat more complex in that the hernia sac must be divided (and left in the mediastinum), and the many fibrous bands that tightly adhere the fundus to the sac must be divided. I advocate the use of a gastrostomy, as described by Koger and Stone [11], to provide further anchorage of the stomach in the subdiaphragmatic position for patients who have a large paraesophageal hernia. Like Cuschieri, I perform a fundoplication in these patients, because it helps prevent recurrence of the hernia, although reflux may not have been a problem preoperatively. I also agree with Stein *et al.* [12], Orr [13], Zucker [14••], and McKernan *et al.* [15], who pointed out in their extensive reviews of laparoscopic applications for treating diseases of the gastrointestinal tract that prospective, controlled studies are needed to determine the final outcome of this new approach. Currently, Hunter from Atlanta and Hinder from Omaha are conducting such studies.

Surgery for benign tumors of the esophagus and mediastinum

Gossot *et al.* [16], Everitt *et al.* [17], and Bardini *et al.* [18], in simultaneous communications, described the use of thoracoscopic techniques to enucleate esophageal leiomyomas. I have used this technique for the same purpose and believe leiomyoma is an ideal indication for this approach. As described by these authors, most patients can be approached from the right side. Port position follows the "diamond shape" approach. The right lung is collapsed, and the esophagus and the tumor are easily visible. An endoscope may help to localize the lesion. The overlying muscularis must be divided and the tumor exposed. The tumor is then dissected from adjacent mucosa until it is completely excised. I place a stitch through the lesion as a handle and have found that this greatly facilitates exposure and manipulation.

Lewis *et al.* [19] described the use of this technique for excising mediastinal cysts. In a very provocative report, Nathanson *et al.* [20••] described the use of thoracoscopy to close an esophageal perforation secondary to balloon dilatation in two patients with achalasia. In these patients, they left the muscularis open, closed the mucosa with a running suture, and drained the chest. I would advocate closure of the disruption using the muscularis as well and performing a myotomy on the other side.

Esophageal resection

Buess [21] first described the use of a long mediastinoscope, especially designed for this purpose, to dissect the esophagus in preparation for resection in patients with cancer. The instrument is introduced through a cervical incision and is advanced through the mediastinum on the side of the esophagus. Dissection and control of the blood supply are accomplished under direct vision and with minimal manipulation. This procedure allows the surgeon to avoid the "blunt" dissection of the esophagus that accompanies a transhiatal esophagectomy. On the other hand, Cuschieri *et al.* [22••] described a right-sided thoracoscopic approach to mobilize the esophagus in the mediastinum. The advantage of this approach is that it allows a more thorough mediastinal dissection that includes lymph nodes, which is almost impossible with Buess's technique. The disadvantage is that it enters the pleural space and requires collapse of the lung (not required during the performance of a routine transhiatal esophagectomy).

References and recommended reading

Papers of particular interest, published within the annual period of review, have been highlighted as:
• Of special interest
•• Of outstanding interest

1. MACK MJ, ARONOFF RJ, ACUFF TE, DOUTHIT MB, BOWMAN RT, RYAN WH: **Present Role of Thoracoscopy in the Diagnosis and Treatment of Diseases of the Chest.** *Ann Thorac Surg* 1992, **54**:403–409.

2. ROVIARO GC, REBUFFAT C, VAROLI F, VERGANI C, MACIOCCO M, GRIGNANI F, SCALAMBRA SM, MARIANI C: **Videoendoscopic Thoracic Surgery.** *Int Surg* 1993, **78**:4–9.

3. •• CUSCHIERI A: **The Spectrum of Laparoscopic Surgery.** *World J Surg* 1992, **16**:1089–1097.
This article gives an excellent review of the spectrum of laparoscopic surgery, particularly in relation to the gastrointestinal tract. It describes briefly the technical aspects of the most commonly practiced operations on the esophagus, stomach, and colon.

4. •• PELLEGRINI CA, WETTER A, PATTI MG, LEICHTER R, MUSSAN G, MORI T, BERNSTEIN G, WAY LW: **Thoracoscopic Esophagomyotomy: Initial Experience With a New Approach for the Treatment of Achalasia.** *Ann Surg* 1992, **216**:291–299.
First detailed description of thoracoscopic esophageal myotomy and the initial results in the treatment of patients with achalasia.

5. SHIMI SM, NATHANSON LK, CUSCHIERI A: **Thoracoscopic Long Oesophageal Myotomy for Nutcracker Oesophagus: Initial Experience of a New Surgical Approach.** *Br J Surg* 1992, **79**:533–536.

6. • DALLEMAGNE B, WEERTS JM, JEHAES C: **Laparoscopic Nissen Fundoplication: Preliminary Report.** *Surg Laparosc Endosc* 1991, **1**:138–143.
Excellent description of the technique. This paper is the first on the subject.

7. FALK GL, BRANCATISANO RP, HOLLINSHEAD J, MOULTON J: **Laparoscopic Fundoplication: A Preliminary Report of the Technique and Postoperative Care.** *Aust N Z J Surg* 1992, **62**:969–972.

8. •• CUSCHIERI A: **Laparoscopic Antireflux Surgery and Repair of Hiatal Hernia.** *World J Surg* 1993, **17**:40–45.
Excellent review of laparoscopic antireflux surgery. This article includes a description of the treatment of patients who have associated large hiatal hernias with the Nissen wrap and the Touppee technique in detail. It has excellent drawings.

9. •• SIEWERT JR, FEUSSNER H, WALKER SJ: **Fundoplication: How To Do It? Peri-Esophageal Wrapping as a Therapeutic Principle in Gastroesophageal Reflux Prevention.** *World J Surg* 1992, **16**:326–334.
This article describes the methodical approach to the work-up of and treatment design for patients with abnormal gastroesophageal reflux. It emphasizes the physiologic principles of antireflux surgery.

10. CUSCHIERI A, SHIMI S, NATHANSON LK: **Laparoscopic Reduction, Crural Repair, and Fundoplication of Large Hiatal Hernia.** *Am J Surg* 1992, **163**:425–430.

11. KOGER KE, STONE JM: **Laparoscopic Reduction of Acute Gastric Volvulus.** *Am Surg* 1993, **59**:325–328.

12. STEIN HJ, FEUSSNER H, SIEWERT JR: **Minimally Invasive Antireflux Procedures.** *World J Surg* 1992, **16**:347–348.

13. ORR KB: **Early Recovery From Laparoscopic Repair of Hiatus Hernia [Letter].** *Med J Aust* 1992, **156**:670.

14. •• ZUCKER KA: **Perceived Future of Laparoscopic General Surgery.** *Am J Surg* 1992, **35**:297–302.
Nice insight into what may be in store for the future in the treatment of gastrointestinal disease with minimally invasive techniques.

15. MCKERNAN JB, WOLFE BM, MACFADYEN BV JR: **Laparoscopic Repair of Duodenal Ulcer and Gastroesophageal Reflux.** *Surg Clin North Am* 1992, **72**:1153–1167.

16. GOSSOT D, FOURQUIER P, METEINI ME, CELERIER M: **Technical Aspects of Endoscopic Removal of Benign Tumors of the Esophagus.** *Surg Endosc* 1993, **7**:102–103.

17. EVERITT NJ, GLINATSIS M, MCMAHON MJ: **Thoracoscopic Enucleation of Leiomyoma of the Oesophagus.** *Br J Surg* 1992, **79**:643.

18. BARDINI R, SEGALIN A, RUOL A, PAVANELLO M, PERACCHIA A: **Videothoracoscopic Enucleation of Esophageal Leiomyoma.** *Ann Thorac Surg* 1992, **54**:576–577.

19. LEWIS RJ, CACCAVALE RJ, SISLER GE: **Imaged Thoracoscopic Surgery: A New Thoracic Technique for Resection of Mediastinal Cysts.** *Ann Thorac Surg* 1992, **53**:318–320.

20. •• NATHANSON LK, GOTLEY D, SMITHERS M, BRANICKI F: **Videothoracoscopic Primary Repair of Early Distal Oesophageal Perforation.** *Aust N Z J Surg* 1993, **63**:399–403.
Provocative article on the use of thoracoscopy to suture esophageal perforations from balloon dilatation.

21. BUESS G: **Thoracoscopic Dissection of the Esophagus.** *Surg Endosc* 1992, **6**:150–151.

22. •• CUSCHIERI A, SHIMI S, BANTING S: **Endoscopic Oesophagectomy Through a Right Thoracoscopic Approach.** *J R Coll Surg Edinb* 1992, **37**:7–11.
Excellent description of the technical aspects of esophageal resection via thoracoscopy.

Carlos A. Pellegrini, MD, Department of Surgery, RF-25, University of Washington, 1959 NE Pacific Street, Seattle, WA 98195, USA.

Peptic ulcer disease, *Helicobacter pylori*, and the surgeon: changing of the guard

Mohammed T. Al-Assi, MD, and David Y. Graham, MD

Veterans Affairs Medical Center and Baylor College of Medicine, Houston, Texas, USA

The ability to assign causative roles to *Helicobacter pylori* and nonsteroidal anti-inflammatory drug use in peptic ulcer disease, and proof that eradication of *H. pylori* infection results in cure of peptic ulcer disease, are resulting in a reassessment of the indications for surgery and the type of surgery to be performed. With only a few exceptions, surgery is rapidly becoming an outdated approach to the management of peptic ulcer disease. We will soon see the day when surgeons with great technical skill in peptic ulcer disease will be rare, just as it happened when chest surgeons were no longer needed for the management of chronic pulmonary infections.

Current Opinion in General Surgery 1994:120–124

Until recently, it would have been unthinkable to suggest that it might be possible to cure peptic ulcer disease. That possibility now deserves serious consideration [1•]. The change in our thinking is a direct result of recent studies linking the seemingly different diseases to an infection with a bacterium, *Helicobacter pylori*. *H. pylori* infection is now accepted as the major cause of gastritis and of the gastritis-associated diseases, gastric and duodenal ulcer disease [2,3].

Until recently, peptic ulcer disease was considered a multifactorial process. Although the pathophysiology of peptic ulcer disease was clearly not understood, it was recognized that duodenal ulcers, ulcers in the pyloric channel, and prepyloric ulcers tended to be acid-related, whereas typical gastric ulcers seemed more related to some undefined defect in the gastric mucosa. It was established that therapy with potent antisecretory drugs resulted in accelerated healing of gastric and duodenal ulcers and that both relapse and complications were infrequent if maintenance ulcer healing therapy was continued [4,5,6••,7,8].

In most medical lectures, after a brief nod to the differences between ulcers in different locations, the same form of therapy was recommended. The only differences in therapy were related to duration and the desirability of maintenance therapy. Surgeons were more likely to tailor their recommendations depending on the location of the ulcer. The effectiveness of modern medical therapy greatly reduced the need for surgical therapy except in patients with complications of ulcer disease. Surgical therapy for ulcer disease is an effective form of therapy but carries a significant price in the form of mortality and morbidity. The excessive long-term morbidity of operations involving gastric resection led to development of less mutilating operations culminating in the highly selective vagotomy. Although the question as to which operation is best for a particular patient continues to be debated, this debate may no longer be relevant. This change is the result of recent work identifying specific causes of ulcer disease.

Causes of peptic ulcer disease

While the pathophysiology of ulcer disease remains unclear, there has been a major revolution in the thinking about ulcer disease, its causes, and therapies [9•]. We have moved away from assigning acid the dominant role in causation and now recognize that there are distinct and identifiable causes of ulcer disease [1•,10••,11]. The most common causes of peptic ulcer are infection with *H. pylori*, nonsteroidal anti-inflammatory drug (NSAID) use, and pathologic hypersecretory states, for example, the Zollinger-Ellison syndrome. *H. pylori* infection and NSAID use account for approximately 99% of ulcers.

The modern approach to ulcer therapy and prevention should be based upon causation. *H. pylori* infection is the most common cause of peptic ulcer, irrespective of whether the ulcer is in the stomach or duodenal bulb [12•,13]. NSAID use is the second most common cause. NSAID use, either overt or covert, in particular, accounts for a sizable proportion of gastric ulcers (Fig. 1) [10••,14]. Ulcers in an unusual location, such as postbulbar ulcers, or ulcer disease of unusual severity suggest the presence of the Zollinger-Ellison syndrome

Abbreviation

NSAID—nonsteroidal anti-inflammatory drug.

 ISBN 1-85922-671-X ISSN 1065–6243

and prompt a request for determination of the serum gastrin concentration.

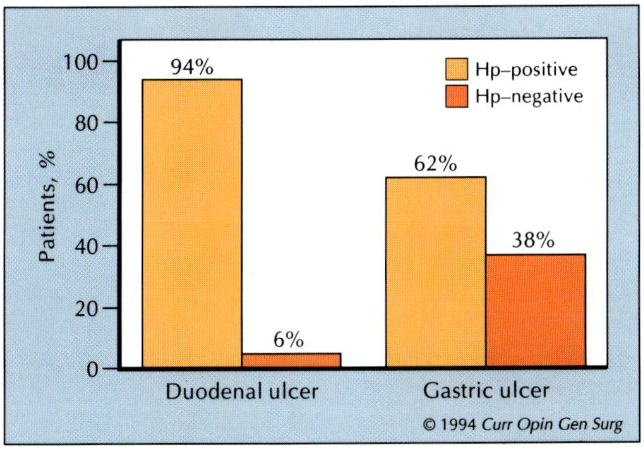

Fig. 1. Prevalence of *Helicobacter pylori* (Hp) infection in 302 consecutive patients with duodenal ulcer and 115 patients with gastric ulcer seen in one private practice. (*Data from* Borody *et al.* [12•,13].)

The organism and epidemiology

Helicobacter pylori is a gram-negative microaerophilic bacterium whose natural host is humans (Fig. 2). *H. pylori* infection may be the most common infection worldwide. The magnitude of the morbidity associated with this infection is only now becoming recognized. For example, infection is associated with a cumulative risk of developing a peptic ulcer of 15% to 20%. In addition, 5% to 10% of those infected eventually develop gastric carcinoma. Overall, the recognized rate of mortality or morbidity related to *H. pylori* infection is 20% to 30% of those infected. *H. pylori* infection precedes development of typical peptic ulcers. For example, in a 10-year study of asymptomatic subjects, only one of the 133 subjects without *H. pylori* gastritis at the initial evaluation developed peptic ulcer compared with 11% of those with infection [15]. Why only a small proportion of infected persons develop ulcers is unexplained. Among the considerations are differences in virulence of *H. pylori* strains of organism, differences in the host response, or both. Work is rapidly progressing in these areas [9•].

Treatment

Conventional medical therapies for peptic ulcer disease with an H_2-receptor antagonist or a proton-pump inhibitor for 4 to 8 weeks result in healing of 90% to 95% of ulcers; however, ulcer recurrence is the rule [10••]. Conventional medical treatment provides symptomatic relief and healing of the ulcer but does not alter the natural history of peptic ulcer disease. In contrast, multiple clinical trials have shown that eradication of *H. pylori* infection cures the ulcer disease; ulcer recurrence is eliminated as are complications of ulcer disease (Fig. 3) [16–18,19••,20–23]. Ulcer recurrence after therapy is associated with failure to eradicate the infection, reinfection, or another cause of ulcer disease, most commonly NSAID use. In the United States, reinfection is rare. Smoking has long been recognized as a major factor influencing duodenal ulcer recurrence. After *H. pylori* eradication smoking is no longer a risk factor [19••,24]. Gastric and duodenal ulcers can now be cured. The old adage "No acid, no ulcer" now becomes "No *Helicobacter pylori*, no ulcer."

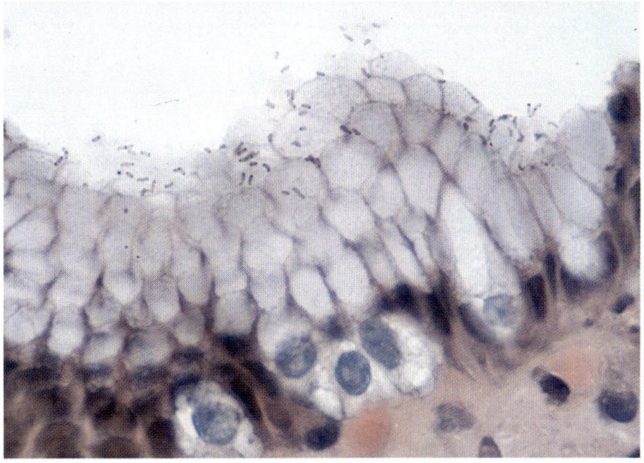

Fig. 2. Genta stain of gastric mucosa showing *Helicobacter pylori* at the luminal surface of the antrum.

Initially *H. pylori* proved difficult to eradicate. We now have several therapies that will yield eradication rates of 90% or greater and new therapies are under investigation. The current best regimens to eradicate *H. pylori* infection are triple therapies (Table 1). Side effects associated with triple therapy are minor and usually do not require discontinuing the treatment. Metronidazole resistance is one of the most common causes of triple therapy failure, which is more common in developing countries and in patients who have been exposed to it previously for treatment of other infections. Clarithromycin can be successfully substituted for metronidazole.

The concept that peptic ulcer disease is an infectious disease and should be treated like any curable infectious disease is becoming increasingly accepted. We believe that an attempt to eradicate *H. pylori* should be made in every patient with peptic ulcer disease and *H. pylori* infection [1•,9•].

The future role of surgery

The recognition that peptic ulcers had identifiable etiologies and that the disease could be cured has led to a reassessment of the role of surgery for ulcer disease [25••]. Traditional gastric surgery has significant short-term and long-term morbidity and in our opinion is no longer an acceptable first-line therapy for a curable dis-

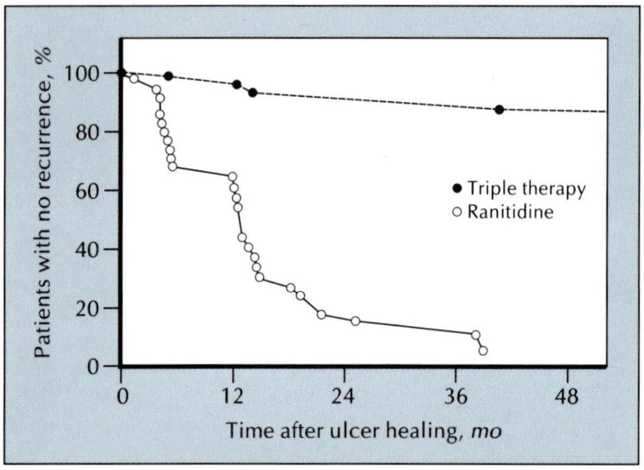

Fig. 3. Patients with duodenal ulcer were randomly assigned to receive 300 mg of ranitidine in the evening or 300 mg of ranitidine plus triple therapy (bismuth subsalicylate, metronidazole, and tetracycline). Triple therapy was given for 2 weeks. Under both regimens, ranitidine was given until ulcer healing or 16 weeks had elapsed. Patients were then followed up without antiulcer therapy. Of those who had received ranitidine alone, 96% suffered ulcer relapse within 40 weeks. Ulcer relapse was rare in the ranitidine plus triple therapy group, and when it occurred, it was associated with failure to eradicate the *H. pylori* infection or use of nonsteroidal anti-inflammatory drugs. (*Adapted from* Graham *et al.* [19••]; with permission.)

Table 1. *Helicobacter pylori* combination therapies
Triple therapy for 14 days*
Bismuth subsalicylate, 2 tablets with meals and at bedtime
Metronidazole†, 250 mg with meals (750 mg)
Tetracycline‡, 500 mg, with meals and at bedtime (2 gm)
Dual therapy
Amoxicillin, 750 mg with meals (2.25 gm)
Metronidazole, 500 mg with meals (1.5 gm)

*Triple therapy is recommended over dual therapies.
†Clarithromycin, 500 mg, can be substituted for metronidazole.
‡Amoxicillin can be substituted for tetracycline.

ease. The effects of being able to categorize, prevent, and even cure ulcer disease will have a major impact on surgery just as antibiotic therapy has changed the surgical practices and indications for management of tuberculosis or complications of pneumonia. We briefly discuss the "traditional" indications for surgical intervention and how they may be influenced by the new knowledge.

Intractability

Intractability is currently equated with clinically severe ulcer disease, which recurs frequently and symptomatically despite maintenance therapy with antisecretory therapy (*eg*, H_2-receptor antagonists), develops complications despite ongoing maintenance antisecretory therapy, or fails to heal despite prolonged therapy with an effective dose of a proton pump inhibitor. The era of the H_2-receptor antagonists resulted in intractability becoming an infrequent indication. Development of proton-pump inhibitors, better understanding of the causes of ulcer disease, and recognition that eradication of *H. pylori* infection could cure the most common form of ulcer has almost eliminated intractability as an indication for surgery. It has become increasingly recognized that covert NSAID use is responsible for ulcers being resistant to healing [26], and *H. pylori* eradication and exclusion of NSAID use should be done before declaring an ulcer intractable.

Hemorrhage

Hemorrhage from peptic ulcer remains a common problem. Bleeding is typically self-limited, and the patient can generally be treated conservatively. The widespread availability of endoscopy hemostasis has further reduced the need for lifesaving surgical intervention [25••]. Patients who have bled from peptic ulcer are at an increased risk of having additional episodes of hemorrhage. It has now been shown that long-term maintenance therapy with H_2-receptor antagonists will markedly reduce this risk [4,5,6••,7,8]. More recent studies have shown that eradication of *H. pylori* infection also essentially eliminates the risk of future bleeding (no ulcer, no complications) (Fig. 4) [27]. Thus, patients who have bled should be investigated for *H. pylori* status and for NSAID use. If *H. pylori* infection is present, it should be eradicated and maintenance H_2-receptor antagonist therapy should not be discontinued until one is confident that eradication has been accomplished. If the patient was receiving NSAIDs (including aspirin), such medications should be prohibited in the future. If, because of severe arthritis, this is not an option, cotherapy with misoprostol (200 μg two or three times daily) should be prescribed. Maintenance therapy with H_2-receptor antagonist is recommended only if the patient cannot tolerate misoprostol and the ulcer was duodenal in location.

Perforation

Perforation is a complication of peptic ulcer disease and both the perforation and the underlying disease must be considered when planning long-term treatment. The primary issue used to be which operation was optimal for a specific patient. A randomized trial comparing nonoperative treatment to emergency surgery showed that an initial period of nonoperative treatment with careful observation revealed an outcome similar to that of emergency surgery, and the decision not to operate should be based on the age and clinical condition of the patient [28]. For those requiring surgery, current evidence suggests that simple closure of the perforation and proximal selective gastric vagotomy is the preferred operation [25••]. The long-term plan for a patient who survived the perforation and is ready to be discharged from the hospital depends on whether the patient received a definitive ulcer operation, had simple closure of the perfo-

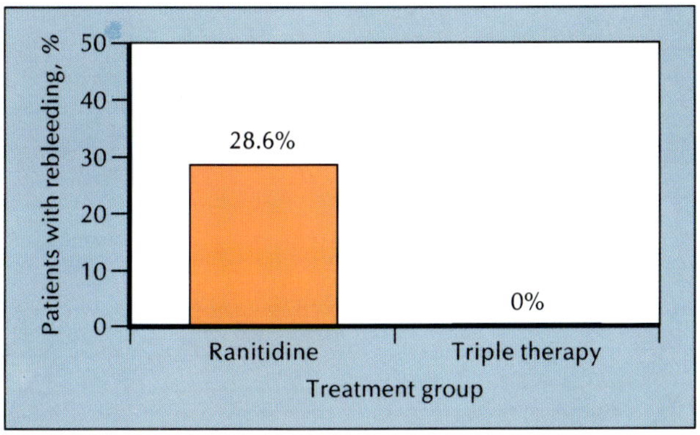

Fig. 4. Patients presenting to hospital with major upper gastrointestinal hemorrhage from peptic ulcer were followed up after ulcer healing with either ranitidine or ranitidine plus triple therapy (bismuth subsalicylate, metronidazole, and tetracycline). There was a marked difference in the incidence of readmission for recurrent upper gastrointestinal bleeding, favoring those who received triple therapy ($P<0.03$). (*Adapted from* Graham *et al.* [27]; with permission.)

ration, or was treated with conservative medical therapy, or whether the perforation was a complication of concomitant NSAID use. In general, *H. pylori* status should be determined, and if present, the infection should be eradicated. Since eradication of *H. pylori* infection cures peptic ulcer disease, we presume that it will also prevent this complication from recurring. This hypothesis has not yet been studied. Even if the patient received a definitive ulcer operation, *H. pylori* should be eradicated if present. As with bleeding, if the perforation is possibly related to NSAID use, further use should be prohibited unless the patient requires NSAIDs. For those patients, misoprostol prophylaxis is recommended.

Penetration

The incidence of penetration is unknown because penetration can be diagnosed reliably only at surgery, by autopsy, when a biopsy of an ulcer reveals liver or pancreatic tissue, or when there is a fistulous communication evident between the stomach or intestine and adjacent structure such as the biliary tree or colon. Data from surgical series reveal that penetration is identified in approximately 20% of patients who required surgery for their peptic ulcer disease. Patients with penetrating ulcer have clinically severe peptic ulcer disease and present as having "intractable" ulcer disease.

Obstruction

Approximately 2% of all ulcer patients develop gastric outlet obstruction; 90% of obstructions are caused by previous or coexistent duodenal or channel ulcers. Active ulcer is present in more than 75% of the cases. Inflammatory swelling surrounding the ulcer, muscular spasm associated with nearby ulcer, or cicatricial narrowing with fibrosis are the factors responsible for the obstruction. Conservative medical management with decompression of the obstructed stomach, correction of fluid, electrolytes, and acid-base abnormalities, plus administration of an intravenous H_2-receptor antagonist are the mainstay of initial resuscitation and therapy. Two events have occurred to reduce the need for surgery of obstruction: endoscopic balloon dilatation and *H. pylori* eradication. Intraoperative dilatation of the stenotic segment combined with highly selective vagotomy is often successful in the long-term management of pyloric stenosis. One would presume that the combination of therapy that cures the disease (*H. pylori* eradication) and endoscopic dilatation of the pyloric ring should be equally effective. Our approach to these patients is resuscitation followed by balloon dilatation of the pylorus, vigorous antisecretory therapy (*eg*, omeprazole, 40 to 60 mg daily) followed by eradication of *H. pylori* infection [25••]. For those in whom the therapy is not successful, one should consider missed cancer.

Conclusions

The discovery of the role of *H. pylori* in peptic ulcer disease and proof that eradication of the infection now allows us to cure peptic ulcer disease are resulting in a reassessment of the indications for surgery and the type of surgery. Patients presenting with a life-threatening complication of ulcer disease such as major hemorrhage or perforation are exceptions to the general rule that surgery is now largely an outdated approach to the management of peptic ulcer disease. Operations that mutilate the normal anatomy and those requiring gastric resection should be avoided if at all possible. In most instances, when an operation is required, a highly selective vagotomy is preferred. We see the day ahead when surgeons with great technical skill in peptic ulcer disease will be rare. This will occur just as it happened when chest surgeons were no longer needed for the management of chronic pulmonary infections.

References and recommended reading

Papers of particular interest, published within the annual period of review, have been highlighted as:
- • Of special interest
- •• Of outstanding interest

1. • Graham DY: **Treatment of Peptic Ulcers Caused by Helicobacter Pylori [Editorial].** *N Engl J Med* 1993, **328**:349–350.
Editorial updating the current thought about the relation between *H. pylori* and ulcer disease.
2. Graham DY: **Helicobacter pylori: Its Epidemiology and Its Role in Duodenal Ulcer Disease.** *J Gastroenterol Hepatol* 1991, 6:105–113.
3. Dixon MF: ***Helicobacter pylori* and Peptic Ulceration: Histopathological Aspects.** *J Gastroenterol Hepatol* 1991, 6:125–130.
4. Penston JG, Wormsley KG: **Asymptomatic Duodenal Ulcers Occurring During Maintenance Treatment With Ranitidine.** *Aliment Pharmacol Ther* 1990, 4:569–576.
5. Penston JG, Wormsley KG: **Review Article: Maintenance Treatment With H_2-Receptor Antagonists for Peptic Ulcer Disease.** *Aliment Pharmacol Ther* 1992, 6:3–29.
6. •• Penston JG, Wormsley KG: **Nine Years of Maintenance Treatment With Ranitidine for Patients With Duodenal Ulcer Disease.** *Aliment Pharmacol Ther* 1992, 6:629–645.
Study showing the efficacy and problems associated with long-term antisecretory therapy to prevent duodenal ulcer recurrence and complications. All in all,

it was very effective and should be the standard of therapy for those patients in whom *H. pylori* eradication is not currently possible.

7. Penston JG, Wormsley KG: **Long-term Maintenance Treatment of Gastric Ulcers With Ranitidine**. *Aliment Pharmacol Ther* 1990, 4:339–355.

8. Van Deventer GM, Elashoff JD, Reedy TJ, Schneidman D, Walsh JH: **A Randomized Study of Maintenance Therapy With Ranitidine to Prevent the Recurrence of Duodenal Ulcer**. *N Engl J Med* 1989, **320**:1113–1119.

9. • Graham DY, Go MF: ***Helicobacter pylori*: Current Status**. *Gastroenterology* 1993, **105**:279–282.
Up-to-date overview of current data concerning *H. pylori* and its relation to disease.

10. •• Soll AH: **Gastric, Duodenal, and Stress Ulcer**. In *Gastrointestinal Disease*. Edited by Sleisenger M, Fordtran J. Philadelphia: WB Saunders; 1993:580–679.
Outstanding and authoritative review of medical approaches to peptic ulcer.

11. Soll AH: **Pathogenesis of peptic ulcer and implications for therapy**. *N Engl J Med* 1990, **322**:909–916.

12. • Borody TJ, Brandl S, Andrews P, Jankiewicz E, Ostapowicz N: ***Helicobacter pylori*-Negative Gastric Ulcer**. *Am J Gastroenterol* 1992, **87**:1403–1406.
Large study showing that *H. pylori* and NSAID use account for most gastric ulcers.

13. Borody TJ, George LL, Brandl S, Andrews P, Ostapowicz N, Hyland L, Devine M: ***Helicobacter pylori*-Negative Duodenal Ulcer**. *Am J Gastroenterol* 1991, **86**:1154–1157.

14. Graham DY: **Prevention of Gastroduodenal Injury Induced by Chronic Nonsteroidal Antiinflammatory Drug Therapy**. *Gastroenterology* 1989, **96**:675–681.

15. Sipponen P, Varis K, Fraki O, Korri UM, Seppala K, Siurala M: **Cumulative 10-Year Risk of Symptomatic Duodenal and Gastric Ulcer in Patients With or Without Chronic Gastritis. A Clinical Follow-up Study of 454 Outpatients**. *Scand J Gastroenterol* 1990, **25**:966–973.

16. George LL, Borody TJ, Andrews P, Devine M, Moore Jones D, Walton M, Brandl S: **Cure of Duodenal Ulcer After Eradication of *Helicobacter pylori***. *Med J Aust* 1990, **153**:145–149.

17. Rauws EA, Tytgat GN: **Cure of Duodenal Ulcer Associated With Eradication of *Helicobacter pylori***. *Lancet* 1990, **335**:1233–1235.

18. Borody T, Andrews P, Mancuso N, Jankiewicz E, Brandl S: ***Helicobacter pylori* Reinfection 4 years Post-eradication [Letter]**. *Lancet* 1992, **339**:1295.

19. •• Graham DY, Lew GM, Klein PD, Evans DG, Evans DJ Jr, Saeed SA: **Effect of Treatment of *Helicobacter pylori* Infection on the Long-Term Recurrence of Gastric or Duodenal Ulcer: A Randomized, Controlled Study**. *Ann Intern Med* 1992, **116**:705–708.
Randomized, controlled trial showing that eradication of *H. pylori* cures gastric and duodenal ulcers.

20. Borody TJ, Cole P, Noonan S, Morgan A, Lenne J, Hyland L, Brandl S, Borody EG, George LL: **Recurrence of Duodenal Ulcer and *Campylobacter pylori* Infection After Eradication**. *Med J Aust* 1989, **151**:431–435.

21. Marshall BJ, Goodwin CS, Warren JR, Murray R, Blincow ED, Blackbourn SJ, Phillips M, Waters TE, Sanderson CR: **Prospective Double-Blind Trial of Duodenal Ulcer Relapse After Eradication of *Campylobacter pylori***. *Lancet* 1988, **2**:1437–1442.

22. Coghlan JG, Gilligan D, Humphries H, McKenna D, Dooley C, Sweeney E, Keane C, O'Morain C: **Campylobacter pylori and Recurrence of Duodenal Ulcers: A 12-Month Follow-up Study**. *Lancet* 1987, **2**:1109–1111.

23. Hentschel E, Brandstatter G, Dragosics B, Hirschl AM, Nemec H, Schutze K, Taufer M, Wurzer H; **Effect of Ranitidine and Amoxicillin Plus Metronidazole on the Eradication on *Helicobacter pylori* and the Recurrence of Duodenal Ulcer**. *N Engl J Med* 1993, **328**:308–312.

24. Borody TJ, George LL, Brandl S, Andrews P, Jankiewicz E, Ostapowicz N: **Smoking Does Not Contribute to Duodenal Ulcer Relapse After *Helicobacter Pylori* Eradication**. *Am J Gastroenterol* 1992, **87**:1390–1393.

25. •• Graham DY: **Ulcer Complications and Their Nonoperative Treatment**. In *Gastrointestinal Disease*. Edited by Sleisenger M, Fordtran J. Philadelphia: WB Saunders; 1993:698–712.
Overview of ulcer complications that begins to integrate the new data about ulcer causation into medical practice.

26. Perrault J, Fleming CR, Dozois RR: **Surreptitious Use of Salicylates: A Cause of Chronic Recurrent Gastroduodenal Ulcers**. *Mayo Clin Proc* 1988, **63**:337–342.

27. Graham DY, Hepps KS, Ramirez FC, Lew GM, Saeed ZA: **Treatment of *H. pylori* Reduces the Rate of Rebleeding in Peptic Ulcer Disease**. *Scand J Gastroenterol* 1993, In press.

28. Crofts TJ, Park KG, Steele RJ, Chung SS, Li AK: **A Randomized Trial of Nonoperative Treatment for Perforated Peptic Ulcer**. *N Engl J Med* 1989, **320**:970–973.

David Y. Graham, MD, Veterans Affairs Medical Center (111D), 2002 Holcombe Boulevard, Houston, TX 77030, USA.

Progress in the management of gastric cancer

Martin S. Karpeh, Jr, MD, and Murray F. Brennan, MD

Memorial Sloan-Kettering Cancer Center, New York, New York, USA

Over the past 30 years, numerous major centers have published analyses of potential factors influencing survival following resection of gastric cancer. The independent significance of depth of tumor penetration and lymph node status has been consistently documented. With proper staging, we know which patients are most likely to die of their disease. Unfortunately, adjuvant treatment in surgical resection has not altered patient outcome. Emphasis should now be on selecting the patients who should receive radical surgery for cure, adjuvant therapy with a hope for cure, or palliation. This brief review concentrates on recent developments in our ability to stage patients preoperatively, developments that may change the way we approach the patient with stomach cancer in the future.

Current Opinion in General Surgery 1994:125–130

The surgical management of adenocarcinoma of the stomach has continued to evolve since Theodore Billroth performed the first subtotal gastrectomy for this disease over a century ago. Today's decisions regarding the management of gastric cancer are based on knowledge of tumor growth patterns, the significance of the depth of tumor infiltration, and the pattern and extent of lymphatic drainage. Initial efforts to improve the survival results of surgical resection led surgeons to seek wider resection margins and a more extensive nodal dissection. In the late 1940s, Brunschwig [1] and McNeer and James [2] at Memorial Sloan-Kettering Cancer Center introduced pancreaticosplenectomy to gastric resection for the management of gastric carcinoma. Appleby [3] later extended the operation to include en bloc resection of the celiac axis and common hepatic artery. By the late 1970s, McNeer in this country and Lartat-Jacob in France had popularized *en principle* total gastrectomy and pancreaticosplenectomy as the standard approach to the management of advanced gastric cancer. Support for this approach was weakened by a failure to demonstrate a clear survival benefit over more conservative resections [4,5]. In the United States and Europe, most surgeons, discouraged by the low rates of patient survival after extensive operations and the higher morbidity [6], now perform a less radical operation [7].

The combination of decreasing incidence of gastric cancer in this country and the fact that 50% of advanced gastric cancer is either inoperable, unresectable, or at best palliatively resectable, has made progress in the treatment of this disease difficult. Surgery remains the only curative option in the treatment of gastric cancer, but the stage of the disease determines survival following a curative operation [8•]. On many occasions, we have been able to identify preoperatively the patient who will benefit from an aggressive operation, the patient who should not be operated on, and the patient who is likely to need more than operation for a chance at improved survival.

Preoperative staging

The prognosis for patients with carcinoma of the stomach depends on the pathologic stage of the disease at the time of presentation. The TNM staging system published in 1988 by the American Joint Committee on Cancer has now been accepted by the Union Internationale Contre le Cancer and the Japanese Research Society for Gastric Cancer [9-11]. While pathologic examination remains the standard for staging stomach cancers, recent improvements in our ability to determine preoperatively the TNM status of a given tumor have aided management decisions [12•].

Sixty-seven percent of 560 gastric cancer patients admitted to our institution during the 6-year period prior to September 1991 had pathologic (p) T3 carcinomas. Of these patients, 90% had metastatic nodal involvement, and 64% had cancers classified as N2 (Fig. 1). Forty-seven percent of these patients had M1 disease. When we looked at patient survival based solely on tumor stage, we found that patients with pT3 disease had a 36-month survival rate of less than 25% (Fig. 2). Jaehne *et al.* [8•] reported a 15% 3-year survival for their patients with pT3 gastric carcinomas following aggressive surgery. Because only 25% of T3 and 1% of M1 patients are alive 3 years after resection, 75% of patients receive no long-term survival benefit by resection alone. Short-term survival following resection is improved over that after no resection, but at 5 years, 80% of resected T3 patients have died. Therefore, in T3 disease, the surgical operation must be considered a palliative procedure for most patients. In these pT3

© 1994 Current Science ISBN 1-85922-671-X ISSN 1065–6243

patients, considering alternatives to operation alone is clearly justified.

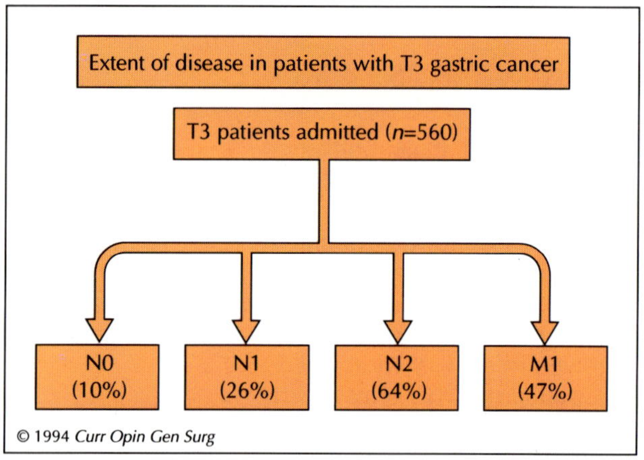

Fig. 1. The distribution of metastatic gastric cancer among patients with pathologic T3 tumors admitted to Memorial Sloan-Kettering Cancer Center from July 1985 to September 1991. Cancer stages are shown according to American Joint Committee on Cancer TNM system.

Improvements in preoperative staging made in the past 20 years have resulted in better 5-year survival. Akoh and Macintyre reviewed all English language publications on survival rate after surgery for gastric cancer from 1970 to 1990 [13]. They showed that the number of patients coming to surgery has fallen from 92% before 1970 to 71% by 1990, whereas the proportion of patients having resection has increased from 37% to 48% over the same time period, suggesting better patient selection. In their review, survival increased significantly for all resected patients, from 21% to 28%, and curatively resected patients demonstrated the most significant change, showing a nearly 18% improvement to 55% by 1990. The authors summarized that better patient selection in addition to better perioperative care have contributed to the decrease in the mortality rate from gastric cancer.

Endoscopic ultrasonography

Preoperative endoscopic ultrasonography is currently the most accurate means of assessing clinical tumor stage (cT). A 7.5- or 12-MHz probe is endoscopically placed into the fluid-filled stomach, allowing the endoscopist to characterize the size and depth of tumor infiltration, with an accuracy of between 71% and 92% [12•,14•,15•,16–19]. The stomach wall is divided into five echographically defined layers that correspond to histologic correlates (Fig. 3) [20]. Early T1 tumors leave the hypoechogenic (dark) muscularis propria intact. T2 lesions infiltrate the muscularis propria, producing a hyperechogenic distortion of this layer. The accuracy of endoscopic ultrasonography is hampered by its inability to distinguish reliably between subserosa and serosa [15•], as a result, some deep T2 tumors may be overstaged.

Rosch *et al.* [14•] recently reviewed their prospectively collected endoscopic ultrasonography staging results in 41 gastric cancer patients. Twenty-nine percent of tumors were misstaged when compared with final pathologic tumor stage. Overstaging was most common, occurring in eight of 12 (67%) of misstaged patients. Half of the overstaged tumors were actually pT2. Fein *et al.* [21] assessed the accuracy of endoscopic ultrasonography in staging ulcerated gastric cancers. Thirty-nine ulcerated gastric cancers were studied, and the linear concordance of endoscopic ultrasonography with pathologic staging was 52%. Ten of these tumors were overstaged (40%), and only two (8%) were understaged. All pathologic T3 tumors were correctly staged by endoscopic ultrasonography; in contrast, all of the nine pathologic T2 tumors were incorrectly staged: eight of nine were called T3 by endoscopic ultrasonography, and one was called T1. Clearly, the difficulties inherent in distinguishing between subserosa and serosa are exacerbated by the presence of inflammation. Enlarged perigastric lymph nodes in the setting of inflammation also contribute to overstaging and must be interpreted with caution.

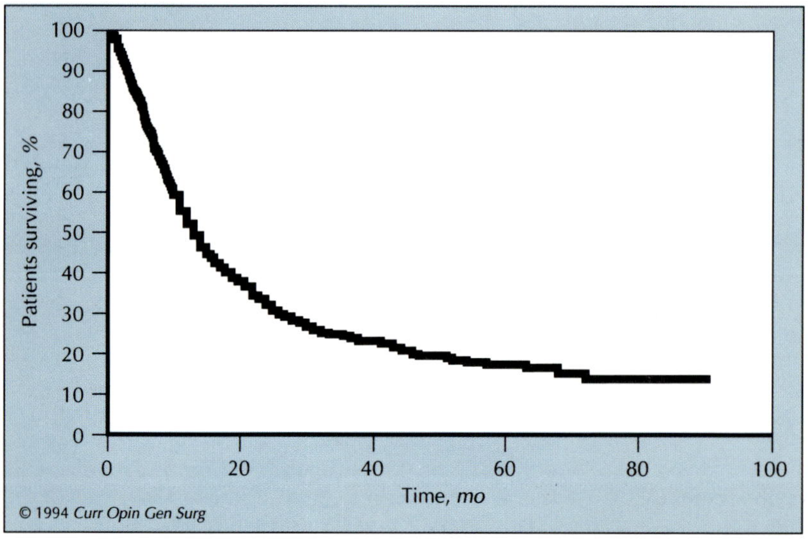

Fig. 2. Kaplan-Meier survival curve of patients with presumed T3 gastric cancer ($n = 573$). Median survival time was 13 months. Data include both resected and nonresected patients. (*Data from* Memorial Sloan-Kettering Cancer Center prospective database, July 1985 to July 1993.)

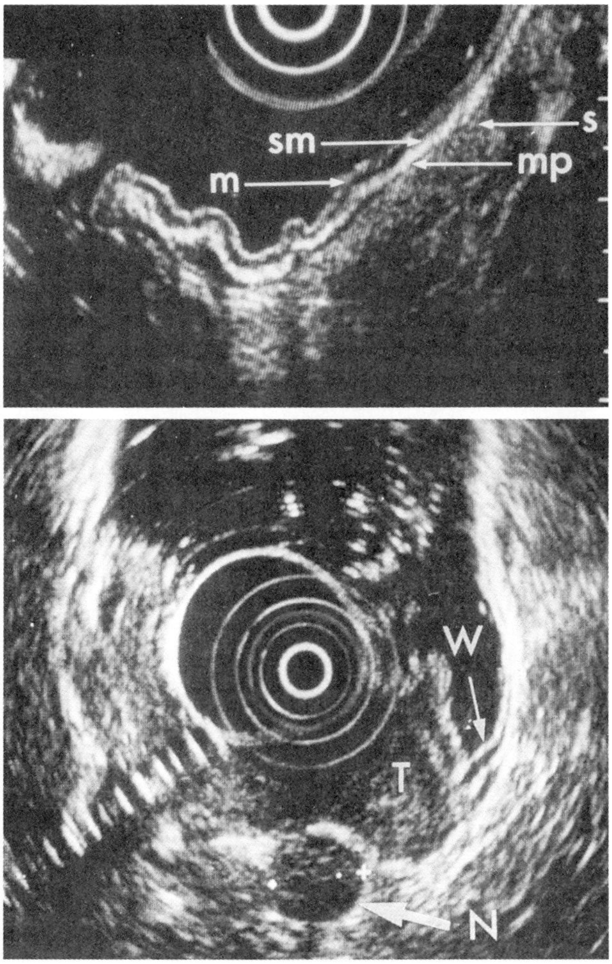

Fig. 3. Endoscopic ultrasonographic images of normal stomach wall (*top panel*) and gastric cancer (*bottom panel*). m—mucosa; sm—submucosa; mp—muscularis propria; N—lymph node; s—serosa; sm—submucosa; T—tumor; W—stomach wall. (*From* Karpeh [47]; with permission.)

By use of endoscopic ultrasonography, metastatic nodal disease is detected by the shape, internal echogenicity, and size of the nodes. Botet and Lightdale [20] described metastatic nodes as more likely to be round than elongated, hypoechoic or isoechoic relative to the primary, and ranging in size from 3 to 5 mm as opposed to larger sizes [20]. The accuracy of endoscopic ultrasonography in detecting positive nodes is generally not as good as in determining tumor depth and ranges between 50% and 88% in recent series [14•,16–19,22], but it is superior to both computed tomography [18,19] and surgical assessment [19].

The exact role endoscopic ultrasonography will play in the surgical management of gastric cancer has yet to be defined [23]. It has been used to assess whether a given gastric cancer resection will be curative versus either palliative or unresectable with an accuracy of 88% [14•]. This kind of information can be useful in selecting treatment. The potential impact of endoscopic ultrasonography in directing the management for this disease depends in part on the development of effective adjuvant and neoadjuvant therapies. Although endoscopic ultrasonography may overstage pT2 tumors, 39% of these tumors will be N1 and an additional 3% will be N2. The data from Rosch *et al.* [14•] showed that 46% of the eight overstaged patients were at risk to have either N1 or N2 involvement and would have been appropriate candidates for investigational treatment. Furthermore, because the risk of nodal metastases is proportional to the depth of invasion, a deep T2 lesion may pose a threat to survival similar to that of the early T3 tumor. An early analysis done at Memorial Sloan-Kettering Cancer Center correlating endoscopic ultrasonography tumor stage with recurrence rates indicated that 14 of 26 patients with endoscopic ultrasonography T3 tumors and three of four patients with endoscopic ultrasonography T4 tumors had recurrences, with a median follow-up of 13 months following surgical resection [24]. This observation has the potential to influence significantly management decisions in the future.

Computed tomography

Recent advances in the use of computed tomography may further enhance our ability to treat gastric cancer patients more selectively. Tumor stage was prospectively determined using incremental dynamic computed tomography on 71 patients with gastric cancer [25•]. Forty-nine of 71 cases (69%) were correctly staged. The detectability rate was 53% for early gastric cancer, 92% for advanced lesions and 81% overall. The specificity and overall accuracy of this method of computed tomographic scanning could not be determined, because no benign lesions were scanned. Unfortunately, the outer musculoserosal layer of the stomach is not reliably visualized with this method, weakening differentiation between T2 and T3 lesions. Computed tomographic scanning provides important information regarding the node and metastasis status of the patient but does not add to endoscopic ultrasonography in determining tumor stage. The most definitive value of computed tomography is in the identification of liver metastases, unsuspected pelvic metastases (ovarian), and ascites.

Laparoscopy

The role of laparoscopy in the management of gastric cancer is still in the developmental stages; however, its potential value in the prelaparotomy assessment of advanced gastric cancers is increasingly evident. In 1986, Possik *et al.* [26] demonstrated the superiority of laparoscopy over abdominal computed tomography scan in detecting peritoneal and hepatic metastases in a study of 360 gastric cancer patients. Although the latest-generation computed tomography scanners are superior to those in use a decade ago, improvements in laparoscopic instrumentation combined with the current availability of laparoscopic ultrasonography have provided the potential for minimally invasive pathologic staging of nodal and metastatic disease and perhaps improved echographic tumor staging.

Intraoperative ultrasonography

Kodama *et al.* [27•] used intraoperative ultrasonography to evaluate the extent of disease during 54 operations for carcinoma of the stomach. They scanned the primary tumor, liver, and lymph nodes in the hepatogastric ligament, omentum, mesocolon, and para-aortic nodes from the diaphragm to the inferior mesenteric artery. Pathologic T1 tumors were diagnosed with an accuracy between 70% and 80%. Subserosal (pT2) and extraserosal (pT3) extension was accurately determined in four of five and five of five cases.

Microscopic examination of excised para-aortic nodes in 30 operations revealed 10 cases with positive nodes (M1 disease). The criteria for detecting positive nodes were well defined [28]. Operative ultrasonography detected para-aortic lymph node metastases with a specificity of 90% and a sensitivity of 100%, for an overall accuracy of 93%. In the absence of gross adenopathy, the para-aortic nodes represent a diagnostic blind spot in preoperative stage assessment. Nodes as small as 3 mm may contain micro metastatic disease [29]. Removing nodes under ultrasonic guidance and assessing them by frozen sectioning eliminates the major limitation of ultrasonographic staging.

Hepatic metastases were detected in five of 30 patients, three of whom had known metastasis preoperatively. The remaining two patients had lesions smaller than 2 cm that were detected only by ultrasonography. Kodama's operative findings are significant because they illustrate the feasibility and potential yield of expanding the use of operative ultrasonography. Current efforts to combine laparoscopy with intra-abdominal ultrasonography may enhance the diagnostic power of each technique and offer the most promise for accurately selecting patients for curative resection.

Surgery

The goal in resecting the stomach for carcinoma is to remove all gross and microscopic disease. In 1984, the British Stomach Cancer Group demonstrated that achieving a clear resection margin improves survival in all patients except those who have T3 tumors or are node positive [30]. Most patients with T3 disease ate node positive and will die of their disease before developing a significant anastomotic recurrence [31]. Therefore, the quest for additional clearance when confronted with a positive margin should be tempered by the clinical stage of disease.

The ideal resection margin depends on size and histology of the tumor [32] but should be at least 5 cm in a curative operation. Bozzetti *et al.* [33] recently investigated the question of whether there is significant variation in the length of the resection margin during operation and after removal of the specimen. They found that the distance, as measured after full mobilization and surgical resection, was the same, confirming the current guidelines that the level of transection should be selected after the stomach has been fully mobilized.

Controversy continues over the best management of distal stomach cancers between proponents of total and subtotal gastrectomy. Analysis of the published series of patients who had undergone an *en principle* total gastrectomy failed to demonstrate any survival advantage of that procedure over subtotal gastrectomy [34•]. Most of these reports were published in the mid to late 1970s [35–37], which complicates meaningful comparisons with today's results. Among the studies comparing the two procedures, mortality tended to be higher for total gastrectomy (0% to 23%) than for subtotal gastrectomy (2.8% to 13%) [34•]. In one recent prospective randomized trial of total versus subtotal gastrectomy for the management of antral cancers, 169 patients were randomly assigned to either subtotal gastrectomy or total gastrectomy. The mortality rate was 3.2% following subtotal gastrectomy and 1.3% for total gastrectomy, with no difference in survival at 3 years. Our approach has been to reserve total gastrectomy for those curative cases in which a lesser procedure would jeopardize a safe margin.

Table 1. Validity of computer predictions of lymph node metastasis to various lymph node stations*

Lymph node stations	Positive predictive value, %	Negative predictive value, %	Accuracy, %
1–6†	80	94	82
7–12‡	83	100	89
13–16§	86	100	96

*Data from Bollschweiler *et al.* [44••].
†Perigastric nodes.
‡Left gastric artery, celiac axis, splenic artery, splenic hylar, and hepatoduodenal lymph nodes.
§Retropancreatic nodes, and mesenteric and para-aortic lymph nodes.

Lymphadenectomy

The surgical management of lymph-node metastases continues to be controversial. It may be of benefit in patients who have a limited number of metastatic lymph nodes in juxtaposition to the primary tumor [8•,38,39]; however, preoperatively identifying who those patients are is problematic. Multivariate analyses have consistently shown that the degree of gastric wall invasion, lymph node status, gross tumor appearance and tumor location are independently predictive of outcome following curative resection [40–42]. Maruyama *et al.* [43] developed a computer program based on their analysis of 3040 resected gastric cancer patients and Bollschweiler *et al.* [44••] tested its validity in a cohort of German patients. The computer-aided predictions were based on the patients' gender and age, and the Borrmann classification, histology, depth of wall penetration, location, and diameter of the tumor. The program proved to be highly accurate in providing information on the expected frequency of metastases in various lymph node positions (Table

1). Predictions were most accurate in determining the presence of metastatic nodes considered to be M1 disease (positions 13 to 16). The program had a powerful negative predictive value of 98%. With this kind of analysis, we can more appropriately select patients most likely to benefit from an R2 node dissection.

Conclusions

Developments in endoscopic ultrasonography, operative ultrasonography, laparoscopy, and dynamic computed tomographic scanning are bringing us closer to reliably determining how to best individualize treatment of gastric cancer. The patient with a T1 tumor can be cured by resection alone. Patients with T3 or T4 tumors should be entered into clinical trials. T2 tumors are a heterogeneous group, with varying potential for metastasis. Until we can better identify the high-risk patients, T2 patients should receive aggressive surgical resection. Studies have now shown that radical surgery can be performed safely [8•,43,45,46•]; however, the question of survival benefit remains to be answered and is currently being addressed in two large European trials.

References and recommended reading

Papers of particular interest, published within the annual period of review, have been highlighted as:

- • Of special interest
- •• Of outstanding interest

1. Brunschwig A: **Pancreato-total Gastrectomy and Splenectomy for Advanced Carcinoma of the Stomach.** *Cancer* 1948, **1**:427–430.

2. McNeer G, James A: **Resection of the Stomach and Adjacent Organs in Continuity for Advanced Cancer.** *Cancer* 1948, **1**:449–454.

3. Appleby LH: **The Coeliac Axis in the Expansion of the Operation for Gastric Carcinoma.** *Cancer* 1953, **6**:704–727.

4. Antonioli DA, Cady B: **Changing Aspects of Gastric Adenocarcinoma [Letter].** *N Engl J Med* 1984, **310**:1538.

5. Cady B: **Lymph Node Metastases: Indicators, but Not Governors of Survival.** *Arch Surg* 1984, **119**:1067–1072.

6. Gilbertson VA: **Results of Treatment of Stomach Cancer: An Appraisal of Efforts for More Extensive Surgery and a Report of 1983 Cases.** *Cancer* 1969, **23**:1305–1308.

7. Cady B, Rossi R, Silverman ML, Piccone W, Heck TA: **Gastric Adenocarcinoma: A Disease in Transition.** *Arch Surg* 1989, **124**:303–308.

8. • Jaehne J, Meyer HJ, Maschek H, Geerlings H, Burns E, Pichlmayr R: **Lymphadenectomy in Gastric Carcinoma: A Prospective and Prognostic Study.** *Arch Surg* 1992, **127**:290–294.
Demonstrates the impact of tumor stage on survival in a cohort of Western patients after thorough pathologic staging.

9. Sherman CD: **Cancer of the Gastrointestinal Tract.** In *The Manual of Clinical Oncology*. Edited by Hossfeld DK, Sherman CD, Love RR, Bosch FX. Berlin: Springer Verlag; 1990:228–252.

10. Beahrs OH, Henson DE, Hutter RVP, Myers MH: **Stomach.** In *The Manual for Staging of Cancer*. Edited by Beahrs OH, Henson DE, Hutter RV, Myers MH. Philadelphia: Lippincott; 1988:69–74.

11. Japanese Research Society for Gastric Cancer: **The General Rules for the Gastric Cancer Study in Surgery and Pathology: I. Clinical Classification.** *Jpn J Surg* 1981, **11**:127–139.

12. • Lightdale CJ: **Endoscopic Ultrasonography in the Diagnosis, Staging and Follow-Up of Esophageal and Gastric Cancer.** *Endoscopy* 1992, **24**(suppl I):297–303.
A thorough review emphasizing the use of endoscopic ultrasonography for preoperative staging.

13. Akoh JA, MacIntyre IM: **Improving Survival in Gastric Cancer: Review of 5-year Survival Rates in English Language Publications From 1970.** *Br J Surg* 1992, **79**:293–299.

14. • Rosch T, Lorenz R, Zenker K, von Wichert A, Dancygier H, Hofler H, Siewert JR, Classen M: **Local Staging and Assessment of Resectability in Carcinoma of the Esophagus, Stomach, and Duodenum by Endoscopic Ultrasonography.** *Gastrointest Endosc* 1992, **38**:460–467.
The most recent series of data from a single center with a large experience in the use of endoscopic ultrasonography in upper gastrointestinal malignancies.

15. • Rosch T: **Endoscopic Ultrasonography.** *Endoscopy* 1992, **24**:144–153.
Excellent general review of endoscopic ultrasonography with a discussion of the clinical relevance of endoscopic ultrasound staging.

16. Akahoshi K, Misawa T, Fujishima H, Chijiiwa Y, Maruoka A, Ohkubo A, Nawata H: **Preoperative Evaluation of Gastric Cancer by Endoscopic Ultrasound.** *Gut* 1991, **32**:479–482.

17. Tio TL, Schouwink MH, Cikot RJLM, Tytgat GNJ: **Preoperative TNM Classification of Gastric Carcinoma by Endosonography in Comparison With the Pathological TNM System: A Prospective Study of 72 Cases.** *Hepatogastroenterology* 1989, **36**:51–56.

18. Botet JF, Lightdale CJ, Zauber AG, Gerdes H, Urmacher C, Brennan MF: **Preoperative Staging of Gastric Cancer: Comparison of Endoscopic US and Dynamic CT.** *Radiology* 1991, **181**:426–432.

19. Ziegler K, Sanft C, Zimmer T, Zeitz M, Felsenberg D, Stein H, Germer C, Deutschmann C, Riecken EO: **Comparison of Computed Tomography, Endosonography, and Intraoperative Assessment in TN Staging of Gastric Carcinoma.** *Gut* 1993, **34**:604–610.

20. Botet JF, Lightdale CJ: **Endoscopic Sonography of the Upper Gastrointestinal Tract.** *AJR Am J Roentgenol* 1991, **156**:63–68.

21. Fein J, Gerdes H, Karpeh MS, Lauers G, Botet JF, Kelsen D, Brennan MF, Lightdale CJ: **Overstaging of Ulcerated Gastric Cancers by Endoscopic Ultrasonography [Abstract].** *Gastrointest Endosc* 1993, **39**:274.

22. Grimm H, Hamper K, Maydeo A, Maas R, Noar M, Soehendra N: **Accuracy of Endoscopic Ultrasound (EUS) and Computed Tomography (CT) in Determining Local/Regional Spread of Gastric Cancer: Results of a Prospective Controlled Study [Abstract].** *Gastrointest Endosc* 1991, **37**:279.

23. Snady H: **Endoscopic Ultrasonography: An Effective New Tool for Diagnosing Gastrointestinal Tumors.** *Oncology* 1992, **6**:63–78.

24. Lightdale CJ, Smith JW, Gerdes H, Botet JF, Brennan MF: **Preoperative Endoscopic Ultrasonography Can Predict Recurrence of Gastric Carcinoma [Abstract].** *Gastrointest Endosc* 1992, **38**:238.

25. • Minami M, Kawauchi N, Itai Y, Niki T, Sasaki Y: **Gastric Tumors: Radiologic-Pathologic Correlation and Accuracy of T Staging With Dynamic CT.** *Radiology* 1992, **185**:173–178.
Emphasizes the limitations of modern computed tomography in evaluating tumor stage.

26. Possik RA, Franco EL, Pires DR, Wohnrath DR: **Sensitivity, Specificity, and Predictive Value of Laparoscopy for the Staging of Gastric Cancer and for the Detection of Liver Metastases.** *Cancer* 1986, **58**:1–6.

27. • Kodama I, Machi J, Tanaka M, Yoshida C, Hashimoto K, Takeda J, Kakegawa T, Sigel B: **The Value of Operative Ultrasonography in Diagnosing Tumor Extension of Carcinoma of the Stomach.** *Surg Gynecol Obstet* 1992, **174**:479–484.
Important for its implications for the future of operative ultrasonography as performed via the laparoscope.

28. Kodama I, Tanaka M, Machi J, *et al.*: **Clinical Evaluation of Perioperative Ultrasonography for Gastric Cancers With Special Reference to Diagnosis of Para-Aortic Lymph Node Metastasis.** *J Jpn Soc Clin Surg* 1990, **51**:2612–2615.

29. Noguchi Y, Imada T, Matsumoto A, Coit D, Brennan MF: **Radical Surgery for Gastric Cancer: A Review of the Japanese Experience.** *Cancer* 1989, **64**:2053–2062.

30. British Stomach Cancer Group: **Resection Line Disease in Stomach Cancer.** *BMJ* 1984, **289**:601–603.

31. Papachristou DN, Karas M, Fortner JG: **Anastomotic Recurrence in the Oesophagus Complicating Gastrectomy for Adenocarcinoma of the Stomach.** *Br J Surg* 1979, **66**:609–612.

32. Cuschieri A: **Gastrectomy for Gastric Cancer: Definitions and Objectives.** *Br J Surg* 1986, **73**:513–514.

33. Bozzetti F, Bonfanti G, Regalia E, Untruly S, Doci R, La Malfa G, Gennari L: **How Long Is a 6 cm Margin of Resection in the Stomach?** *Eur J Surg Oncol* 1992, **18**:481–483.

34. • Bozzetti F: **Total Versus Subtotal Gastrectomy in Cancer of the Distal Stomach: Facts and Fantasy.** *Eur J Surg Oncol* 1992, **18**:572–579.

A current and complete discussion of the issues surrounding a long-standing debate.

35. McNeer G, Bowden L, Booher RJ, McPeak JC: **Elective Total Gastrectomy for Cancer of the Stomach: End Results.** *Ann Surg* 1974, **180**:252–256.

36. Lartat-Jacob JL, Giuli R, Estenne B, Clot PH: **Interpret de la gastrectomie totale pour le traitement des cancers de l'estomac: etude des 482 interventions radicales.** *Chirurgie* 1975, **101**:59–67.

37. Pichlmayr R, Meyer HJ: **Value of the Gastrectomy de Principe.** In *Gastric Cancer.* Edited by Herfarth CH, Schlag P. Berlin: Springer Verlag; 1979:196–204.

38. Shiu MH, Moore E, Sanders M, Huvos A, Freedman B, Goodbold J, Chaiyaphruk S, Wesdrop R, Brennan MF: **Influence of the Extent of Resection on Survival After Curative Treatment of Gastric Carcinoma: A Retrospective Multivariate Analysis.** *Arch Surg* 1987, **122**:1347–1351.

39. Maehara Y, Okuyama T, Moriguchi S, Orita H, Kusumoto H, Korenaga D, Sugimachi K: **Prophylactic Lymph Node Dissection in Patients With Advanced Gastric Cancer Promotes Increased Survival Time.** *Cancer* 1992, **70**:392–395.

40. Arveux P, Faivre J, Boutron M-C, Piard F, Dusserre-Guion L, Monnet E, Hillon P: **Prognosis of Gastric Carcinoma After Curative Surgery: A Population-Based Study Using Multivariate Crude and Relative Survival Analysis.** *Dig Dis Sci* 1992, **37**:757–763.

41. Maruyama K: **The Most Important Prognostic Factors for Gastric Cancer Patients: A Study Using Univariate and Multivariate Analyses.** *Scand J Gastroenterol* 1987, **22(suppl 133)**:63–68.

42. Moriguchi S, Maehara Y, Korenaga D, Sugimachi K, Hayashi Y, Nose Y: **Prediction of Survival Time After Curative Surgery for Advanced Gastric Cancer.** *Eur J Surg Oncol* 1992, **18**:287–292.

43. Maruyama K, Okabayashi K, Kinoshita Y: **Progress in Gastric Cancer Surgery in Japan and Its Limits of Radicality.** *World J Surg* 1987, **11**:418–425.

44. Bollschweiler E, Boettcher K, Hoelscher AH, Sasako M, Kinoshita
•• T, Maruyama K, Siewert JR: **Preoperative Assessment of Lymph Node Metastases in Patients With Gastric Cancer: Evaluation of the Maruyama Computer Program.** *Br J Surg* 1992, **79**:156–160.

An important study that evaluates an exciting new method of preoperatively assessing extent of nodal metastasis. It is also an excellent comparison of presentation of this disease in Japanese and German patients.

45. Smith JW, Shiu MH, Kelsey L, Brennan MF: **Morbidity of Radical Lymphadenectomy in the Curative Resection of Gastric Carcinoma.** *Arch Surg* 1991, **126**:1469–1473.

46. Bonenkamp JJ, van de Velde CJ, Sasako M, Hermans J: **R2 Compared
• With R1 Resection for Gastric Cancer: Morbidity and Mortality in a Prospective, Randomized Trial.** *Eur J Surg* 1992, **158**:413–418.

The latest update from a large, well-controlled randomized trial that emphasizes the importance of proper instruction in maintaining an acceptable morbidity and mortality following an R2 resection.

47. Karpeh M: **Adenocarcinoma of the Stomach.** In *Current Practice of Surgery.* Edited by Levine BA, Copeland EN, Howard RJ, Sugarman HJ, Warshaw AL. New York: Churchill Livingstone; 1993:1–24.

Martin S. Karpeh, Jr, MD, and Murray F. Brennan, MD, Department of Surgery, Memorial Sloan-Kettering Cancer Center, 1275 York Avenue, New York, NY 10021, USA.

Recent advances in the localization and surgical management of duodenal gastrinomas

Gary P. Lawton, MD, and Irvin M. Modlin, MD, PhD

Yale University School of Medicine, New Haven, Connecticut, USA

Duodenal gastrinomas are now more frequently recognized as the source of hypergastrinemia in patients with Zollinger-Ellison syndrome. The cell lineage of duodenal gastrinomas may differ from that of pancreatic gastrinomas, which accounts for variations in their clinical behavior. Attempts to localize the submucosal tumors are difficult and are limited by their small size. Intraoperative endoscopic transillumination, selective intra-arterial secretin injection, and duodenotomy with mucosal eversion are currently the most sensitive and reliable methods of localization. Endoscopic ultrasonography and somatostatin scintigraphy further enhance the accuracy of preoperative localization of these tumors. Current information based on cure rates and survival data mandates a primary surgical approach in patients with either the sporadic or the multiple endocrine neoplasia type 1–associated form of the disease. Thus, wide local resection of duodenal gastrinomas with removal of all tumor-bearing lymphatic tissue and acid inhibitory pharmacotherapy (proton pump inhibition) may yield 5-year survival rates of 80% to 90%. Similarly, in patients with pancreatic and duodenal gastrinomas as a manifestation of multiple endocrine neoplasia type 1, the additional enucleation of pancreatic lesions with or without distal pancreatectomy has resulted in cure rates of 67% to 100%.

Current Opinion in General Surgery 1994:131–137

In 1955, Zollinger and Ellison [1] initially described the association of gastric hypersecretion, hyperacidity, atypical peptic ulceration, and non–insulin-producing islet cell tumors of the pancreas. The resection of these pancreatic tumors has failed to result in a reliable cure because the lesions present late and are often metastatic or multicentric. Of particular interest is the more recent recognition that 20% to 77% of the gastrinomas responsible for the Zollinger-Ellison syndrome (ZES) may be located in the submucosa of the duodenum [2•,3,4••,5,6,7••]. In 1958, Oberhelman, *et al.* [8] reported the first cure of ZES by the resection of a primary duodenal gastrinoma. In the succeeding two decades, total gastrectomy was used in the treatment of ZES to obviate the complications of the hypersecretion of gastric acid. Surgical cures of ZES (achievement of eugastrinemia) during this period may, in fact, have been largely the result of inadvertent resection of duodenal tumors as a component of the total gastrectomy [9]. The recent experience with the identification and resection of duodenal gastrinomas has supported this possibility. Over the past three decades, the development of the gastrin radioimmunoassay has enhanced the early diagnosis of ZES [10]. Similarly, the introduction of histamine$_2$ receptor antagonists has revolutionized the medical management of the disease (Table 1). With the further development of specific parietal cell proton pump inhibitor pharmacotherapy, the surgical control of acid hypersecretion has become relatively obsolete.

These therapeutic advances, combined with the increasing awareness of the variable malignant potential of the gastrinoma, have resulted in a major medical shift in the emphasis of treatment. The role of surgery has become focused more on the identification and resection of solitary or focal lesions. This change has been particularly evident in the emphasis placed on recognition of primary duodenal wall gastrinomas. The increased awareness that this component of ZES is encountered with greater frequency than was originally reported has been of considerable therapeutic relevance. Attempts at resection for cure have resulted in eugastrinemia in up to 82% of patients [11], with 5- and 10-year survival rates of greater than 85% [2•]. The high clinical profile of this disease and the widespread availability of the gastrin radioimmunoassay have resulted in an increasing number of patients presenting earlier,

Abbreviations

MEN-1—multiple endocrine neoplasia type 1; **ZES**—Zollinger-Ellison syndrome.

 ISBN 1-85922-671-X ISSN 1065–6243

Table 1. Significant events in the history of the localization and treatment of the duodenal gastrinoma

Year	Event
1955	Original description of Zollinger-Ellison syndrome [1]
1958	Excision of duodenal gastrinoma; cure rates of 2% to 5% reported [8]
1960	Identification of gastrin as the secretory product of the islet-cell tumor in Zollinger-Ellison syndrome
1968	Development of the gastrin radioimmunoassay [10]
1972	Introduction of the secretin injection test [35]
1976	Histamine$_2$ receptor antagonists shift the focus to the medical management of patients with Zollinger-Ellison syndrome
1977	Description of portal venous gastrin sampling [31]
1980	Intraoperative identification of duodenal gastrinomas
1982	Identification of biologic differences in gastrinomas from different locations
1984	Introduction of proton pump inhibition (omeprazole)
1988	Definition of the gastrinoma triangle; augmented localization of duodenal tumors [33]
1990	Description of intraoperative endoscopic transillumination [3]; reports of increased cure rates of 30% to 82% [2•,4••,11,13]

with smaller tumors that are more difficult to locate. Thus, preoperative localization of the gastrinoma has become a critical adjunct to successful resection of the tumor. Imaging techniques capable of visualizing the duodenum and the head of the pancreas have been used in attempts to establish topographic localization. Recent advances in the use of endoscopic ultrasonography and somatostatin scintigraphy to localize both primary gastrinomas and metastases have amplified the likelihood of preoperative localization and successful surgical resection of the lesion. The importance of accurate identification of all components of the tumor has been accentuated by recent information suggesting that resection of primary duodenal gastrinomas in patients with either sporadic or multiple endocrine neoplasia type 1 (MEN-1)–associated ZES may be curative.

Epidemiology

In 1964, Ellison and Wilson [12] reported that 20% of patients with ZES exhibited duodenal gastrinomas. More recently, this figure has been reported to be much larger, as high as 77% in patients exhibiting the sporadic form of the disease [2•,3,4••,5,6,7••]. Of note is the observation that duodenal gastrinomas occur in up to 100% of patients with ZES as a manifestation of MEN-1 [13]. The characteristics of the patients with duodenal gastrinomas are not inconsistent with the general epidemiology of ZES.

Biologic behavior

The clinicopathologic characteristics of duodenal gastrinomas appear to differ in some respects from those of pancreatic gastrinomas. Imamura *et al.* [14•] reported a statistically significant difference in the incidence of hepatic and lymphatic metastases between patients with duodenal and those with pancreatic primary tumors. Multiple liver metastases were more often found in patients with pancreatic gastrinomas, whereas lymphatic metastases were more common in patients with duodenal tumors. Immunohistochemical analysis of the tumors and their associated metastases revealed some differences in the peptide secretory profile of the tumors. This difference in molecular pathology was interpreted by the authors as evidence of a different process of cellular differentiation or lineage in the respective tumors.

The biologic variation between pancreatic and duodenal gastrinomas was further illustrated by Howard *et al.* [15], who noted that a majority of tumors to the right of the superior mesenteric artery exhibited lymph node metastasis (64%). This finding contrasted with the incidence of hepatic metastases in tumors to the left of the superior mesenteric artery (56%). The tumors to the right of the superior mesenteric artery were more often resectable (73% vs 25%), and resulted in cure rates of 43% (right) and 6% (left). On the basis of these differences, the authors concluded that gastrinomas to the right of the superior mesenteric artery, which are more frequently extrapancreatic, duodenal, and within the lymph nodes, behave in a more benign fashion and can be adequately treated by local excision. Conversely, gastrinomas to the left of the superior mesenteric artery, which are always pancreatic in origin, rarely involve the lymph nodes and are frequently metastatic to the liver, behave in a more malignant fashion, and have a poor long-term prognosis, regardless of the nature of the operation.

Duodenal gastrinomas in multiple endocrine neoplasia type 1

Although there is a recognized benefit to the resection of sporadic gastrinomas in ZES, controversy still surrounds the surgical treatment of patients who have gastrinomas as a component of MEN-1. Hypergastrinemia in patients with ZES due to MEN-1 was previously believed to represent multiple pancreatic gastrinomas scattered throughout the gland. Surgical attempts at cure using partial pancreatectomy were unsuccessful [16]. Farley *et al.* [2•], Delcore *et al.* [17], and Grama *et al.* [18] reported only transient, if any, eugastrinemia in patients treated surgically, with a high incidence of subsequent metastases and death from progression of the disease. However, recent evidence has suggested that an aggressive surgical approach may be warranted. Pipeleers-Marichal *et al.* [13] reported successful cure (eugastrinemia) in up to two thirds of patients with MEN-1 and duodenal gastrinomas who underwent tumor resection. Similarly, Thompson [19•] reported the surgical cure of 10 of 11 (91%) patients with ZES and MEN-1 who were subjected to an extensive exploration and resection of duodenal and pancreatic gastrinomas.

Localization techniques

A myriad of techniques, some routine and widely available and others highly specialized and invasive, have been used in attempts to localize the elusive submucosal gastrinoma of the duodenum. Overall, preoperative imaging studies successfully localize duodenal gastrinomas in some 10% to 50% of cases [2•,3,4••,5,7••,20]. Preoperative localization is thus unreliable, and negative imaging findings should not deter operative exploration and recognition of the possibility that an undetected duodenal gastrinoma may be present.

Noninvasive

Noninvasive localization techniques include transabdominal ultrasonography, computed tomography, magnetic resonance imaging, and radionuclide scintigraphy. Transabdominal ultrasonography [21], computed tomography [22], and magnetic resonance imaging [20] have been used with very limited success in the localization of duodenal gastrinomas because none of these techniques is able to image tumors less than 1 cm in diameter reliably.

In 1987, Reubi *et al.* [23], using *in vitro* techniques, demonstrated somatostatin receptors on gastrinomas. Subsequently, ^{123}I-labeled octreotide and more recently ^{111}In-labeled pentatreotide radionuclide scanning techniques for gastrinomas have been developed. Lamberts *et al.* [24] reported successful localization of all three pancreatic gastrinomas studied. Furthermore, they were able to identify tumors with somatostatin receptors that were as small as 1 cm in diameter. The exquisite sensitivity of somatostatin receptor imaging makes it of considerable promise in the localization of gastrinomas.

Invasive

Although intraoperative ultrasonography has been reported to be sensitive enough to detect tumors smaller than 0.5 cm in diameter, as well as tumors of the duodenal wall, in a recent prospective analysis of 44 patients with islet cell tumors, it failed to image 56% of the primary duodenal gastrinomas [25]. This result was confirmed by Sugg *et al.* [7••], who found only 26% of 31 surgically confirmed duodenal gastrinomas using intraoperative ultrasonography.

Angiography has also been shown to be of limited use in localizing duodenal gastrinomas. Even when an extrahepatic gastrinoma has been imaged, it is reported to be impossible to determine the tumor's precise location. This was recently shown in 70 consecutive patients: angiography exhibited a sensitivity of 68%, a specificity of 94%, and a negative predictive value of 53% [26]. Of note, 66% of the primary gastrinomas of the duodenum, all of which were less than 1 cm in diameter, were not identified.

Endoscopic ultrasonography has been shown to be a highly sensitive and specific tool for the localization of pancreatic endocrine tumors. With its high-frequency resolution, endoscopic ultrasonography may be used to identify structures as small as 2 to 3 mm in diameter in the pancreas. Rosch, *et al.* [27] reported the successful localization of 82% of pancreatic gastrinomas using this technique. Endoscopic ultrasonography has also been successfully used to localize pancreatic and extrapancreatic gastrinomas in 60% of patients [28], but it was not adequate in imaging either pedunculated tumors or those less than 1 cm in diameter. Only limited information is available on the use of endoscopic ultrasonography to specifically identify gastrinomas of the duodenal wall. Lightdale, *et al.* [29] reported the detection of two tumors in one patient, but Ruszniewski, *et al.* [30] failed to image the two duodenal tumors present in 13 patients with gastrinoma.

Intraoperative endoscopic transillumination of the duodenum may prove to be the most effective way to identify the usually small (less than 1 cm in diameter) gastrinomas in this location (Fig. 1). In a prospective analysis of 26 patients, Frucht *et al.* [3] reported a sensitivity of 83%. Identification was achieved by preoperative imaging studies or by intraoperative ultrasonography and direct palpation in only a fraction of these patients (25% and 42%, respectively). Seventy-five percent of the tumors less than 1 cm in diameter were located, and 80% of the lesions between 1 and 1.5 cm and 100% of the tumors greater than 1.5 cm were identified. Although a specific percentage was not reported, the authors stated that most tumors located by transillumination were not palpable until a duodenotomy had been performed.

In 1977, Ingemansson *et al.* [31] reported the first successful localization of a gastrinoma by gastrin assay of venous blood obtained by direct catheterization of a branch of the portal vein. To date, selective sampling of portal venous tributaries has been used extensively in an attempt to localize gastrinomas. However, because of the shared venous drainage, discrimination cannot be made between the duodenum and the pancreatic head. Consequently, some controversy exists as to the efficacy of this method. In a recent study, localization was provided in 64% of patients [32] with tumors in the gastrinoma triangle [33]. Vinik *et al.* [34] reported a sensitivity of 94% in localizing the tumor either to the gastrinoma triangle or to the body or tail of the pancreas.

The direct intra-arterial injection of secretin with hepatic venous gastrin measurement was described by Imamura [35] in 1987. Subsequently, the sensitivity of the procedure was confirmed by several authors [36–38]. Recently, intra-arterial secretin injection sampling was prospectively studied in 36 consecutive patients. An overall localization success of 89% was achieved [39•]. No patients with a duodenal tumor had negative findings with intra-arterial secretin injection but 25% exhibited negative findings with portal venous sampling.

Intraoperative intra-arterial methylene blue injection has been used to successfully identify a small (6 mm) duodenal gastrinoma that was not imaged by any of the previously mentioned techniques [40]. However, the mechanism of this method has not been elucidated.

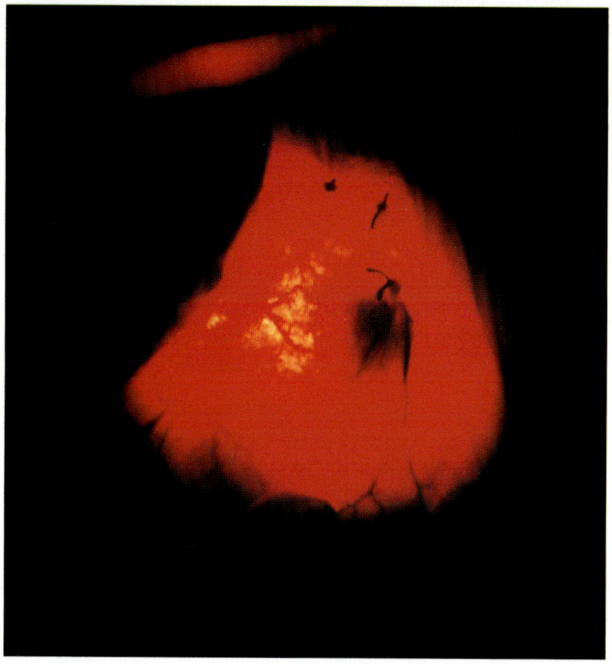

Fig. 1. The serosal surface of the second part of the duodenum, transilluminated during surgery to define structures within the duodenal wall. The area that failed to transilluminate was excised and histologically proven to be a gastrinoma. (*From* Frucht *et al.* [3]; with permission.)

Duodenotomy has been advocated for localization of primary duodenal gastrinomas in all patients undergoing laparotomy for resection and cure [4••,19•,41]. Thompson [19•] and Sugg *et al.* [7••] described the localization of tumors that were otherwise not identified until a duodenotomy with meticulous evaluation of the mucosa by eversion and direct palpation was performed. The technique is not without morbidity. Complications, which were observed in 17% of Sugg *et al.*'s patients, included pancreatitis, duodenal leak, and intra-abdominal abscess.

Surgical treatment

It has been reported that more than 50% of patients with unresected gastrinomas will die of the disease [42–44]. Because chemotherapy and radiation therapy had been shown to be ineffective in halting this progression [45], surgical resection was advocated as early as 1961 [46]. Surgical treatment options range from local excision, with or without lymph node dissection, to pancreatoduodenectomy. The role of pancreatoduodenectomy in the treatment of primary duodenal wall gastrinomas has always been controversial. When the procedure was first recommended, the operative morbidity and mortality were prohibitively high [46]. Now that experience with the procedure has lowered the attendant morbidity, it may be entertained as a viable surgical option for the widespread ablation of gastrinoma tissue. Pancreatoduodenectomy was recommended for patients with extensive pancreatioduodenal gastrinoma by Delcore and Friesen [47] in 1992, based both on their surgical results in three patients treated over a 30-year period, and on a review of the literature, which yielded an additional 16 cures (eugastrinemia). This proposal has not been widely accepted.

The most reasonable surgical approach to the patient with gastrinoma is an extensive exploratory laparotomy with local resection of all identifiable disease (Fig. 2). Inspection of the liver for metastases is performed first. Although Cherner and Sawyers [48] and Norton *et al.* [49] have reported liver resections for hepatic gastrinoma in a total of four patients, only two were disease-free 1 year after resection. Patients with metastatic gastrinoma to the liver exhibit a 5-year survival rate of less than 20% [4••]. It is generally accepted, therefore [2•,4••,11,19•,41], that in the presence of hepatic metastases, the patient should be treated medically. If no hepatic disease is identified, the entire pancreas is exposed and examined. Masses in the head and body of the pancreas should be enucleated if possible. Lesions in the tail should be resected by distal pancreatectomy. Evaluation of the duodenum should be undertaken initially by palpation, followed by endoscopic transillumination. Thereafter, a duodenotomy should be performed and all other duodenal gastrinomas identified. The lesions should then be locally resected with a wide margin, after the ampulla of Vater has been identified. Careful sampling of pancreaticoduodenal lymph nodes should be undertaken, with a wide dissection of this area. This aggressive surgical approach is advocated for patients with sporadic ZES and those with MEN-1–associated ZES.

Endoscopic treatment

Endoscopic treatment of a duodenal gastrinoma was reported in a patient who had previously undergone a partial gastrectomy, a vagotomy, and a Billroth II reconstruction for duodenal ulcer disease [50]. Within 24 hours, the patient underwent laparotomy with duodenorrhaphy for a 1.5-cm full-thickness perforation. This two-stage procedure is probably suboptimal because even if the endoscopic removal is successful, other duodenal gastrinomas might not be identified and lymph node deposits would be left in place.

Outcome

Although historically, rates of cure (defined as eugastrinemia) have been reported to be only 2% to 5%, rates of 10% to 82% have more recently been reported for patients undergoing surgical resection of duodenal gastrinomas [2•,4••,11].

Despite the presence of metastatic disease to the lymph nodes, duodenal gastrinomas overall seem to be associated with a somewhat better survival rate than that seen with pancreatic gastrinomas. Farley, *et al.* [2•] reported a survival rate after resection of duodenal gastrinomas of 87% at 5 years and 85% at 10 years. Norton *et al.* [4••] also reported, in a mixed population

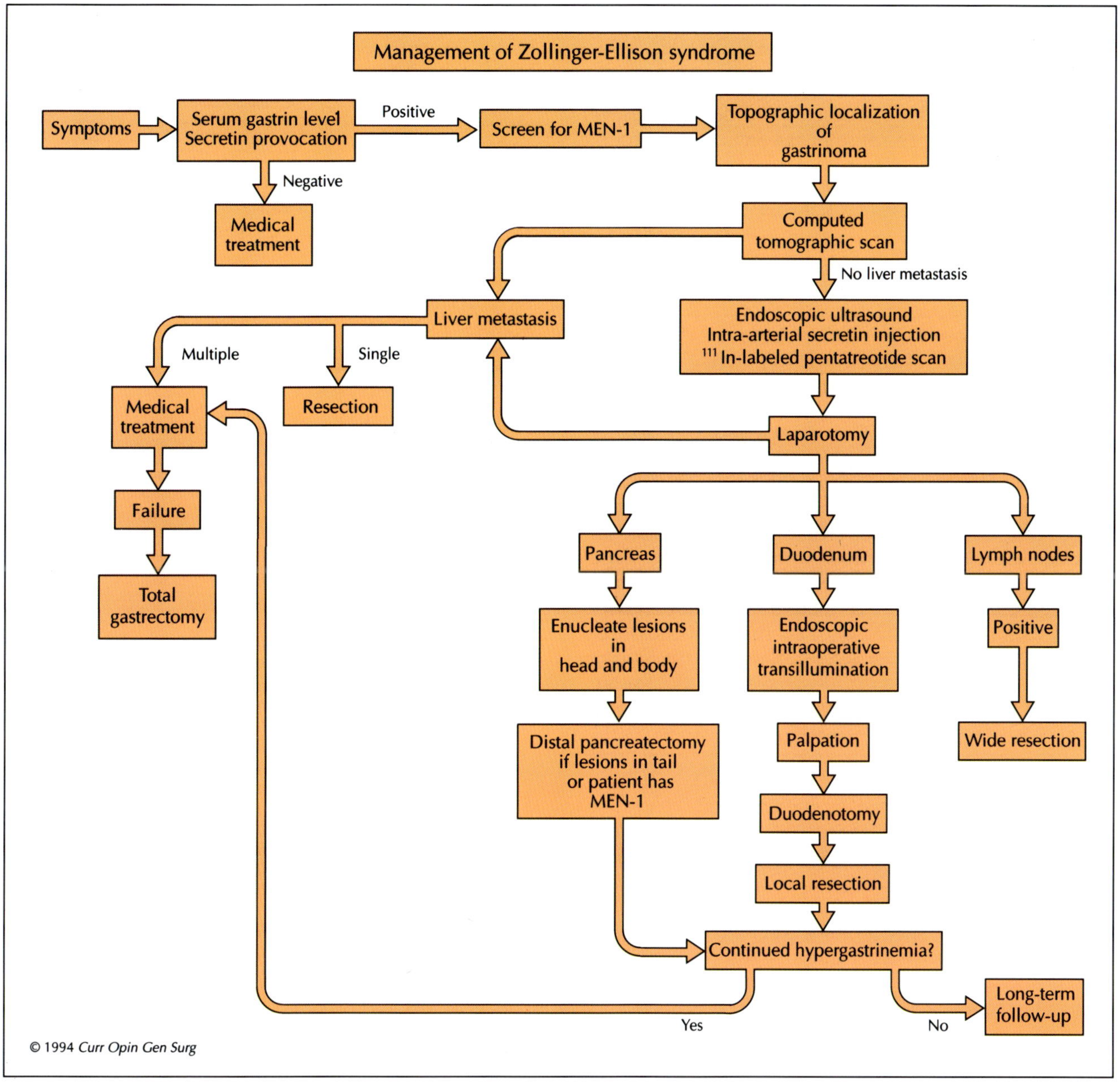

Fig. 2. Management of Zollinger-Ellison syndrome. MEN-1—multiple endocrine neoplasia type 1.

of patients with duodenal and pancreatic gastrinomas without evidence of hepatic metastases, a 5-year survival rate of greater than 90% after tumor resection. In a retrospective analysis of 90 patients with ZES treated surgically over a 32-year period, a significant correlation was noted by Farley *et al.* [2•] between long-term survival and tumor size, location, and the presence of metastases. Tumors less than 1 cm in diameter and those located in the duodenum rather than in the pancreas were associated with a better survival. The presence of metastatic disease was an indicator of poor prognosis. Outcome in patients with hepatic tumors was significantly worse than that in patients with lymphatic disease. No correlation was noted between survival and the preoperative gastrin level, patient age, patient gender, the operative procedure, or disease etiology (MEN-1 or sporadic).

Conclusions

Duodenal gastrinomas have become more frequently recognized as a source of hypergastrinemia in patients with ZES. Patients with MEN-1 are likely to have multiple duodenal gastrinomas in association with pancreatic lesions. The peptide secretory profile, pattern of metastatic spread, and long-term prognosis differ somewhat between duodenal and pancreatic primary tumors.

Imaging techniques are limited in their ability to localize the tumors, which are commonly less than 1 cm in diameter. Currently, intraoperative endoscopic transillumination of the duodenum and selective intra-arterial secretin injection testing are the most sensitive and reliable methods of localizing duodenal gastrinomas. Careful palpation through the intact duodenum, as well as visual inspection and palpation via a limited duodenotomy, are useful intraoperative methods for identifying small submucosal tumors. In the future, ^{111}In-labeled pentatreotide scanning will probably be of significant benefit in successfully localizing duodenal gastrinomas.

Because the complications of acid hypersecretion are significantly less common given the potency of the antisecretory drugs, a large proportion of patients with unresected tumors now die as a consequence of the malignant progression of their disease. For this reason, an aggressive surgical approach is advocated. Resection of duodenal tumors, with a rim of normal tissue when possible, or by pancreatoduodenectomy if necessary, is the recommended treatment for patients with sporadic disease and for those with MEN-1–associated disease. It is difficult to summarize the cure rates because of differences in the definition of cure (either eugastrinemia or negative findings on provocative secretin testing) and in the length of follow-up among the many studies. However, eugastrinemia after surgical resection is reported in 40% to 82% of patients with the sporadic form of the disease at various intervals. Early attempts to cure patients with gastrinomas as a manifestation of MEN-1 failed. Recently, an aggressive surgical approach resulted in eugastrinema in 91% of the 11 patients studied. Despite the recurrence of hypergastrinemia in a significant proportion of patients, survival rates are excellent after resection of duodenal tumors and have been reported to be as high as 85% at 10 years. Duodenal gastrinomas, whether sporadic or a manifestation of MEN-1, are more amenable to surgical resection than are pancreatic gastrinomas.

References and recommended reading

Papers of particular interest, published within the annual period of review, have been highlighted as:

- • Of special interest
- •• Of outstanding interest

1. Zollinger RM, Ellison EH: **Primary Peptic Ulcerations of the Jejunum Associated With Islet Cell Tumors of the Pancreas.** *Ann Surg* 1955, **142**:709–728.

2. • Farley DR, van Heerden JA, Grant CS, Miller LJ, Ilstrup DM: **The Zollinger-Ellison Syndrome: A Collective Surgical Experience.** *Ann Surg* 1992, **215**:561–570.

In a retrospective study of 90 surgically treated patients with ZES, the epidemiology, localization, pathology, and management were evaluated with respect to patient outcome. Significant correlations were observed between survival and small tumor size, extrapancreatic primary tumor location, and absence of metastatic disease. Complete resection of tumor burden was recommended for patients without liver metastases. An aggressive surgical approach to patients with ZES and MEN-1 was also advocated.

3. Frucht H, Norton JA, London JF, Vinayek R, Doppman JL, Gardner JD, Jensen RT, Maton PN: **Detection of Duodenal Gastrinomas by Operative Endoscopic Transillumination: A Prospective Study.** *Gastroenterology* 1990, **99**:1622–1627.

4. •• Norton JA, Doppman JL, Jensen RT: **Curative Resection in Zollinger-Ellison Syndrome: Results of a 10-Year Prospective Study.** *Ann Surg* 1992, **215**:8–18.

In this 10-year prospective study of the diagnosis and treatment of patients with ZES without liver metastases (n=73), the results of the recent focus on the identification of duodenal gastrinomas were evaluated. Significantly more gastrinomas were found and resected after the institution of routine duodenal transillumination and duodenotomy. The difference between disease-free interval (eugastrinemia) and survival is underscored. An evaluation of the disease-free interval reported for the duodenal and "nodal" primary tumors must take into account that the latter are considered by many to be metastases from missed or previously resected duodenal tumors.

5. Thom AK, Norton JA, Axiotis CA, Jensen RT: **Location, Incidence, and Malignant Potential of Duodenal Gastrinomas.** *Surgery* 1991, **110**:1086–1093.

6. Delcore R, Cheung LY, Friesen SR: **Characteristics of Duodenal Wall Gastrinomas.** *Am J Surg* 1990, **160**:621–624.

7. •• Sugg SL, Norton JA, Fraker DL, Mets DC, Pisegna JR, Fishbeyn V, Benya RV, Shawker TH, Doppman JL, Jensen RT: **A Prospective Study of Intraoperative Methods to Diagnose and Resect Duodenal Gastrinomas.** *Ann Surg* 1993, **218**:138–144.

In a prospective study of 35 consecutive patients with ZES who underwent surgical exploration for gastrinomas, the identification of duodenal tumors was attempted by palpation, intraoperative ultrasonography, intraoperative endoscopic transillumination, and duodenotomy. The sensitivities were 61%, 26%, 64%, and 100%, respectively. Duodenotomy identified five duodenal tumors (16%) that were not imaged by any of the other techniques. Postoperative complications ranging from pancreatitis to duodenal leak and intra-abdominal abscess were observed in 17.1% of the patients. The authors recommend the combination of intraoperative endoscopic transillumination and routine duodenotomy for all patients undergoing exploration for gastrinoma.

8. Oberhelman HA Jr, Nelson TS, Dragstedt LR: **Peptic Ulcer Associated With Tumors of the Pancreas.** *Arch Surg* 1958, 77:402–415.

9. Delcore R, Friesen SR: **Zollinger-Ellison Syndrome: A New Look at Regression of Gastrinomas.** *Arch Surg* 1991, **126**:556–558.

10. McGuigan JE, Trudeau WL: **Immunochemical Measurement of Elevated Levels of Gastrin in the Serum of Patients With Pancreatic Tumors of the Zollinger-Ellison Variety.** *N Engl J Med* 1968, **278**:1308–1313.

11. Howard TJ, Zinner MJ, Stabile BE, Passaro E Jr: **Gastrinoma Excision for Cure: A Prospective Analysis.** *Ann Surg* 1990, **211**:9–14.

12. Ellison EH, Wilson SD: **The Zollinger-Ellison Syndrome: Reappraisal and Evaluation of 260 Registered Cases.** *Ann Surg* 1964, **160**:512–530.

13. Pipeleers-Marichal M, Somers G, Willems G, Foulis A, Imrie C, Bishop AE, Polak JM, Hacki WH, Stamm B, Heitz PU, Kloppel G: **Gastrinomas in the Duodenums of Patients With Multiple Endocrine Neoplasia Type 1 and the Zollinger-Ellison Syndrome.** *N Engl J Med* 1990, **322**:723–727.

14. • Imamura M, Kanda M, Takahashi K, Shimanda Y, Miyahara T, Wagata T, Hashimoto M, Tobe T, Soga J: **Clinicopathological Characteristics of Duodenal Microgastrinomas.** *World J Surg* 1992, **16**:703–710.

A retrospective analysis of 114 patients with ZES but not MEN-1 revealed a significant difference in the incidence of hepatic and lymph node metastases between patients with primary duodenal gastrinomas and those with pancreatic gastrinomas. Immunohistochemical analysis of the primary and metastatic tumors revealed some differences in the peptide secretory profiles. The authors interpreted this information as evidence for a different process of cellular differentiation or lineage in the respective tumors.

15. Howard TJ, Sawicki MP, Stabile BE, Watt PC, Passaro E Jr: **Biologic Behavior of Sporadic Gastrinoma Located to the Right and Left of the Superior Mesenteric Artery.** *Am J Surg* 1993, **165**:101–106.

16. Deveney CW, Deveney KE, Stark D, Moss A, Stein S, Way LW: **Resection of Gastrinomas.** *Ann Surg* 1983, **198**:546–553.

17. Delcore R, Hermreck AS, Friesen SR: **Selective Surgical Management of Correctable Hypergastrinemia.** *Surgery* 1989, **106**:1094–1102.

18. Grama D, Skogseid B, Wilander E, Eriksson B, Martensson H, Cedermark B, Ahren B, Kristofferson A, Oberg K, Rastad J, Akerstrom G: **Pancreatic Tumors in Multiple Endocrine Neoplasia Type 1: Clinical Presentation and Surgical Treatment.** *World J Surg* 1992, **16**:611–619.

19. • Thompson NW: **Surgical Treatment of the Endocrine Pancreas and Zollinger-Ellison Syndrome in the MEN-1 Syndrome.** *Henry Ford Hosp Med J* 1992, **40**:195–198.

Patients with MEN-1 and ZES without liver metastases (n=11) were subjected to an extensive exploration including duodenotomy, peripancreatic lymph node dissection, enucleation of pancreatic head tumors, resection of duodenal tumors, and distal pancreatectomy. Duodenal gastrinomas were identified in 64% of the patients. A surgical cure (eugastrinemia) was achieved in 91% of patients. An aggressive surgical approach to patients with gastrinomas as a manifestation of MEN-1 was advocated.

20. FRUCHT H, DOPPMAN JL, NORTON JA, MILLER DL, DWYER AJ, FRANK JA, VINAYEK R, MATON PN, JENSEN RT: **Gastrinomas: Comparison of MR Imaging With CT, Angiography, and US.** *Radiology* 1989, **171**:713–717.

21. LONDON JF, SHAWKER TH, DOPPMAN JL, FRUCHT HH, VINAYEK R, STARK HA, MILLER LS, MILLER DL, NORTON JA, JENSEN RT, GARDNER JD, MATON PN: **Zollinger-Ellison Syndrome: Prospective Assessment of Abdominal US in the Localization of Gastrinomas.** *Radiology* 1991, **178**:763–767.

22. WANK SA, DOPPMAN JL, MILLER DL, COLLEN MJ, MATON PN, VINAYEK R, SLAFF JI, NORTON JA, GARDNER JD, JENSEN RT: **Prospective Study of the Ability of Computed Axial Tomography to Localize Gastrinomas in Patients With Zollinger-Ellison Syndrome.** *Gastroenterology* 1987, **92**:905–912.

23. REUBI JC, HACKI WH, LAMBERTS SWJ: **Hormone-Producing Gastrointestinal Tumours Contain a High Density of Somatostatin Receptors.** *J Clin Endocrinol Metab* 1987, **65**:1127–1134.

24. LAMBERTS SWJ, BAKKER WH, REUBI JC, KRENNING EP: **Somatostatin Receptor Imaging in the Localization of Endocrine Tumors.** *N Engl J Med* 1990, **323**:1246–1249.

25. NORTON JA, CROMACK DT, SHAWKER TH, DOPPMAN JL, COMI R, GORDEN P, MATON PN, GARDNER JD, JENSEN RT: **Intraoperative Ultrasonic Localization of Islet Cell Tumors: A prospective Comparison to Palpation.** *Ann Surg* 1988, **207**:160–168.

26. MATON PN, MILLER DL, DOPPMAN JL, COLLEN MJ, NORTON JA, VINAYEK R, SLAFF JI, WANK SA, GARDNER JD, JENSEN RT: **Role of Selective Angiography in the Management of Patients With Zollinger-Ellison Syndrome.** *Gastroenterology* 1987, **92**:913–918.

27. ROSCH T, LIGHTDALE CJ, BOTET JF, BOYCE GA, SIVAK MV, YASUDA K, HEYDER N, PALAZZO L, DANCYGIER H, SCHUSDZIARRA V, CLASSEN M: **Localization of Pancreatic Endocrine Tumors by Endoscopic Ultrasonography.** *N Engl J Med* 1992, **326**:1721–1726.

28. PALAZZO L, ROSEAU G, SALMERON M: **Endoscopic Ultrasonography in the Preoperative Localization of Pancreatic Endocrine Tumors.** *Endoscopy* 1992, **24**(suppl 1):350–353.

29. LIGHTDALE CJ, BOTET JF, WOODRUFF JM, BRENNAN MF: **Localization of Endocrine Tumors of the Pancreas With Endoscopic Ultrasonography.** *Cancer* 1991, **68**:1815–1820.

30. RUSZNIEWSKI P, AMOUYAL P, COMBES R: **Endoscopic Ultrasonography Is Useful for the Localization of Primary Gastrinomas [Abstract].** *Gastroenterology* 1991, **100**(suppl A):297.

31. INGEMANSSON S, LARSSON L, LUNDERQUIST A, STADIL F: **Pancreatic Vein Catheterization With Gastrin Assay in Normal Patients and in Patients With the Zollinger-Ellison Syndrome.** *Am J Surg* 1977, **134**:558–563.

32. MILLER DL, DOPPMAN JL, METZ DC, MATON PN, NORTON JA, JENSEN RT: **Zollinger-Ellison Syndrome: Technique, Results, and Complications of Portal Venous Sampling.** *Radiology* 1992, **182**:235–241.

33. STABILE BE, MORROW DJ, PASSARO E JR: **The Gastrinoma Triangle: Operative Implications.** *Am J Surg* 1984, **147**:25–31.

34. VINIK AI, MOATTARI AR, CHO K, THOMPSON N: **Transhepatic Portal Vein Catheterization for Localization of Sporadic and MEN Gastrinomas: A Ten Year Experience.** *Surgery* 1990, **107**:246–255.

35. IMAMURA M, TAKAHASHI K, ADACHI H, MINEMATSU S, SHIMADA Y, NAITO M, SUZUKI T, TOBE T, AZUMA T: **Usefulness of Selective Arterial Secretin Injection Test for Localization of Gastrinoma in the Zollinger-Ellison Syndrome.** *Ann Surg* 1987, **205**:230–239.

36. IMAMURA M, TAKAHASHI K, ISOBE Y, HATTORI Y, SATOMURA K, TOBE T: **Curative Resection of Multiple Gastrinomas Aided by Selective Arterial Secretin Injection Test and Intraoperative Secretin Test.** *Ann Surg* 1989, **210**:710–718.

37. DOPPMAN JL, MILLER DL, CHANG R, MATON PN, LONDON JF, GARDNER JD, JENSEN RT, NORTON JA: **Gastrinomas: Localization by Means of Selective Intraarterial Injection of Secretin.** *Radiology* 1990, **174**:25–29.

38. ROSATO FE, BONN J, SHAPIRO M, BARBOT DJ, FURNARY AM, GARDINER GA: **Selective Arterial Stimulation of Secretin in Localization of Gastrinomas.** *Surg Gynecol Obstet* 1990, **171**:196–200.

39. • THOM AK, NORTON JA, DOPPMAN JL, MILLER DL, CHANG R, JENSEN RT: **Prospective Study of the Use of Intraarterial Secretin Injection and Portal Venous Sampling to Localize Duodenal Gastrinomas.** *Surgery* 1992, **112**:1002–1009.

Intra-arterial secretin injection was prospectively compared with portal venous sampling in 36 consecutive patients with ZES. Localization was provided with intra-arterial secretin injection in 89% of the patients. Portal venous sampling resulted in localization in only 60% of the patients. None of the patients with duodenal tumors found at surgery had a negative intra-arterial secretin injection , but 25% had a negative portal venous sampling. Intra-arterial secretin injection was advocated over portal venous sampling for the localization of occult tumors in patients with ZES.

40. KO TC, FLISAK M, PRINZ RA: **Selective Intra-arterial Methylene Blue Injection: A Novel Method of Localizing Gastrinoma.** *Gastroenterology* 1992, **102**:1062–1064.

41. THOMPSON NW, VINIK AI, ECKHAUSER FE: **Microgastrinomas of the Duodenum: A Cause of Failed Operations for the Zollinger-Ellison Syndrome.** *Ann Surg* 1989, **209**:396–404.

42. FOX PS, HOFMANN JW, WILSON SD, DECOSSE JJ: **Surgical Management of the Zollinger-Ellison Syndrome.** *Surg Clin North Am* 1974, **54**:395–407.

43. HOFMANN JW, FOX PS, WILSON SD: **Duodenal Wall Tumors and the Zollinger-Ellison Syndrome: Surgical Management.** *Arch Surg* 1973, **107**:334–339.

44. ZOLLINGER RM, ELLISON EC, FABRI PJ, JOHNS J, SPARKS J, CAREY LC: **Primary Peptic Ulcerations of the Jejunum Associated With Islet Cell Tumors: Twenty-five Year Appraisal.** *Ann Surg* 1980, **192**:422–430.

45. VON SCHRENCK T, HOWARD JM, DOPPMAN JL, NORTON JA, MATON PN, SMITH FP, VINAYEK R, FRUCHT H, WANK SA, GARDNER JD, JENSEN RT: **Prospective Study of Chemotherapy in Patients With Metastatic Gastrinoma.** *Gastroenterology* 1988, **94**:1326–1334.

46. OBERHELMAN HA JR, NELSEN TS, JOHNSON AN JR, DRAGSTEDT LR II: **Ulcerogenic Tumors of the Duodenum.** *Ann Surg* 1961, **153**:214–227.

47. DELCORE R, FRIESEN SR: **Role of Pancreatoduodenectomy in the Management of Primary Duodenal Wall Gastrinomas in Patients With Zollinger-Ellison Syndrome.** *Surgery* 1992, **112**:1016–1023.

48. CHERNER JA, SAWYERS JL: **Benefit of Resection of Metastatic Gastrinoma in Multiple Endocrine Neoplasia Type-1.** *Gastroenterology* 1992, **102**:1049–1053.

49. NORTON JA, SUGARBAKER PH, DOPPMAN JL, WESLEY RA, MATON PN, GARDNER JD, JENSEN RT: **Aggressive Resection of Metastatic Disease in Selected Patients With Malignant Gastrinoma.** *Ann Surg* 1986, **203**:352–359.

50. STRAUS E, RAUFMAN JP: **The Brooklyn Gastrinomas.** *Mt Sinai J Med* 1992, **59**:125–128.

Gary P. Lawton, MD, and Irvin M. Modlin, MD, PhD, Department of Surgery, Yale University School of Medicine, FMB 136, P.O. Box 3333, 333 Cedar Street, New Haven, CT 06510, USA.

Mucosal healing and adaptation in the small intestine

Marc D. Basson, MD, PhD

Yale University School of Medicine, New Haven, Connecticut, USA

The closely related processes of healing and adaptation in the intestinal mucosa are of substantial clinical significance in patients after injury, intestinal surgery, and inflammatory or infectious ulceration, as well as all patients who are fasting. Recent investigations demonstrate that mucosal healing and adaptation are complex processes that seem likely to be regulated by a variety of autocrine and juxtacrine growth factors as well as conventional gut peptides. Further studies of the biology of mucosal healing may permit pharmacological intervention to promote healing and adaptation in the future.

Current Opinion in General Surgery 1994:138–146

Although the healing of the intestine resembles dermal healing in many ways, there exist important differences between healing in the gut and the skin, including the spontaneous motility of the gut after resolution of ileus and differences in patterns of collagen metabolism [1•]. Such differences are associated with substantial variations between dermis and gut in the speed and character of wound healing [2]. The small intestinal mucosa responds to injury by a combination of restitution, proliferation, and phenotypic modulation (Fig. 1). The distinct modulation of these processes has been known for a century, but much remains to be learned about the relative contribution of each to intestinal pathobiology and the mechanisms that modulate them. This review describes new information about the genesis of small intestinal injury in inflammatory bowel disease and after nonsteroidal anti-inflammatory drug (NSAID) therapy, outlines recent efforts to develop better models for the study of mucosal healing, and summarizes new information about the role of polyamines and growth factors in regulating mucosal healing and adaptation. The role of *Helicobacter pylori* in the genesis of duodenal ulcer disease represents a separate subject and is not considered here.

Mechanisms of mucosal injury

One paradigm of study for gastrointestinal mucosal disease is offered by peptic ulcer disease, in which the

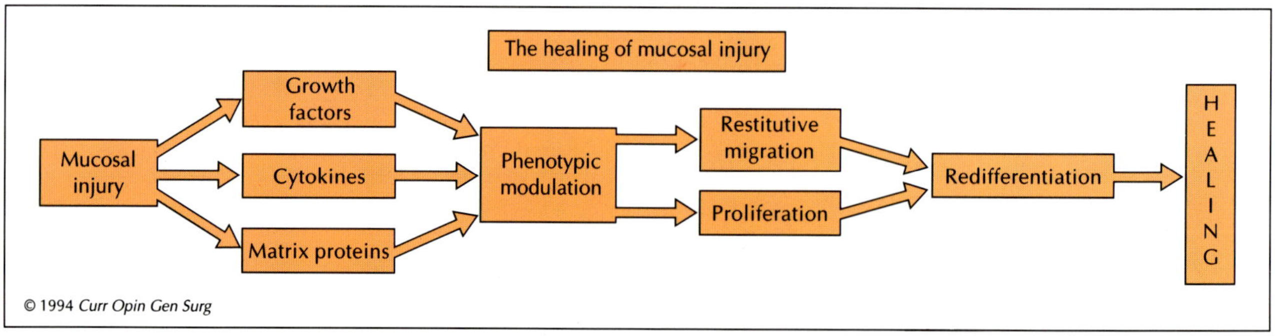

Fig. 1. Mucosal injury triggers the release of growth factors and cytokines and exposes matrix proteins from the basement membrane and interstitial matrix. These factors cause enterocytes at the edge of a mucosal defect to assume a squamous phenotype and to migrate across the defect in restitution. Enterocytic proliferation is also stimulated during mucosal healing, but it appears to be a secondary phenomenon.

Abbreviations

EGF—epidermal growth factor; **NSAID**—nonsteroidal anti-inflammatory drug; **TGF**—transforming growth factor.

study of underlying causes has facilitated pharmacological and surgical therapy specifically targeted against known pathogenic factors including acid, pepsin, and *H. pylori*. Indeed, the development of therapy based on pathobiology in this disease has been so successful that peptic ulcer is decreasingly a surgical problem. Students of mechanisms of mucosal injury have now begun to consider the genesis of inflammatory bowel disease and mucosal lesions associated with NSAIDs with a view toward similar progress.

Inflammatory bowel disease

It has been clear since the earliest histologic descriptions of inflammatory bowel disease that flares of disease are accompanied by a mononuclear cell infiltration. Isaacs *et al.* [3•] used polymerase chain reaction amplification to suggest that these infiltrating mononuclear cells may not only increase in density but may also exhibit an abnormal profile of interleukin cytokine secretion. Although Isaacs *et al.* have demonstrated an increase in messenger RNA levels without clear evidence of an increase in bioactive protein, other investigators have evaluated bioactive protein levels as well. For instance, Pullman *et al.* [4••] compared lamina propria mononuclear cells isolated from the colons of patients with Crohn's disease and ulcerative colitis with mononuclear cells from "normal" control subjects (patients with a variety of nonmalignant, noninflammatory conditions). This study demonstrated increased granulocyte colony-stimulating factor and interleukin 1 at the protein and messenger RNA level in patients with inflammatory bowel disease but decreased production of interleukin 3 and granulocyte-macrophage colony-stimulating factor. That these changes were at least somewhat biologically significant was demonstrated by increased colony-stimulating factor activity in the conditioned media derived from the inflammatory bowel disease mononuclear cells. Pullman *et al.* further demonstrated that hydrocortisone and 5-aminosalicylic acid (but not cyclosporin A) inhibit mononuclear cell cytokine production, suggesting that this suppression may contribute to their clinical effect in patients with inflammatory bowel disease. Pullman *et al.* propose that cytokine release represents an intermediate step in the pathogenesis of inflammatory bowel disease, as an initial mucosal injury permits endotoxin absorption that might then stimulate the cytokine production demonstrated in this paper. In this model, such enhanced cytokine production might result in a positive feedback loop in which these cytokines cause further inflammation, increasing mucosal injury and leading to increased endotoxin absorption and additional injury. This promising hypothesis awaits further evaluation.

Nonsteroidal anti-inflammatory drug–associated mucosal injury

New data (Table 1) have also recently been developed on the pathogenesis of the mucosal injury associated with NSAIDs, a problem of increasing clinical significance [5,6•]. Therapy with these drugs is clearly associated with mucosal injury *in vivo* [7,8], as well as an inhibition of the healing of experimental gastroduodenal ulcers [9]. However, we have recently observed in a cell culture model of mucosal healing [10•] that even at suprapharmacologic doses indomethacin does not substantially inhibit intestinal epithelial sheet migration. The contrast between these observations may be explained by increasing evidence that the NSAIDs interfere with the normal balance between mucosal cell loss into the lumen and the proliferation necessary to replace lost mucosal cells. Levi *et al.* [11•] have attacked this problem directly, dissecting out duodenal crypts adjacent to NSAID-associated duodenal ulcers and duodenal ulcers in the absence of NSAID therapy. Duodenal crypts from non-NSAID ulcers exhibited a mitotic index of over twice that of adjacent normal mucosa, whereas duodenal crypts from NSAID-associated ulcers did not exhibit increased proliferation. Levi *et al.* speculate that NSAID-associated inhibition of injury-stimulated enterocyte proliferation may contribute to NSAID-associated delays in ulcer healing. By contrast, Uribe [12•] reported that a single intraperitoneal injection of indomethacin accelerates the clearance of ^{3}H-methyl-thymidine–labeled cells from rat antral, duodenal, and jejunal mucosa by an unclear mechanism. To the extent to which data in the well-differentiated human Caco-2 enterocyte line may be extrapolated to normal mucosal enterocytes, it seems unlikely that this increased clearance relates to decreased enterocyte adhesion to matrix proteins because we have not been able to demonstrate changes in either Caco-2 adhesion or Caco-2 integrin expression after indomethacin treatment [10•]. Uribe suggests that indomethacin may therefore injure the mucosa by increasing the normal exfoliation of mucosal enterocytes into the lumen beyond the capacity of mucosal renewal. In contrast to the observations of Levi *et al.* [11•], Uribe also observed a delayed increase in mucosal DNA synthesis after indomethacin treatment, perhaps stimulated by a primary mucosal injury. The differences between the results of Levi *et al.* and Uribe may reflect species differences or (more likely) important differences in proliferative kinetics after a single experimental dose [12•] or chronic NSAID therapy [11•].

Table 1. Possible causes of nonsteroidal anti-inflammatory drug–associated mucosal injury

Failure to increase proliferation after injury [11•]
Increased clearance of enterocytes into the lumen [12•]
Decreased epidermal growth factor release [9,13•]
Decreased mucosal blood flow [14]

In addition to direct effects on the gut mucosa, aspirin and NSAIDs may also interfere with the physiological feedback loops that stimulate mucosal healing after injury. Indeed, this may partially explain the failure of duodenal crypts to increase proliferation in response to NSAID-associated ulcers observed by Levi *et al.* [11•]. Indomethacin has been reported to inhibit epidermal growth factor (EGF) release [9,13•] and also appears to decrease gastric blood flow [14], although its effect on intestinal mesenteric blood flow remains to be established.

Models of mucosal healing

Investigations such as those described previously are beginning to elucidate the pathobiology responsible for mucosal injury. However, normal gut mucosa exhibits rapid turnover and efficient healing. It may therefore be important to consider not only how the mucosa is injured but how it heals. Recent efforts to study gut mucosal healing *in vivo* have ranged from the application of sophisticated immunohistochemical and molecular techniques to conventional ulcer models [15•,16•] to the development of new models that mimic the mucosal lesions of ischemia rather than ulcerogenesis [17•]. *In vivo* models continue to demonstrate the primacy of epithelial sheet migration over cell proliferation in the initial phase of mucosal healing.

In vivo studies

Park *et al.* [17•] evaluated the histologic reconstitution of the small intestinal mucosa after standardized ischemic injury, demonstrating that rapid restoration of the mucosa occurs without any increase in mucosal cell mitotic rate. These results are consistent with the observations of Riegler *et al.* [18•] in the human and rabbit colon. These investigators have described a novel technique for real-time morphometry during mucosal healing that has quantitated colonic epithelial migration during restitution at 2 to 3 μm/min. *In vivo* studies using the cryoprobe-ulcer model (which creates a mucosal ulcer secondary to ischemia when the cryoprobe is applied to the serosa of the gut) and direct surgical trauma to the gut have also been useful in providing tissue for biochemical and immunohistochemical assessment of levels of growth factors and matrix proteins [16•,19,20].

In vitro studies

Although *in vivo* studies usefully characterize the phenomenon of mucosal restitution, other researchers have studied cultured cells for more detailed investigation of the cellular mechanisms that contribute to mucosal healing. We have previously characterized the differential modulation of sheet migration, proliferation, and differentiation in Caco-2 cells [21••], a human cell line derived from a well-differentiated colonic adenocarcinoma that shares many characteristics of normal human adult small intestinal mucosa or fetal colonic mucosa. These studies have used a "fence" migration assay, in which epithelial cells are cultured to confluence on matrix-coated plastic dishes within a constraining steel ring (Fig. 2). When the ring is removed, the expansion of the epithelial sheet across the matrix resembles mucosal restitution and may be quantitated by staining and measurement after 6 days. Proliferation may be quantitated in this system by ^{3}H-thymidine uptake, and differentiation by assay for digestive enzymes by hydrolysis of synthetic substrates. Johnson *et al.* [22•] have similarly studied the processes of migration and cell proliferation in the rat small intestinal epithelial crypt cell line (IEC-6), scratching the monolayer with a razor blade to generate a "wound" in the epithelial sheet. In another study using the IEC-6 cell line, Olson [23••] evaluated the contraction of collagen gels seeded with IEC-6 cells and proposed that the speed of this contraction may be used to evaluate the tractional forces generated by intestinal epithelial cells during mucosal wound contraction and demonstrate that actin microfilament function may be required for such contraction. In recent papers using the human Caco-2 and T-84 enterocyte-like cell lines, Bement *et al.* [24••] and Nusrat *et al.* [25•] offer elegant histological descriptions of monolayer wound contraction and provide additional inferential support for the view that mucosal wounds may heal not only by restitution but also by actin-based wound contraction.

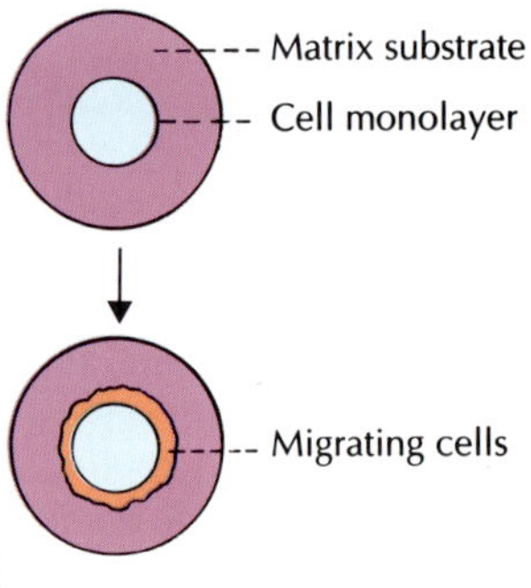

Matrix	Caco-2 migration
Plastic	1.00 ± 0.09
Fibronectin	1.12 ± 0.17
Laminin	1.28 ± 0.11
Collagen I	1.59 ± 0.11

Fig. 2. Migration assay adapted to the study of Caco-2 sheet migration. Using a confining stainless steel "fence" (not shown), a sharply circumscribed confluent monolayer of cells is created within a sterile dish precoated with a purified matrix protein substrate. The constraining "fence" is then removed, and the monolayer expands radially as the cells migrate outward over 6 days. The area of migration may be determined by subtracting the area of the original constrained monolayer from the total monolayer area at the conclusion of the experiment. The *table* shows the relative speed of migration of Caco-2 cells over purified matrix protein substrates; data are normalized to the rate of migration over tissue culture plastic, represented as mean ±95% CI. (*From* Basson *et al.* [21••]; with permission.)

Studies of cultured cells such as those from our laboratory and that of Johnson *et al.* continue to yield interesting and potentially important results, but must be interpreted with care. Extrapolation from cell culture studies to *in vivo* pathophysiology requires close analysis and cautious inference, both because of abnormalities inherent in the cell culture milieu and because they require the use of transformed cell lines inherently different from normal mucosal enterocytes [26•].

Two different approaches have recently been used to develop cell populations that can be maintained and studied in culture but which more closely resemble normal enterocytes. Whitehead *et al.* [27••] have established conditionally immortalized epithelial cell lines from the colon and small bowel of novel transgenic mice. These mice contain a temperature-sensitive mutation that produces a reversible malignant transformation. Cells derived from the gut mucosa of these mice proliferate continuously at 33°C but cease proliferating and express low levels of digestive enzymes (markers of enterocytic differentiation) at 39.5°C. Such cell lines offer the possibility of establishing large numbers of cells that may be induced by manipulation of the temperature-sensitive oncogene to revert to a more differentiated phenotype for study. In a different approach, Fukamachi [28•] has taken advantage of the greater adaptability of fetal enterocytes, developing a system for the study of the proliferation and differentiation of primary fetal rat intestinal epithelial cells in serum-free culture. Such techniques offer the promise of large numbers of relatively normal enterocytes for study in culture, but require further refinement because the cells they provide for study are in many ways less differentiated than some of the established cell lines currently under study.

Polyamine metabolism and mucosal healing

Recent studies in two different animal models have implicated mucosal polyamine metabolism in the process of mucosal healing. Fujimoto *et al.* [29•] have used a model of superior mesenteric artery ischemia and reperfusion in the rat to demonstrate increases in jejunal mucosal histamine and histidine decarboxylase activity, which could be ablated by an ornithine decarboxylase inhibitor with consequent delays in mucosal healing. Similarly, Wang and Johnson [30] used a rat immersion stress ulcer model to demonstrate that the ornithine decarboxylase inhibitor, difluoromethyl ornithine, inhibits mucosal repair and that replacement with exogenous luminal polyamines restores healing. The precise manner in which polyamine metabolism modulates mucosal restitution after ischemia remains unclear, however. As Johnson *et al.* [22•] have begun to characterize these effects *in vitro*, perhaps more mechanistic insights will be forthcoming.

Growth factors and mucosal healing

Increasing evidence suggests that a variety of growth factors exert complex regulatory influences on gut mucosal healing (Fig. 3). Recent data is summarized here for several of the most important factors.

Epidermal growth factor

Epidermal growth factor is a 53-amino-acid polypeptide, secreted in large amounts by the salivary glands and Brunner's glands of the duodenal mucosa. Echoing previous links between EGF and gastroduodenal ulcer healing, increasing evidence now implicates EGF in the stimulation of intestinal mucosal healing and regeneration. EGF appears to stimulate not only cell proliferation [31•] but also enterocyte sheet migration (restitution). For instance, Saxena *et al.* [32•] have demonstrated increased uptake of radiolabeled EGF during the healing of a full-thickness ileal defect, whereas Luck and Bass [33••] have described amelioration by systemic EGF treatment of rat colonic ulcerations induced by rectal administration of a noxious agent. Interestingly, Luck and Bass found EGF efficacious when given parenterally, but not via the rectum. This mirrors previous observations that oral EGF does not promote mucosal hyperplasia in the intact gut [34], although some observations suggest that luminal EGF may become bioactive in the setting of mucosal injury [35].

Basson *et al.* [36••] recently explored the mechanisms of the EGF effect in the Caco-2 cell culture model described previously. We observed that in addition to stimulating Caco-2 proliferation, EGF separately stimulated the actual migration of Caco-2 cells across a laminin substrate, and that this effect appeared to be caused by an upregulation and alteration in organiza-

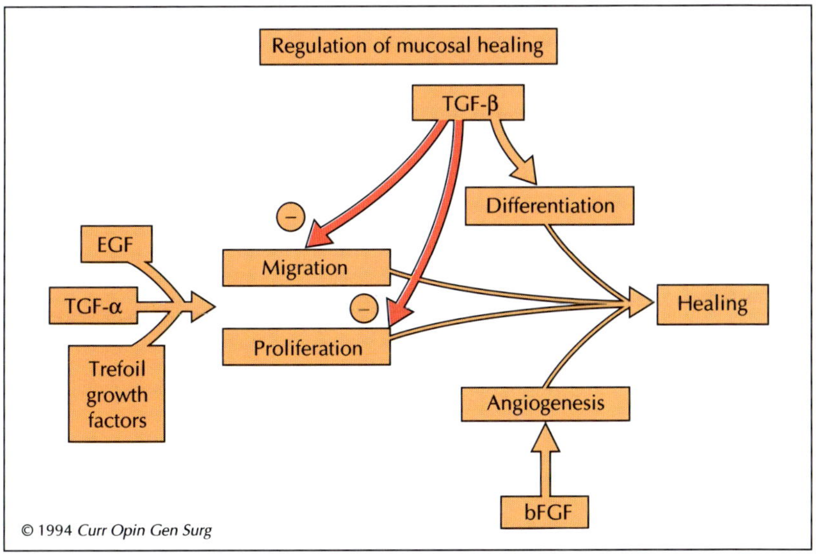

Fig. 3. Growth factors act to regulate mucosal healing. In particular, growth factors ligating the epidermal growth factor (EGF) receptor (EGF, transforming growth factor [TGF]–α, and the trefoil growth factors) appear to stimulate enterocyte migration and proliferation. TGF-β may downmodulate these processes (*minus signs*), although this awaits further investigation. Although basic fibroblast growth factor (bFGF) has not been clearly demonstrated to regulate enterocytic migration or proliferation directly, it is likely to support mucosal healing by promoting angiogenesis.

tion of β1α2 integrin heterodimer which serves as a Caco-2 laminin receptor (Fig. 4).

It is important to recognize in the interpretation of studies of EGF that EGF and transforming growth factor (TGF)–α share the same receptor. Beauchamp *et al.* [37] have demonstrated that TGF-α is also active in the gut, perhaps in an autocrine fashion [38], similar to that which has elsewhere been suggested for EGF [39]. Thus, studies demonstrating the efficacy of EGF (or TGF-α) or changes in the "EGF" receptor may not exclude the other of these two agents.

Trefoil growth factors

The EGF receptor is activated not only by EGF and TGF-α, but also by a novel class of "trefoil" growth factors that have recently been described [19], named after their unique three-lobed tertiary structure. These growth factors have been demonstrated to be increased in the setting of chronic ulcer disease and inflammatory bowel disease [19,40••]. Among the most interesting of these is human intestinal trefoil factor, which has recently been cloned [41••]. Human intestinal trefoil factor and its rat homologue appear to be localized specifically to the mucosal goblet cells [15•,41••] and appear to increase locally in the setting of mucosal injury [16•]. It seems increasingly likely that mucosal injury results in upregulation of mucosal synthesis of one or more peptides that ligates the EGF receptor, including EGF, TGF-α, and trefoil growth factors, and that these peptides then stimulate mucosal healing in an autocrine or juxtacrine fashion.

Transforming growth factor-β

Transforming growth factor-β also appears to be active in the regulation of mucosal biology, but its actions are less clearly defined. Unrelated to TGF-α despite its similar name, TGF-β has been demonstrated to accelerate seromuscular healing in the gut [42] but its effects on mucosal healing in the gut are less well characterized. Basson *et al.* [10•] observed that TGF-β promotes Caco-2 migration over laminin, but inhibits Caco-2 migration

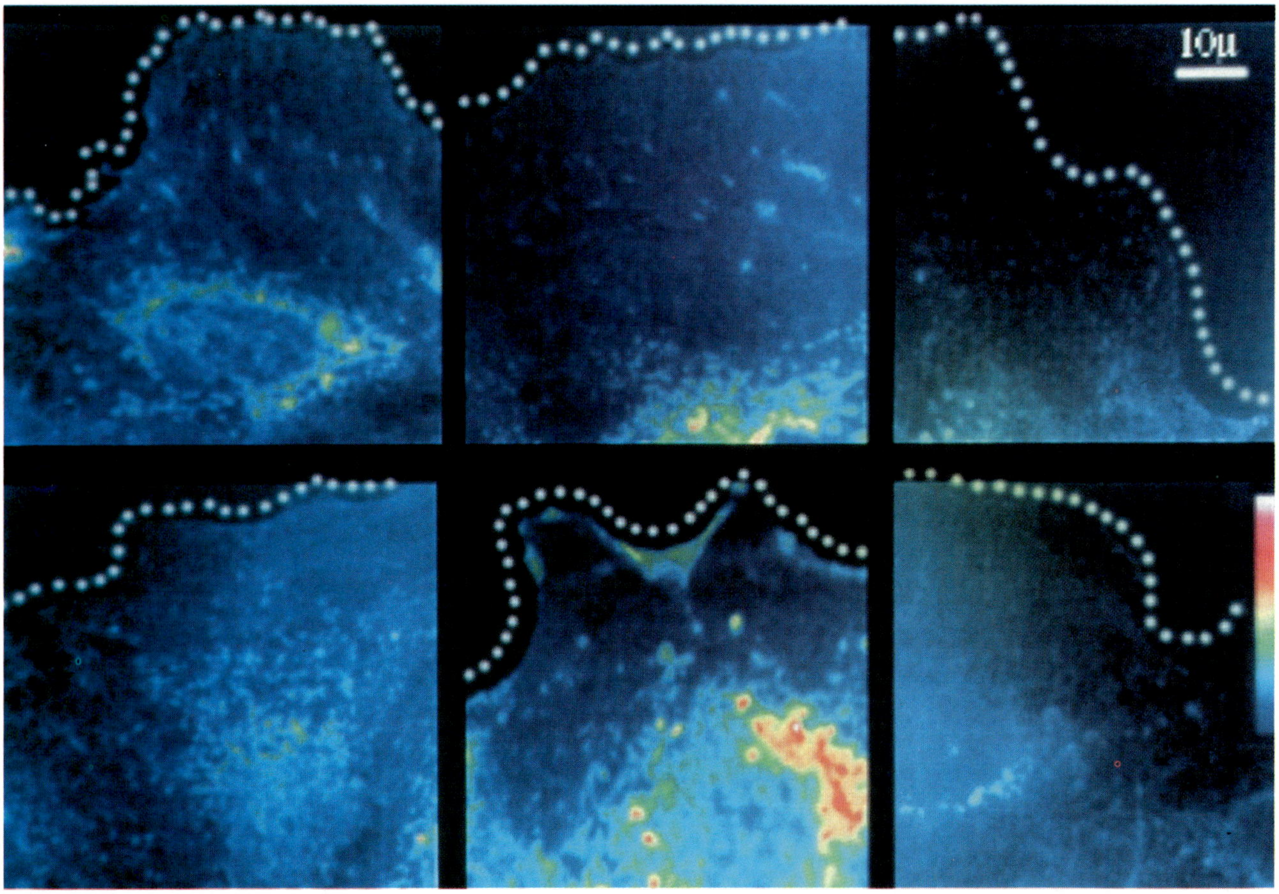

Fig. 4. Patterns of α2 integrin immunostaining in migrating Caco-2 cells imaged by laser scanning confocal microscopy are shown on collagen I (*top left panel*), collagen I after treatment with 30 ng/mL of epidermal growth factor (EGF) (*top center panel*) or transforming growth factor (TGF)–β1 (*top right panel*), laminin (*bottom left panel*), and laminin after treatment with 30 ng/mL EGF (*bottom center panel*) or TGF-β1 (*bottom right panel*). All cells are migrating toward the top of the figure. The *scale bar* represents 10 μm, and the pattern of pseudocolor staining is represented in the *color wedge* shown in *bottom right panel*. (*From* Basson *et al.* [10•]; with permission.)

over collagen I, and appears to downregulate Caco-2 α2 integrin subunit expression (Fig. 4). Podolsky *et al.* [43••] allude in a recent review to unpublished observations of similar stimulation of IEC-6 cell migration to reconstitute wounded cell monolayers, although the substrate over which this migration occurred is not specified. TGF-β appears to inhibit proliferation in some moderately well-differentiated cell lines derived from colonic carcinomas [44], but not proliferation of primary human keratinocytes [45] or Caco-2 cells [10•]. Podolsky [43••] has proposed a model for the regulation of enterocyte proliferation in which TGF-α or TGF-β exert opposing autocrine feedback loops, but validation of this model awaits investigation of the effects of TGF-β on the proliferation of normal enterocytes *in vivo*.

Fibroblast growth factor

Although little data implicate fibroblast growth factor directly in the regulation of enterocyte migration, differentiation,or proliferation, the healing of deep intestinal wounds may require the development of a new capillary bed to perfuse the neomucosa. The subject of angiogenesis has recently been reviewed in detail [46•] and is not discussed in depth here. However, Folkman *et al.* [46•,47] have clearly demonstrated that basic fibroblast growth factor is critical for the angiogenetic support of gastroduodenal ulcer healing. Indeed, at least part of the activity of sucralfate in this regard appears secondary to its ability to bind basic fibroblast growth factor,protecting it from luminal gastric acid and presenting it to the mucosal wound. It seems likely that angiogenic factors such as basic fibroblast growth factor play a role in the healing of deep intestinal wounds elsewhere in the gut.

Matrix proteins and mucosal healing

Restitutive migration is likely to be regulated not only by the growth factors to which mucosal cells may be exposed but also by the extracellular matrix substrate over which migration occurs. We have demonstrated substantial variation in the rate of Caco-2 sheet migration between matrix proteins [36••] (Fig. 2). McCormack *et al.* [22•] have similarly observed that Matrigel (a heterogeneous matrix derived from Engelbreth-Holm-Swarm [EHS] tumor cells) promotes the migration of cells of the rat intestinal epithelial crypt cell line IEC-6 after a cell monolayer has been wounded by a razor blade, although interpretation of such data must consider the complex composition of Matrigel and the possible release of growth factors and cytokines from injured cells in such a model [48]. Nevertheless, such data may be interpreted as further supporting the regulation of enterocyte migration by matrix proteins.

Moore *et al.* [49] have studied the relevance of matrix to restitution after superficial injury to isolated guinea pig ileal mucosa in Ussing chambers. Although antibodies to individual matrix components did not alter the rate of reconstitution of the mucosal barrier, restitution was inhibited by the blockade of protein synthesis in combination with antibodies to collagen III and collagen IV. The specificity of this observation was enhanced by the further demonstration that restitution was also inhibited by these antibodies when collagen synthesis was specifically inhibited using the proline analogue *cis*-hydroxyproline.

If matrix is important for enterocyte migration, it is perhaps not surprising that mucosal healing is more rapid in superficial lesions that leave the basement membrane intact than in deep ulcers that penetrate the basal lamina. The healing of deep ulcers therefore requires not only epithelial migration but also the synthesis and reorganization of a new matrix. The synthesis and organization of a new basement membrane is demonstrable by immunohistochemical techniques within 48 hours of acute transmural duodenal injury [16•], but the mechanisms that regulate matrix synthesis after mucosal injury remain largely unexplored at this time. Studies of gut mucosal enterocytes in culture suggest that matrix production may be most prominent in undifferentiated cells [50]. It is tempting to speculate that increased matrix synthesis might also be characteristic of the less-specialized mucosal enterocytes involved in migration and repair of mucosal injuries. However, few data are available to resolve this issue.

Growth factors and mucosal adaptation

Mucosal adaptation to compensate for decreased nutrient absorption following massive bowel resection, bypass, or prolonged fasting is an area of substantial clinical relevance for the critically ill fasted patient, and for the patient suffering from a short gut syndrome. The importance of nutrition for maintenance of the gut mucosal barrier function and the evidence that manipulation of nutrition can support the gut have both been extensively reviewed in the previous volume in this series [51••,52••]. The scope of this discussion is therefore limited to a brief sketch of recent evidence that growth factors may also be used to support the gut and stimulate adaptation.

Although mucosal adaptation is as yet poorly understood, it appears to be stimulated by growth factors and bioactive peptides in a manner similar to the regulation of mucosal restitution. The subject has recently been extensively reviewed [53••]. Intestinal mucosal adaptation is characterized by hyperplasia of the mucosal villi and crypts, increasing absorptive capacity on a macroscopic level [53••] as well as by some modulation of the expression of brush-border digestive enzymes within individual villi [54••]. Surprisingly, rat enterocytes do not seem to uniformly increase brush-border enzyme expression during adaptation, although this might seem teleologically desirable, and it has been suggested that strategies to stimulate digestive enzyme expression may be useful to augment natural adaptive changes [54••].

Logic suggests that adaptation is stimulated by changes in nutrient absorption rather than by the sequelae of gut resection, because these phenomena are reproduced after intestinal bypass and reversed by fasting even during total parenteral nutrition. However, the mechanism by which decreased nutrient absorption results in intestinal adaptation awaits elucidation. Polyamine synthesis appears to play some role in the process [55•]. Recent research has emphasized the possibility of parenteral supplementation with nutrients or growth factors to augment adaptation or prevent the changes associated with fasting. In particular, EGF has been reported to acutely increase enterocyte brush-border area by redistribution of existing preformed microvillus plasma membrane via a verapamil-sensitive mechanism in New Zealand white rabbit blind jejunal loops [56•]. In more long-term studies, Salleh and Ardawi [57•] observed that EGF supplementation in septic fasting rats receiving parenteral nutrition improves glutamine utilization, increases jejunal wet weight, stimulates mucosal enterocyte proliferation, and slightly improves survival (from 80% in controls to 85% in EGF-treated rats). Neurotensin [58•,59•] and insulin-like growth factor 1 [60••,61•,62••] have also been reported to exert beneficial effects after small bowel resection or bypass in animal models. Albiston *et al.* [60••] proposed that insulin-like growth factor 1 may stimulate ileal adaptation not by increased levels of the growth factor itself but by decreased levels of a binding protein, which prevents its bioactivity. Because many studies of a putative stimulatory agent have previously focused exclusively on the expression of the agent itself in adapting or injured tissue, the concept that bioavailable levels of a growth factor may change without modulation of the growth factor itself may prove important for future studies of adaptive mechanisms.

Conclusions

Important progress has been made in the past year in understanding the mechanisms that regulate mucosal healing and adaptation. These appear to be complex processed regulated by growth factors, cytokines, and matrix proteins. Animal studies suggest that the exogenous administration of relevant growth factors may actually stimulate healing and adaptation after injury and in settings of sepsis and fasting. Extension of these findings to the clinical arena may significantly improve treatment of patients with such syndromes in the future.

References and recommended reading

Papers of particular interest, published within the annual period of review, have been highlighted as:

- • Of special interest
- •• Of outstanding interest

1. • MARTENS MFWC, HUYBEN CMLC, HENDRIKS TH: **Collagen Synthesis in Fibroblasts From Human Colon: Regulatory Aspects and Differences With Skin Fibroblasts.** *Gut* 1992, **33**:1664–1670.
An important demonstration of differences in the biology of healing between the gut and the skin.

2. ADAMSONS RJ, KAHAN SA: **The Rate of Healing of Incised Wounds of Different Tissues in Rabbits.** *Surg Gynecol Obstet* 1970, **130**:837–846.

3. • ISAACS KL, SARTOR RB, HASKILL S: **Cytokine Messenger RNA Profiles in Inflammatory Bowel Disease Mucosa Detected by Polymerase Chain Reaction Amplification.** *Gastroenterology* 1992, **103**:1587–1595.
Observes that cytokine messenger RNA profiles are altered in inflammatory bowel disease.

4. •• PULLMAN WE, ELSBURY S, KOBAYASHI M, HAPEL AJ, DOE WF: **Enhanced Mucosal Cytokine Production in Inflammatory Bowel Disease.** *Gastroenterology* 1992, **102**:529–537.
Demonstrates that altered cytokine production is not only present but also bioactive in the mucosa of patients with inflammatory bowel disease.

5. LANGMAN MJS: **Epidemiologic Evidence on the Association Between Peptic Ulceration and Anti-inflammatory Drug Use.** *Gastroenterology* 1989, **96**:640–646.

6. • HAYLLAR J, MACPHERSON A, BJARNASON I: **Gastroprotection and Non-steroidal Anti-inflammatory Drugs (NSAIDS): Rationale and Clinical Implications.** *Drug Safety* 1992, **7**:86–105.
A recent review of the relationship between NSAIDs and mucosal injury.

7. MCCARTHY D: **Non-steroidal Anti-inflammatory Drug Induced Ulcers: Management by Traditional Therapies.** *Gastroenterology* 1989, **96**:662–674.

8. HAWKEY CJ: **Non-steroidal Anti-inflammatory Drugs and Peptic Ulcers.** *BMJ* 1990, **300**:278–284.

9. KONTUREK SJ, BRZOZOWSKI T, DROZDOWICZ D, DEMBINSKI A, NAUERT C: **Healing of Chronic Gastroduodenal Ulcerations: Role of Prostaglandins and Epidermal Growth Factor.** *Dig Dis Sci* 1990, **35**:1121–1129.

10. • BASSON MD, MODLIN IM, FLYNN SD, JENA BP, MADRI JA: **Independent Modulation of Enterocyte Migration and Proliferation by Growth Factors, Matrix Proteins and Pharmacologic Agents in an In Vitro Model of Mucosal Healing.** *Surgery* 1992, **112**:299–308.
A cell-culture model for the study of enterocyte migration and proliferation in which effects of growth factors and matrix proteins may be evaluated.

11. • LEVI S, GODLAD RA, LEE CY, STAMP G, WALPORT MJ, WRIGHT NA, HODGSON HJ: **Non-steroidal Anti-inflammatory Drugs Inhibit the Processes of Mucosal Cell Proliferation Associated With Duodenal Ulcer Healing.** *Digestion* 1992, **53**:129–133.
An attempt to demonstrate a mechanism for NSAID inhibition of mucosal healing.

12. • URIBE A: **Indomethacin Accelerates Clearance of Labeled Cells and Increases DNA Synthesis in Gastrointestinal Mucosa of the Rat.** *Dig Dis Sci* 1992, **37**:403–408.
Another mechanistic study of the effect of NSAIDs on mucosal healing, perhaps demonstrating a complementary mechanism to that described by Levi *et al.* (*Digestion* 1992, 53:129–133).

13. • ZANDOMENEGHI R, SERRA L, PAVESI C, BAUMGARTL U, POPPI C, MONTANARI P: **Effect of Aspirin and Indomethacin on Epidermal Growth Factor Secretion in Duodenal Tissue Fragments Cultivated In Vitro.** *Digestion* 1992, **51**:37–41.
The authors suggest a third indirect mechanism for the effects of aspirin and NSAIDs, which are no doubt multifaceted.

14. HIROSE H, TAKEUCHI K, OKABE S: **Effect of Indomethacin on Gastric Mucosal Blood Flow Around Acetic Acid-Induced Gastric Ulcers in Rats.** *Gastroenterology* 1991, **100**:1259–1265.

15. • CHINERY R, POULSOM R, ROGERS LA, JEFFERY RE, LONGCROFT JM, HANBY AM, WRIGHT NA: **Localization of Intestinal Trefoil-Factor mRNA in Rat Stomach and Intestine by Hybridization In Situ.** *Biochem J* 1992, **85**:5–8.
Demonstration of specific tissue localization of a novel trefoil growth factor in the rat stomach and intestine.

16. • MODLIN IM, BASSON MD, SOROKA CJ, WRIGHT N, POULSOM R, CHINNERY R, HANBY A, PATEL K, ROGERS L, ALISON M: **Ulcer-Induced Alterations in Cell Phenotype and Growth Factor Expression.** *Eur J Gastroenterol*, in press.
A description of the modulation of cell phenotype and the expression of growth factors and matrix proteins in a rat model of duodenal ulcer healing.

17. • PARK P, HAGLUND U: **Regeneration of Small Bowel Mucosa After Intestinal Ischemia.** *Crit Care Med* 1992, **20**:125–139.
Another model of intestinal mucosal injury, reflecting the pathophysiology of ischemia rather than ulcer disease or wounding. This paper nicely demonstrates the significance of restitution in the mucosal response to injury.

18. • RIEGLER M, FEIL W, LINDROTH J, WONG M: **MIPSY: Real-Time Morphometry to Quantify the Time Course of Rapid Epithelial Restitution.** *Pathol Res Pract* 1992, **188**:443–448.
An interesting technique that permits real-time visualization of epithelial restitution *in vivo* and may prove useful for the evaluation of potential pharmacologic promoters of mucosal healing.

19. WRIGHT NA, PIKE C, ELLIA G: **Induction of a Novel Epidermal Growth Factor-Secreting Cell Lineage by Mucosal Ulceration in the Human Gastrointestinal Stem Cells.** *Nature* 1990, **343**:82–85.

20. LEE H, HANSON H-A, NORSTROM E, HELANDER HF: **Immunoreactivities for Epidermal Growth Factor (EGF) and for EGF Receptors in Rats With Gastric Ulcers.** *Cell Tissue Res* 1991, **265**:211–218.

21. BASSON MD, MODLIN IM, TUROWSKI G, MADRI JA: **Enterocyte-Matrix**
•• **Interactions in the Healing of Mucosal Injury.** *Eur J Gastroenterol,* in press.
A detailed review of the regulation of enterocyte phenotype by extracellular matrix proteins and the evidence that these enterocyte-matrix interactions are important in mucosal healing.

22. MCCORMACK SA, VIAR MJ, JOHNSON LR: **Migration of Rat IEC-6 Cells:**
• **A Model for Mucosal Healing.** *Am J Physiol* 1992, **263**:G426–G435.
A cell culture study that evaluates monolayer healing after "wounding."

23. OLSON AD: **Contraction of Collagen Gels by Intestinal Epithelial Cells**
•• **Depends on Microfilament Function.** *Dig Dis Sci* 1993, **38**:388–395.
An interesting approach to the quantitation of the traction forces generated by intestinal epithelial cells during mucosal wound contraction, and perhaps during restitutive migration as well.

24. BEMENT WM, FORSCHER P, MOOSEKER MS: **A Novel Cytoskeletal Struc-**
•• **ture Involved in Purse String Wound Closure and Cell Polarity Maintenance.** *J Cell Biol* 1993, **121**:565–578.
Replication of mucosal wound contracture in a cell culture system and linkage of this process to cytoskeletal organization within the enterocyte.

25. NUSRAT A, DELP C, MADARA JL: **Intestinal Epithelial Restitution: Char-**
• **acterization of a Cell Culture Model and Mapping of Cytoskeletal Elements in Migrating Cells.** *J Clin Invest* 1992, **89**:1501–1511.
Description of cytoskeletal changes in migrating enterocytes in culture.

26. MADRI JA, BASSON MD: **Extracellular Matrix-Cell Interactions: Dynamic**
• **Modulators of Cell, Tissue and Organism Structure and Function.** *Lab Invest* 1992, **66**:519–521.
A brief exploration of the role of matrix-cell interactions in determining biology at the cellular level and above which also discusses problems in the extrapolation of cell culture data to the whole organism.

27. WHITEHEAD RH, VANEEDEN PE, NOBLE MD, ATALIOTIS P, JAT PS: **Es-**
•• **tablishment of Conditionally Immortalized Epithelial Cell Lines From Both Colon and Small Intestine of Adult H-2Kb-tsA58 Transgenic Mice.** *Proc Natl Acad Sci U S A* 1993, **90**:587–591.
A unique approach directed at avoiding the necessity for studying transformed cells in culture, using a transgenic mouse model to establish conditionally transformed cell lines via a temperature-sensitive oncogene.

28. FUKAMACHI H: **Proliferation and Differentiation of Fetal Rat Intesti-**
• **nal Epithelial Cells in Primary Serum-Free Culture.** *J Cell Sci* 1992, **103**:511–519.
A model for the study of primary fetal intestinal epithelial cells in serum-free culture that avoids the use of transformed cells but uses fetal cells, which themselves differ from the adult enterocyte.

29. FUJIMOTO K, IMAMURA I, GRANGER DN, WADA H, SAKATA T, TSO P:
• **Histamine and Histidine Decarboxylase Are Correlated With Mucosal Repair in Rat Small Intestine After Ischemia-Reperfusion.** *J Clin Invest* 1992, **89**:126–133.
Linkage of histamine metabolism to mucosal repair after ischemic injury.

30. WANG J-Y, JOHNSON LR: **Luminal Polyamines Substitute for Tissue Polyamines in Duodenal Mucosal Repair After Stress in Rats.** *Gastroenterology* 1992, **102**:1109–1117.

31. GOODLAD RA, LEE CY, WRIGHT NA: **Cell Proliferation in the Small**
• **Intestine and Colon of Intravenously Fed Rats: Effects of Urogastrone-Epidermal Growth Factor.** *Cell Prolif* 1992, **25**:393–404.
Evaluation *in vivo* of the effects of EGF on mucosal enterocyte proliferation.

32. SAXENA SK, THOMPSON JS, SHARP JG: **Role of Epidermal Growth Factor**
• **in Intestinal Regeneration.** *Surgery* 1992, **111**:318–325.
Another *in vivo* study of the effect of EGF on intestinal mucosal healing.

33. LUCK MS, BASS P: **Effect of Epidermal Growth Factor on Experimental**
•• **Colitis in the Rat.** *J Pharmacol Exp Ther* 1993, **264**:984–990.
This demonstration that exogenous administration of EGF is effective *in vivo* in ameliorating experimental colitis may foreshadow future treatment of colitis with growth factors.

34. GOODLAD RA, WILSON TJG, LENTON W, GREGORY H, MCCULLOGH KG, WRIGHT NA: **Intravenous But Not Intragastric Urogastrone-EGF is Trophic to the Intestine of Parenterally Fed Rats.** *Gut* 1987, **28**:573–582.

35. KONTUREK SJ, DEMBINSKI A, WARZECHA Z, BRZOZZOSKI T, GREGORY H: **Role of Epidermal Growth Factor in Healing of Chronic Gastroduodenal Ulcers in Rats.** *Gastroenterology* 1988, **94**:1300–1307.

36. BASSON MD, MODLIN IM, MADRI JA: **Human Enterocyte (Caco-2) Mi-**
•• **gration is Modulated In Vitro by Extracellular Matrix Composition and Epidermal Growth Factor.** *J Clin Invest* 1992, **90**:15–23.
Cell culture studies suggesting a novel mechanism for the stimulation of restitution by EGF.

37. BEAUCHAMP RD, BARNARD JA, MCCUTCHEN CM, CHERNER JA, COFFEY RJ JR: **Localization of Transforming Growth Factor α and Its Receptor in Gastric Mucosal Cells: Implications for a Regulatory Role in Acid Secretion and Mucosal Renewal.** *J Clin Invest* 1989, **84**:1017–1023.

38. COFFEY RJ, GOUSTIN AS, SODERQUIST AM, SHIPLEY GD, WOLFSHOHOL J, CARPENTER G, MOSES HL: **Transforming Growth Factor α and β Expression in Human Colon Cancer Lines: Implications for an Autocrine Model.** *Cancer Res* 1987, **47**:4590–4594.

39. WAN CW, MCKNIGHT MK, BRATTAIN DE, BRATTAIN MG, YEOMAN LC: **Different Epidermal Growth Factor Growth Responses and Receptor Levels in Human Colon Carcinoma Cell Lines.** *Cancer Lett* 1988, **43**:139–143.

40. WRIGHT NA, POULSOM R, STAMP G, VAN NORDEN S, SARRAF C, ELIA
•• G, AHNEN D, JEFFERY R, LONGCROFT J, PIKE C, *ET AL.*: **Trefoil Peptide Gene Expression in Gastrointestinal Epithelial Cells in Inflammatory Bowel Disease.** *Scand J Gastroenterol* 1992, **193(suppl)**:76–82.
Demonstrates that trefoil growth factor expression is altered in the gut mucosa in the setting of inflammatory bowel disease.

41. PODOLSKY DK, LYNCH-DEVANEY K, STOW JL, OATES P, MURGUE B,
•• DEBEAUMONT M, SANDS BE, MAHIDA YR: **Identification of Human Intestinal Trefoil Factor: Goblet Cell-Specific Expression of a Peptide Targeted for Apical Secretion.** *J Biol Chem* 1993, **268**:6694–6702.
The cloning of intestinal trefoil growth factor and evaluation of its expression *in vivo.*

42. MUSTOE TA, LANDES A, CROMACK DT, MISTRY D, GRIFFIN A, DEUEL TF, PIERCE GF: **Differential Acceleration of Healing of Surgical Incisions in the Rabbit Gastrointestinal Tract by Platelet-Derived Growth Factor and Transforming Growth Factor, Type Beta.** *Surgery* 1990, **108**:324–330.

43. PODOLSKY DK: **Regulation of Intestinal Epithelial Proliferation: A Few**
•• **Answers, Many Questions.** *Am J Physiol* 1993, **264**:G179–G186.
A thoughtful review of what is known of the regulation of intestinal epithelial proliferation.

44. HOOSEIN NM, MCKNIGHT MK, LEVINE AE, MULDER KM, CHILDRESS KE, BRATTAIN DE, BRATTAIN MG: **Differential Sensitivity of Subclasses of Human Colon Carcinoma Cell Lines to the Growth Inhibitory Effects of Transforming Growth Factor-β1.** *Exp Cell Res* 1989, **181**:442–453.

45. REISS M, SARTORELLI AC: **Regulation of Growth and Differentiation of Human Keratinocytes by Type β Transforming Growth Factor and Epidermal Growth Factor.** *Cancer Res* 1987, **47**:6705–6709.

46. FOLKMAN J, SHING Y: **Angiogenesis.** *J Biol Chem* 1992, **267**:10931–
• 10934.
A brief but careful review of current knowledge about angiogenic factors by investigators who have made seminal contributions to the field.

47. FOLKMAN J, SZABO S, STOVROFF M, MCNEIL P, LI W, SHING Y: **Duodenal Ulcer: Discovery of a New Mechanism and Development of Angiogenic Therapy That Accelerates Healing.** *Ann Surg* 1991, **214**:414–425.

48. MCNEIL PL, ITO S: **Molecular Traffic Through Plasma Membrane Disruptions of Cells In Vivo.** *J Cell Sci* 1990, **96**:549–556.

49. MOORE R, CARLSON S, MADARA J: **Rapid Barrier Restitution in an In Vivo Model of Intestinal Epithelial Injury.** *Lab Invest* 1989, **60**:237–244.

50. HAHN U: **Extracellular Matrix Proteins in Small-Intestinal Cell Cultures.** *Scand J Gastroenterology* 1988, **23(suppl 151)**:70–78.

51. DEITCH EA: **Nutrition and the Gut Mucosal barrier.** *Curr Opin Gen*
•• *Surg* 1993, **1**:85–91.
A thorough review of the modulation of the gut mucosal barrier by nutritional support in fasting patients.

52. GALLAGHER HJ, DALY JM: **Malnutrition, Injury, and the Host Immune**
•• **Response: Nutrient Substitution.** *Curr Opin Gen Surg* 1993, 1:92–104.
Complementary to the review by Deitch (*Curr Opin Gen Surg* 1993, 1:85–91), this is a detailed analysis of the effects of nutritional substitution on the host immune response.

53. DOWLING RH: **Cellular and Molecular Basis of Intestinal and Pancre-**
•• **atic Adaptation.** *Scand J Gastroenterol* 1992, **27(suppl 293)**:64–67.
An excellent summary of available data on the biology of intestinal and pancreatic adaptation.

54. ALBERT V, YOUNG GP: **Differentiation Status of Rat Enterocytes After**
•• **Intestinal Adaptation to Jejunoileal Bypass.** *Gut* 1992, **33**:1638–1643.
Quantitates the phenotypic changes in rat enterocytes during adaptation to jejunoileal bypass using digestive enzyme expression as a quantitative marker.

55. CHUNG DH, EVERS M, TOWNSEND CM, HUANG KF, HERNDON D,
• THOMPSON JC: **Role of Polyamine Biosynthesis During Gut Mucosal Adaptation After Burn Injury.** *Am J Surg* 1993, **165**:144–149.
An investigation into one phase of possible intracellular regulation during mucosal adaptation.

56. HARDIN JA, BURET A, MEDDINGS JB, GALL DG: **Effect of Epidermal**
• **Growth Factor on Enterocyte Brush-Border Surface Area**. *Am J Physiol* 1993, **264**:G312–G318.
Epidermal growth factor not only stimulates enterocyte proliferation but also modulates the area of the brush border available for absorption.

57. SALLEH M, ARDAWI M: **Effects of Epidermal Growth Factor and**
• **Glutamine-Supplemented Parenteral Nutrition on the Small Bowel of Septic Rats**. *Clin Sci* 1992, **82**:573–580.
Parenteral epidermal growth factor also ameliorates the effects of fasting and sepsis.

58. IZUKURA M, EVERS BM, PAREKH D, YOSHINAGA K, UCHIDA T, TOWNSEND
• CM, THOMPSON JC: **Neurotensin Augments Intestinal Regeneration After Small Bowel Resection in Rats**. *Ann Surg* 1992, **215**:520–527.
Neurotensin is demonstrated to support mucosal adaptation to short gut syndrome after small bowel resection.

59. CHUNG DH, EVERS BM, SHIMODA I, TOWNSEND CM, RAJARAMAN S,
• THOMPSON JC: **Effect of Neurotensin on Gut Mucosal Growth in Rats With Jejunal and Ileal Thiry-Vella Fistulas**. *Gastroenterology* 1992, **103**:1254–1258.
Complementary to the paper by Izukura *et al.* (*Ann Surg* 1992, 215:520–527), this paper by the same group demonstrates the effects of neurotensin on the adaptation to fasting in defunctionalized small bowel loops.

60. ALBISTON AL, TAYLOR RG, HERINGTON AC, BEVERIDGE DJ, FULLER PJ:
•• **Divergent Ileal IGF-I and IGFBP-3 Gene Expression After Small Bowel Resection: A Novel Mechanism to Amplify IGF Action?** *Mol Cell Endocrinol* 1992, **83**:R17–R20.
An interesting paper suggesting that investigators of growth factor effects may need to consider bioavailability as well as absolute levels of a bioactive agent.

61. VANDERHOOF JA, MCCUSKER RH, CLARK R, MOHAMMADPOUR H,
• BLACKWOOD DJ, HARTY RF, PARK JHY: **Truncated and Native Insulinlike Growth Factor I Enhance Mucosal Adaptation After Jejunoileal Resection**. *Gastroenterology* 1992, **102**:1949–1956.
Another demonstration of the ability of a growth factor (in this case insulinlike growth factor 1) to support mucosal adaptation to the short gut syndrome.

62. OLANREWAJU H, PATEL L, SEIDEL ER: **Trophic Action of Local Intraileal**
•• **Infusion of Insulin-Growth Factor I: Polyamine Dependence**. *Am J Physiol* 1992, **263**:E282–E286.
Intraluminal infusion of insulin-like growth factor appears to exert its trophic effects via modulation of polyamine metabolism.

Marc D. Basson, MD, PhD, Department of Surgery, Yale University School of Medicine, 310 Cedar Street, New Haven, CT 06510, USA.

Liver, biliary tract, and pancreas*

Editorial overview

John R. T. Monson, MD, FRCS, Josef E. Fischer, MD, FRCSE, and Howard A. Reber, MD

Castle Hill Hospital, Cottingham, UK, University of Cincinnati Medical Center, Cincinnati, Ohio, and University of California Los Angeles Medical Center, Los Angeles, California, USA

* The articles on the liver in this section were edited by Dr. Monson; those on the biliary tract, by Dr. Fischer; and those on the pancreas, by Dr. Reber.

Current Opinion in General Surgery 1994:147–150

Liver

To anyone involved in the management of patients suffering from multifocal malignant disease of the liver, one thing is abundantly clear: the wide range of therapeutic options available indicates a lack of consensus that has resulted from the lack of a single clearly beneficial therapy. The review by Peter McCullough (pp 151–155) on nonsurgical treatment of liver metastases illustrates this point most vividly. In practical terms, the majority of patients with malignant liver disease in the West will have metastatic disease, although bilobar primary hepatocellular carcinoma remains a clinical challenge in the Far East in particular. Furthermore, the majority of metastatic disease will originate in the gastrointestinal tract; fewer will come from the breast, the lung, and melanoma. There is widespread agreement surgical resection, when possible, affords the best prospect for long-term survival. Sadly, it is rarely possible, and for a large cohort of patients, the therapeutic options are at the same time unencouraging and widely varied. Is there any light at the end of the tunnel?

For patients with metastatic colorectal carcinoma, systemic chemotherapy using some combination of 5-fluorouracil and folinic acid may provide palliation and a modest increase in survival. Similar results may be achieved with a regional perfusion system, but at the cost of increased toxicity and expense. What must be clear at this stage is that if progress is to be made, a new approach must be adopted. Chemotherapeutic trials of 5-fluorouracil have been done for more than 20 years, and regardless of whatever manipulation of this agent is used, the results remain unimpressive. The benefits to a small group of patients have been achieved at considerable cost. Indeed, Scheithauer *et al.* [1] recently asked whether there is any benefit to be gained over a regimen of simple supportive care. In a randomized trial, they concluded some benefit was apparent and that good palliation was associated with a slight increase in overall survival. Although encouraging for patients, this conclusion doesn't alter the fact that new agents are needed, both for adjuvant therapy and for the treatment of advanced disease. In his excellent review, McCullough deals largely with regional perfusion and targeted therapy. Both of these approaches have shown improved results in recent years and clearly should be continued in the future. Where does that leave us for other directions?

In recent years, monoclonal antibodies have enjoyed somewhat of a resurgence of interest. Several studies have demonstrated good localization of colorectal tumors—both primary and metastatic—by murine and chimeric antibodies. A trial has just been completed of adjuvant therapy in colorectal cancer, in which murine 17-1A was administered as a single agent; the results are awaited with interest. For advanced disease, it is possible to target isotope therapy (both ^{131}I and ^{90}Y) with significant reduction in tumor mass, at least in animal models [2]. The 17-1A antibody is now used increasingly for tumor detection. Its toxicity profile is gratifyingly low, thus making it an ideal agent for adjuvant therapy. A recent clinical trial of OK432 combined with adoptive lymphocyte immunotherapy was reported in patients with advanced colorectal cancer. Of 24 patients treated, two showed complete response, and a further four achieved partial responses [3]. Toxicity was low, although the addition of lymphocyte transfer must make this approach somewhat restrictive. However, antibody delivery remains difficult. A pretherapeutic study of dose recovery using ^{131}I-labelled and anti-carcinoembryonic antigen monoclonal antibody was rather disappointing. Although bone marrow dosage was acceptable, tumor recovery was limited, leading the authors to suggest that this antibody may be ineffective as a single approach [4]. Overall, therefore, the antibody story remains alive but not ready for center stage.

Newer biological response modifiers are being evaluated. The Tulane group recently studied the somatostatin analogue RC-160 in animal models of metastatic colon cancer. True tumor regression is not clearly evident, although inhibition of growth has been suggested—somewhat like the experience with RC-160 in pancreatic cancer [5]. For this approach to be viable, it is likely that new receptor modifiers will be required. Nonspecific immunostimulation continues to be evaluated, most recently in combination with chemotherapy.

Abbreviation

ERCP—endoscopic retrograde cholangiopancreatography.

 ISBN 1-85922-671-X ISSN 1065–6243

In a mouse model, liposomal muramyl tripeptide administered together with 5-fluorouracil and leucovorin significantly increased response rates over those achieved by chemotherapy alone [6].

Leaving aside these more experimental approaches for a moment, the more direct attack of intralesional therapy continues to offer promise. Tumor destruction may be brought about by either heating or cooling. Extensive experience of direct cryotherapy of liver metastases is now available. This approach is both time-consuming and difficult to assess; few controlled data are available. The results in selected patients, recently reviewed by Morris *et al.* [7], are nonetheless reasonable. Largely limited by the number and size of lesions that can be treated by current equipment, this approach requires a full laparotomy and may take up to 4 hours to complete. The size of the area to be frozen may be accurately determined by real-time intraoperative ultrasonography, thus preventing unnecessary tissue destruction. Toxicity is low, although not inconsequential; coagulopathy, sepsis, and liver and renal failure were all documented in recent series. Essentially, the incidence of these side effects rises with the volume of tissue destroyed during therapy. In addition, the larger the lesion frozen, the greater the risk of fracture of the ice ball, which may lead to subsequent hemorrhage. Despite these drawbacks, cryotherapy requires limited hospital stay as a single-episode therapy. As with those patients undergoing hepatic resection, it has primarily been offered to patients with disease limited to the liver, although recent work has suggested it may be combined with regional chemotherapy for patients with disease limited to the liver substance and nodes within the porta hepatis.

In contrast to cryotherapy, the role of hyperthermia is less clear. Animal studies have been reported using extracorporeally generated shock waves to bring about focal tissue destruction. Although this technique has the advantage of being noninvasive, accurate localization of the tumor with existing external ultrasound scanners is difficult [8], and collateral tissue damage remains a concern during therapy. Computer-aided guidance systems may help in this regard. Interstitial hyperthermia has been more widely studied. In a pilot clinical study using a neodymium:yttrium-aluminum-garnet laser guided by ultrasound localization of the target lesion, 11 patients with 16 liver metastases were treated. Twelve of these lesions were radically ablated, an outcome that was accurately predicted with real-time ultrasonography and interstitial temperature monitoring. However, the effect on patient survival following this approach remains unknown [9].

Using a similar method of access, interstitial high-dose radiotherapy of colorectal hepatic metastases with ^{192}Ir was recently reported. A single dose was administered to 22 patients with an afterloader. Median actuarial local control was 8 months with 26% actuarial local control at 26 months as judged by computed tomography [10]. Despite these apparently encouraging results, the authors concluded that further study is required to determine whether this therapy will have any effect on the natural history of the disease.

In conclusion, it seems clear that the problem of metastatic liver disease remains beyond the reach of current therapies. Current chemotherapeutic agents are unlikely to provide the answers, regardless of the method of administration. Newer agents are required, and some are on the horizon. For the majority of patients, meanwhile, the outlook remains gloomy.

Biliary tract

In the three articles on biliary surgery, distinguished authors and experts in their own areas investigate some of the vagaries and mysteries of the bile ducts. Bile ducts appear to be relatively simple structures made up of a group of metabolically active cells with connections to the hepatic parenchyma, the reticuloendothelial system, Kupffer cells, and hepatocytes, which undoubtedly are much more complicated than we realize. These simple structures, however, bedevil the liver in a series of diseases that are difficult to comprehend and even more difficult to deal with clinically at times.

The difficulties with the bile ducts do not end in infancy or childhood; later in life, sclerosing cholangitis makes an appearance. These patients tend to be younger, generally in their 20s or 30s. The association between sclerosing cholangitis and inflammatory bowel disease, notably ulcerative colitis, is an intriguing one and has been often commented on. Indeed, in some series, 80% of the patients with sclerosing cholangitis have coexistent ulcerative colitis. I have seen a patient with sclerosing cholangitis who presented with cirrhosis and only on determined investigation proved to have a very mild case of ulcerative colitis. It is also interesting that surgeons dealing with patients with ulcerative colitis have come to accept that if patients do not have the changes of sclerosing cholangitis prior to colectomy, it is likely that they will never get sclerosing cholangitis. However, once sclerosing cholangitis has begun, colectomy does not change the outcome, and a number of patients who have had successful colectomies and pull-through procedures have subsequently gone on to liver transplantation. What does this tell us about the nature of the disease? Does it not suggest either an infectious or an immunological etiology, as some authors have argued? Is it possible to hypothesize that the initial lesion, that of early sclerosing cholangitis, is the response to some infectious agent arising in the colon, making its way in the portal circulation, or along the lymphatics, to infect, as it were, the bile ducts and elicit a desmoplastic and other type of response? Then, the argument would carry forward, once the infection "is established," an immunological process takes over in which the resulting scarring fibrosis, swelling, and distortion in bile duct architecture are ongoing even though the initial stimulus has been removed. This, of course, is a viable hypothesis, but it remains largely unproven. Finally, John Braasch (pp 156–160) does point out some interesting diagnostic criteria by which he proposes that a manifestation of more than one narrowing constitutes an absolute diagnostic criterion for sclerosing cholangitis. On casual inspection, that would not be my conclusion from clinical experience, in which I believe I have seen several patients who are exceptions to this proposed rule, but it is good to bear in mind.

The obvious difficulty in patients with sclerosing cholangitis is telling the difference between sclerosing cholangitis and adenocarcinoma of the bile ducts, the so-called

Klatskin tumor. It is interesting that my predecessor, Altemeier [11], was probably the first to describe the tumor. However, there were a number of authors on the paper, and so a single-authored paper, that authored by Klatskin, is the paper by which the name of the syndrome was popularized. Like sclerosing cholangitis, Klatskin tumors tend to be insidious, infiltrating lesions that are probably indolent for a long period of time. I am convinced that I have seen patients in whom 8 to 10 years had to elapse before the entire full-blown nature of the Klatskin tumor became apparent. Certainly, patients with ulcerative colitis have a pronounced tendency toward bile duct complications not only of sclerosing cholangitis but also of carcinomas. Thus, it seems likely that the same stimulus that results in sclerosing cholangitis can, under certain circumstances, result in neoplastic disease of the bile ducts.

The important message from Keith Lillemoe's review (pp 161–167) and the contribution from the Hopkins group to this difficult disease is that it ultimately lends itself to the same type of meticulous surgical care that we associate with other neoplastic disease. What I derive from the Hopkins group's contribution to the area of Klatskin tumors is that although one cannot always effect cure, the surgical approach is worthwhile and results in significant palliation and improved quality of life. My guess is that in most patients, even those in whom we think we have a clean surgical resection for cure, there exist foci of disease elsewhere, and that Klatskin tumors constitute a multifocal disease with a single prominent manifestation rather than a disease localized in one segment of the bile duct. Be that as it may, it appears as if a vigorous surgical approach will result in significant palliation and improvement in outcome.

The final review, by Jay Grosfeld (pp 168–172), deals with an illness that begins *in utero*, which, if we really understood it, might unlock the doors to some understanding of significant bile duct pathophysiology. What is the nature of the disease of bile duct hypoplasia? It is a structural disease? Is it secondary to ischemia? Is it the response to a series of noxious stimuli *in utero*? Is it an immunological disease, and if it is, how is it possible that an immunological disease results at a time when immunology is theoretically privileged, as *in utero*? What type of disease is it once it gets established? Grosfeld argues strongly for intervention in the first 3 months of life, and the statistics he summons to back up his case are impressive indeed. What is the nature of change that takes place after 3 months that leads to failure of the Kasai operation in these patients? Is it immunologic? If so, how do these cells provoke an autoimmune stimulus in a privileged situation? Is it infectious? Bacteriologic and other infectious techniques have been used in an attempt to localize a noxious agent. Nothing has been forthcoming, but that does not mean that such an agent is not present. Or is it simply a series of ongoing injuries that, once begun, are self-progressive and cannot be interrupted by any form of therapy, including the provision of adequate drainage? These questions are tantalizing, but there is little information on which to base the answers. It does appear, however, that if one can interrupt the damage process early on, long-term survival may be possible.

Taken together, the three reviews cover a spectrum of interesting, technically challenging, and difficult disease for even the most masterful surgeons. The reviews are the result of a distillation of extensive experience in their areas, for which we are grateful.

Pancreas

Charles Yeo (pp 173–178) has provided a valuable update on a number of advances in the management of pancreatic pseudocysts, pancreatic ascites, and pancreatic fistulas. He begins with the definition of several terms, including "pseudopseudocyst," which has been used to describe the peripancreatic fluid collections that may accompany an episode of severe acute pancreatitis. This is a cumbersome term and should probably be discarded. Instead, the term *acute fluid collection* should be used.

Yeo points out that newly evolving information about the natural history of pseudocysts is important and is changing long accepted principles of management. For example, we now know that pseudocysts resolve in up to 50% of cases and that the complication rate is quite low. Therefore, many cysts may not require treatment. It is also clear that in certain situations, percutaneous pseudocyst drainage and endoscopic approaches can be effective alternatives to surgery. Nevertheless, as in a variety of other areas where nonsurgical interventional techniques are being introduced, their role and effectiveness are still being determined.

Yeo stresses appropriately that one of the concerns about nonoperative management of pseudocysts is the possibility that cystic neoplasms may be overlooked. Although analysis of cyst fluid is of some interest, the diagnosis of the type of cyst and, in particular, whether a cyst is malignant still must depend upon clinical findings and pathologic information obtained at surgery. Efforts to select more intelligently those patients who should have surgery are evolving. New techniques include the use of endoscopic retrograde cholangiopancreatography (ERCP) to determine whether the cyst communicates directly with the pancreatic duct.

In regard to the management of pancreatic ascites, Yeo stresses the importance of preoperative demonstration of the site of leak from the pancreatic duct by ERCP. He discusses the use of octreotide in the treatment of both pancreatic ascites and pancreatic fistulas. Anecdotal evidence continues to accumulate that octreotide may hasten the resolution of these problems, but there are still no prospective studies that have addressed the problem.

In the article on pancreatic transplantation, F. Charles Brunicardi and Christopher Shackleton (pp 179–185) compare the risks, benefits, and problems associated with whole-pancreas and islet transplantation for the treatment of diabetes mellitus. They point out that while whole-organ transplantation reliably achieves insulin independence and euglycemia in many patients, the complications are nevertheless significant. At present, the overall 1-year patient survival is 85%, and the 1-year graft survival is 63%. When they are successful, the quality of life is improved significantly, because patients are free from the need for glucose monitoring, dietary restrictions, and injections of insulin. While prevention of the long-term complications of diabetes is a likely benefit, it remains to be proven whether established complications such as retinopathy and nephropathy are alleviated following transplantation. Islet transplantation has been plagued by difficulties associated with isolation of human islets and, of course, rejection. The overall success rate for islet transplants has been much less, about 11%. Although many of the patients are still not insulin-independent, they may have reduced insulin requirements. The review represents a useful update and describes the state of the art in this exciting but challenging field by two acknowledged experts.

Jennifer Meko and Jeffrey Norton (pp 186–194) have provided a superb update on endocrine tumors of the pancreas. Although these lesions are rare, they cause significant morbidity, and many of them are malignant, eventually resulting in the demise of the patient. The authors discuss the altered approach to the treatment of patients with Zollinger-Ellison syndrome as a result of potent new acid antisecretory drugs. A significant number of patients with gastrinoma now undergo resection of the tumor and appear to be cured. The availability of the drug octreotide, which reduces the plasma concentration of many of these hormones, has also been valuable in controlling symptoms and preparing patients for surgery. The use of intraoperative ultrasonography is also reviewed. It too represents a significant advance in the intraoperative identification and management of many of these lesions.

References

1. Scheithauer W, Rosen H, Kornek G-V, Sebesta C, Depisch D: **Randomised Comparison of Combination Chemotherapy Plus Supportive Care With Supportive Care Alone in Patients With Metastatic Colorectal Cancer.** *BMJ* 1993, **306**:752–755.
2. Buchsbaum DJ, Lawrence TS, Roberson PL, Heidorn DB, Ten Haken RK, Steplewski Z: **Comparison of ^{131}I- and ^{90}Y-labeled Monoclonal Antibody 17-1A for Treatment of Human Colon Cancer Xenografts.** *Int J Radiat Oncol Biol Phys* 1993, **25**:629–638.
3. Satoh K, Kan N, Okino T, Mise K, Yamasaki S, Harada T, Hori T, Ohgaki K, Tobe T: **The Therapeutic Effect of OK-432-Combined Adoptive Immunotherapy Against Liver Metastases From Gastric or Colorectal Cancers.** *Biotherapy* 1993, **6**:41–49.
4. Ychou M, Ricard M, Lumbroso J, Rougher P, Mach J-P, Buchegger F, Saccavini JC, Lasser P, Elias D, Eschwege F: **Potential Contribution of ^{131}I-Labelled Monoclonal Anti-CEA Antibodies in the Treatment of Liver Metastases From Colorectal Carcinomas: Pretherapeutic Study With Dose Recovery in Resected Tissues.** *Eur J Cancer* 1993, **29A**:1105–1111.
5. Qin Y, Van Cauteren M, Osteaux M, Schally AV, Willems G: **Inhibitory Effect of Somatostatin Analogue RC-160 on the Growth of Hepatic Metastases of Colon Cancer in Rats: A Study With Magnetic Resonance Imaging.** *Cancer Res* 1992, **52**:6025–6030.
6. Asao T, Shibata HR, Batist G, Brodt P: **Eradication of Hepatic Metastases of Carcinoma H-59 by Combination Chemoimmunotherapy With Liposomal Muramyl Tripeptide, 5-Fluorouracil, and Leucovorin.** *Cancer Res* 1992, **52**:6254–6257.
7. Morris DL, Horton MDA, Dilley AV, Warlters A, Clingan PR: **Treatment of Hepatic Metastases by Cryotherapy and Regional Cytotoxic Perfusion.** *Gut* 1993, **34**:1156–1157.
8. Darzi A, Chartier-Kestler E, Valencien G, Goldin R, Guillou PJ, Monson JRT: **High Energy Extracorporeal Shock Wave Thermotherapy: A New Anti-Tumour Option?** *Surg Oncol* 1993, **2**:197–203.
9. Nolsoe CP, Torp-Pedersen S, Burcharth F, Horn T, Pedersen S, Christensen S, Olldag ES, Anderson PH, Karstrup S, Lorentzen T: **Interstitial Hyperthermia of Colorectal Liver Metastases With a US-Guided Nd-YAG Laser With a Diffuser Tip: A Pilot Clinical Study.** *Radiology* 1993, **187**:333–337.
10. Thomas DS, Nauta RJ, Rodgers JE, Popescu GF, Ngumen H, Lee TC, Petrucci PE, Harter KW, Holt RW, Dritschilo A: **Intraoperative High-Dose Rate Interstitial Irradiation of Hepatic Metastases From Colorectal-Carcinoma: Results of a Phase I-II Trial.** *Cancer* 1993, **71**:1977–1981.
11. Altemeier WA, Gall EA, Zinninger MM, Hoxworth PI: **Sclerosing Carcinoma of the Major Intrahepatic Bile Ducts.** *Arch Surg* 1957, **75**:450–461.

John R. T. Monson, MD, FRCS, University of Hull, Academic Surgical Unit, Castle Hill Hospital, Castle Road, Cottingham, North Humberside HU16-5JQ, UK.

Josef E. Fischer, MD, University of Cincinnati Medical Center, Department of Surgery, 231 Bethesda Avenue, Cincinnati, OH 45267-0558, USA.

Howard A. Reber, MD, Division of General Surgery, UCLA Medical Center, 10833 Le Conte Avenue, Los Angeles, CA 90024-1749, USA.

Nonsurgical treatment of liver metastases

Peter McCulloch, MD

University of Liverpool, Liverpool, UK

Experimental studies demonstrate that angiotensin II and somatostatin analogues have some ability to redirect hepatic arterial blood flow toward liver metastases. Albumin microspheres and liposomes are both effective to animal models in enhancing intra-arterial drug delivery to tumor tissue. Clinical studies show that such strategies can also improve drug targeting in humans. Clinical trials of intrahepatic arterial chemotherapy demonstrate definite response and survival benefits, but toxicity can be considerable, and progression of extrahepatic disease remains an unsolved problem. Selective means of delivering radiation, biologic therapy, and thermal energy to liver metastases are possible alternative nonsurgical treatments that merit further investigation.

Current Opinion in General Surgery 1994:151–155

This review concentrates on therapy for metastatic disease in the liver. The literature on nonresectional therapy for primary hepatoma concentrates largely on different issues and has recently been well reviewed by Ellis *et al.* [1].

Regional intra-arterial chemotherapy

Experimental studies

The rationale for hepatic arterial infusion of chemotherapy is to maximize the ratio of drug delivery between tumor and normal tissue. This approach can logically be refined further by manipulating hepatic blood flow. Pharmacologic and physical manipulation have been described in a rat model, through the use of angiotensin II, a somatostatin analogue, and albumin microspheres [2•,3]. Microspheres of average diameter 40 μm were preferentially directed toward tumor tissue to a greater extent than predicted by arterial blood flow ratios. This effect may result from transient vasoconstriction in normal vessels. Once injected, they cause obstruction to flow, resulting in an 80% drop in the tumor/normal arterial flow ratio [2•]. Angiotensin II caused a 30% increase in the tumor/normal distribution ratio of microspheres, but this effect did not reach statistical significance. Hepatic arterial injection of the somatostatin analogue octreotide reduced hepatic arterial flow but increased the tumor/normal blood flow ratio. The net arterial flow through tumor tissue was therefore unaffected [3]. Somatostatin has been shown to have potent cytostatic effects *in vitro* [4], and to prolong host survival *in vivo*, so its influence is clearly complex. The potential of microsphere therapy was demonstrated in animal studies [5•], in which hepatic arterial doxorubicin-loaded microspheres reduced tumor mass by 38%, whereas intra-arterial doxorubicin alone was ineffective (Fig. 1). Liposome encapsulation may also maximize the selectivity of hepatic arterial drugs by permitting slow release of the active drug in the correct site. A phase I clinical study of systemic liposome–incorporated doxorubicin demonstrated reduced toxicity but did not make clear whether efficacy was also lost [6]. Regionally administered liposomal therapy is a logical development, and there is experimental evidence that this therapy may improve response and survival while retaining the low toxicity of systemic treatment [7•]. Hepatic arterial doxorubicin liposomes in rats produced systemic doxorubicin levels several times lower, and tumor levels four times higher, than did systemic administration. The intraportal route has also been under study, but recent results have not been particularly encouraging. Intraportal chemotherapy alone proved of no value in animal studies, and combined intraportal and intra-arterial infusion was no better than arterial treatment alone [8]. After hepatic artery ligation, vasopressin analogues reduce normal liver but not tumor blood flow [9]. The attractions of intraportal therapy do not seem convincing enough to warrant major clinical studies at present.

The essential message from these experimental studies seems to be that therapy may be optimized by a combination of intra-arterial administration, pharmacologic manipulation of flow toward the tumor, and the use of slow-release preparations, such as microspheres or liposomes. The clinical benefits of such approaches will depend on the tumor/normal drug ratios that can be achieved.

Clinical studies

Clinical pharmacokinetic studies have used laser Doppler techniques to demonstrate the effects of angiotensin II on blood flow in patients with hepatic metastases [10]. Tumor blood flow was increased in lesions under 5 cm in diameter, but not in larger metastases. This finding is consistent with that of previous work showing that the arterial predominance of blood supply to metastases disappears as lesions enlarge. The dual nature of liver tumor blood supply was demonstrated by a study of bromodeoxyuridine uptake after intra-arterial or intraportal injection during liver resection [11•]. Both routes gave high levels of nuclear uptake, but only on the periphery of the tumor. Intra-arterial injection of bromodeoxyuri-

Abbreviation

LAK—lymphokine-activate killer.

 ISBN 1-85922-671-X ISSN 1065–6243

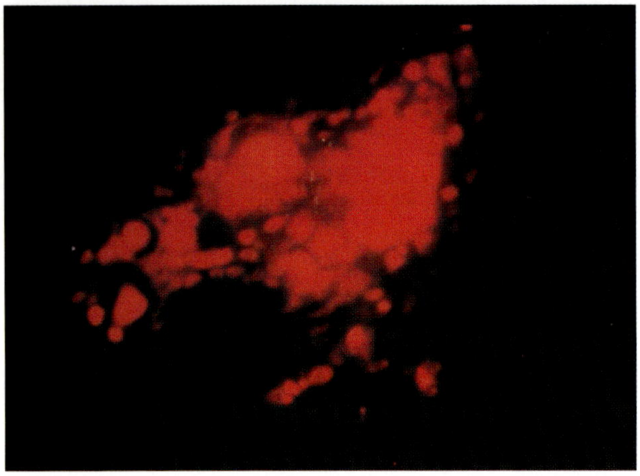

Fig. 1. Fluorescent micrograph of tumor tissue from an animal treated with doxorubicin-loaded albumin microspheres 4 days previously. Intravascular fragments of drug-loaded particles can be seen containing a high concentration of doxorubicin, which is intensely fluorescent. The background fluorescence indicates the presence of drug within the tissue at an intracellular level. Similar micrographs from animals treated with doxorubicin in simple solution showed no evidence of any drug. (*From* Goldberg *et al.* [5•]; with permission.)

dine suspended in Lipiodol (Guerlet, Aulnay-sur-Bois, France), however, resulted in uptake right through the tumor. The effect of Lipiodol is to retain the drug in the tumor vessels, allowing greater cellular uptake. Liver-to-lung shunting of blood may cause systemic toxicity following intra-arterial therapy, and this effect has been investigated in patients being treated with microsphere chemotherapy [12]. Although shunting increased with tumor burden, it never exceeded 4.4% of total drug dose, so its importance is likely to be small.

Minimally invasive means of administering regional hepatic chemotherapy have become popular in situations in which the opportunity to insert a catheter at open operation does not arise. The remarkable advance of interventional radiology is illustrated by a report of eight patients whose liver metastases were treated by percutaneous isolated liver perfusion with 5-fluorouracil [13••]. A perfusion catheter was placed in the hepatic artery via a femoral artery, while a special balloon catheter was introduced into the vena cava via the opposite femoral vein. This method placed balloons fore and aft of a middle fenestrated section that were used to isolate the hepatic veins (Fig. 2). The effluent was filtered via an extracorporeal charcoal hemoperfusion system before reinfusion via the internal jugular vein. 5-fluorouracil extraction was over 85%, with minimal drug leakage. The technical expertise required clearly limits this procedure to the specialist, but for those with the facilities it has exciting potential.

Several major reports of the outcome of regional chemotherapy were published recently. The largest of these is a German report on 221 regionally treated patients [14]. Unfortunately, the variety of approaches used, the lack of direct randomized comparisons, and the lack of clear data on the comparability of the treatment groups make interpretation of the results somewhat difficult. Response rates and the incidence of chemical hepatitis varied widely between regimens. Additional systemic treatment did not delay extrahepatic recurrence, and leucovorin treatment was associated with an increase in treatment-limiting stomatitis and diarrhea.

A nonrandomized comparative study of systemic versus intra-arterial mitomycin C versus intra-arterial mitomycin C with *cis*-platin in patients with liver metastases from gastric cancer showed greatly improved response and survival duration in the third group. Both adjuvant therapy after liver resection and primary treatment of unresected metastases were included [15], and the resultant heterogeneity may compromise the significance of the large difference in response rate (4% vs 29%) between the first and second groups. The superiority of combined intra-arterial therapy versus systemic mitomycin C (response rates, 4% and 73%; median survivals, 2.9 and 11.8 months) seems unlikely to be artifactual. A phase II study of combination intra-arterial therapy with 5-fluorouracil and carboplatin in metastases from colorectal cancer produced encouraging median survival (23.5 months) and response rates (52%) without serious systemic or regional toxicity [16]. This approach merits development in phase III comparisons with monotherapy.

The long-term results of intrahepatic arterial monotherapy with floxuridine for metastases from colorectal cancer were reported by Rougier *et al.* [17••]. The large study population (166 patients) and long follow-up (median, 54 months) allowed accurate evaluation, although the control population was given either no treatment or systemic 5-fluorouracil (at the clinician's discretion), whereas systemic 5-fluorouracil was given for progression in the floxuridine group. The results correlate well with those of other reports of this type of treatment. Intra-arterial chemotherapy achieved a modest but significant increase in mean survival, from 11 to 15 months. Those with a good response often survived considerably longer, so 2-year survival rates in the floxuridine and control groups were 23 and 13 months, respectively (Fig. 3). These rates were achieved at the cost of considerable local toxicity: 58% of the floxuridine group suffered either chemical hepatitis or biliary sclerosis, and the incidence of sclerosing cholangitis after 1 year of treatment was 255%. As floxuridine is largely metabolized in the liver, systemic toxicity was minimal, but the drug provided no therapeutic effect against progression of extrahepatic metastases, the commonest cause of death in these patients. The authors therefore concluded that intra-arterial floxuridine requires combination with an active regimen of systemic chemotherapy. A second trial using the same floxuridine regimen considered addition of intra-arterial dexamethasone [18]. This study suffered from its smaller sample size (25 patients/arm), which prevented statistically sound conclusions from being drawn. Patients receiving dexamethasone apparently did better in terms of serum bilirubin levels, response rate, and survival, but only the response rate reached statistical significance (complete response and partial response = 71% vs 40%). Another randomized trial compared intrahepatic arterial floxuridine with a combination regimen of mitomycin, carmustine, and floxuridine in pretreated patients [19]. The group was split between those who had failed systemic treatment and those who had only had adjuvant therapy. In the former group, the combination yielded a better response

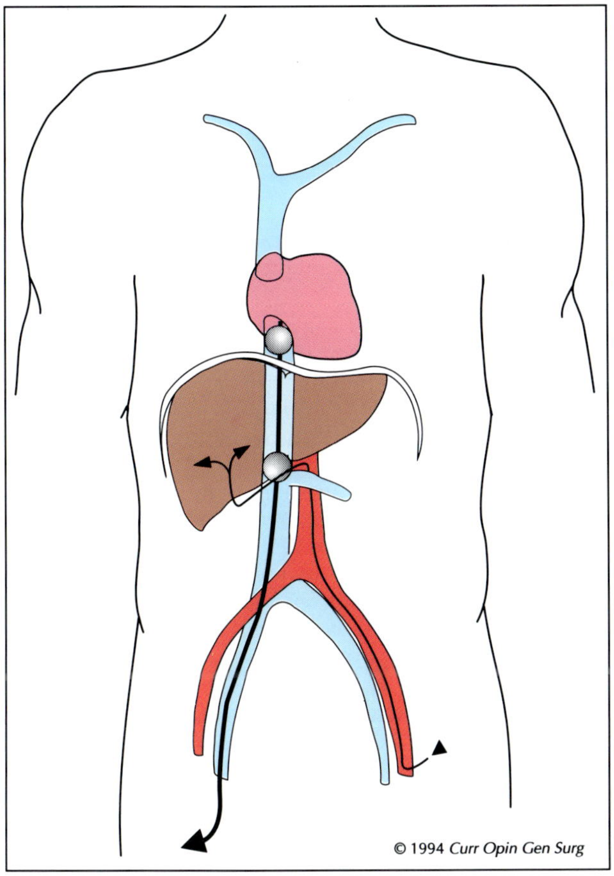

Fig. 2. Percutaneous isolated liver perfusion. A perfusion catheter is shown entering the hepatic artery (*small arrows*) via the left femoral artery and celiac axis (*wedge*). A double-balloon fenestrated catheter is shown draining the hepatic veins via the right femoral vein (*large arrow*). The two balloons provide effective isolation of the intrahepatic section of the inferior vena cava.

rate (47% vs 23%). The overall median survival was 16 months, and there was no significant survival advantage for the patients receiving combination therapy.

The number of questions which remain in this field, the relatively small patient population, and the long time scale of clinical trials make it difficult to conduct powerful trials leading to definitive results. Even the largest research centers must resist the temptation to divide their efforts. Cooperation and agreement between centers is the best way to avoid wasted activity. In the context of what we already know, these results emphasize the need for better drugs or combinations, better targeting to tumor tissue, and the limitations of regional chemotherapy in diseases in which concomitant metastasis to other organs is the rule.

Biologic therapy

The evident need to refine regional therapy and the equally clear need to limit the systemic toxicity of some forms of biologic therapy have resulted in several studies of their regional or local use for metastases in the liver. An interesting case report suggests that high local concentrations of lymphokine-activated killer (LAK) cells may be required for response [20]. This patient responded only in lesions in which direct intra-arterial or intralobar infusion of LAK cells was given: systemic infusion was ineffective. Tumor necrosis factor is too toxic for systemic administration but has theoretical attractions in cancer therapy. A recent animal study illustrated that a dose (40 μg/kg) that is fatal when given intravenously is highly effective in reducing tumor growth when injected directly into the tumor [21]. Phase I studies were then performed in patients with inoperable liver metastases [22]. Side effects included pyrexia and vomiting, but no evidence of serious cardiac, renal, or biochemical complications, which would have occurred with the same dose given systemically. A phase II study of tumor necrosis factor therapy via the hepatic artery showed a relatively disappointing response rate of 14% in patients who had become refractory to chemotherapy but confirmed the low toxicity of regional therapy [23•]. A retrospective Japanese report documented the beneficial effect of the immunostimulant OK432 and expanded autologous T lymphocytes via the hepatic artery in advanced breast cancer with liver metastases [24]. The response rate was high (65%), and survival was 22 months in responders versus only 2.8 months in nonresponders.

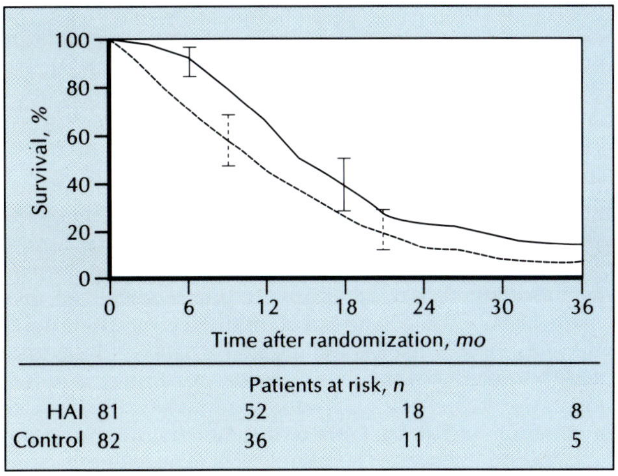

Fig. 3. Survival of patients with liver metastases according to treatment assignment to either hepatic arterial infusion (HAI) with floxuridine (*solid line*) or control treatment (*broken line*) (CI=95%). Control treatment was either observation or systemic 5-fluorouracil, at clinician's discretion. The survival advantage of HAI is significant by log-rank test ($P<0.02$). (*From* Rougier *et al.* [17••]; with permission.)

Targeted radiation therapy

Radiation has not had a major role in the treatment of liver tumor because of the well-established toxicity of whole-liver irradiation. Novel ideas on improving selectivity are however being developed. A Chinese group has developed an ingenious animal model involving first transcatheter intrahepatic arterial embolization, then intrahepatic arterial injection of the radiosensitizer misonidazole, and finally, external electron beam irradiation [25]. Pretreatment was successful in concentrating radiation damage in tumor tissue, and clinical studies may now be justified. Another radiosensitizer, razoxane, has been used in a phase II study of whole-liver irradiation [26]. A more than 50% decline in tumor volume was recorded in half of 25 patients. The overall response rate of 62% was comparable to that of regional chemotherapy. A third approach to selective irradiation has been the intra-arterial injection of yttrium-90 microspheres, with direction toward tumor tissue by the use of angiotensin II. In a phase I study with a calculated uniform liver dose of 150 Gy, there was evidence of some response in six of seven patients [27], but not of adverse effects. A phase II study [28•] showed that 48% of patients had a more than 50% reduction in tumor volume at 3 months after treatment. These studies show that it is possible, using selective methods, to achieve significant tumor responses by irradiation without unacceptable immediate morbidity. Whether these responses translate into improved survival and whether the risk-benefit ratio will be sufficient to compete with other treatment strategies remain uncertain.

Other regional approaches

The use of intraperitoneal drugs to target therapy to the liver is based on the hepatofugal lymphatic and venous drainage of much of the membrane. Intermittent 5-fluorouracil infusion into the peritoneal cavity by implantable port [29] caused no major side effects. The median survival of the 13 patients with metastases from colon cancer was only 4 months, so the efficacy of the treatment seems questionable.

Infusion of mixtures of Lipiodol, hemostatic agents, and chemotherapeutic drugs via the hepatic artery is a popular treatment modality in hepatocellular carcinoma. A cautionary report of its use in metastatic liver disease warns of the considerable side effects experienced when the whole liver is treated [30], chiefly fatigue and hepatitis with jaundice. The authors recommended sequential treatment of each lobe. Percutaneous injection of alcohol into the tumor is another technique commonly used in primary hepatoma that is now being evaluated in metastatic diseases [31]. A large survival advantage was obtained in an elaborate rat model, and the procedure was carried out with minimal side effects in six patients, whose median survival was 20 months. The principal attractions of the technique are its simplicity, low morbidity, and safety, as well as its track record in primary hepatoma. Larger studies to evaluate clinical survival benefit are justified.

The use of photodynamic therapy in the liver is restricted by selective uptake of photosensitizer by normal liver tissue. This can, however, be overcome by direct targeting of the laser light energy to the tumor tissue [32]. Although apparently successful and relatively selective, this approach requires considerable development. A clinical trial dispensing with the use of photosensitizer reported on interstitial laser hyperthermia for unresectable metastases in 10 patients [33]. This early study showed that the procedure was feasible, safe, and simple. The objective response rate of 44% was useful rather than dramatic. One might question whether the treatment could be made even simpler by dispensing with the laser. Low-energy diathermy current via an insulated needle and microwave therapy have both been used in this situation and might prove equally effective but cheaper. Percutaneous cryotherapy also has potential, and more publications on this topic can be expected. The use of the laparoscope to direct percutaneous injectional therapy will probably become a focus of interest in the near future, although it is unlikely to replace computed tomographic scanning as the workhorse of therapy targeting.

Conclusions

Much remains to be done, but much has been achieved: it is worth reflecting on how recently complete therapeutic nihilism held sway in cases of liver metastasis. The ability of regional chemotherapy to produce survival advantages over no treatment is now established. It also seems clear that regional therapy is superior to systemic therapy, but questions remain about the practical value and cost-benefit ratio of what can be achieved. We can be at least moderately hopeful that clinically worthwhile improvements in outcome can be gained from drug combinations and the use of techniques to target more therapy to the tumor tissue for longer periods of time. It is encouraging to see that chemotherapy is being challenged by regional and selective approaches to immunotherapy and radiotherapy, and by techniques for the percutaneous delivery of energy directly to the tumor deposit. The elements of a future strategy for much more effective treatment seem to be visible, but is too early to predict the final pattern or the degree to which it will fulfill our hopes. The problem of extrahepatic disease and the inability of any therapy other than resection to provide curative treatment remain the greatest challenges to future work in this field.

References and recommended reading

Papers of particular interest, published within the annual period of review, have been highlighted as:
- • Of special interest
- •• Of outstanding interest

1. Ellis LM, Demers ML, Roh MS: **Current Strategies for the Treatment of Hepatocellular Carcinoma.** *Curr Opin Oncol* 1992, 4:741–751.

2. • Anderson JH, Angerson WJ, Willmott N, Kerr DJ, McArdle CS, Cooke TG: **Is There a Relationship Between Regional Microsphere Distribution and Hepatic Arterial Blood Flow?** *Br J Cancer* 1992, 66:287–289.
Microspheres are preferentially directed to tumor tissue by mechanisms that remain unclear. The benefits for directed therapy may be very useful.

3. Hemingway DM, Jenkins SA, Cooke TG: **The Effects of Sandostatin (Octreotide, SMS 201-995) Infusion on Splanchnic and Hepatic Blood Flow in an Experimental Model of Hepatic Metastases.** *Br J Cancer* 1992, 65:396–398.

4. Qin Y, van Cauteren M, Osteaux M, Schally AV, Willems G: **Inhibitory Effect of Somatostatin Analogue RC-160 on the Growth of Hepatic Metastases of Colon Cancer in Rats: A Study With Magnetic Resonance Imaging.** *Cancer Res* 1992, 52:6025–6030.

5. • Goldberg JA, Willmott N, Kerr DJ, Sutherland C, McArdle CS: **An *In Vivo* Assessment of Adriamycin-Loaded Albumin Microspheres.** *Br J Cancer* 1992, 65:393–395.
Intra-arterial therapy using doxorubicin-loaded microspheres produced a 38% reduction in tumor volume in a model in which simple arterial infusion of the same dose was completely ineffective. Such vehicles may improve the efficacy of clinical intra-arterial therapy.

6. OWEN RR, SELLS RA, GILMORE IT, NEW RR, STRINGER RE: **A Phase I Clinical Evaluation of Liposome-Entrapped Doxorubicin (Lip-Dox) in Patients With Primary and Metastatic Hepatic Malignancy.** *Anticancer Drugs* 1992, 3:101–107.

7. • ZOU Y, HORIKOSHI I, UENO M, GU X, PEREZ-SOLER R: **Targeting Liver Tumors by Administering Liposomal Doxorubicin Into the Hepatic Artery.** *Int J Cancer* 1992, **51**:232–237.

Regional liposome-incorporated doxorubicin produced a fourfold increase in liver concentration, a 3.8-fold decrease in cardiac concentration, and a 16-fold decrease in systemic plasma concentration compared with systemic therapy. Tumor growth was abolished for 5 days after regional but not systemic therapy.

8. RIEMENSCHNEIDER T, RUF C, KRATZSCH HC, ZIEGLER M, SPATH G: **Arterial, Portal or Combined Arterio-Portal Regional Chemotherapy in Experimental Liver Tumours?** *J Cancer Res Clin Oncol* 1992, **118**:597–600.

9. NAREDI P, LINDNER P, HOLMBERG SB, SODERBERG R, CARLSSON G, GUSTAVSSON B, JACOBSSON L, HAFSTROM L: **The Influence of Hepatic Artery Ligation and/or Vasopressin on Liver Tumour Blood Flow in Rats.** *J Surg Oncol* 1992, **50**:70–76.

10. HEMINGWAY DM, ANGERSON WJ, ANDERSON JH, GOLDBERG JA, MCARDLE CS, COOKE TG: **Monitoring Blood Flow to Colorectal Liver Metastases Using Laser Doppler Flowmetry: The Effect of Angiotensin II.** *Br J Cancer* 1992, **66**:958–960.

11. • TANIGUCHI H, DAIDOH T, SHIOAKI Y, TAKAHASI T: **Blood Supply and Drug Delivery to Primary and Secondary Human Liver Cancers Studied With *In Vivo* Bromodeoxyuridine Labelling.** *Cancer* 1993, **71**:50–55.

This study provides clear evidence for the superiority of Lipiodol-associated drugs over conventional arterial infusions in penetrating to all areas of hepatic lesions.

12. HENNIGAN TW, EARLAM S, ALLEN-MERSH TG: **Is Liver to Lung Shunting in Colorectal Liver Metastasis the Cause of Toxicity Following Treatment With Cytotoxic Microsphere Aggregates?** *Br J Cancer* 1992, **66**:1169–1170.

13. •• BEHESHTI MV, DENNY DF JR, GLICKMAN MG, BODDEN W, MARSH JC, STRAIR R, RAVIKUMAR TS: **Percutaneous Isolated Liver Perfusion for Treatment of Hepatic Malignancy: Preliminary Report.** *J Vasc Intervent Radiol* 1992, 3:453–458.

This report of a completely percutaneous method for isolated liver perfusion represents a remarkable technical achievement with great clinical potential.

14. LORENZ M, HOTTENROTT C, MAIER P, REIMANN M, INGLIS R, ENCKE A: **Continuous Regional Treatment With Fluoropyrimidines for Metastases From Colorectal Carcinomas: Influence of Modulation With Leucovorin.** *Semin Oncol* 1992, **19**(suppl 3):163–170.

15. YONEMURA Y, MATUKI N, SAKUMA H, KATAYAMA K, SAWA T, FUJIMURA T, OHYAMA S, MIWA K, MIYAZAKI I, TANAKA M, *ET AL.*: **Effect of Intra-hepatoarterial Infusion of MMC and CDDP for Gastric Cancer Patients With Liver Metastases.** *Surg Today* 1992, **22**:253–259.

16. HIDALGO OF, REBOLLO J, VIEITEZ JM, BILBAO I, TANGCO E, ABUCHAIBE O, PARDO F: **Intra-arterial Hepatic Treatment With Carboplatin (CBDCA) and 5-Fluorouracil (5-FU) in Metastases From Colorectal Carcinoma.** *Am J Clin Oncol* 1993, **16**:30–35.

17. •• ROUGIER P, LAPLANCHE A, HUGUIER M, HAY JM, OLLIVIER JM, ESCAT J, SALMON R, JULIEN M, ROULLET-ANDY JC, GALLOT D, *ET AL.*: **Hepatic Arterial Infusion of Floxuridine in Patients With Liver Metastases From Colorectal Carcinoma: Long-Term Results of a Prospective Randomized Trial.** *J Clin Oncol* 1992, **10**:1112–1118.

This large, prospective, randomized trial with a long follow-up gives a clear picture of the outcome of regional floxuridine treatment. Survival is slightly but definitely prolonged, but hepatic toxicity is considerable, and extrahepatic disease is not affected.

18. KEMENY N, SEITER K, NIEDZWIECKI D, CHAPMAN D, SIGURDSON E, COHEN A, BOTET J, ODERMAN P, MURRAY P: **A Randomized Trial of Intrahepatic Infusion of Fluorodeoxyuridine With Dexamethasone Versus Fluorodeoxyuridine Alone in the Treatment of Metastatic Colorectal Cancer.** *Cancer* 1992, **69**:327–334.

19. KEMENY N, COHEN A, SEITER K, CONTI JA, SIGURDSON ER, TAO Y, NIEDZWIECKI D, BOTET J, BUDD A: **Randomized Trial of Hepatic Arterial Floxuridine, Mitomycin, and Carmustine Versus Floxuridine Alone in Previously Treated Patients With Liver Metastases From Colorectal Cancer.** *J Clin Oncol* 1993, **11**:330–335.

20. KEILHOLZ U, SCHLAG P, TILGEN W, BRADO B, GALM F, GORICH J, KAUFFMANN GW, MOLLER P, SCHNEIDER S, HUNSTEIN W: **Regional Administration of Lymphokine-Activated Killer Cells Can Be Superior to Intravenous Application.** *Cancer* 1992, **69**:2172–2175.

21. IZERMANS JN, SCHERINGA M, VAN DER SCHELLING GP, GEERLING RA, MARQUET RL, JEEKEL J: **Injection of Recombinant Tumor Necrosis Factor Directly Into Liver Metastases: An Experimental and Clinical Approach.** *Clin Exp Metastasis* 1992, **10**:91–97.

22. VAN DER SCHELLING GP, IZERMANS JN, KOK TC, SCHERINGA M, MARQUET RL, SPLINTER TA, JEEKEL J: **A Phase I Study of Local Treatment of Liver Metastases With Recombinant Tumour Necrosis Factor.** *Eur J Cancer* 1992, **28A**:1073–1078.

23. • MAVLIGIT GM, ZUKIWSKI AA, CHARNSANGAVEJ C, CARRASCO CH, WALLACE S, GUTTERMAN JU: **Regional Biologic Therapy: Hepatic Arterial Infusion of Recombinant Human Tumor Necrosis Factor in Patients With Liver Metastases.** *Cancer* 1992, **69**:557–561.

Important for its demonstration that this approach can limit toxicity. The response rate remains relatively disappointing.

24. YAMASAKI S, OKINO T, KAN N, SATOH K, MISE K, TERAMURA Y, HARADA T, KODAMA H, HORI T, OHGAKI K, *ET AL.*: **Factors Influencing the Response and Survival of Patients With Liver Metastases From Breast Cancer Receiving OK-432-Combined Adoptive Immunotherapy.** *J Cancer Res Clin Oncol* 1992, **118**:157–162.

25. WANG Y, TIAN J, WANG Q, XING Z, YANG L, WANG S, YANG D, CHENG G: **Intra-hepatic-arterial Infusion of Misonidazole: An Experimental Study of Regional Radiosensitization by Intraarterial Embolization.** *Br J Cancer* 1992, **66**:1131–1134.

26. HELLMANN K, GOOLD M, HIGGINS N, PHILLIPS RH: **Responses of Liver Metastases to Radiotherapy and Razoxane.** *J R Soc Med* 1992, **85**:136–138.

27. ANDERSON JH, GOLDBERG JA, BESSENT RG, KERR DJ, MCKILLOP JH, STEWART I, COOKE TG, MCARDLE CS: **Glass Yttrium-90 Microspheres for Patients With Colorectal Liver Metastases.** *Radiother Oncol* 1992, **25**:137–139.

28. • GRAY BN, ANDERSON JE, BURTON MA, VAN HAZEL G, CODDE J, MORGAN C, KLEMP P: **Regression of Liver Metastases Following Treatment With Yttrium-90 Microspheres.** *Aust N Z J Surg* 1992, **62**:105–110.

This study reports response rates from intra-arterial microsphere delivery of radiotherapy that are comparable to those of regional chemotherapy.

29. ANDERSSON R, HOLMBERG A: **Intraperitoneal 5-Fluorouracil in the Management of Colorectal Liver Cancer.** *Eur J Surg Oncol* 1992, **18**:152–155.

30. BORNER M, CASTIGLIONE M, TRILLER J, BAER HU, SOUCEK M, BLUMGART L, BRUNNER K: **Considerable Side Effects of Chemoembolization for Colorectal Carcinoma Metastatic to the Liver.** *Ann Oncol* 1992, **3**:113–115.

31. SALIM AS: **Chemonecrosis for Localized Dynamic Destruction of Hepatic Metastases of Colonic Cancer: A New Approach.** *Oncology* 1993, **50**:18–21.

32. VAN HILLEGERSBERG R, MARIJNISSEN JP, KORT WJ, ZONDERVAN PE, TERPSTRA OT, STAR WM: **Interstitial Photodynamic Therapy in a Rat Liver Metastasis Model.** *Br J Cancer* 1992, **66**:1005–1014.

33. MASTERS A, STEGER AC, LEES WR, WALMSLEY KM, BOWN SG: **Interstitial Laser Hyperthermia: A New Approach for Treating Liver Metastases.** *Br J Cancer* 1992, **66**:518–522.

Peter McCulloch, MD, Department of Surgery, University of Liverpool, Box 147, Liverpool L69 3BX, UK.

Surgery for sclerosing cholangitis

John W. Braasch, MD

Lahey Clinic, Burlington, Massachusetts, USA

The diagnosis of primary sclerosing cholangitis is made radiologically in patients with extrahepatic obstructive jaundice. This condition lacks a known cause and another method of diagnosis, and its treatment is palliative-mechanical, with bypasses, dilation, or orthotopic liver transplantation. Recent progress has been seen in stratifying patients with respect to prognosis. Stratification is important for conducting clinical trials and for predicting which patients should receive a transplant at an earlier, less risky stage in the course of the disease. Expandable metal stents are on trial in patients with benign or malignant strictures. These newer stents seem to be better than polyethylene stents, although their use has not been reported in sclerosing cholangitis. With survival data used as a measuring point, relief of jaundice does not appear to correlate with increased survival. Of concern has been the association of cholangiocarcinoma with sclerosing cholangitis. Cholangiocarcinoma is difficult to recognize clinically and has a negative impact on the results of transplantation.

Current Opinion in General Surgery 1994:156–160

Sclerosing cholangitis, a condition known only for the past 70 years [1], is a disease of the biliary tract in which focal proliferation and obliteration of the bile ducts are associated with periductal fibrosis (Fig. 1), copper deposition, and cholestasis. Because this condition is rare and poorly understood, it is important to review its characteristics as a baseline for the consideration of more recent progress.

General considerations

In essence, sclerosing cholangitis is a pathologic entity with radiologic requirements for diagnosis [2••]. It is usually a disease of middle-aged men. The clinical presentation may be asymptomatic, with recognition only from the profile of liver function test results. Usually, the serum alkaline phosphatase level is greatly elevated, with or without modest rises in the levels of serum bilirubin and serum glutamic-oxaloacetic transaminase. Conversely, the disease may be marked clinically by the onset of jaundice with recurrent bouts of cholangitis, sometimes with abdominal pain.

The rate of progression of the disease varies: it may progress to cirrhosis and death over a few years, or a slow progression of gradually increasing disability may be apparent, with the result that liver function tests become increasingly abnormal over many years.

The distribution of disease is usually both intrahepatic and extrahepatic, although some patients may have a greater degree of stricturing and dilation either within the liver (Fig. 2) or extrahepatically (Fig. 3). Occasionally, the disease may be concentrated in the common hepatic, right hepatic, and left hepatic ducts (Fig. 4, *left*) or obstruction of the common bile duct may be seen in some portion of its extrahepatic course, at times within the pancreas (Fig. 4, *right*).

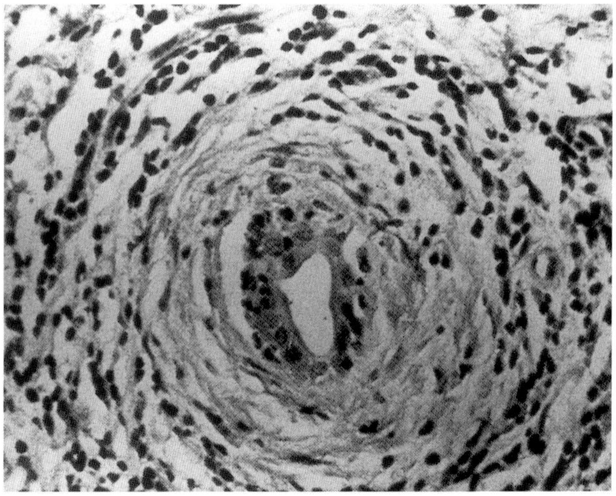

Fig. 1. High-power microscopic view of fibrous tissue surrounding a bile duct with sclerosing cholangitis involvement.

The cause of sclerosing cholangitis is unknown. The disease is closely associated with inflammatory bowel disease, predominantly with chronic ulcerative colitis but occasionally with regional enteritis. Antibody-mediated diseases and altered lymphocyte mechanisms suggest a strong autoimmune cause. The frequency of certain specific HLA antigens in patients with primary sclerosing cholangitis appears to be increased. Riedel's thyroiditis, retroperitoneal fibrosis, glomerulonephritis, immune thrombocytopenic purpura, dysgammaglobulinemia, and IgA deficiency have been reported to be associated with sclerosing cholangitis.

Other conditions and treatments can produce changes in the biliary tract that mimic sclerosing cholangitis.

 ISBN 1-85922-671-X ISSN 1065–6243

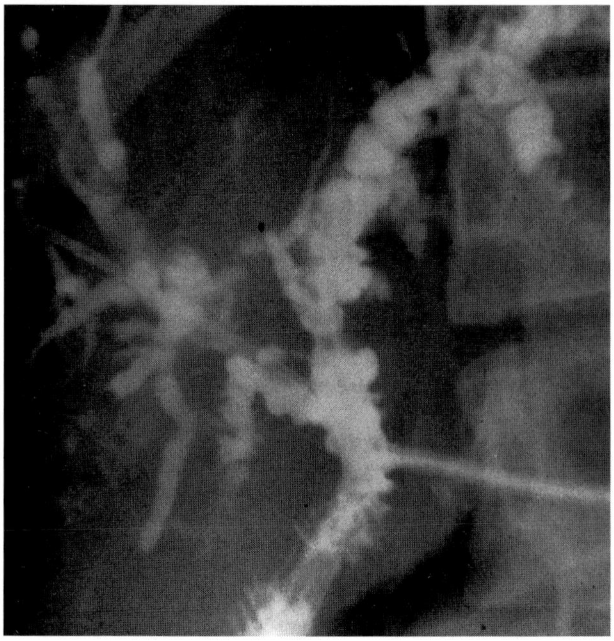

Fig. 2. T-tube cholangiogram shows considerable intrahepatic duct involvement by sclerosing cholangitis. Stricturing and dilation are visible. (*From* Martin and Braasch [2••]; with permission.)

They include AIDS, intrahepatic artery chemotherapy, bone marrow transplantation, and hepatic artery thrombosis after liver transplantation. Certainly, a prominent cause of a cholangiographic picture similar to that of sclerosing cholangitis can be repeated bouts of cholangitis caused by calculus or other partially obstructing mechanisms in the biliary tract.

The requirements for the diagnosis of sclerosing cholangitis have gradually changed. Initially, primary sclerosing cholangitis was marked by the absence of inflammatory bowel disease and the absence of calculi within the biliary system. Because secondary stone formation is fairly common in this disease, many true cases of sclerosing cholangitis were not included. The type of sclerosing cholangitis that accompanies inflammatory bowel disease is similar, if not identical, to that which is not complicated by ulcerative colitis. Therefore, it has become customary to diagnose patients with calculi and with inflammatory bowel disease as having sclerosing cholangitis, provided the biliary tract has the usual radiologic appearance and the calculi are of the stasis type.

Cholangiocarcinoma is associated with sclerosing cholangitis in about 10% to 15% of all patients, and it is a difficult complication to recognize and to manage. Previously, the treatment of patients with sclerosing cholangitis was limited to bypass procedures, dilation, and stenting. It was recently recognized that these procedures are associated with a high incidence of failure and that the most logical treatment is liver transplantation. With regard to the nontransplantation procedures, it is evident that patients with extrahepatic concentrated disease, for whom these procedures are suitable, do not survive longer than other patients (Fig. 5), and relief of jaundice does not correlate with increased survival.

Recent progress

Medical and adjuvant treatment

Medical treatment has not been effective [2••]. Responses to steroids, immunosuppression, and copper-binding agents have been less than satisfactory. In patients with inflammatory bowel disease, colectomy has no impact on the overall progress of biliary tract disease [2••].

Further experience with the use of ursodeoxycholic acid therapy for primary sclerosing cholangitis has been reported on by Lebovics *et al.* [3]. One patient with diffuse primary sclerosing cholangitis first had choledochoduodenostomy, which did not result in much improvement, and then was started on a treatment regimen of ursodeoxycholic acid, 300 mg orally three times a day. These authors noted the resolution of pruritus and improvements with respect to nausea, fatigue, and anorexia. The patient gained 11.25 kg, and all liver function test results gradually and consistently improved. The serum bilirubin concentration, which was as high as 6.3 mg/dL, was normalized within 4 months.

Improvement was also noted on cholangiographic studies in that previously seen abnormalities in the liver were almost completely resolved and the pancreatic duct strictures, which had been noted before treatment, were less severe. However, two consecutive liver biopsy samples revealed progression of disease. This report of one case is interesting, but it does not permit generalizations. The reported follow-up time was 16 months, and given the known proclivity of this condition for remissions and exacerbations, this positive response to ursodeoxycholic acid should not be given too much weight.

Differential diagnosis

Of interest in the differential diagnosis of sclerosing cholangitis that mainly involves the common hepatic duct and the right and left ducts is an article by Wetter *et al.* [4]. These authors described the variation between the preoperative and postoperative diagnoses of Klatskin tumor: 98 patients were thought to have Klatskin tumor preoperatively, but microscopic examination showed neoplasm in only 68 of the 98 patients. Confused with Klatskin tumor were three cases of granuloma involving the common hepatic duct and three other cases of idiopathic benign focal stenosis. Because focal sclerosing lesions are known to occur in the biliary tract at sites other than the common hepatic duct, any focal stenotic lesion may be sclerosing cholangitis or a variant rather than carcinoma. The differential diagnosis rests partially on the appearance of the intrahepatic biliary tract. If the intrahepatic ducts show alternating dilations and constrictions instead of a uniform dilation, the diagnosis is almost always sclerosing cholangitis.

When an area of stenosis exists only in the intrahepatic or distal bile duct, the differential diagnosis becomes taxing. It is difficult to obtain histologic tissue from these portions of the duct. When the distal duct lies mostly external to the pancreas, biopsy samples can be obtained preoperatively or during surgery, either by needle aspiration or by direct incision. However, when the diagnosis is reported to be an inflammatory stenosing lesion, enough doubt exists in the accuracy of the

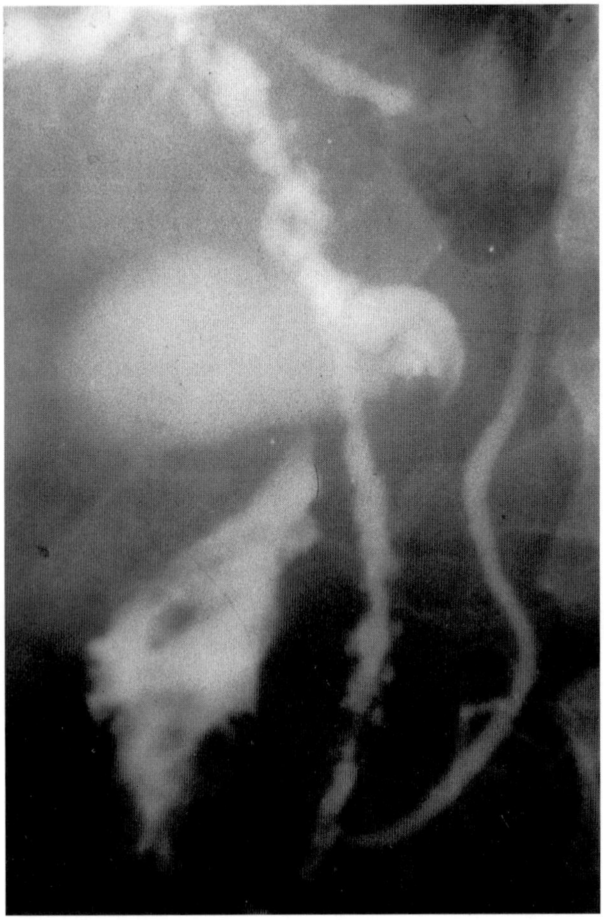

Fig. 3. Cholangiogram of a distal bile duct involved with sclerosing cholangitis shows a nodular appearance. (*From* Braasch and Martin [16]; with permission.)

diagnosis to force resection of the area, possibly by pancreatoduodenectomy. Some benign focal sclerosing lesions have been categorized as benign, nontraumatic, inflammatory strictures: many have mucosal ulcerations that are thought to differentiate them from sclerosing cholangitis [5].

Surgical treatment

Dilation, stenting, and bypass

Although the presence of major strictures at the hilus of the liver that can be bypassed or dilated does not seem to have an impact on long-term survival, it is important to provide symptomatic relief when possible. The relatively recent development of expandable metallic stents has raised hopes that percutaneous or even endoscopic retrograde stenting of the major strictures in patients with sclerosing cholangitis would enable patients to avoid operative surgery to the hilus of the liver but yet give good palliation.

The major thrust behind the development of expandable metallic stents is the palliation of nonresectable carcinomas that are obstructing the biliary tract. Lee *et al.* [6] described their experience with the use of these stents in 34 patients who had malignant obstruction. In 105 patients reported on by Davids *et al.* [7••], 49 of whom received a metallic stent and 56 of whom received a polyethylene stent, metallic stents were clearly an improvement over polyethylene stents. In this randomized, prospective trial of first stents, metal stents were free of complications for a median of 273 days, versus 126 days for the polyethylene stents. The expandable nature of these stents made them less likely to migrate, and if tumor ingrowth occurred, it could be managed by various methods, without removal of the stent.

The application of metallic stents to benign biliary strictures was reported by Maccioni *et al.* [8] in 18 patients: the Z-stent (Cook, Bloomington, IN) was used in 17 patients, and the Wall stent (Schneider [USA], Minneapolis, MN) was used in one patient. The follow-up time was 30 to 41 months, at the end of which 56% of patients had no symptoms of biliary obstruction and 28% had recurrent symptoms (in three patients because of tissue ingrowth and in one patient because of migration). No trials of metallic stents have been reported in patients with sclerosing cholangitis, but such trials are expected in the future.

Transplantation

Stratification of patients at presentation with respect to prognosis is important for conducting clinical trials and for deciding on the proper timing of liver transplantation. Farrant *et al.* [9] reported on a series of 126 patients who were studied carefully with univariate and multivariate analyses. Hepatomegaly, splenomegaly, serum alkaline phosphatase levels, liver histologic stage, and patient age were found to be of prognostic significance. Of note in the multivariate analysis in this study was that the serum bilirubin level could not be correlated with prognosis independent of the histologic stage. Ismail *et al.* [10] identified male gender, cirrhosis, disease duration of longer than 3 years, and a serum bilirubin level of greater than 100 μmol/L as being associated with a worse outcome.

Both studies provided some evidence that earlier transplantation can be undertaken in patients in whom many factors indicate a poor prognosis. If transplantation is performed, these patients can expect a better survival result than patients who have transplantation after multiple operative procedures at the biliary hilus and who have worse liver function. Furthermore, the risk of cholangiocarcinoma, which is a real risk in patients who have undergone transplantation (found in 23% of patients in the series of Farrant *et al.* [9]), might be lessened with earlier transplantation.

Three extremely important considerations relative to the use of liver transplantation in treating patients with sclerosing cholangitis and those with primary biliary cirrhosis have been addressed by Wiesner *et al.* [11•]. Using univariate and multivariate analyses and worldwide data from other transplantation centers, these authors concluded that liver transplantation realistically prolongs survival in patients with sclerosing cholangitis. Furthermore, patients who received transplants at an earlier stage of disease without waiting for life-threatening complications to develop had a much better immediate course after transplantation and better long-term survival than patients who received a transplant when they were about to die of complications. In addition, these authors believe that the present system in the United

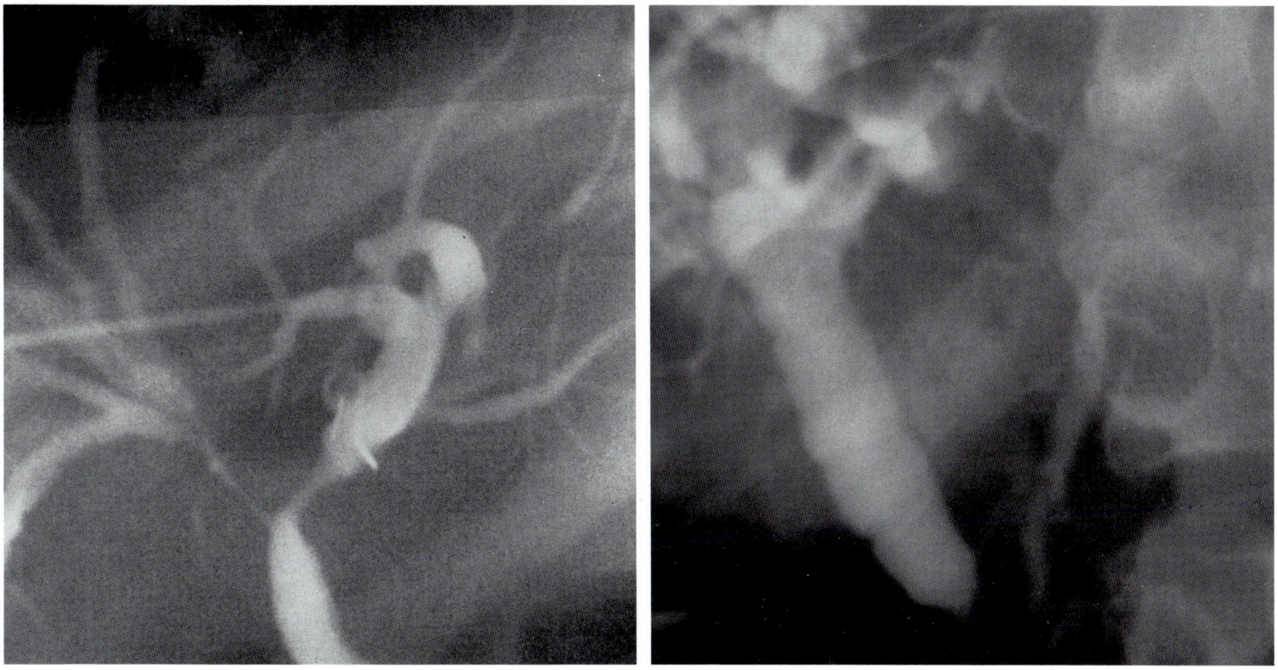

Fig. 4. Cholangiograms show possible Klatskin adenocarcinoma of the common, right, and left hepatic ducts (*left panel*) and possible distal bile duct adenocarcinoma (*right panel*), both of which proved to be benign fibrosing strictures on resection and microscopic examination. (*From* Martin and Braasch [2••]; with permission.)

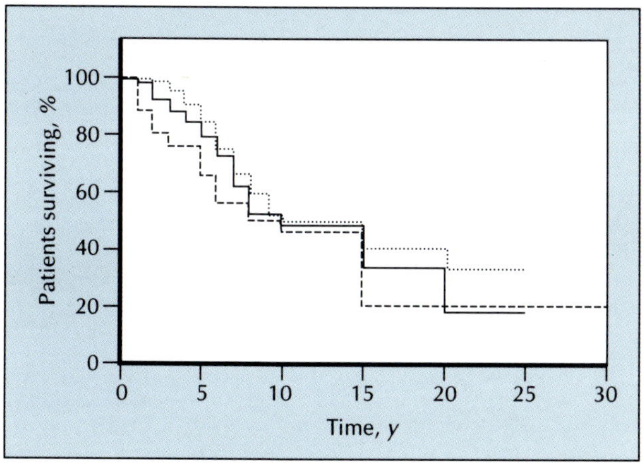

Fig. 5. Survival related to the distribution in the biliary tract of the major lesions of sclerosing cholangitis. *Solid line* indicates patients with diffuse lesions; *dotted line* indicates patients with intrahepatic lesions; *dashed line* indicates patients with extrahepatic lesions. Median survival times were 9.5 years for those with diffuse lesions, 9.9 years for those with intrahepatic lesions, and 9.1 years for those with extrahepatic lesions. $P = 0.65$. (*From* Martin *et al.* [17]; with permission.)

States for the allocation of scarce donor organs is not optimal for getting the best result as far as survival, lifestyle, and cost in dollars are concerned. They pointed out that it might be preferable in the future, based on the studies mentioned, to use the scarce donor material for patients who are in better condition but who have a worse prognosis in the short and medium term.

Associated cholangiocarcinoma

Four recent papers deal with the complication of cholangiocarcinoma in patients with sclerosing cholangitis. Rosen *et al.* [12,13] noted the poor prognostic implication of the presence of cholangiocarcinoma and the usual rapid death of patients after liver transplantation. They called attention to the clear need for heightened clinical awareness and for methods of earlier detection of the carcinoma. In their experience, the development of cholangiocarcinoma was heralded by rapid clinical deterioration with jaundice, weight loss, and abdominal discomfort. They proposed that the potential for the development of cholangiocarcinoma in patients with primary sclerosing cholangitis might indicate that liver transplantation should be considered earlier in the course of the disease.

Strangely enough, Rosen *et al.* noted that in the more than 50 patients who had undergone liver transplantation at the Mayo Clinic for primary sclerosing cholangitis, not a single instance of cholangiocarcinoma was found. Furthermore, they noted that patients with chronic ulcerative colitis were at risk for both sclerosing cholangitis and independent cholangiocarcinoma.

In another report, Miros *et al.* [14] suggested that patients with cholangiocarcinoma presented with a rapid onset of persistent jaundice, pruritus, and weight loss. Study of the transplanted livers revealed multiple areas of carcinoembryonic antigen–positive epithelial cells with atypia and carcinoma *in situ*.

Abu-Elmagd *et al.* [15••], from the Pittsburgh Transplant Center, reported on 169 patients with primary sclerosing cholangitis who received liver allografts. Of their patients, 18 (10.6%) were found to have cholangiocarcinoma. Of these 18 patients, seven were known to have carcinoma preoperatively. These authors recorded age, gender, duration of liver disease, presence or absence and duration of inflammatory bowel disease, and liver histologic stage of primary sclerosing cholangitis, and they found that these factors were similar in patients with and in those without the development of cholangiocarcinoma. In addition, no significant difference was found between the two groups when laboratory values of liver function were compared. The authors also noted that the histologic stage of primary sclerosing cholangitis did not correlate with the presence of cholangiocarcinoma.

Abu-Elmagd *et al.* agreed, however, with other investigators that the survival of patients who underwent transplantation for primary sclerosing cholangitis and who had cholangiocarcinoma was greatly diminished. In their experience, the 1-year survival rate for patients with just primary sclerosing cholangitis was 85%, and the 5-year survival rate was 75.8%. The 1- and 5-year survival rates for patients with the combination of cholangiocarcinoma and primary sclerosing cholangitis were 72% and 26.7%, respectively. It is apparent from these reports that it is difficult to recognize the presence of cholangiocarcinoma in patients with sclerosing cholangitis, and the results of liver transplantation in these circumstances are worse than usual. It seems clear that earlier liver transplantation is desirable, which implies dilitation and stenting and bypass procedures.

References and recommended reading

Papers of particular interest, published within the annual period of review, have been highlighted as:

- • Of special interest
- •• Of outstanding interest

1. Delbet P: **Rétrécissement du Cholédoque: Cholécysto-duodénostomie.** *Bull Mem Soc Natl Chir* 1924, **20**:1144–1146.

2. •• Martin FM, Braasch JW: **Primary Sclerosing Cholangitis.** *Curr Probl Surg* 1992, **29**:135–193.

Recent comprehensive review of all aspects of sclerosing cholangitis.

3. Lebovics E, Salama M, Elhosseiny A, Rosenthal WS: **Resolution of Radiographic Abnormalities With Ursodeoxycholic Acid Therapy of Primary Sclerosing Cholangitis.** *Gastroenterology* 1992, **102**:2143–2147.

4. Wetter LA, Ring EJ, Pellegrini CA, Way LW: **Differential Diagnosis of Sclerosing Cholangiocarcinomas of the Common Hepatic Duct (Klatskin Tumors).** *Am J Surg* 1991, **161**:57–63.

5. Dhiman RK, Choudhuri G, Agarwal DK, Tandon P, Sahi RP: **Benign Non-traumatic Inflammatory Stricture of the Common Bile Duct.** *Indian J Gastroenterol* 1992, **11**:174–175.

6. Lee MJ, Dawson SL, Mueller PR, Krebs TL, Saini S, Hahn PF: **Palliation of Malignant Bile Duct Obstruction With Metallic Biliary Endoprostheses: Technique, Results, and Complications.** *J Vasc Intervent Radiol* 1992, **3**:665–671.

7. •• Davids PHP, Groen AK, Rauws EAJ, Tytgat GNJ, Huibregtse K: **Randomised Trial of Self-expanding Metal Stents Versus Polyethylene Stents for Distal Malignant Biliary Obstruction.** *Lancet* 1992, **340**:1488–1492.

This report of a rare randomized trial of stenting for malignant biliary obstruction describes a clear advantage for metal stents. Stents might have an advantage in patients with sclerosing cholangitis because their use does not cause problems for the surgeon who performs liver transplantation.

8. Maccioni F, Rossi M, Salvatori FM, Ricci P, Bezzi M, Rossi P: **Metallic Stents in Benign Biliary Strictures: Three-Year Follow-Up.** *Cardiovasc Intervent Radiol* 1992, **15**:360–366.

9. Farrant JM, Hayllar KM, Wilkinson ML, Karani J, Portmann BC, Westaby D, Williams R: **Natural History and Prognostic Variables in Primary Sclerosing Cholangitis.** *Gastroenterology* 1991, **100**:1710–1717.

10. Ismail T, Angrisani L, Powell JE, Hübscher S, Buckels J, Neuberger J, Elias E, McMaster P: **Primary Sclerosing Cholangitis: Surgical Options, Prognostic Variables and Outcome.** *Br J Surg* 1991, **78**:564–567.

11. • Wiesner RH, Porayko MK, Dickson ER, Gores GJ, LaRusso NF, Hay JE, Wahlstrom HE, Krom RAF: **Selection and Timing of Liver Transplantation in Primary Biliary Cirrhosis and Primary Sclerosing Cholangitis.** *Hepatology* 1992, **16**:1290–1299.

An in-depth consideration of stratification and survival and impact of and on liver transplantation by a group of authors who have been prominent in the field for many years.

12. Rosen CB, Nagorney DM, Wiesner RH, Coffey RJ Jr, LaRusso NF: **Cholangiocarcinoma Complicating Primary Sclerosing Cholangitis.** *Ann Surg* 1991, **213**:21–25.

13. Rosen CB, Nagorney DM: **Cholangiocarcinoma Complicating Primary Sclerosing Cholangitis.** *Semin Liver Dis* 1991, **11**:26–30.

14. Miros M, Kerlin P, Walker N, Harper J, Lynch S, Strong R: **Predicting Cholangiocarcinoma in Patients With Primary Sclerosing Cholangitis Before Transplantation.** *Gut* 1991, **32**:1369–1373.

15. •• Abu-Elmagd KM, Selby R, Iwatsuki S, Fung J, Tzakis A, Todo S, Demetris AJ, Baddour N, Irish W, Van Thiel DH, Starzl T: **Cholangiocarcinoma and Sclerosing Cholangitis: Clinical Characteristics and Effect on Survival After Liver Transplantation.** *Transplant Proc* 1993, **25**:1124–1125.

A report from the world's most experienced liver transplantation center on current results of transplantation in 169 patients with sclerosing cholangitis. The 1- and 5-year survival rates were 85% and 76%, respectively, for patients who had just sclerosing cholangitis; in the 11% of patients who had cholangiocarcinoma, the results were considerably worse.

16. Braasch JW, Martin FM: **Strictures and Benign Obstructive Disorders of the Bile Ducts.** In *Shackelford's Surgery of the Alimentary Tract*, vol 3. Edited by Zuidema GD, Turcotte JG. Philadelphia: WB Saunders; 1991:228–237.

17. Martin FM, Rossi RL, Nugent FW, Scholz FJ, Jenkins RL, Lewis WD, Gagner M, Foley E, Braasch JW: **Surgical Aspects of Sclerosing Cholangitis: Results in 178 Patients.** *Ann Surg* 1990, **212**:551–558.

John W. Braasch, MD, Department of General Surgery, Lahey Clinic, 41 Mall Road, Burlington, MA 01805, USA.

Current status of surgery for Klatskin tumors

Keith D. Lillemoe, MD

The Johns Hopkins Medical Institutions, Baltimore, Maryland, USA

Klatskin tumors, or hilar cholangiocarcinomas, are an uncommon cause of obstructive jaundice. With the advent of sophisticated imaging studies and cholangiography, these tumors can be preoperatively identified in most patients, and a treatment plan can be outlined before operative exploration. Surgical resection of the hepatic bifurcation with the addition of a hepatic lobectomy as indicated by tumor extension is the treatment of choice. Although complete surgical resection improves survival over that achieved with palliative procedures, the 5-year survival rate remains less than 20%. Postoperative radiation therapy may increase long-term survival.

Current Opinion in General Surgery 1994:161–167

Carcinoma of the hepatic duct bifurcation was first described by Altemeier *et al.* [1] in 1957, and subsequently, a series of 13 patients with this diagnosis was reported on by Klatskin [2] in 1965. Since then, cholangiocarcinomas at this location have been called Klatskin tumors. Approximately 15,000 new cases of liver and biliary tract carcinoma are diagnosed annually in the United States, with roughly 10% of these cases being Klatskin tumors. Although these tumors are considered to be slow-growing malignancies, death due to progressive hepatic failure occurs quickly unless adequate biliary decompression is achieved. Therefore, current techniques for diagnosis and treatment with either nonoperative stenting or surgical resection should be applied to optimize the management of obstructive jaundice and in some cases offer the opportunity for long-term survival.

Pathology and etiology

Klatskin tumors are adenocarcinomas, usually with a diffuse or nodular pattern, that result in fibrosis and obliteration of the bile duct lumen. Although papillary features can be found with cholangiocarcinomas at some locations, this pattern is uncommon at the hepatic duct bifurcation. The etiology of Klatskin tumors is unknown, but a number of etiologic factors have been linked to this diagnosis. Strong associations have been found between cholangiocarcinoma and cystic abnormalities of the bile duct, infection with the liver fluke *Clonorchis sinensis*, gallstones, sclerosing cholangitis, use of the radiocontrast agent thorium dioxide, and ulcerative colitis. A common theme with many of these associated conditions is bile stasis and chronic inflammation of the biliary tree. Despite these recognized associations, most Klatskin tumors occur sporadically, without an associated etiologic factor.

Presentation

Most patients with Klatskin tumors are between 50 and 70 years of age, and there is a slight male predominance. Progressive jaundice is the presenting complaint in more than 90% of patients. Pruritus, weight loss, and abdominal pain are seen less frequently. Cholangitis is uncommon unless prior biliary tract manipulation has occurred. Rarely, either the right or the left hepatic duct may be obstructed before progressive involvement at the bifurcation leads to jaundice. Such patients may experience mild abdominal discomfort, unilobular liver enlargement, and elevation of serum alkaline phosphatase or γ-glutamyltransferase levels. In such cases, thorough evaluation with computed tomography and cholangiography may lead to the diagnosis at an earlier stage.

Diagnosis and staging

The evaluation of the jaundiced patient should begin with either abdominal ultrasonography or computed tomography. The findings on either study suggestive of a Klatskin tumor include a dilated intrahepatic biliary tree, a normal or collapsed gallbladder and extrahepatic biliary tree, and a normal pancreas. The primary tumor mass is rarely visualized. Early experience suggests that magnetic resonance imaging may be somewhat more sensitive in detecting these tumors.

After biliary ductal dilatation has been demonstrated by imaging studies, it is imperative that cholangiography be performed for biliary tumors. Cholangiography should not only define the location of the tumor but also visualize its uppermost extent to determine the limits of resectability. Percutaneous transhepatic cholangiography is favored over endoscopic

 ISBN 1-85922-671-X ISSN 1065–6243

retrograde cholangiography because it better defines the proximal extent of tumor involvement and allows placement of percutaneous transhepatic catheters (Fig. 1). In most patients with Klatskin tumors, both the right and left hepatic ducts must be intubated to establish adequate biliary drainage.

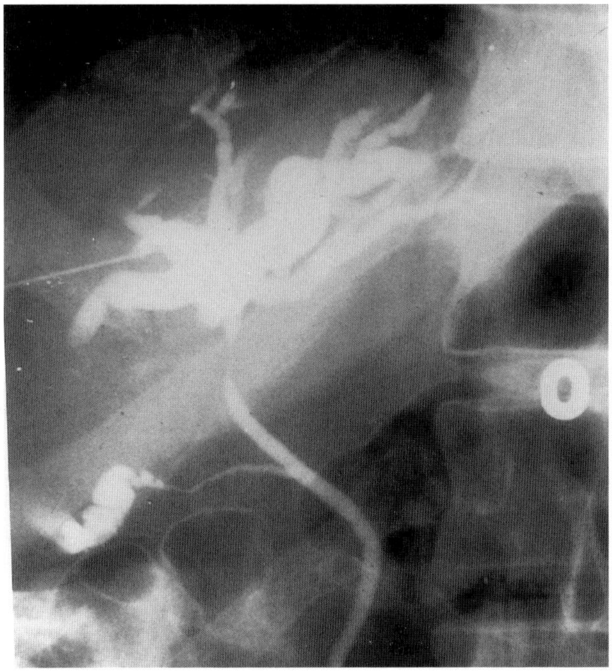

Fig. 1. A percutaneous transhepatic cholangiogram in a patient with hilar cholangiocarcinoma. (*From* Yeo *et al.* [24]; with permission.)

Preoperatively placed biliary catheters are used primarily to assist in the identification and dissection of the hepatic duct bifurcation and the individual right and left hepatic ducts [3]. In addition, in operative techniques in which large-bore silastic stents are used for reconstruction, biliary catheters greatly facilitate their placement. Finally, although prolonged biliary decompression to relieve jaundice is not indicated routinely [4], patients with significant malnutrition, biliary sepsis, or medical problems such as renal failure may benefit from biliary drainage to allow an opportunity for recovery before a planned surgical procedure.

Techniques available for obtaining a preoperative tissue diagnosis include percutaneous fine-needle biopsy, direct cholangioscopic biopsy of the tumor, scrape biopsy or brushings of the stricture obtained via the transhepatic biliary catheter, and cytologic examination of bile. Success rates for these modalities are only approximately 50%; therefore, unless the patient is not considered a candidate for surgery, diagnostic efforts should not be prolonged at the expense of delaying surgery. An exception to this is with the patient who has advanced primary sclerosing cholangitis with a dominant bifurcation stricture. In such patients, who might otherwise be considered candidates for liver transplantation, malignancy should be ruled out before operative management is undertaken.

In patients who are candidates for surgical resection, preoperative staging should be completed. Findings on computed tomography such as extrahepatic disease or bilobar liver metastasis preclude curative resection. Extensive bilobar proximal extension into the hepatic parenchyma on cholangiography also indicates unresectability. Finally, involvement of the major hepatic portal vessels (hepatic artery and portal vein) with tumor encasement or occlusion precludes resection. Currently, hepatic arteriography with venous phase studies is the standard for determining major vessel involvement. Magnetic resonance imaging and spiral computed tomography with bolus contrast hold promise as noninvasive tools for assessing tumor extent and the invasion of major portal vascular structures.

A recent retrospective review from the Johns Hopkins Hospital compared the results of cholangiography and angiography over an 8-year period in patients with pathologically proven Klatskin tumors. Overall, 28 of the 65 patients (43%) underwent curative resection. Cholangiographic involvement of four or more ductal systems or extensive right intrahepatic ductal encasement was observed in 12 patients, and none of these tumors were resectable. Cholangiography predicted the clinical management in 62% of the patients. Angiographic findings of arterial or venous encasement were observed in 38% of patients and only one of these patients, who had a left portal vein encasement, underwent curative resection. Angiography predicted the clinical management in 80% of the patients. When combined, cholangiography and angiography predicted the clinical management in 86% of patients, emphasizing that these studies should be performed routinely in the preoperative staging of perihilar cholangiocarcinomas (Dooley, Personal communication).

Operative management

At the completion of preoperative staging, approximately two thirds of patients with Klatskin tumors will be considered candidates for surgery. Tumor resectability is further assessed at operation by careful exploration for peritoneal implants, hepatic metastases, and regional lymph node involvement. Finally, the extent of tumor along the bile duct must be carefully assessed. The operative approach at the Johns Hopkins Hospital for bifurcation tumors includes hilar resection with reconstruction as a bilateral hepaticojejunostomy using transhepatic silastic stents [5–7]. Typically, the abdomen is entered by a right subcostal or midline vertical incision. After thorough exploration is performed, dissection of the hepatic duct bifurcation can be facilitated by two maneuvers. First, early mobilization of the gallbladder helps to expose the extrahepatic biliary tree and the hepatic duct bifurcation, which can be palpated using the preoperatively placed transhepatic catheters. Second, early division of the distal extrahepatic biliary tree below the tumor aids in the technical aspects of the proximal hepatic bile duct dissection (Fig. 2). The distal extrahepatic biliary tree is sutured closed, and the proximal bile duct is reflected cephalad, freeing the biliary tree from the portal vein and hepatic artery under direct vision. Once the hepatic duct bifurcation has been visualized, the surgeon palpates the transhepatic catheters and the hepatic ducts above the tumor to determine if a tumor-free segment is present. If it is, the right and left hepatic ducts are then divided, leaving the transhepatic catheters exiting through each of the lobar hepatic ducts. If gross tumor extends along either the right or left hepatic duct and into the hepatic parenchyma, appropriate hepatic lobectomy can be considered.

After resection of the tumor at the hepatic duct bifurcation, the previously-placed transhepatic catheters are used to pull progressively larger coudé catheters and eventually silastic transhepatic biliary stents into each of the lobar hepatic ducts (Fig. 3). The silastic transhepatic stents are in proper position when all of their side holes reside in the intrahepatic biliary tree and in the upper portion of a 50-cm retrocolic Roux-en-Y jejunal limb that is used for the biliary enteric anastomosis. Normally, two separate end-to-side hepaticojejunostomies are performed over the silastic stents. Interrupted 4-0 or 5-0 polypropylene or synthetic absorbable sutures are used for the hepaticojejunal anastomoses. The free ends of the stents exit through the upper aspect of the liver capsule and then brought out through separate stab wounds in the abdominal wall.

In cases in which hilar cholangiocarcinoma extends along either the left or right hepatic duct into the hepatic parenchyma, appropriate hepatic lobectomy can be considered in addition to hilar resection. Several published series have included patients undergoing hepatic resection for hilar cholangiocarcinoma [7–11,12••,13••]. The major indication for hepatic lobectomy can be suspected at the time of preoperative cholangiography, with proximal tumor involvement extending into the hepatic parenchyma in either the right or left hepatic duct. The hepatic resection is performed with standard techniques. After resection of the hepatic duct bifurcation, biliary enteric continuity is restored with a hepaticojejunostomy performed over a silastic transhepatic stent.

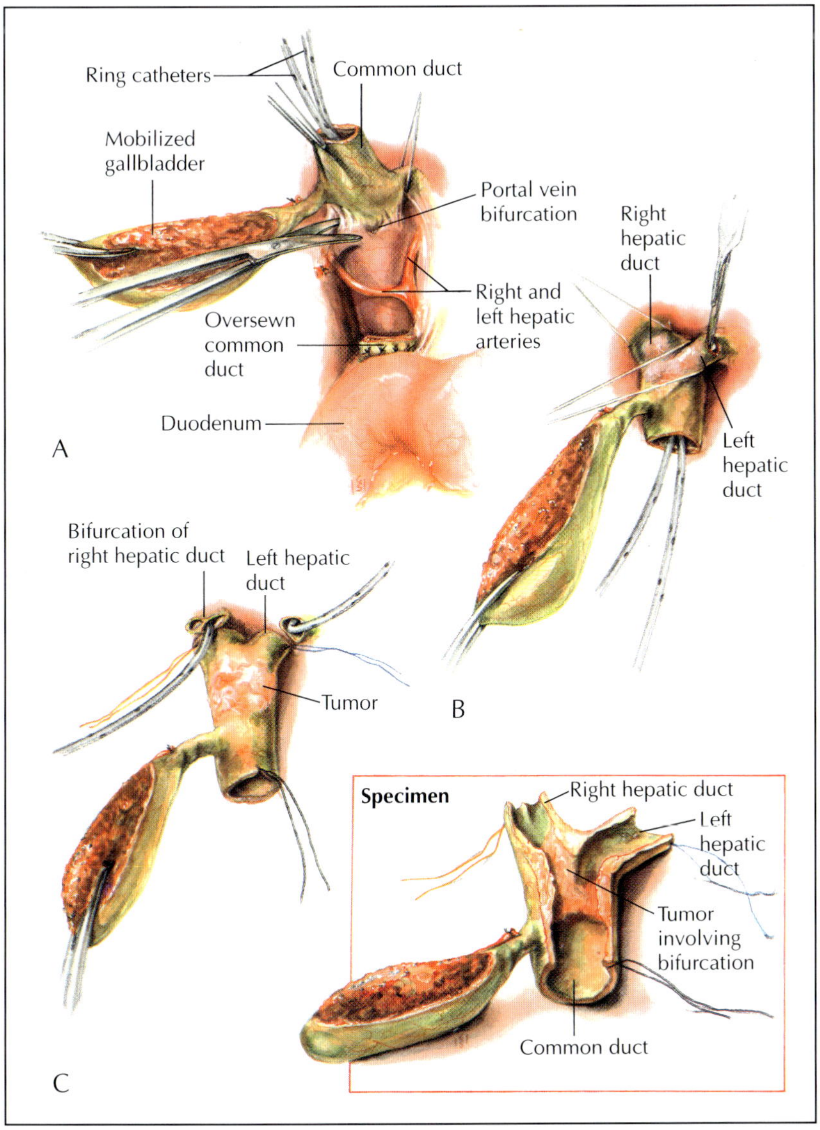

Fig. 2. A, During exploration and resection of a hilar carcinoma, early gallbladder mobilization and transection of the distal common bile duct are recommended. This allows cephalad reflection of the common bile duct using the preoperatively placed transhepatic (Ring) catheters for traction and facilitates hilar dissection of the common hepatic duct and tumor off the portal vein. **B**, The right and left hepatic ducts are then identified by palpation of the Ring catheters and divided above the tumor. **C**, The specimen is resected and all margins are identified and submitted to pathologic examination. **Inset**, Resected specimen. (*From* Cameron [25]; with permission.)

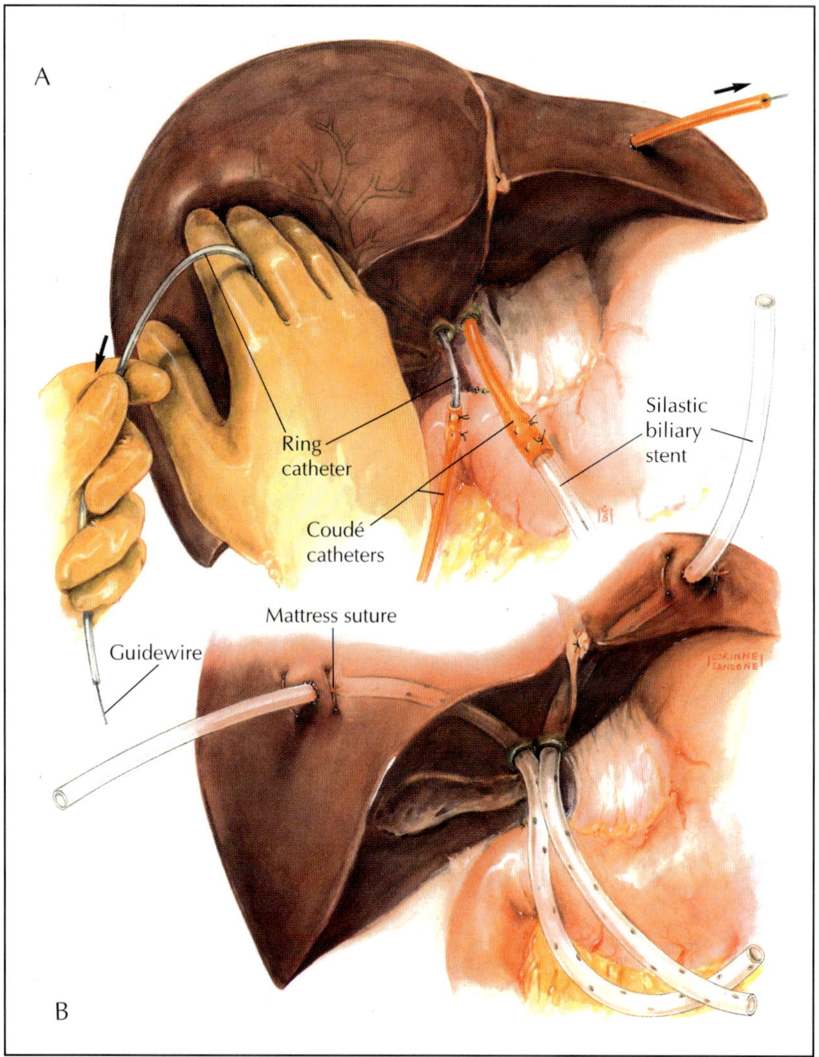

Fig. 3. A, After resection of the tumor at the hepatic duct bifurcation, the preoperatively placed percutaneous catheters are used to place the silastic transhepatic stents. A 14-F coudé catheter is first sutured to the 8-F Ring catheter, and this catheter is withdrawn through the top of the liver, leaving the coudé in the transhepatic tract. This dilates the transhepatic tract and corrects the size discrepancy between the 8-F preoperative catheter and the 16-F to 18-F silastic transhepatic stent. The silastic transhepatic stent is sutured to the widened flange of the coudé catheter and then pulled out the top of the liver. **B**, The silastic stents are positioned so that the portion of the stent with the side holes lies entirely within the hepatic parenchyma and extends outside the porta hepatis to be placed through the anastomosis. (*From* Cameron [25]; with permission.)

Recently, a more aggressive approach to hepatic resection has been advocated by groups in Europe and Japan [12••,14]. These groups recognized by anatomic and pathologic studies that tumor involvement at or above the bifurcation is almost always accompanied by extension into the biliary ducts draining the caudate lobe (segment I). These groups, therefore, advocate resection of segment I for all tumors involving the hepatic bifurcation. Furthermore, these authors advocate caudate lobe resection and formal hepatic lobectomy for any tumor extension above the bifurcation because of concerns about secondary ductal involvement on the involved side. In a recent report from Japan, curative resection was accompanied by 3- and 5-year survival rates of 55% and 41%, respectively [14].

A final, more controversial resectional option for patients with hilar cholangiocarcinoma is total hepatectomy and liver transplantation. Although initially the presence of a bile duct cancer was considered a contraindication for liver transplantation [15,16], some centers consider transplantation an option in selected patients [12••,17]. The indication for this approach is bilateral extension of the tumor into the hepatic parenchyma or involvement of the main trunk of the hepatic artery or portal vein. Most protocols also include aggressive preoperative chemotherapy and radiation therapy. The results of liver transplantation for perihilar cholangiocarcinoma have been disappointing, however, with early and widespread recurrence precluding tumor-free survival in the vast majority of patients. Survival rates of less than 10% have been reported among all patients who undergo liver transplantation for cholangiocarcinoma [18,19]. Liver transplantation should, therefore, be considered primarily as an option only as part of an investigative protocol.

Palliative therapy

Palliative therapy in patients with Klatskin tumors can consist of either nonoperative therapy or biliary enteric bypass. If preoperative staging suggests the presence of unresectable disease or if the patient is not a suitable surgical candidate, a nonoperative approach is indicated. Although endoscopically placed biliary catheters are preferred for mid and distal bile duct malignant obstruction, proximal cholangiocarcinomas at the bifurcation usually require intubation of both the right and left ducts to avoid complications of recurrent cholangitis, liver abscess, or both. Therefore, percutaneous transhepatic catheters provide the best long-term palliation for inoperable Klatskin tumors. These catheters are readily exchangeable in the event of catheter sludging and can easily be externalized to treat biliary sepsis, which frequently accompanies the advanced stages of this disease.

In patients who do undergo abdominal exploration for attempted surgical resection but are found to have unresectable tumors, there are two options. In patients with widespread intraperitoneal tumor, minimal operative manipulation should be performed. Transhepatic catheters placed preoperatively are left in position for palliation of biliary obstruction. Cholecystectomy should be performed to prevent the development of acute cholecystitis from cystic duct obstruction, either from tumor or related to the indwelling catheter. Postoperatively, the transhepatic catheter can be exchanged fluoroscopically for a larger-diameter soft silastic catheter. After the patient is discharged from the hospital, the catheters should be exchanged at periodic intervals to prevent sludging and sepsis.

In patients with locally advanced unresectable tumor at the porta hepatis, biliary enteric bypass can be performed. Cholecystectomy is performed, and the bile duct distal to the tumor is divided. The malignant stricture can be dilated using progressively larger coudé catheters, and eventually a silastic transhepatic stent is positioned into the right and left ductal systems. A choledochojejunostomy to a Roux-en-Y jejunal limb is completed. The advantages of this approach over simply leaving the percutaneous stents include 1) removal of the gallbladder, 2) placement of larger stents, and 3) positioning of the stents into a Roux-en-Y jejunal limb. Although it is difficult to document, larger stents that drain into a defunctionalized limb with jejunum should reduce the incidence of cholangitis.

A second palliative surgical approach is biliary enteric bypass to the segment III branch of the left hepatic duct. This technique involves identifying this duct in its superficial location in the umbilical fissure. The anastomosis can be performed either with or without intubation of the duct with a silastic transhepatic stent. This left-sided bypass can provide good palliation in most patients, even those with predominantly right-sided ductal obstruction.

In a recent retrospective review from the Johns Hopkins Hospital, 65 patients with unresectable Klatskin tumors were treated for biliary obstruction [20]. Twenty-one patients were treated completely nonoperatively, and 44 underwent laparotomy. The mean survival time in the nonoperative group was 5 months, and that in the operative groups was 8 months. A significant difference in survival rates at 6 months was found between the nonoperative group (30%) and the operative group (64%). The incidence of cholangitis following initial treatment was 50% in each of the two groups. No differences between the two groups were found in the number of readmissions to the hospital: however, fewer unscheduled emergency stent changes were needed in the operative group than in the nonoperative group. These results tend to favor an operative approach to unresectable hilar carcinoma, but these differences may reflect bias in patient selection in this retrospective analysis.

Adjuvant therapy

Chemotherapy alone, using 5-fluorouracil and other drugs, has not been known to improve survival in patients with either resected or unresected Klatskin tumors. Radiotherapy has been evaluated by many investigators using a variety of methods, including external beam radiotherapy, intraoperative radiotherapy, internal radiotherapy, and radioimmunotherapy. External beam therapy is most frequently delivered through multiple fields with a total dose of 50 to 60 Gy [21]. Internal radiotherapy is normally delivered by either percutaneous or endoscopically placed biliary stents, with ^{192}Ir or ^{60}Co used as the radiation source [22]. Radiotherapy is believed to be useful in this disease because of the high incidence of microscopic tumor found at the resection margins and the tendency of the tumor to invade through the ductal wall into the surrounding portal structures. Prospective trials designed to evaluate the role of radiotherapy as an adjuvant are currently under way. A troublesome complication of duodenal obstruction from severe post-irradiation peptic ulceration has been noted.

Survival

Survival in patients with Klatskin tumors is highly dependent on whether the patient is treated with palliative stenting or tumor resection. At the Johns Hopkins Hospital, between 1973 and 1989, 96 patients with Klatskin tumors were operated on with curative intent [7]. At the time of laparotomy, 15% of patients had disseminated tumors, 30% had locally unresectable tumors, and the remaining 55% had tumors initially believed to be resectable. At the end of the resection, 14 of the 53 patients who underwent resection had obvious gross tumors remaining, and 39 of the 53 were believed to have undergone curative resection. Eight of these 39 patients had a hepatic lobectomy in addition to their bifurcation resection. Postoperative mortality was 4%. All deaths resulted from biliary sepsis. Postoperative radiotherapy to a total dose of 50 to 60 Gy was delivered to 63 patients (66%). In addition, internal radiotherapy using ^{192}Ir was delivered via silastic transhepatic stents to the area of the hepaticojejunostomy to a total boosting dose of 20 Gy. The 1-, 2-, 5-, and 10-year actuarial survival rates for all 96 patients were 49%, 20%, 15%, and 2%, respectively. If only the 53 patients treated with resection are considered, the 39 patients who had a complete resection had higher survival rates than the 14 patients who underwent only a partial resection (Fig. 4). The patients who had a partial resection had a course similar to that of the patients who underwent palliative stenting alone.

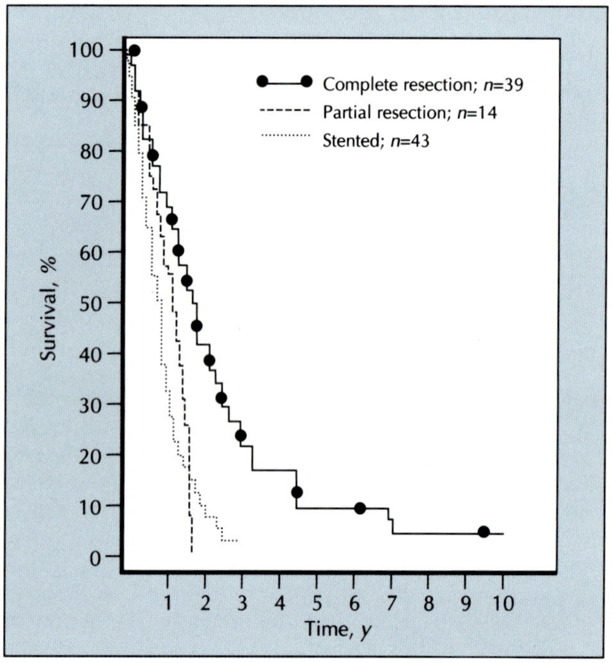

Fig. 4. Actuarial survival curves for patients undergoing partial and complete tumor resection. Patients undergoing partial resection followed a clinical course closer to that of those who were merely stented than to that of patients who underwent complete resection. (*From* Cameron *et al.* [7]; with permission.)

In the 43 patients who underwent palliative stenting alone, the 25 patients who received postoperative radiotherapy survived longer than the 18 patients who did not receive radiotherapy. One- and 2-year survival rates were 38% and 9%, respectively, for the irradiated group versus 10% and 0%, respectively, for the patients who did not receive radiotherapy. The benefits of radiotherapy were also seen in the group of 53 patients who underwent tumor resection: the patients who received radiotherapy had a 5-year survival rate of 11%, compared with a 0% 5-year actuarial survival rate in patients who did not receive radiotherapy. Although this difference in survival rates did not achieve statistical significance, all of the patients who were alive 5 years after tumor resection had received postoperative radiotherapy. These results in both the unresected and the resected groups suggest a benefit from postoperative radiotherapy, although it is important to note that the patients were not randomly assigned to receive postoperative radiotherapy. Prospective, randomized trials of the adjuvant treatment of cholangiocarcinoma with radiotherapy are in progress. In patients not undergoing operative exploration at Johns Hopkins, the 1- and 2-year actuarial survival rates were 25% and 5%, respectively, with a median survival of 5 months.

Recent reports advocating more aggressive surgical therapy, including liver resection, have suggested improved survival with this treatment. A 5-year survival rate of greater than 40% was reported by Nimura *et al.* [14] with this approach. However, a collective review analyzing cases since 1980 did not clearly observe such differences in outcomes in patients undergoing local resection versus major liver resection for hilar cholangiocarcinomas [23]. In 201 patients undergoing local resection of hilar carcinoma, the operative mortality rate was 8%, the mean survival time was 21 months, and the percentages of patients alive 1, 3, and 5 years after resection were 76%, 21%, and 7%, respectively. In contrast, in 188 patients undergoing major liver resection for hilar carcinoma, the operative mortality was 15%, the mean survival time was 24 months, and the percentages of patients alive 1, 3, and 5 years after resection were 61%, 28%, and 17%, respectively. These results indicate that mean survival time is not improved by the addition of a major liver resection for hilar cholangiocarcinoma. In addition, operative mortality rates can be expected to nearly double in association with liver resection.

Conclusions

Klatskin tumors are an uncommon but clinically significant cause of obstructive jaundice. The diagnosis is confirmed by cholangiography, and the tumor is staged by a combination of cholangiography and angiography. To patients with unresectable disease, either nonoperative or operative palliation can be offered. In approximately 35% to 45% of patients, curative resection is possible. Noncontrolled studies suggest that postoperative adjuvant radiotherapy can improve long-term survival.

References and recommended reading

Papers of particular interest, published within the annual period of review, have been highlighted as:
• Of special interest
•• Of outstanding interest

1. Altemeier WA, Gall EA, Zinninger MM, Hoxworth PI: **Sclerosing Carcinoma of the Major Intrahepatic Bile Ducts.** *Arch Surg* 1957, 75:450–461.

2. Klatskin G: **Adenocarcinoma of the Hepatic Duct at Its Bifurcation Within the Porta Hepatis: an Unusual Tumor With Distinctive Clinical and Pathologic Features.** *Am J Med* 1965, 38:241–256.

3. Crist DW, Kadir S, Cameron JL: **Proximal Biliary Tract Reconstruction: the Value of Preoperatively Placed Percutaneous Biliary Catheters.** *Surg Gynecol Obstet* 1987, 165:421–424.

4. Pitt HA, Gomes AS, Louis JF, Mann LL, Deutsch LS, Longmire WP: **Does Preoperative Percutaneous Biliary Drainage Reduce Operative Risk or Increase Hospital Cost?** *Ann Surg* 1985, 201:545–553.

5. Cameron JL, Broe P, Zuidema GD: **Proximal Bile Duct Tumors: Surgical Management With Silastic Transhepatic Biliary Stents.** *Ann Surg* 1982, 196:412–419.

6. Cameron JL, Gayler BW, Zuidema GD: **The Use of Silastic Transhepatic Stents in Benign and Malignant Biliary Strictures.** *Ann Surg* 1978, 188:552–561.

7. Cameron JL, Pitt HA, Zinner MJ, Kaufman SL, Coleman J: **Management of Proximal Cholangiocarcinoma by Surgical Resection and Radiotherapy**. *Am J Surg* 1990, **159**:91–98.

8. Iida S, Tsuzuki T, Ogata Y, Yonoyama K. Iri H, Watanabe K: **The Long-Term Survival of Patients With Carcinoma of the Main Hepatic Duct Junction**. *Cancer* 1987, **60**:1612–1619.

9. Bengmark S, Ekberg H, Evander A, Klofver-Stahl B, Tranberg KG: **Major Liver Resection for Hilar Cholangiocarcinoma**. *Ann Surg* 1988, **207**:120–125.

10. Fortner JG, Vitelli CE, Maclean BJ: **Proximal Extrahepatic Bile Duct Tumors: Analysis of a Series of 52 Consecutive Patients Treated Over a Period of 13 Years**. *Arch Surg* 1989, **124**:1275–1279.

11. Reding R, Buard J-L, Lebeau G, Launois B: **Surgical Management of 552 Carcinomas of the Extrahepatic Bile Ducts (Gallbladder and Periampullary Tumors Excluded): Results of the French Surgical Association Survey**. *Ann Surg* 1991, **213**:236–241.

12. •• Bismuth H, Nakache R, Diamond T: **Management Strategies in Resection for Hilar Cholangiocarcinoma**. *Ann Surg* 1992, **215**:31–38.
This paper defines a management strategy for Klatskin tumors based on tumor location. The authors advocate an aggressive surgical approach with the addition of hepatic resection in most cases.

13. •• Nagorney DM, Donohue JH, Farnell MB, Scleck CD, Ilstrum DM: **Outcomes After Curative Resections of Cholangiocarcinoma**. *Arch Surg* 1993, **128**:871–876.
This paper provides a retrospective review of the outcome after curative surgical resection of cholangiocarcinoma.

14. Nimura Y, Hayakawa N, Kamiya J, Konda S, Shionoya S: **Hepatic Segmentectomy With Caudate Lobe Resection for Bile Duct Carcinoma of the Hepatic Hilus**. *World J Surg* 1990, **14**:535–544.

15. Caine RY: **Liver Transplantation for Liver Cancer**. *World J Surg* 1982, **6**:76–80.

16. MacDougall BRD, Williams R: **Indications for and Results of Liver Transplantation**. In *Liver Surgery*. Edited by Caine RY. Padua: Piccin Medical Books; 1982:187–194.

17. Pichlmayr R, Ringe B, Luchart W, Bechstein WO, Gubernatis G, Wagner E: **Radical Resection and Liver Grafting as the Two Main Components of Surgical Strategy in the Treatment of Proximal Bile Duct Cancer**. *World J Surg* 1988, **12**:68–77.

18. Iwatsuki S, Gordon RD, Shaw BW, Starzl TS,: **Role of Liver Transplantation in Cancer Therapy**. *Ann Surg* 1985, **202**:401–407.

19. Ringe B, Wittekind C, Bechstein WO, Bunzendahl H, Pichlmayr R: **The Role of Liver Transplantation in Hepatobiliary Malignancy: A Retrospective Analysis of 95 Patients With Particular Regard to Tumor Stage and Recurrence**. *Ann Surg* 1989, **209**:88–98.

20. Nordbach IH, Coleman JC, Veubrux A, Dooley WC, Cameron JL, Pitt HA: **Palliative Treatment of Biliary Obstruction in Unresectable Hilar Cholangiocarcinomas**. *Surgery* 1993, in press.

21. Hayes JK Jr, Sapozink MD, Miller FJ: **Definitive Radiation Therapy in Bile Duct Carcinoma**. *Int J Radiat Oncol Biol Phys* 1988, **15**:735–744.

22. Meyers WC, Jones RS: **Internal Radiation for Bile Duct Cancer**. *World J Surg* 1988, **12**:99–104.

23. Boerma EJ: **Research Into the Results of Resection of Hilar Bile Duct Cancer**. *Surgery* 1990, **108**:572–580.

24. Yeo CJ, Pitt HA, Cameron JL: **Cholangiocarcinoma**. *Surg Clin North Am* 1990, **70**:1429–1447.

25. Cameron JL: **Resection of a Proximal Cholangiocarcinoma With Reconstruction Utilizing Silastic Transhepatic Biliary Stents and Bilateral Hepaticojejunostomies**. In *Atlas of Surgery*, vol 1. Edited by Cameron JL. Toronto: BC Decker; 1990:58–71.

Keith D. Lillemoe, MD, Department of Surgery, Blalock 603, 600 N. Wolfe Street, Baltimore, MD 21287-4603, USA.

Is there a place for the Kasai procedure in biliary atresia?

Jay Grosfeld, MD

Indiana University School of Medicine, Indianapolis, Indiana, USA

The survival of infants with biliary atresia has improved significantly during the past two decades as a result of modification of the Kasai hepatoportenterostomy procedure complemented by advances in liver transplantation. Recent reports suggest that the long-term success rate of the Kasai procedure is 40%. Failures are salvaged by liver transplantation. Advances in organ preservation, the use of reduced-sized grafts, and newer immunosuppressive agents (cyclosporine, FK 506) have strongly influenced these improved results. Unfortunately, liver transplantation is associated with a high complication rate, the risk of opportunistic infection, and an increased rate of malignancy due to immunosuppression. Until immunotolerance can be achieved, the Kasai procedure remains the procedure of choice for infants with biliary atresia. Liver transplantation is a life-saving complementary procedure for patients who fail to drain bile following the Kasai procedure, who are older than 3 to 4 months of age at diagnosis, or who have advanced cirrhosis. In the current era, the overall survival should exceed 80%.

Current Opinion in General Surgery 1994:168–172

Before 1960, most infants with biliary atresia met their demise as a result of progressive liver disease by 18 months to 2 years of age. Although Professor Mario Kasai, of Sendai, Japan, introduced the hepatic-portoenterostomy procedure to achieve bile drainage in babies with "uncorrectable" biliary atresia in 1959, the report was published in Japanese, and most English-speaking pediatric surgeons were unaware of this important contribution until almost a decade later [1]. Kasai *et al.*'s [2] follow-up report in 1968 stimulated a significant amount of interest in this topic. Over the past two decades, there has been steady but gradual improvement in survival for infants with biliary atresia as a result of modification of Kasai's original technique and the development of new immunosuppressive agents that permit liver transplantation. Some of the best results in liver transplantation have occurred in patients with biliary atresia. Because the Kasai procedure is successful in only 25% to 40% of reported cases, some transplant enthusiasts have recommended that liver transplantation be the primary procedure of choice. The purpose of this report is to review the most current literature concerning biliary atresia and reassess the role of the Kasai procedure for this condition.

Recent results of hepatoportoenterostomy

Suruga *et al.* [3••] reported on 38 of 93 (40.9%) patients treated by Suruga II modification of the Kasai procedure. These patients survived for more than 5 years following portoenterostomy. The authors evaluated age and histologic changes in the liver at the time of the initial operation. Twenty-seven of 30 patients (90%) who survived for more than 5 years without jaundice or cirrhosis had only a minimal degree of liver fibrosis or a mild degree of bile duct degeneration. Those who had severe fibrosis or bile duct degeneration did not survive more than 5 years. Based on these observations, the authors recommended operation before 3 months of age, before the development of severe histologic changes in the liver.

Losty and Guiney [4] also emphasized the importance of early referral of infants with biliary atresia. They documented long-term survival in 27% of infants following the Kasai procedure and 50% following liver transplantation.

Jolley *et al.* [5] reported on the long-term jaundice-free survival of an infant that underwent a Kasai procedure as a neonate. The operation was done in conjunction with repair of an associated small-bowel atresia. Lin *et al.* [6] reported on a 38.3% long-term success rate following portoenterostomy for infants operated on when they were younger than 3 months of age and noted that most performed normal activities appropriate for their age.

Although most authors experienced in the care of infants with biliary atresia recommended surgical intervention before the infants are 90 days of age, Bielam-

© 1994 Current Science ISBN 1-85922-671-X ISSN 1065–6243

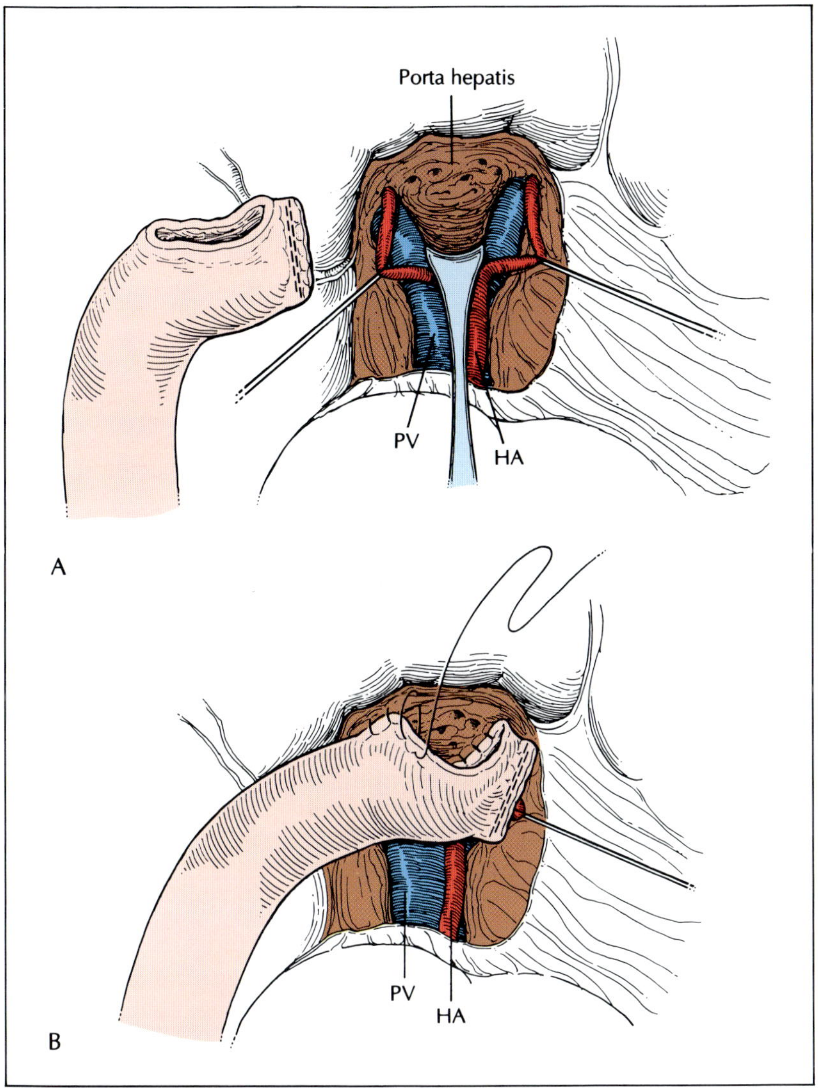

Fig. 1. A, Dissection of the porta hepatis is facilitated by mobilization of the bifurcation of the portal vein (PV). Downward traction on the vein allows identification of one or two small tributaries that are divided to expose the entire porta hepatis. **B**, The entire area of the fibrous porta hepatis containing tiny biliary ductules is included in a single layer "fishmouth" anastomosis to a Roux-Y loop of jejunum using a fine (5-0) absorbable suture. HA—hepatic artery.

owicz *et al.* [7] reported a successful outcome following portoenterostomy in a 132-day-old infant. These results emphasize that there can be variability in presentation.

Nietgen *et al.* [8] demonstrated that failure of portoenterostomy may be related to ongoing intrahepatic bile duct loss. Periodic wedge biopsies of the liver studied by histologic and immunohistochemical characterization showed a progressive loss of intrahepatic bile ducts (vanishing bile duct syndrome) with a geographic anatomic distribution that in some instances was limited to one hepatic lobe.

Late complications, including cholangitis, portal hypertension, hypersplenism, esophageal varices, and gastrointestinal bleeding, can occur more than 5 years after portoenterostomy. Chiba *et al.* [9••] indicated that factors associated with late complications included a past history of cholangitis soon after the initial operation, advanced age of the patient at the time of diagnosis, high portal pressure at the initial procedure, and a long interval of time before the jaundice disappeared following operation. They suggested that early operation and intense postoperative treatment (steroids, chloretics, antibiotics) were important management considerations.

Ohtomo *et al.* [10] noted that 44% of babies with biliary atresia had hematuria, proteinuria, or both. They reviewed renal biopsies from 28 patients with biliary atresia who died and documented a good correlation between glomerular alterations and the period of reduced hepatic function. All kidney specimens showed mesangial proliferation, and IgA was present in the mesangium. Elevated serum IgA and circulating IgA-containing immune complex levels were found in babies with prolonged obstructive jaundice.

Operative technique

The operative technique in performing the portoenterostomy procedure is important. Adequate exposure of the porta hepatis is essential and is facilitated by division of the left triangular ligament, falciform ligament, and a portion of the right triangular ligament. Careful identification of structures in the hepatoduodenal ligament is important. The hepatic arteries should be protected from injury to reduce the risk of liver and bile duct ischemia. The remnant of the often obliterated gallbladder and fibrous common bile duct cord is dissected up to the porta hepatis. The level of transection is superior to the bifurcation of the portal vein. To ensure the entire porta hepatis is included in the anastomosis, the portal vein bifurcation is gently retracted inferiorly, and one or two tiny portal venous branches may require division to further facilitate adequate exposure (Fig. 1*A*).

After biopsy to document the presence of microscopic bile ductules, a Roux-Y loop of jejunum is brought up to the porta hepatis and a fish-mouth anastomosis (which includes the entire porta hepatis area) is accomplished with interrupted 5-0 or 6-0 absorbable suture (Maxon: Davis and Geck, Norwalk, CT; or PDS: Ethicon, Sommerville, NJ) with the knots placed on the outside (Fig. 1*B*).

Ohi recently reported a trend of earlier referral of patients and a change in operative technique by the addition of an intussuscepted valve in the Roux-Y limb in an effort to prevent cholangitis (Paper presented at session of World Federation of Associations of Pediatric Surgeons, International Surgical Week, Hong Kong, 1993). These changes resulted in a reduction in the rate of cholangitis from 46% to 28%. The authors noted that the presence of a biliary stoma reduced the severity of cholangitis but not the incidence. Ohi's group recommended the routine use of postoperative choleretic agents, including phenobarbital, dehydrocholic acid and ursodeoxycholic acid. Patients are also given prednisolone and parenteral antibiotics (a cephalosporin and an aminoglycoside) early on and are subsequently switched to oral antibiotics. Vitamins D, E, A, and K and fatty acid supplements are also given.

The results following portoenterostomy in the recent Sendai experience have improved from 35% jaundice-free patients in 1972 to 63% (68 patients) in 1993. Long-term success (> 10 years) is 72% in patients who were younger than 90 days of age at diagnosis, compared with 14% in patients older than 90 days. Six patients died after 10 years. Seventeen of the patients have been alive and jaundice-free more than 20 years.

Of the 68 long-term survivors, eight required endosclerosis for bleeding esophageal varices, and 16 developed hypersplenism. Nine responded to splenic artery embolization, and seven underwent splenectomy. Five patients required a splenorenal shunt for portal hypertension. Only one patient required liver transplantation.

Ohi's report suggested that with the current changes in management, perhaps 50% of patients with biliary atresia could achieve long-term, jaundice-free success following portoenterostomy and thereby avoid or delay liver transplantation with its associated hazards related to immunosuppression (infection and cancer).

Results of liver transplantation for biliary atresia

The results of liver transplantation have improved significantly following the development of improved organ preservation, cyclosporine, FK 506, and alternate surgical techniques, including reduced-sized grafts and, in some instances, the use of the living related donors (University of Chicago and Japanese experience). In most major pediatric liver transplant centers, the 1-year survival following liver transplantation ranges from 75% to 85%. Salt *et al.* [11] reported the results in 100 children following liver transplantation in the United Kingdom. He noted a 71% 1-year actuarial patient survival and 51% 1-year graft survival. In the past 2 years, these numbers have improved to 86% and 63%, respectively.

Ryckman *et al.* [12••] reported an actuarial patient survival of 89% at 1 year and 80% at 2 years. Since the introduction of reduced-size grafts, the 2-year survival has increased to 91%. Badger *et al.* [13], however, reported only a 62% 1-year survival and 25% retransplantation rate following reduced-sized allograft liver transplantation. Despite the improved results, liver transplantation is not an innocuous procedure and is associated with significant morbidity and some mortality. The important question is not whether a liver transplantation patient will develop a complication postoperatively; it is how many and which complications will occur.

Complications following liver transplantation

Numerous reports have documented significant infectious, noninfectious, and surgical complications following liver transplantation. Bilik *et al.* [14••] described a series of surgical complications following liver transplantation in children. Sixty transplants were carried out in 48 children. The retransplantation rate was 20%. Excluding retransplantation, 48 other abdominal procedures were required for postoperative bleeding, vascular complications, (portal venous occlusions and hepatic artery thrombosis), bowel perforation, splenic infarcts, bile leaks, pancreatitis, and intra-abdominal abscess.

In a recent report from the University of Wisconsin, Kalayoglu *et al.* [15] reported a 25% retransplantation rate, a 49% reoperative rate for other intra-abdominal complications, a 14% mortality at 7 years, and a 62% graft survival. In addition, a risk of four potentially life-threatening infections existed per immunosuppressed pediatric patient.

George *et al.* [16•] documented a 72% rate of infection following liver transplantation. During the first 2 weeks after surgery, most infections (52 cases) were bacterial and were noted in an intra-abdominal site, the bloodstream, or a wound. The next most frequent infection was viral (*n*=16), with cytomegalic virus being the most common virus cultured. Eleven patients had fungal infections (*Candida albicans*).

The Achilles heel of liver transplantation is bile duct ischemia leading to a spectrum of biliary complications from a bile leak, biliary stricture, or diffuse biliary tract injury. Many of these events follow hepatic artery thrombosis. Heffron *et al.* [17] reported on 20 biliary leaks occurring in 13.6% of patients after liver transplantation. In 50% of these cases, the etiology was traced to hepatic artery thrombosis. There was no difference in bile duct complications in whole-graft or reduced-sized grafts. Colonna *et al.* [18] suggested that biliary stricture may be a significant factor in the genesis of sepsis and allograft failure. Most strictures followed hepatic artery thrombosis or prolonged cold ischemia time. Li *et al.* [19] described a diffuse biliary tract injury characterized by multiple intrahepatic biliary strictures in liver transplant recipients.

Other, less common complications include hepatic artery pseudoaneurysms [20] and supracaval vascular rings [21]. Numerous treatment-related complications resulting from the use of certain immunosuppressive drugs, including hirsutism, renal insufficiency, skin rash, seizures, and hypertension, have also been observed. One of the most serious long-term complications related to administration of immunosuppressive drugs is the occurrence of lymphoproliferative disease, which may progress to an aggressive and lethal form of non-Hodgkin's lymphoma.

Martinez and Ahdab-Barmada [22••] compared at autopsy the neuropathy of liver transplantation in children and adults who died following transplantation. There was an increased rate of cerebrovascular accidents in children: intracranial hemorrhage was noted in 27%, a cerebral ischemic lesion in 32%, and global brain ischemia in 49% of pediatric cases, versus 20%, 28%, and 20% of adult cases, respectively.

Conclusions

The fact that the Kasai procedure is successful in up to 40% of babies with biliary atresia suggests that many of these patients can achieve long-term jaundice-free survival without requiring liver transplantation with its attendant morbidity, potential risks of opportunistic infection, and increased rate of malignancy. Furthermore, an unsuccessful portoenterostomy does not adversely influence the subsequent success of liver transplantation. Hepatoportoenterostomy therefore remains the primary procedure of choice for infants with biliary atresia who are less than 3 months of age. Patients referred at an older age because of late diagnosis and those with advanced cirrhosis may be candidates for primary liver transplantation. Liver transplantation is a life-saving complementary procedure for patients with biliary atresia who fail to drain bile following portoenterostomy or show evidence of progressive liver disease. Until our understanding of the interaction of the immune system and the donor graft improves and we can perfect immunomodulation to achieve donor graft immunotolerance, the suggestion that liver transplantation be the primary method of therapy for all cases of biliary atresia cannot be accepted. The Kasai procedure continues to play an important role in the treatment of biliary atresia and when complimented by liver transplantation, should result in the survival of most infants with this condition (Fig. 2).

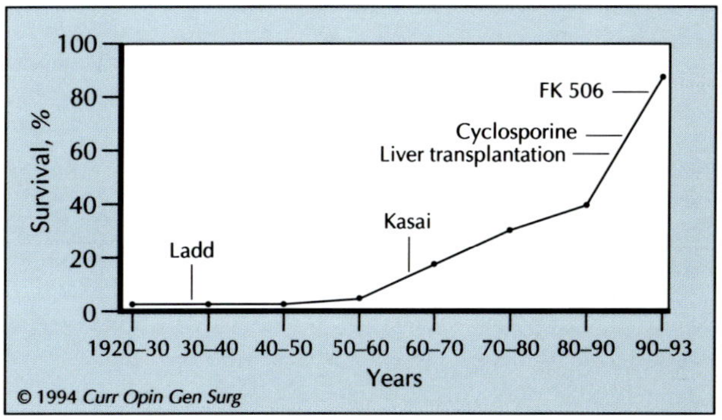

Fig. 2. Impact of Kasai procedure and liver transplantation on survival of infants with biliary atresia. The improvement has been dramatic. The first successful operation for biliary atresia was performed by Dr. Ladd in 1928.

References and recommended reading

Papers of particular interest, published within the annual period of review, have been highlighted as:
- • Of special interest
- •• Of outstanding interest

1. Kasai M, Suzuki S: **A New Operation for Noncorrectable Biliary Atresia: Hepatic Porto-enterostomy.** *Shijijsu* 1959, **13**:733–739.
2. Kasai M, Kimura S, Asakura Y, Suzuki H, Taira Y, Ohashi E: **Surgical Treatment of Biliary Atresia.** *J Pediatr Surg* 1968, 3:665–675.
3. •• Suruga K, Tsunoda S, Deguchi E, Kimura K, Miyano T: **The Future Role of Hepatic Portoenterostomy as Treatment of Biliary Atresia.** *J Pediatr Surg* 1992, **27**:707–709.

This interesting report evaluating age of the patient at diagnosis and histopathology demonstrates that early age (less than 3 months of age at diagnosis), minimal liver fibrosis, and a mild degree of bile duct degeneration were associated with an improved outcome following hepatoportoenterostomy.

4. Losty P, Guiney E: **Biliary Atresia: Lessons From the Dublin Experiences.** *Ir Med J* 1992, **85**:144–147.
5. Jolley SG, Kurlinski JP, Unger JL: **Simultaneous Correction of Biliary Atresia and Small Bowel Atresia in the Neonate.** *J Pediatr Surg* 1992, **27**:1565–1568.
6. Lin JN, Wang KL, Chuang JH: **The Efficacy of the Kasai Operation for Biliary Atresia: A Single Institutional Experience.** *J Pediatr Surg* 1992, **27**:704–706.
7. Bielamowicz A, Weitzman JJ, Alshak NS, Rosenthal P: **Successful Late Kasai Portoenterostomy.** *J Pediatr Gastroenterol Nutr* 1992, **14**:232–236.
8. Nietgen GW, Vacanti JP, Perez-Atayde AR: **Intrahepatic Bile Duct Loss in Biliary Atresia Despite Portoenterostomy: A Consequence of Ongoing Obstruction.** *Gastroenterology* 1992, **102**:2126–2133.
9. •• Chiba T, Ohi R, Nio M, Ibrahim M: **Late Complications in Long-Term Survivors of Biliary Atresia.** *Eur J Pediatr Surg* 1992, 2:22–25.

This report evaluates the long-term complications (longer than 4 years) following portoenterostomy for biliary atresia. Complications were more common in patients of advanced age at diagnosis who also had a history of cholangitis, high portal pressure, and slow reduction of bilirubin level.

10. Ohtomo Y, Fukuda Y, Yabuta K, Miyano T, Tomino Y, Shirai T: **Glomerular Alterations in Children With Biliary Atresia.** *J Pediatr* 1992, **120**:404–408.

11. SALT A, NOBLE-JAMIESON G, BARNES ND, MOWAT AP, ROLLES K, JAMIESON N, JOHNSTON P, FRIEND P, CALNE RY: **Liver Transplantation in 100 Children: Cambridge and King's College Hospital Series.** *BMJ* 1992, **304**:416–421.

12. •• RYCKMAN F, FISHER R, PEDERSEN S, DITTRICH V, HEUBI J, FARRELL M, BALISTRERI W, ZIEGLER M: **Improved Survival in Biliary Atresia Patients in the Present Era of Liver Transplantation.** *J Pediatr Surg* 1993, **28**:382–386.

This excellent report shows the improvement in survival in children following liver transplantation after the development of the reduced-size graft concept. The authors suggest that the Kasai procedure and liver transplantation are complementary and not competitive procedures.

13. BADGER IL, CZERNIAK A, BEATH S, TISONE G, DEAKIN M, SHERLOCK DJ, KELLY DA, MCMASTER P, BUCKLES JA: **Hepatic Transplantation in Children Using Reduced-Size Allografts.** *Br J Surg* 1992, **79**:47–49.

14. •• BILIK R, YELLEN M, SUPERINA RA: **Surgical Complications in Children After Liver Transplantation.** *J Pediatr Surg* 1992, **27**:1371–1375.

This study carefully documents the myriad of surgical complications following orthotopic liver transplantation in children.

15. KALAYOGLU M, D'ALESSANDRO AM, KNECHTLE SJ, ECKHOFF DE, PIRSH JB, JUDD R, SOLLINGER HN, HOFFMAN RM, BELZER FO: **Long-Term Results of Liver Transplantation for Biliary Atresia.** *Surgery* 1993, **114**: 711–718.

16. • GEORGE DL, ARNOW PM, FOX A, THISTLEWAITE JR, EMOND JC, BROELSCH CE, WHITINGTON PF: **Patterns of Infection After Pediatric Liver Transplantation.** *Am J Dis Child* 1992, **146**:924–929.

This report indicates that most early infections following liver transplantation are bacterial in origin. The second most common pathogens are viruses, and the third are fungi.

17. HEFFRON TG, EMOND JL, WHITINGTON PF, THISTLEWAITE JR, STEVENS L, PIPER J, WHITINGTON S, BROELSCH CE: **Biliary Complications in Pediatric Liver Transplantation: A Comparison of Reduced-Size and Whole Graft.** *Transplantation* 1992, **53**:391–395.

18. COLONNA JO, SHAKED A, GOMES AS, COLQUHOUN SD, JURIM O, MCDIARMID SV, MILLIS JU, GOLDSTEIN LI, BUSITTIL RW: **Biliary Strictures Complicating Liver Transplantation: Incidence, Pathogenesis, Management and Outcome.** *Ann Surg* 1992, **216**:344–350.

19. LI S, STRATTA RJ, LANGNAS AN, WOOD RP, MARVJO W, SHAW BW JR: **Diffuse Biliary Tract Injury After Orthotopic Liver Transplantation.** *Am J Surg* 1992, **164**:536–540.

20. MADARIAGA J, TZAKIS A, ZAJKO AB, TZORACOLEFTHERAKIS E, TEPETES K, GORDON R, TODO J, STARZL TE: **Hepatic Artery Pseudoaneurysm Ligation After Orthotopic Liver Transplantation: A Report of 7 Cases.** *Transplantation* 1992, **54**:824–828.

21. WECHSLER RJ, FELD R, MUNOZ SJ, DELAURENTIS M, LEV-TOAFF AS, HELINIK TG, RUBIN R, MORITZ MJ: **Suprahepatic Circumcaval Ring: CT Findings After Orthotopic Liver Transplantation.** *Radiology* 1992, **183**:545–548.

22. •• MARTINEZ AJ, AHDAB-BARMADA M: **The Neuropathology of Liver Transplantation: Comparison of Main Complications in Children and Adults.** *Mod Pathol* 1993, **6**:25–32.

This important autopsy study shows that in children who received an orthotopic liver transplant, there was a distinct increase in the rate of cerebrovascular accidents as compared with adults. Lesions observed included intracranial hemorrhage, cerebral ischemia lesion, and global brain ischemia.

Jay Grosfeld, MD, Department of Surgery, Indiana University Medical Center, 545 Barnhill Drive, Emerson Hall 244, Indianapolis, IN 46202-5124, USA.

Pancreatic pseudocysts, ascites, and fistulas

Charles J. Yeo, MD

Johns Hopkins Medical Institutions, Baltimore, Maryland, USA

Recent publications dealing with pancreatic pseudocysts, pancreatic ascites, and pancreatic fistulas are reviewed. Terminology relevant to pancreatic pseudocysts and other complications of acute pancreatitis is clarified. The natural history of pseudocysts is examined. Newer management strategies for these complications of pancreatic inflammatory disease are discussed, including percutaneous drainage of pseudocysts and the use of octreotide in the management of pancreatic ascites and pancreatic fistulas.

Current Opinion in General Surgery 1994:173–178

In recent years the terminology applied to acute pancreatitis and its many complications has become diverse, conflicting, and confusing. Definitions from a recent international symposium may assist in the clinical classification of acute pancreatitis and assessment of treatment modalities for acute pancreatitis [1••]. Particularly relevant to the topics of this review are the consensus definitions of pancreatic pseudocyst, pseudo-pseudocyst (acute fluid collection), and pancreatic abscess. A *pseudocyst* is a localized collection of pancreatic juice enclosed by a wall of fibrous or granulation tissue, arising as a consequence of pancreatitis or pancreatic trauma. Pseudocysts contain high concentrations of pancreatic enzymes, lack an epithelial lining, and typically require at least 4 weeks from the onset of acute pancreatitis for formation. A *pseudo-pseudocyst* (acute fluid collection) forms early in the course of acute pancreatitis and lacks a wall of fibrous or granulation tissue. More than one half of these lesions resolve spontaneously. A *pancreatic abscess* is a circumscribed collection of pus, containing little to no pancreatic necrosis, caused by acute pancreatitis or pancreatic trauma. Based on this terminology, an infected pancreatic pseudocyst is best termed a pancreatic abscess.

Pancreatic pseudocysts

Diagnosis

Two recent papers have dealt with the issue of the analysis of pseudocyst fluid. Lewandrowski *et al.* [2] performed an analysis of the fluid aspirated intraoperatively from 26 peripancreatic cystic structures being treated surgically. Of these structures, nine were pseudocysts and 17 were cystic neoplasms. Pseudocyst fluid was found to contain a high concentration of amylase, negative cytology, low viscosity, and low concentrations of the tumor markers carcinoembryonic antigen (CEA) and CA 125 (Table 1). Fluid from mucinous neoplasms (such as cystadenoma or cystadenocarcinoma) had variable amylase concentration, positive cytology, high viscosity, and variably high values for the tumor markers CEA and CA 125. Analysis of fluid from serous neoplasms showed intermediate results, with variable amylase concentration, negative cytology, low viscosity, low CEA, and variable CA 125. These data demonstrate that analysis of cyst fluid by a panel of diagnostic parameters can differentiate between the various types of pancreatic cystic lesions. This cyst fluid analysis may be useful, in selected cases, to assist in diagnosis prior to therapeutic decision making. However, in most patients the clinical setting is most important in differentiating between pseudocyst and neoplasm.

Duvnjak *et al.* [3] correlated the amylase concentration in pseudocysts and pseudo-pseudocysts with the success of therapeutic aspiration. In their experience, 24 patients had pseudocysts (amylase concentration of fluid greater than upper limit of normal for amylase in serum), with percutaneous aspiration successfully leading to pseudocyst resolution in only three of the patients (12.5%). In contrast, of 19 patients with pseudo-pseudocysts (amylase concentration of fluid not elevated), percutaneous aspiration successfully resolved and fluid collection in 17 patients (89.5%). These data, combined with past reports of percutaneous therapy for pseudocysts [4–6], suggest that 1) percutaneous aspiration alone for pseudocysts is rarely successful and is not indicated; 2) percutaneous aspiration of pseudo-pseudocysts is likely to be successful, although is rarely indicated, since most resolve spontaneously and cause few symptoms; and 3) percutaneous drainage of pseudocysts requires placement of in-dwelling catheters to improve the results of these percutaneous interventions.

Natural history

Appropriate management of pancreatic pseudocysts requires knowledge of their natural history. In the past,

Abbreviations

CEA—carcinoembryonic antigen; **ERCP**—endoscopic retrograde cholangiopancreatography.

© 1994 Current Science ISBN 1-85922-671-X ISSN 1065–6243

Table 1. Cyst fluid parameters useful in diagnosis*

Diagnosis	Amylase	Cytology	Viscosity	CEA	CA 125
Pseudocyst	High	Negative	Low	Low	Low
Serous cystic neoplasm	Variable	Negative	Low	Low	Variable
Mucinous cystic neoplasm	Variable	Usually positive	Usually high	High	Variable

**Adapted from* Lewandrowski *et al.* [2•]; with permission.
CEA—carinoembryonic antigen.

spontaneous resolution of pseudocysts was thought to be uncommon (<10%), and pseudocyst-related complications were believed to occur in up to 50% of patients. Hence, in the past the mere presence of a pseudocyst was thought to mandate intervention. With the advent of sophisticated imaging techniques (ultrasonography, computed tomography, magnetic resonance imaging), pseudocysts are now discovered more frequently in association with acute pancreatitis and pancreatic trauma. Recent evidence suggests that the spontaneous resolution rate of pseudocysts may approach 50% and that complications occur less commonly than was once observed [7,8]. As a result of these findings, a nonoperative, noninterventional, expectant approach to selected patients with pseudocysts has been proposed by several groups [7,8,9••]. In the report by Vitas and Sarr [9••], 68 patients with asymptomatic pseudocysts were initially treated via an expectant approach. In only six patients (9%) did a severe complication occur, and in only 24 patients (35%) was operative treatment required. One patient with intracystic hemorrhage was treated with angiographic embolization. Forty-three patients (63%) were successfully treated without any form of intervention. Pseudocyst diameter correlated with resolution and the need for eventual operative treatment (Table 2), although no strict size criterion predicted the absolute need for intervention. With careful clinical and radiographic follow-up, the application of this expectant approach to pseudocysts appears to be appropriate in asymptomatic patients without evidence of pseudocyst-related complications.

Table 2. Natural history of patients with pancreatic pseudocyst managed by a primary nonoperative expectant approach*

Pseudocyst size, *cm*	Patients, *n*	Pseudocysts resolved, %	Eventual operative treatment, %
<5	25	83	28
5–10	29	50	38
>10	7	50	57

**From* Vitas and Sarr [9••]; with permission.

Management

The recommended management strategies for pancreatic pseudocysts have changed dramatically over recent years. Surgery is no longer the only option for therapy, having been joined by percutaneous and endoscopic approaches. The mere presence of a pseudocyst no longer mandates intervention.

The role of endoscopic retrograde cholangiopancreatography (ERCP) in pseudocyst management has evolved to the point where it may predict the success of surgical versus percutaneous treatment. For many years ERCP has been considered of value in defining pancreatic ductal anatomy, and in choosing the most effective operative management [10,11]. Now, Ahearne *et al.* [12•] have suggested that ERCP may additionally serve to determine the optimal means of pseudocyst treatment, *ie*, surgical versus percutaneous drainage. In their analysis, they made the assumption (unproven and not entirely supported by percutaneous drainage data) that pseudocysts associated with main pancreatic duct obstruction or main pancreatic duct communication require surgical treatment, while those without such ERCP findings could be managed via percutaneous drainage. A treatment algorithm was constructed (Fig. 1) based on these assumptions. The authors then retrospectively analyzed their treatment of 40 patients with pseudocysts and found that the 26 patients treated in a fashion consistent with the algorithm had only a 12% incidence of adverse outcome, while the 14 patients treated in a fashion inconsistent with the algorithm had a significantly higher (43%) incidence of adverse outcome. This retrospective study supports the use of ERCP in decision making regarding pseudocyst treatment. The authors acknowledged that a prospective analysis is needed.

Several series of pseudocyst treatment have recently been published [13–15]. In the report by Huizinga and Baker [14] from Durban, South Africa, pseudocysts were identified in 241 (12.7%) of 1895 patients admitted with acute pancreatitis during a 4-year period (1986–1990). Over 75% of patients were treated expectantly or with percutaneous aspiration, while only 59 patients (24.5%) required operation. Operative procedures performed included internal drainage in 35 patients (23 to stomach, 10 to jejunum, two to duodenum), external drainage in 20 patients, pancreatic resection in two patients, and biliary-enteric bypass in

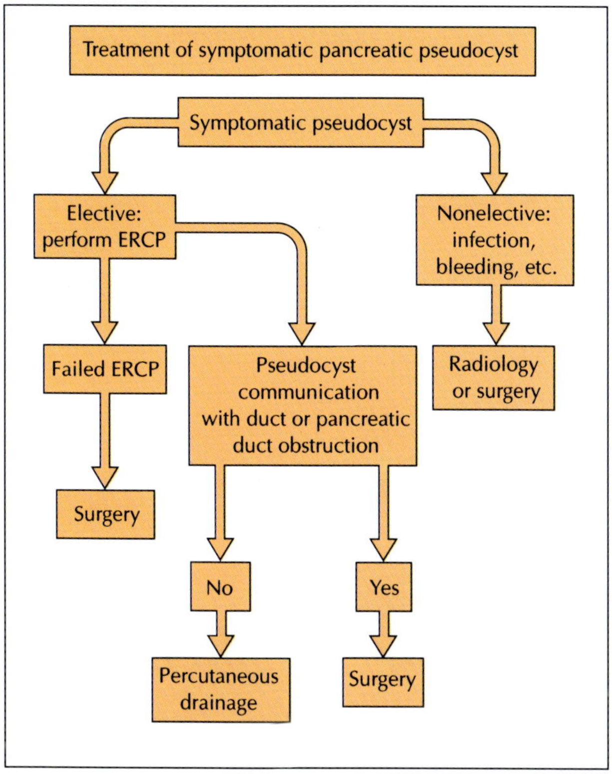

Fig. 1. Algorithm used in the retrospective assignment of treatment in the management of 40 cases of pancreatic pseudocyst. ERCP—endoscopic retrograde cholangiopancreatography. (*From* Ahearne *et al.* [12•]; with permission.)

eight patients. There were six (10.2%) postoperative deaths and three (5.1%) recurrent pseudocysts; major postoperative morbidity occurred in an additional five patients (8.5%). The report by Adams and Anderson [15] from Charleston, South Carolina, reviews the surgical treatment of 92 patients with pseudocysts, comprising largely a referral practice, treated between 1982 and 1990. The largest proportion of patients (42 patients, 46%) were treated by percutaneous catheter drainage, with 22 patients (24%) treated via longitudinal pancreaticojejunostomy, 15 patients (16%) by internal drainage and six patients (6%) by operative external drainage. The overall morbidity rate was 28%, with one patient death (1%). Direct comparisons between these two reports [14,15] are not possible, based on differences in patient population, underlying disease, and selection criteria. Nonetheless, two recent trends in pseudocyst management are clear: increased use of percutaneous drainage and increased use of longitudinal pancreaticojejunostomy (Peustow procedure) in properly selected patients.

Percutaneous approaches to pseudocyst drainage have been reported for nearly two decades. Modifications of technique continue to be reported [16,17]. A recent article by Freeny [18•] reviews the technique and results of percutaneous catheter drainage of pseudocysts. Therapeutic aspiration (without catheter drainage) is not discussed and should no longer be used because of high complication and recurrence rates. The indications for percutaneous catheter drainage include symptomatic pseudocysts (pain), pseudocyst complications (infection, obstruction), and pseudocyst enlargement. The "involvement of contiguous organs or structures" is stated by Freeny as an indication for percutaneous catheter drainage, but it should *not* be so considered; many pseudocysts have their walls composed of adjacent structures (*eg*, stomach, spleen, kidney, transverse mesocolon) and may nonetheless be successfully managed expectantly, without intervention. Contraindications to percutaneous catheter drainage include the presence of pancreatic necrosis or a solid or nondrainable pancreatic mass, lack of a safe access route, pseudocyst hemorrhage, and (arguably) obstruction of the main pancreatic duct. After catheter placement, follow-up imaging is required to document pseudocyst resolution prior to catheter removal. Catheter removal occurs on average after 34 days of drainage, with the length of drainage being extended (up to many months) in patients with demonstrable fistulas. The overall short-term success rate in this review, encompassing 270 patients from 11 series, was 79%, with a complication rate of 15% [18•].

At present there are no prospective randomized data to guide the choice between operative and percutaneous catheter drainage of pseudocysts. The role of percutaneous catheter drainage seems most strongly supported for treatment of infected pseudocysts (pancreatic abscess), where laparotomy for external drainage appears to have little to no benefit [19,20], and perhaps is attended by increased morbidity and mortality. Some data have suggested higher success rates for percutaneous catheter drainage of infected pseudocysts, as compared with noninfected pseudocysts [21•]. Successful percutaneous drainage of pseudo-pseudocysts continues to be reported [22], although the indications for drainage of these acute fluid collections without ductal communication remain too broad. Size criteria alone (some authors use 5 cm, some 6 cm, some 8 cm) should no longer be considered an indication for drainage [7,9••].

The long-term results of percutaneous catheter drainage of pseudocysts have been only infrequently reported. A report by Criado *et al.* [21•] cautions against the widespread application of percutaneous catheter drainage. In their experience, 42 patients with pseudocysts underwent percutaneous catheter drainage and were followed for a mean of 10 months, with only nine patients (21%) having successful drainage leading to pseudocyst resolution. Three factors that favored success of percutaneous catheter drainage included pseudocyst infection, alcohol-related etiology, and duration of catheter placement greater than 7 days. Statistical significance was not achieved for all three factors because of the small numbers in each group.

Percutaneous catheter drainage of pseudocysts is associated with the development of pancreaticoenteric fistulas in a small number of cases. Catheter erosion in the face of ongoing pancreatitis may be the cause of these fistulas. Recently Wolfsen *et al.* [23•] presented their experience with the treatment of seven patients with pancreaticoenteric fistula (four to duodenum, three to colon). Five patients were successfully treated without operation, three by catheter removal alone, and two by catheter removal plus endoscopic transpapillary stenting of the disrupted pancreatic duct. Two patients with pancreaticocolonic fistula required surgery (one diverting colostomy and one distal pancreatectomy) for healing. This report underscores one of the potential complications of percutaneous catheter drainage and outlines a rational approach to management of catheter-induced fistulas.

Complications

The commonly recognized complications of pseudocysts are infection, hemorrhage, obstruction, and rupture. In a retrospective review of a 25-year experience, Adams *et al.* [24] identified 13 (7.2%) of 180 patients with pseudocysts as having arterial hemorrhage. Angiographic embolotherapy has gained increasing acceptance and utility in the management of many of these arterial bleeding sources, which often originate in pseudoaneurysms from branches of the splenic or gastroduodenal arteries. Patients with unstable vital signs and massive hemorrhage should continue to be treated with emergency operation [25]. Obstruction of the gastrointestinal tract (most typically distal stomach or duodenum) by a pseudocyst is a common indication for intervention. Browman *et al.* [26] have reported an uncommon obstructive occurrence: pseudocyst compression of the inferior vena cava, leading to leg edema. The patient's pseudocyst was drained percutaneously, and the edema resolved.

Pseudocysts in the pediatric population

Pancreatic trauma is the leading cause of pseudocysts in children, and traumatic disruption of the pancreatic duct is the presumed mechanism of pseudocyst formation. Computed tomography is the recommended imaging study; ERCP may be impossible because of the small size of the patient. Operative internal drainage has had universally favorable outcome [27]. Successful percutaneous catheter drainage has also been reported [28]. It may be anticipated that a high percentage of pediatric pseudocysts will show pancreatic ductal communication on sinography via the drainage catheter. Longer durations of catheter drainage may be required to allow ductal healing.

Pancreatic ascites

Pancreatic ascites results when inflammatory pancreatic disease causes a disruption of the main pancreatic duct, allowing inactive pancreatic exocrine secretions to freely extravasate into the peritoneal cavity. Lipsett and Cameron [29•] reviewed 41 patients with pancreatic ascites treated over a 27-year period. Alcohol-related pancreatitis was believed to be the cause of the pancreatic ascites in 59% of cases. Most patients presented with painless abdominal swelling. Initial nonoperative therapy, including parenteral nutrition and repeat paracentesis, was successful in 17 (47%) of 36 patients. Surgical management included pancreatic resection, internal drainage via cystojejunostomy or cystogastrostomy, or longitudinal pancreaticojejunostomy, with two deaths. Preoperative pancreatography via ERCP is essential in planning operative strategy (Fig. 2).

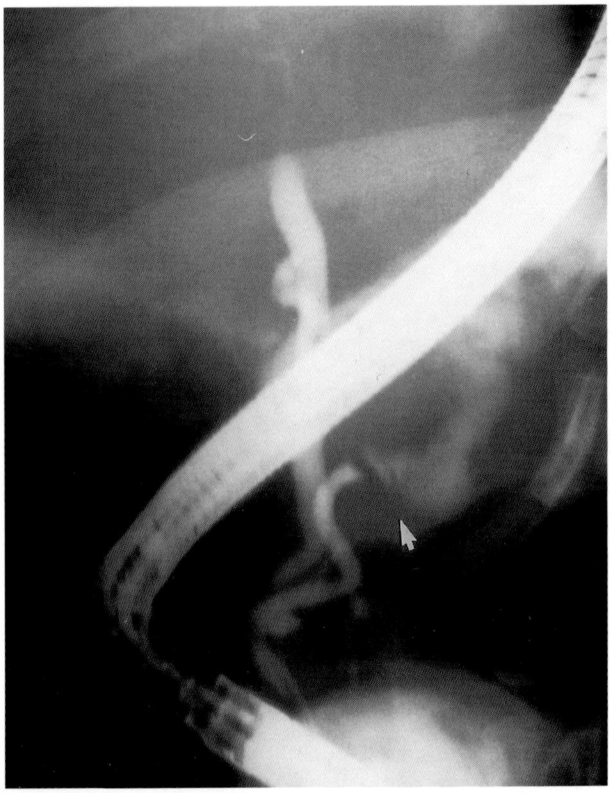

Fig. 2. Endoscopic retrograde cholangiopancreatogram in a patient with pancreatic ascites. The pancreatic duct disruption is well visualized, demonstrating an abrupt cutoff with contrast extravasating into the lesser sac (*arrow*). The patient, whose nonoperative therapy failed, was treated successfully by pancreaticojejunostomy to the site of the ductal disruption. (*From* Yeo and Cameron [36]; with permission.)

Anecdotal reports have suggested that administration of the long-acting somatostatin analogue, octreotide, may improve the success of nonoperative therapy for pancreatic ascites [30,31]. A recent report by Parekh and Segal [32•] evaluated the treatment of 23 patients with pancreatic ascites or pancreatic pleural effusion over a 7.5 year period. Standard nonoperative therapy was initially instituted and 10 patients (43%) responded and were cured after a mean of 30 days of treatment. Standard nonoperative therapy failed in five additional patients, but they were cured when octreotide was added to the treatment regimen. Factors associated with failure of nonoperative therapy included low total serum protein and severe pancreatic ductal disease as visualized by ERCP. ERCP early in the course of nonoperative treatment may be useful to identify patients with severe ductal disease, who may be best served by early operative intervention.

Pancreatic fistulas

The importance of appropriately timed catheter removal in cases of catheter-related pancreaticoenteric fistula has been previously discussed [23•]. Octreotide continues to be evaluated for its role in the management of pancreatic fistula. Octreotide has been shown to decrease the volume, amylase content, and bicarbonate content of pancreatic juice in human external pancreatic fistulas seen after pancreatic resection [33] or pancreatic transplantation [34]. A recently reported multicenter trial from Spain and Italy evaluated the role of continuously administered intravenous somatostatin in 40 patients being treated with total parenteral nutrition for closure of gastrointestinal fistulas [35]. Seven patients had pancreaticocutaneous fistulas. Twenty patients were randomly assigned to receive total parenteral nutrition alone, while 20 received total parenteral nutrition plus somatostatin (250 μg/h). Unfortunately, the randomization yielded groups with significant pretreatment differences (both age and pretreatment fistula output were higher in the somatostatin group), biasing the data against the somatostatin treatment arm. The results indicated no difference in eventual fistula closure rate. They did reveal significantly shorter time to 75% reduction of fistula output and significantly fewer complications in the total parenteral nutrition plus somatostatin group. It is uncertain if these preliminary results using intravenous somatostatin will be reproduced by studies using more conventional therapy such as subcutaneous octreotide administration in doses up to 250 μg three times daily.

Acknowledgment

Thanks are extended to Ms. Donna Taylor for her assistance in the preparation of this review.

References and recommended reading

Papers of particular interest, published within the annual period of review, have been highlighted as:
- • Of special interest
- •• Of outstanding interest

1. •• BRADLEY EL III: **A Clinically Based Classification System for Acute Pancreatitis.** *Arch Surg* 1993, **128**:586–590.
Summary of an international symposium on acute pancreatitis, providing consensus definitions and a clinically based classification system for acute pancreatitis.

2. • LEWANDROWSKI KB, SOUTHERN JF, PINS MR, COMPTON CC, WARSHAW AL: **Cyst Fluid Analysis in the Differential Diagnosis of Pancreatic Cysts.** *Ann Surg* 1993, **217**:41–47.
Presents fluid analysis for tumor markers, amylase content, amylase isoenzymes, viscosity, and cytology on 26 cystic lesions of the pancreas.

3. DUVNJAK M, VUCELIC B, ROTKVIC I, SIKIRIC P, BRKIC T, BANIC M, TSOSKOT B, SUPANC V: **Assessment of Value of Pancreatic Pseudocyst Amylase Concentration in the Treatment of Pancreatic Pseudocysts by Percutaneous Evacuation.** *JCU J Clin Ultrasound* 1992, **20**:183–186.

4. VAN SONNENBERG E, WITTICH GR, CASOLA G, BRANNIGAN TC, KARNEL F, STABILE BE, VARNEY RR, CHRISTENSEN RR: **Percutaneous Drainage of Infected and Noninfected Pancreatic Pseudocysts: Experience in 101 Cases.** *Radiology* 1989, **170**:757–761.

5. GROSSO M, GANDINI G, CASSINIS MC, REGGE D, RIGHI D, ROSSI P: **Percutaneous Treatment (Including Pseudocystogastrostomy) of 74 Pancreatic Pseudocysts.** *Radiology* 1989, **173**:493–497.

6. SACHS D, ROBINSON ML: **Transgastric Percutaneous Drainage of Pancreatic Pseudocysts.** *AJR Am J Roentgenol* 1988, **151**:303–306.

7. YEO CJ, BASTIDAS JA, LYNCH-NYHAN A, FISHMAN EK, ZINNER MJ, CAMERON JL: **The Natural History of Pancreatic Pseudocysts Documented by Computed Tomography.** *Surg Gynecol Obstet* 1990, **170**:411–417.

8. WILLIAMS KJ, FABIAN TC: **Pancreatic Pseudocyst: Recommendations for Operative and Nonoperative Management.** *Am Surg* 1992, **58**:199–205.

9. •• VITAS GJ, SARR MG: **Selected Management of Pancreatic Pseudocysts: Operative Versus Expectant Management.** *Surgery* 1992, **111**:123–130.
These data support a nonoperative, noninterventional approach to the treatment of a selected majority of patients with pancreatic pseudocysts.

10. NEALON WH, TOWNSEND CM, THOMPSON JC: **Preoperative Endoscopic Retrograde Cholangiopancreatography (ERCP) in Patients With Pancreatic Pseudocysts Associated With Resolving Acute and Chronic Pancreatitis.** *Ann Surg* 1989, **209**:532–540.

11. LAXSON LC, FROMKES JJ, COOPERMAN M: **Endoscopic Retrograde Cholangiopancreatography in the Management of Pancreatic Pseudocysts.** *Am J Surg* 1985, **150**:683–686.

12. • AHEARNE PM, BAILLE JM, COTTON PB, BAKER ME, MEYERS WC, PAPPAS TN: **An Endoscopic Retrograde Cholangiopancreatography (ERCP)-Based Algorithm for the Management of Pancreatic Pseudocysts.** *Am J Surg* 1992, **163**:111–116.
An algorithm was retrospectively applied to 40 patients with pseudocysts, allocating therapy based on the findings of pancreatic duct obstruction or pseudocyst-duct communication. Patients whose treatment followed the algorithm had significantly fewer adverse outcomes.

13. JONES DR, VAUGHAN RA, TIMBERLAKE GA: **Pancreatic Pseudocyst: Diagnosis and Management.** *South Med J* 1992, **85**:729–734.

14. HUIZINGA WKJ, BAKER LW: **Treatment of Persistent and Complicated Pancreatic Pseudocysts.** *J R Coll Surg Edinb* 1992, **37**:373–376.

15. ADAMS DB, ANDERSON MC: **Changing Concepts in the Surgical Management of Pancreatic Pseudocysts.** *Am Surg* 1992, **58**:173–180.

16. DAS KM, KOCHHAR R: **Pancreatic Pseudocysts: Treated With Dual Drainage.** *Clin Radiol* 1992, **45**:92–93.

17. DAS K, KOCHHAR R, KAUSHIK SP, GUPTA NM, MEHTA SK, SURI S, WIG JD: **Double Pigtail Cystogastric Stent in the Management of Pancreatic Pseudocyst.** *JCU J Clin Ultrasound* 1992, **20**:11–17.

18. • FREENY PC: **Percutaneous Management of Pancreatic Fluid Collections.** *Baillieres Clin Gastroenterol* 1992, **6**:259–272.
A review of percutaneous drainage techniques and results.

19. HIMAL HS, CUSIMANO RJ: **Pancreatic Pseudocysts: The Role of Percutaneous Catheter Drainage.** *Can J Surg* 1992, **35**:403–406.

20. ADAMS DB, ANDERSON MC: **Percutaneous Catheter Drainage Compared With Internal Drainage in the Management of Pancreatic Pseudocyst.** *Ann Surg* 1992, **215**:571–578.

21. • CRIADO E, DESTEFANO AA, WEINER TM, JAQUES PF: **Long-Term Results of Percutaneous Drainage of Pancreatic Pseudocyst.** *Surg Gynecol Obstet* 1992, **175**:293–298.
Patients were followed up for a mean of 10 months after percutaneous catheter drainage of pseudocysts. Of 42 patients who received percutaneous drainage, only nine (21%) had ultimately successful outcomes.

22. D'EGIDIO A, SCHEIN M: **Percutaneous Drainage of Pancreatic Pseudocysts: A Prospective Study.** *World J Surg* 1992, **16**:141–146.

23. • WOLFSEN HC, KOZAREK RA, BALL TA, PATTERSON DJ, TRAVERSO LW, FREENY PC: **Pancreaticoenteric Fistula: No Longer a Surgical Disease?** *J Clin Gastroenterol* 1992, **14**:117–121.
Discussion of the treatment of seven patients with catheter-related pancreaticoenteric fistula.

24. ADAMS DB, ZELLNER JL, ANDERSON MC: **Arterial Hemorrhage Complicating Pancreatic Pseudocysts: Role of Angiography.** *J Surg Res* 1993, **54**:150–156.

25. SANTOS JCM JR., FERES O, ROCHA JJR, ARACAVA MM: **Massive Lower Gastrointestinal Hemorrhage Caused by Pseudocyst of the Pancreas Rupture Into the Colon: Report of Two Cases.** *Dis Colon Rectum* 1992, **35**:75–77.

26. BROWMAN MW, LITIN SC, BINKOVITZ LA, MOHR DN: **Pancreatic Pseudocyst That Compressed the Inferior Vena Cava and Resulted in Edema of the Lower Extremities.** *Mayo Clin Proc* 1992, **67**:1085–1088.

27. Hall KN: **Pediatric Pancreatic Pseudocyst: A Case Report and Review of the Literature.** *J Emerg Med* 1992, **10**:573–576.

28. Corbally MT, Blake NS, Guiney EJ: **Management of Pancreatic Pseudocyst in Childhood: An Increasing Role for Percutaneous External Drainage.** *J R Coll Surg Edinb* 1992, **37**:169–171.

29. Lipsett PA, Cameron JL: **Internal Pancreatic Fistula.** *Am J Surg* 1992,
• **163**:216–220.
A review of 50 patients with internal pancreatic fistula, including 41 patients with pancreatic ascites.

30. Rushforth JA, Beck JM, McMahon M, Puntis JWL: **Resolution of Pancreatic Ascites With Octreotide.** *Arch Dis Child* 1993, **68**:135–136.

31. Hartley JE, Hershman MJ, Glazer G: **Ruptured Pancreatic Pseudocyst.** *J R Soc Med* 1992, **85**:107–108.

32. Parekh D, Segal I: **Pancreatic Ascites and Effusion: Risk Factors for**
• **Failure of Conservative Therapy and the Role of Octreotide.** *Arch Surg* 1992, **127**:707–712.
Low total serum protein and severe pancreatic ductal disease are associated with failure of nonoperative therapy for pancreatic ascites.

33. Ohta T, Nagakawa T, Mori K, Kanno M, Kayahara M, Veno K, Miyazaki I: **Effect of SMS-995 on Exocrine Pancreatic Secretion in a Patient With External Pancreatic Fistula.** *Int J Pancreatol* 1992, **11**:185–189.

34. Secchi A, DiCarlo V, Martinenghi S, LaRocca E, Caldara R, Staudacher C, Ferrari G, Castoldi R, Torri G, Pozza G: **Octreotide Administration in the Treatment of Pancreatic Fistulae After Pancreas Transplantation.** *Transpl Int* 1992, **5**:201–204.

35. Torres AJ, Landa JI, Moreno-Azcoita M, Arguello JM, Silecchia G, Castro J, Hernandez-Merlo F, Jover JM, Moreno-Gonzalez E, Balibrea JL: **Somatostatin in the Management of Gastrointestinal Fistulas: A Multicenter Trial.** *Arch Surg* 1992, **127**:97–100.

36. Yeo CJ, Cameron JL: **The Pancreas.** In *Textbook of Surgery: The Biological Basis of Modern Surgical Practice*, edn 14. Edited by Sabiston DC Jr. Philadelphia: WB Saunders; 1992:1076–1107.

Charles J. Yeo, MD, Department of Surgery, Johns Hopkins Medical Institutions, 600 North Wolfe Street, Baltimore, MD 21287–4606, USA.

Whole-organ versus islet pancreatic transplantation

F. Charles Brunicardi, MD, and Christopher R. Shackleton, MD

University of California at Los Angeles School of Medicine, Los Angeles, California, USA

The goals of pancreatic transplantation are to improve the quality of life for the diabetic patient, reverse the metabolic abnormalities of diabetes, and prevent the dreaded secondary complications. Although transplantation of the whole pancreas is the only therapy that reliably achieves euglycemia, the complications associated with this procedure and the need for immunosuppression make it undesirable except to a select subpopulation of type I diabetic patients. Islet cell transplantation is the exciting alternative; however, insulin independence has been achieved in only 10% to 20% of patients. Although advances in technology could make islet transplantation the treatment of choice for type I diabetic patients, islet transplantation currently remains an experimental procedure. Diabetes is not commonly considered a surgical disease, but surgeons have made major contributions to its treatment and must remain active in the development of new treatment modalities for this debilitating disease.

Current Opinion in General Surgery 1994:179–185

Pancreatic transplantation represents the most exciting treatment for the type I diabetic patient by providing the patient with functioning endocrine pancreatic tissue. With the subsequent improvement in glucose homeostasis, many of the complications of diabetes should be prevented [1••]. Although transplantation of the whole organ reliably achieves insulin independence and euglycemia, the complications associated with the procedure are significant [2•]. Transplantation of the islets of Langerhans has a negligible morbidity and mortality; however, insulin independence is achieved in only a small percentage of the patients [3••]. In the following discussion, the essentials of whole-pancreas transplantation will be compared with those of islet transplantation.

Diabetes exists in all countries. In Western countries, the prevalence is 2%, and approximately 1.5% of the population dies of diabetes-related complications [4,5]. Diabetes reduces quality and duration of life by affecting the brain, heart, eyes, kidneys, arteries, legs, and the nervous system. Myocardial infarctions and kidney failure are the most common causes of death in these patients. Diabetes is one of the most common causes of blindness, and 10% of diabetic patients undergo a major amputation during their lifetime. Furthermore, the annual cost in health care dollars for this disease runs in the billions of dollars. Because strict metabolic control of glucose has been shown to lower the incidence of blindness, renal failure, and amputations, there is an obvious need for improvement in treatments for this debilitating disease [1••,4,5].

History

Researchers have been led to several of the major advances in the treatment of diabetes through surgical procedures [6]. In 1890, a pancreatectomy performed in a dog resulted in the causal relationship of the pancreas to glucose homeostasis. In 1922, an orthopedic surgeon and physiology science student extracted a pancreatic hormone that demonstrated the ability to lower the blood glucose of pancreatectomized dogs. These studies resulted in the discovery of insulin, which became the mainstay of treatment for type I diabetics in this century. Insulin was hailed for its ability to save the lives of patients suffering from this lethal disease. It was realized in the decades that followed that although these patients could live a nearly normal lifespan, they would suffer the long-term sequelae of diabetes, namely retinopathy, nephropathy, neuropathy, and cardiovascular disease. In an attempt to find a better treatment for diabetes, the first whole-organ pancreas transplantation was performed at the University of Minnesota in 1966 by Kelly *et al.* [7]. With similar intent, the first successful human islet transplantations were performed at the University of Pittsburgh, the Washington University in St. Louis, and the University of Alberta in 1990 [8–10]. Surgeons should be familiar with the basic concepts involved in these procedures, because their continued input may help to improve the current treatments for diabetes.

Whole-organ transplantation

Whole-pancreas transplantation is currently the only reliable method of establishing a constant euglycemic state in the type I diabetic patient. Immediately following implantation of the whole pancreas, euglycemia and insulin independence is achieved. The patient no longer requires constant glucose monitoring and insulin supplementation to achieve glucose homeostasis. However, because the patients require immunosuppression, only those receiving another solid organ transplant or those with unmanageably labile diabetes can receive a whole-organ pancreas transplant. Therefore, this form of treatment is limited to a subpopulation of type I diabetic patients [11].

Successful pancreas transplantation begins with prudent patient selection [11,12]. The two major groups of patients receiving whole-organ pancreas transplantation are those that have diabetic nephropathy and end-stage renal disease who require a kidney transplant, and those that have already received a renal allograft. A third category of patients are those who have unmanageable glucose regulation, in particular, who have labile hypoglycemic unawareness and require numerous hospitalizations for metabolic control. Most patients receiving a pancreas-kidney transplant range in age from 25 to 47 years, with the median age being 36 years. On average, these patients have had diabetes for approximately 25 years, with a range of 4 to 42 years. Such patients require a thorough evaluation for other complications of diabetes, including the extent of the retinopathy, neuropathy, and cardiovascular disease. The cardiovascular evaluation is especially important, as this patient population has a very high incidence of occult but clinically significant coronary artery disease. Many centers include a psychiatric evaluation prior to the transplantation.

The proper donor must also be carefully selected to optimize success with this procedure. Pancreas donor factors have been reviewed with respect to graft function following transplantation [13]. The effect of multiple donor variables on function and survival of 307 cadaveric pancreas allograft transplanted into 253 recipients was examined at the University of Minnesota. This study concluded that donor hyperglycemia and HLA-DR mismatch are risk factors for loss of the pancreas graft.

Figure 1 demonstrates the whole-organ pancreatic graft. The pancreas is taken with a segment of duodenum. It is also possible to transplant only a segment of the pancreas, usually the body and tail.

Most whole-organ pancreas donors are also liver donors. For an understanding of procurement surgery, special consideration must be given to the arterial supply, and in variations thereof, to both organs. In most cases, the gastroduodenal and splenic arteries are divided, and the celiac axis hepatic artery complex is maintained in continuity with the liver. The superior mesenteric artery origin remains with the pancreas, and thus the head of the pancreas and the duodenal segment are dependent for their blood supply on the inferior pancreaticoduodenal circuit. The portal vein is divided at its confluence with the splenic vein. Reconstruction of the superior mesenteric artery and splenic artery is accomplished with a "Y" graft of donor iliac arteries, and the splenic vein can be elongated with donor external iliac vein.

Following vascular isolation, the pancreas is flushed with a cold preservation solution, either Belzer's solution or Eurocollin's solution. Most of the successful centers are now using the Belzer's solution for preservation of the pancreas [14,15]. Preservation periods of up to 28 hours can be achieved with good graft function following transplantation; however, many centers prefer to minimize the old storage time.

The implantation of the pancreas can be performed with one of several techniques, including whole-pancreas transplantation with bladder drainage (Fig. 2), whole-pancreas transplantation with enteric drainage (Fig. 3), segmental pancreas transplantation with enteric drainage, and segmental pancreas transplantation with polymer obliteration of the ducts. Venous drainage is usually routed via the external iliac vein [13–16]. Although there may be certain physiologic advantages to portal venous drainage, this approach has proved problematic surgically. From a metabolic standpoint, systemic venous drainage has yielded satisfactory results.

The postoperative management of the patient following pancreas and kidney transplantation includes vital sign monitoring and early detection of graft failure due to either rejection or technical problems. In most centers, the patients remain in the intensive care unit for several days for intensive monitoring of vital signs, urinary amylase, blood glucose levels, and creatinine clearance. The immunosuppressive regimen is the same as that for the other solid-organ transplantations and at most centers includes cyclosporine, azathioprine, steroids, and antilymphocyte globulin [14]. However, the kidney-pancreas combination has proved itself to be quite immunostimulatory, and quadruple immunosuppression with mono- (OKT3) or polyclonal antilymphocyte preparations is used in most major centers. Patients are usually maintained on parenteral nutrition for 1 week, and oral nutrition is started as soon as possible. Long-term monitoring includes measuring blood levels of cyclosporine, C-peptide, glucose, hemoglobin A_1C, urinary amylase, and creatinine clearance. Unfortunately, monitoring rejection in the pancreas graft is difficult and any evidence of rejection must be aggressively treated to avoid complete rejection of the pancreas graft.

To date, 4285 pancreas transplants have been performed worldwide (Sutherland, Personal communication). Most of these are cadaveric pancreas transplants that have been performed in kidney-transplant recipients. The overall 1-year patient survival is 85%, but the overall 1-year graft survival since 1983 is 63%. These are forbidding statistics, because they indicate that one in every six patients receiving this operation will die within the 1st year and that almost half of all patients

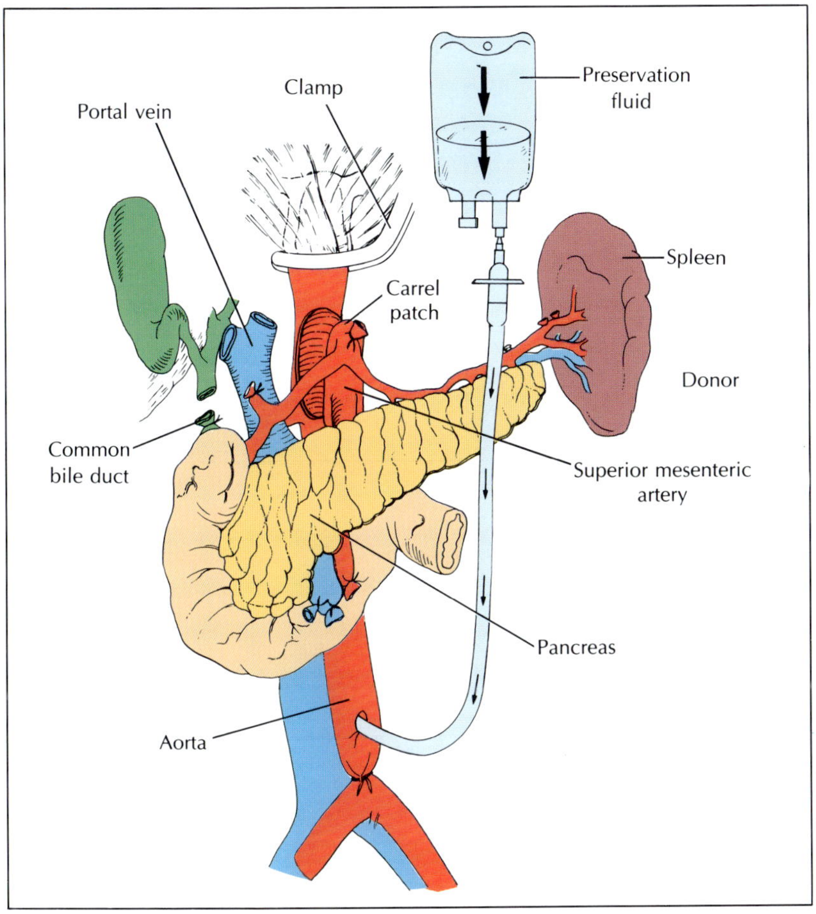

Fig. 1. The isolation of the whole-organ pancreatic graft. The pancreas is taken with a cuff of duodenum, and its blood supply from the celiac and superior mesenteric arteries is preserved. The cold preservation fluid is infused into the aorta, which is crossclamped at the diaphragm. (*From* Starzl and Tzakis [35]; with permission.)

will lose their graft at the end of that year. Fortunately, the results have greatly improved over the past 5 years and approach that of kidney transplantation: 1-year graft survival has been 71% to 85%, and 1-year patient survival has been 91% to 96% for simultaneous pancreas-kidney transplants [2•,15].

Although pancreas transplantation establishes a euglycemic, insulin-independent state, the clinician must determine whether the benefits are worth the risk. The major benefit is the improvement of quality of life [2•,14,16]. The patients are free from constant glucose monitoring, multiple insulin injections, and dietary restrictions. Most patients agree that they have an improved quality of life. Retinopathy and nephropathy also appear to be reduced or stabilized following pancreas transplantation. In the University of Minnesota study, patients with long-term functioning pancreas grafts had stability of retinopathy, whereas those with failed grafts had progression of retinopathy [2•,16]. Their study also showed improvements in neuropathy following pancreas transplantation. Preliminary results suggest an improvement in nephropathy; however, beneficial results are often masked by the detrimental effects of cyclosporine on renal function. With the recent landmark study indicating that long-term complications are prevented by meticulous glucose control, it is reasonable to assume that whole-pancreas transplantation should prevent many of these complications [1••].

Although the full benefits have yet to be realized, the risks of pancreas transplantation are quite serious [2•,14,17]. The most significant risk is loss of life, which occurs in up to 4% to 18% of patients during the 1st year following transplantation. Secondly, the patients risk a 15% to 36% chance of losing the graft within the 1st year. They also face a 10% to 20% complication rate associated with the procedure. Most of the complications are related to the presence of pancreatic exocrine tissue and include pancreatitis, pancreatic ascites, fistulae, abscesses, and wound infections. Another complication is vascular thrombosis, requiring removal of the graft. Anticoagulation may decrease the thrombosis rate; however, bleeding complications are then encountered. Gastrointestinal complications, such as bowel obstruction, perforation, or ileus, can occur following pancreas transplantation and require exploration. Finally, complications related to immunosuppression, such as cancer and opportunistic infections, may occur. Although pancreas transplantation is the most reliable means of achieving euglycemia and insulin independence in the type I diabetic patient, and although the success of this modality continues to increase, it remains a form of therapy limited to selected diabetic patients because of the need for immunosuppression and the significant morbidity associated with the procedure.

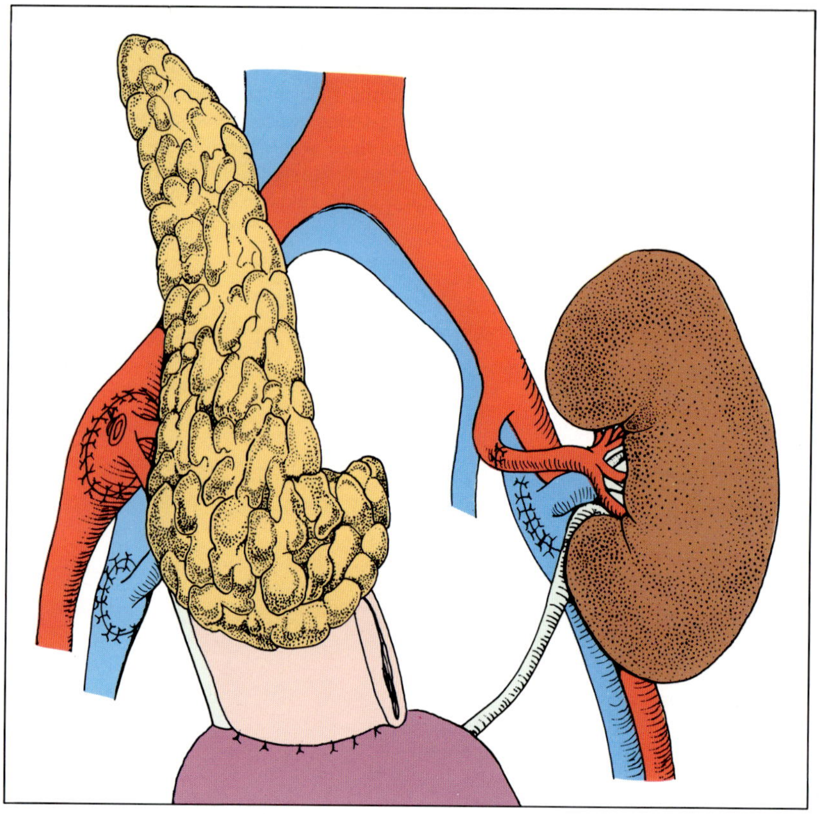

Fig. 2. The most common pancreas transplant procedure performed. The vessels of the kidney are anastomosed to the iliac artery and vein on one side; the pancreas is anastomosed to the contralateral iliac artery and vein, and a cuff of duodenum is sewn to the bladder. (*From* Corry [36]; with permission.)

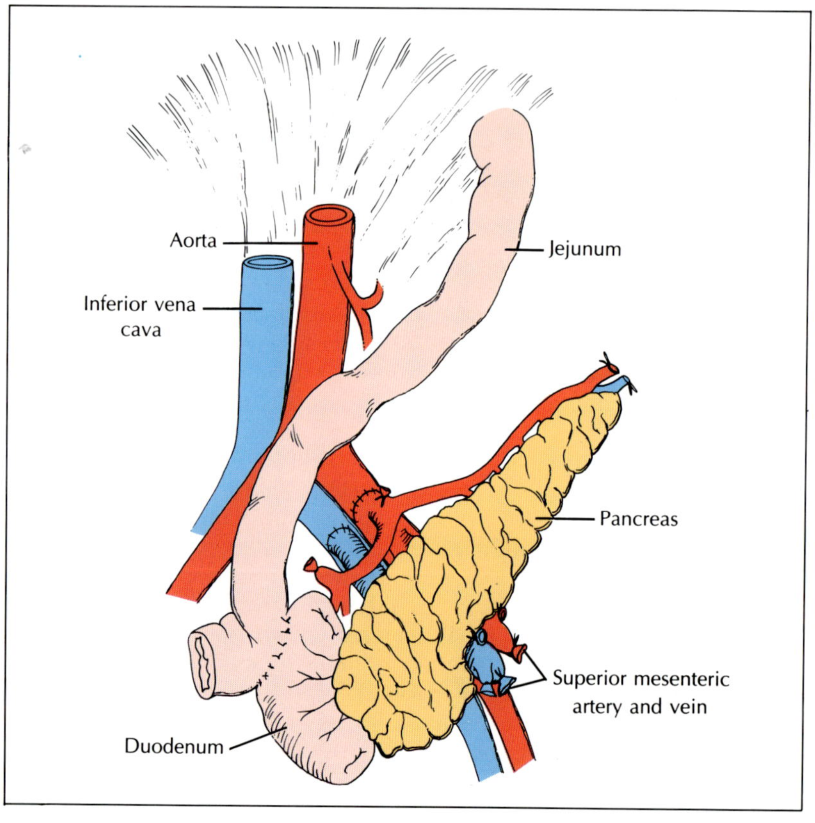

Fig. 3. The enteric drainage of the pancreatic exocrine secretion. The pancreatic vessels are anastomosed to the iliac artery and vein, and the duodenum is anastomosed to a Roux-en-Y loop of jejunum. (*From* Starzl and Tzakis [35]; with permission.)

Islet transplantation

The alternative is transplantation of the endocrine pancreas. Because most of the complications of pancreas transplantation are related to the exocrine pancreas, its exclusion greatly reduces the complication rate associated with whole-organ transplantation. However, clinical success with islet transplantation has been difficult to achieve. Isolation of human islets and rejection of the islet graft have been the two major obstacles preventing the success of islet transplantation [3••,18].

Donor factors governing successful islet isolation have been studied [19]. The success of islet transplantation begins with procurement of the pancreas, and the important predictors of successful isolation are donor blood glucose level, cold ischemia time, and length of donor hospitalization.

The human pancreas is procured and preserved in a manner similar to that used in the whole-organ procedure; the pancreas is then returned to the laboratory for separation and purification of the islets of Langerhans. The most successful isolation technique was developed by Ricordi *et al.* [20] in 1988 as an automated modification of the technique described by Lacy in 1967 (Fig. 4). A digestive enzyme, collagenase, is forcefully injected into the pancreatic duct, thereby destroying the architecture of the pancreas, but leaving many islets intact. The type of collagenase used is a significant factor in determining successful islet retrieval [21]. The islets are then separated from the rest of the pancreatic elements using Ficoll-gradient centrifugation.

Through this technique, approximately 50% of the islet mass, or 500,000 islets, can be recovered from a single pancreas. However, viable islets are recovered from only 60% of the pancreata, and the average yield per pancreas is approximately 230,000 [19].

Because an estimated 500,000 islets are required to achieve euglycemia in diabetics, most of the clinical successes were achieved by transplanting islets procured from multiple pancreata [8–10,22•]. The necessity for multiple pancreata, however, limits the practicality of clinical success with purified islet transplantation.

In an attempt to use only one pancreas, one center has transplanted the dispersed pancreas, *ie*, unpurified islets [23•]. Following collagenase digestion, the entire dispersed pancreas (30- to 60-mL pellet) is infused into the portal vein, and the portal vein pressure is constantly monitored. Two patients have achieved insulin independence with this technique. Because the major advantage of this technique is that one dispersed pancreas can result in insulin independence, two schools of islet transplantation have emerged, one using purified islets and one using unpurified islets.

Once isolated, the islets can be cultured, cryopreserved, or transplanted immediately, depending on the

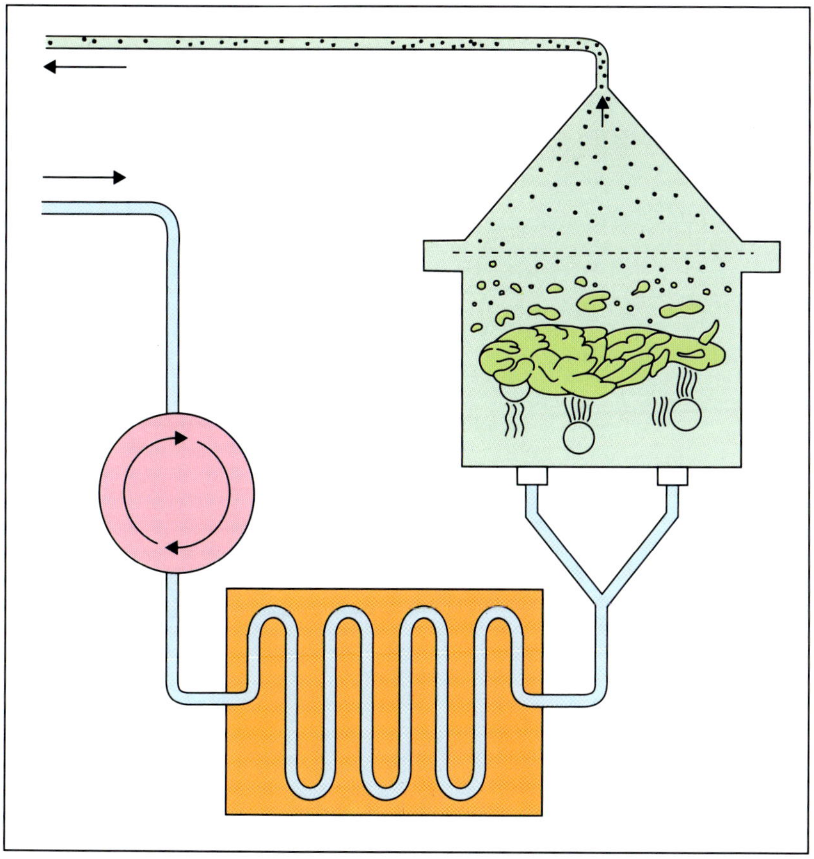

Fig. 4. The automated method for pancreatic islet isolation. A peristaltic pump propels the fluid through a heating circuit to the digestion chamber, in which the pancreas is progressively dispersed into fragments of decreasing size, and the continuously released islets are saved from further digestion. (*From* Ricordi [37]; with permission.)

technique preferred. The islets can be transplanted into many locations, such as the portal vein, kidney capsule, spleen, and omentum; however, infusion into the portal vein is the most common technique. This procedure can be done through either a mesenteric vein catheter, an umbilical vein catheter, or a percutaneous transhepatic portal vein catheter [8–10,22•].

Postoperative management of these patients is simpler than that of whole-pancreas transplantation, and patients need not be monitored in an intensive care unit. However, the islet transplant patients need 2 weeks of intense glucose monitoring and an intravenous insulin drip to protect the islet graft from exhaustion [24]. The patients require quadruple immunosuppression; therefore, only diabetic patients with kidney or liver grafts are receiving islet transplants. Other immunosuppressive agents, such as FK 506 or deoxyspergualin, have been tried; however, the experience with these agents is too limited to determine if greater benefit results from this technique than from standard quadruple immunosuppression regimens [8,23•].

A recent analysis on the clinical adult islet transplants performed worldwide through June 1992 was recently reported by the Islet Transplant Registry [3••]. One hundred sixty-seven attempts at adult islet transplantation were performed at 25 institutions, and 19 patients are currently insulin-independent, indicating an 11% success rate. Fortunately, a significant improvement in the clinical results has occurred in the 1990 to 1992 era; 69 cases were performed, with a 20% insulin-independent rate. Further analysis of these patients indicate that 64% of the patients have circulating C-peptide levels, therefore representing partial success. Although many of these patients are not insulin independent following islet transplantation, they have demonstrated improved glucose control and reduced insulin requirements. Partial successes are most likely important in light of the recent study indicating that the improved glucose homeostasis results in fewer complications [1••]. However, although prevention of diabetic complication by islet transplantation has been demonstrated in animal studies, there is no clear proof that these patients are protected from the complications of diabetes.

The following advantages of islet transplantation are theoretical but represent exciting advances in this field. The islets can be cryopreserved and stored indefinitely in a bank, whereas whole pancreata can be preserved for only hours [25,26]. The islets can thus be accumulated and transplanted at a convenient time [10]. The cryopreserved islets can also be easily transported from one institution to another. Islets can also be altered immunologically before transplantation, thus eliminating or reducing the need for immunosuppression [27–30]. Ideally, xenograft islets could be altered immunologically and used to treat patients [31]. The use of xenograft islets, such as pig or fish islets, would permit the treatment of thousands of diabetic patients, [32], and tolerance to the islet graft could also be achieved. One of the most significant advances is the finding that transplanting islets to the rat thymus followed by a short course of antilymphocyte globulin results in tolerance to a subsequent islet allograft without the need for immunosuppression [33••]. Preliminary work in larger animals is also encouraging [34].

Conclusions

The goals of pancreatic transplantation are to improve the quality of life for the diabetic patient, reverse the metabolic abnormalities of diabetes, and prevent the dreaded secondary complications. Although transplantation of the whole pancreas is the only therapy that reliably achieves euglycemia, the complications associated with this procedure and the need for immunosuppression make it suitable for a select subpopulation of type I diabetic patients. Islet cell transplantation is the exciting alternative; however, insulin independence has been achieved by only 10% to 20% of the patients. Although improvements could make islet transplantation the treatment of choice for type I diabetic patients, this procedure remains experimental. Although diabetes is not commonly considered a surgical disease, surgeons must remain active in the development of treatments for this debilitating disease.

References and recommended reading

Papers of particular interest, published within the annual period of review, have been highlighted as:

• Of special interest
•• Of outstanding interest

1. •• Richard P, Nilsson BY, Rosenqist U: **The Effect of Long-Term Intensified Insulin Treatment on the Development of Microvascular Complications of Diabetes Mellitus.** *N Engl J Med* 1993, **329**:304–309.

This landmark study demonstrates that improved glucose control helps to prevent the long-term complications of diabetes. Although physicians suspected that this was true for many years, this study gave scientific proof to the hypothesis.

2. • Sutherland DER, Gruessner A, Moudry-Munns K: **Analysis of United Network for Organ Sharing "UNOS" in the United States of America "USA" Pancreas Transplantation Registry Data According to Multiple Variables.** In *Clinical Transplants*. Edited by Terasaki P. Los Angeles: UCLA Tissue Typing Laboratory; 1992:45–59.

Sutherland continues to be a leader in the field of pancreas transplantation and is to be congratulated for maintaining a pancreas transplantation registry. This article reviews the results of pancreas transplantation.

3. •• Hering BJ, Browatzki CC, Schultz A, Bretzel RG, Federlin KF: **Clinical Islet Transplantation: Registry Report, Accomplishments in the Past and Future Research Needs.** *Cell Transplantation* 1993, 2:269–282.

Hering has compiled all of the data pertaining to clinical islet transplantation and has published a comprehensive article concerning the current status of islet cell transplantation. In his analysis of these data, he demonstrates that the clinical results of islet cell transplantation have improved over the past 2 years.

4. National Diabetes Data Group: **Diabetes in America.** Washington, DC: NIH Publisher; 1985.

5. Deckert T: **Insulin-Dependent Diabetes Mellitus and Its Complications.** In *Pancreatic Transplantation*. Edited by Groth CG. Philadelphia: WB Saunders; 1988:1–14.

6. Bliss M: **The Discovery of Insulin.** Toronto: McClelland and Stewart; 1982.

7. Kelly WD, Lillehei RC, Merkel RK, Idezuki Y, Goetz FC: **Allotransplantation of the Pancreas and Duodenum Along With the Kidney in Diabetic Nephropathy.** *Surgery* 1967, **61**:827–837.

8. Tzakis AG, Riccordi C, Alejandro R, Zeng Y, Fung JJ, Tadcio S, Demetris AJ, Mints OH, Starzl TE: **Pancreatic Islet Transplantation After Upper Abdominal Exenteration and Liver Replacement.** *Lancet* 1990, **336**:402–405.

9. Scharp DW, Lacy PE, Santiago JV, McCullough CS, Weide LG, Falgire L, Marchetti P, Gingerich RL, Jaffe AS, Cryer PE, Anderson CB, Flye MW: **Insulin Independence After Islet Transplantation Into Type I Diabetic Patient.** *Diabetes* 1990, **39**:515–518.

10. Warnock GL, Kneteman NM, Ryan E, Seelis REA, Rabinovitch A, Rajotte RV: **Normoglycemia After Transplantation of Freshly Isolated and Cryopreserved Pancreatic Islets in Type I (Insulin-Dependent) Diabetes Mellitus.** *Diabetologia* 1991, 34–55.

11. Sutherland DER: **Who Should Get a Pancreas Transplant?** *Diabetes Care* 1988, **11**:681–685.

12. Groth CG: **Patient Selection.** In *Pancreatic Transplantation.* Edited by Groth CG. Philadelphia: WB Saunders; 1988:37–48.

13. Gores PF, Gillingham KJ, Dunn DL, Moudry-Munns KC, Najarian JS, Sutherland DER: **Donor Hyperglycemia as a Minor Risk Factor and Immunologic Variables as Major Risk Factors for Pancreas Allograft Loss in a Multivariate Analysis of a Single Institution's Experience.** *Ann Surg* 1992, **215**:217–230.

14. Sollinger HW, Knechtle SJ, Reed A, *et al.*: **Experience With 100 Consecutive Simultaneous Kidney-Pancreas Transplants With Bladder Drainage.** *Ann Surg* 1991, **214**:703–711.

15. Elahi D, McAllon-Dyke M, Clark B, Kahn B, Weinref J, Minaker KL, Wong G, Morse L, Brown R, Shapiro M, Gingerich RL, Rosenlof L, Pruitt T, Ancersen DK, Hanks JB: **Sequential Evaluation of Islet Cell Responses to Glucose in the Transplanted Pancreas in Humans.** *Am J Surg* 1993, **165**:15–22.

16. Robertson P: **Pancreas Transplantation in Humans With Diabetes Mellitus.** *Diabetes* 1991, **40**:1085–1089.

17. Groth CG: **Surgical Complications Following Pancreatic Transplantation.** In *Pancreatic Transplantation.* Edited by Groth CG. Philadelphia: WB Saunders; 1988:219–238.

18. Mullen Y, Clare-Saltzler M, Stein E, Clark W: **Islet Transplantation for the Cure of Diabetes.** *Pancreas* 1989, **4**:123–135.

19. Watt PC, Mullen Y, Benhamore PY, Hober C, Nomura Y, Watanabe Y, Kleinman R, Miyamoto M, Passaro EP, Zinner MJ, Brunicardi FC: **Donor Factors Affecting Successful Isolation of Islets From the Human Pancreas.** *Transplant Proc* 1993, in press.

20. Ricordi C, Lacy PE, Finke EH, Olack B, Scharp DW: **An Automated Method for the Isolation of Human Pancreatic Islets.** *Diabetes* 1984, **33**:1055–1061.

21. Watt PC, Mullen Y, Benhamore PY, Hober C, Nomura Y, Watanabe Y, Kleinman R, Miyamoto M, Passaro EP, Zinner MJ, Brunicardi FC: **Technical Factors Affecting Successful Isolation of Islets From the Human Pancreas.** *Transplant Proc* 1993, in press.

22. • Socci C, Falqui L, Davalli AM, Ricordi C, Maffi P, Secchi A, DiCarlo V, Pozza G: **Substitution of the Endocrine Pancreatic Function in IDDM Patients: The Milan Experience.** In *Pancreatic Islet Cell Transplantation.* Edited by Ricordi C. Austin: Landes; 1992:414–422.

Currently, Socci has the best results using islet transplantation in patients with type I diabetes. He and his group have achieved insulin independence in approximately 70% of the patients receiving islet transplants.

23. • Gores PF, Najarian JS, Stephanian E, Loveras JJ, Kelley SL, Sutherland DER: **Insulin Independence in Type I Diabetes After Transplantation of Unpurified Islets From Single Donor With 15-Deoxyspergualin.** *Lancet* 1993, **341**:19–21.

This exciting article demonstrates that insulin independence can be achieved with a dispersed pancreas from a single donor. This group used a new immunosuppressive regimen to achieve this exciting success.

24. Alejandro R, Burke G, Shapiro ET, Stresser S, Nery J, Ricordi C, Esquenazi V, Miller J, Mintz DH: **Long-Term Survival of Intraportal Islet Allografts in Type I Diabetes Mellitus.** In *Pancreatic Islet Cell Transplantation.* Edited by Ricordi C. Austin: Landes; 1992:410–413.

25. Rajotte RV, Scharp DW, Downing R, Preston R, Molnar GD, Ballinger WF: **Pancreatic Islet Banking: The Transplantation of Frozen-Thawed Rat Islets Transported Between Centers.** *Cryobiology* 1981, **18**:357–369.

26. Miyamoto M, Mullen Y, Stein E, Watt PC, Benhamou PY, Kemmochi T, Brunicardi FC: **Cryopreservation of Human Islets by a Fully Automated Cryounit.** *Transplant Proc* 1993, in press.

27. Lim F, Sun AM: **Microencapsulated Islets as a Bioartificial Endocrine Pancreas.** *Science* 1980, **210**:908.

28. Stein E, Mullen Y, Benhamou PY, Watt PC, Hober C, Watanabe Y, Nomura Y, Brunicardi FC: **Reduction in Immunogenicity of Human Islets by 24°C Culture.** *Transplant Proc* 1993, in press.

29. Oluwole SF, Hardy MA: **Immunomodulation by UV-B Irradiation.** In *Pancreatic Islet Cell Transplantation.* Edited by Ricordi C. Austin: Landes; 1992:158–167.

30. Faustman D: **Graft Modification Prior to Transplantation.** In *Pancreatic Islet Cell Transplantation.* Edited by Ricordi C. Austin: Landes; 1992:150–157.

31. Weber CJ, Costanzo MK, Zabinski S, Krekum S, Koschitzky T, D'Agati V, Rajotte R, Reentsma K: **Xenografts of Microencapsulated Rat, Canine, Porcine and Human Islets.** In *Pancreatic Islet Cell Transplantation.* Edited by Ricordi C. Austin: Landes; 1992:177–189.

32. Wright JR Jr: **Experimental Transplantation Using Principal Islets of Teleost Fish.** In *Pancreatic Islet Cell Transplantation.* Edited by Ricordi C. Austin: Landes; 1992:336–351.

33. •• Posselt AM, Barker CF, Tomaszewski JE, Markmann JF, Choti MA, Naji A: **Induction of Donor-Specific Unresponsiveness by Intrathymic Islet Transplantation.** *Science* 1990, **249**:1293–1295.

This landmark article demonstrates that tolerance to an allograft can be achieved in a small animal model. Because tolerance is the ultimate achievement in transplantation, this work represents one of the one of the most exciting advances in the field.

34. Watt P, Mullen Y, Nomura Y, Watanabe Y, Brunicardi FC, Andersen C, Zinner M, Passaro EP: **Successful Engraftment of Autologous and Allogeneic Islets Into the Porcine Thymus.** *J Surg Res* 1993, in press.

35. Starzl TE, Tzakis AG: **Pancreatico-duodenal Transplantation With Enteric Exocrine Drainage.** *Pancreatic Transplantation.* Edited by Groth CG. Philadelphia: WB Saunders; 1988:113–129.

36. Corry RJ: **Pancreatico-duodenal Transplantation With Urinary Tract Drainage.** In *Pancreatic Transplantation.* Edited by Groth CG. Philadelphia: WB Saunders; 1988:147–153.

37. Ricordi C: **The Automated Method for Islet Isolation.** In *Pancreatic Islet Cell Transplantation.* Edited by Ricordi C. Austin: Landes; 1992:99–107.

F. Charles Brunicardi, MD, UCLA School of Medicine, Division of General Surgery, 10833 Le Conte Avenue, 72-244 CHS, Los Angeles, CA 90024-6904, USA.

Endocrine tumors of the pancreas

Jennifer B. Meko, MD, and Jeffrey A. Norton, MD

Washington University School of Medicine, St. Louis, Missouri, USA

Pancreatic endocrine tumors are rare, yet can cause significant morbidity due to excessive secretion of hormones. Octreotide is effective in reducing the plasma concentrations of many of these hormones. The availability of potent H_2-receptor antagonists and omeprazole has altered the emphasis in patients with Zollinger-Ellison syndrome away from total gastrectomy and towards resection of the gastrinoma for potential cure. Fifty percent of insulinomas and gastrinomas are not evident on preoperative imaging studies, despite their sophistication. Calcium angiography, endoscopic ultrasonography, isotope-labeled octreotide scanning, and injection of methylene blue during secretin angiography are recent imaging modalities that have shown promise in the localization of these tumors. Intraoperative ultrasound has emerged as the best method for operative detection of insulinomas. Duodenotomy and intraoperative endoscopic transillumination are especially important in the surgical management of Zollinger-Ellison syndrome because 30% to 40% of gastrinomas are located in the duodenum. The management of patients with multiple endocrine neoplasia type 1 and Zollinger-Ellison syndrome continues to be controversial. Some advocate an aggressive surgical approach, whereas others have had little success in rendering patients eugastrinemic.

Current Opinion in General Surgery 1994:186–194

Incidence

Endocrine tumors of the pancreas are rare, exhibiting an annual incidence of less than 1 per 100,000 [1]. Insulinomas comprise the most common islet cell tumor [2], with an incidence of approximately one per million population per year, followed by gastrinoma with an incidence of 0.1 to 0.4 per million population per year [3]. The remaining neuroendocrine tumors of the pancreas include VIPoma, glucagonoma, somatostatinoma, GRFoma, ACTHoma, PTH-like-oma, neurotensinoma, and nonfunctional islet cell tumor or PPoma. These tumors occur in less than 0.2 per million population per year.

Diagnosis

Pancreatic endocrine tumors can cause significant morbidity due to excessive secretion of specific hormones. Although greater than 50% of pancreatic islet cell tumors contain more than one hormone as evidenced by immunocytochemistry [4–10], in most instances, patients exhibit symptoms characteristic of only one of these peptides.

The symptoms, diagnosis, and treatment of 85 patients with endocrine pancreatic tumors from 1973 to 1986 are discussed in a recent review article [11•]. The majority (63%) of patients with insulinomas presented with neuroglycopenic symptoms, including episodes of clouded consciousness, attacks of unconsciousness, and personality changes. Seizures have been reported in up to 30% of patients [12]. The biochemical diagnosis is confirmed by fasting hypoglycemia (glucose ≤ 40 mg/dL) and inappropriately high serum insulin values (>5 μU/mL) during a supervised 72-hour fast. C-peptide values are elevated in 73% to 91% of patients, and proinsulin values are elevated in 75% to 80% of patients [11•,12,13]. Proinsulin may be a marker of a malignant tumor [14].

Patients with Zollinger-Ellison syndrome classically present with severe peptic ulcer disease associated with profound gastric acid hypersecretion. Epigastric pain is the most common symptom, and approximately 90% of patients have evidence of duodenal ulcer disease at the time of diagnosis [15,16,17•,18]. Patients may experience recurrent and atypically located ulcers, such as ulcers of the distal duodenum or jejunum. However, it should be noted that some pa-

Abbreviations

ACTH—adrenocorticotropic hormone; **CT**—computed tomography;
MEN-1—multiple endocrine neoplasia type 1; **MR**—magnetic resonance.

 ISBN 1-85922-671-X ISSN 1065–6243

tients with Zollinger-Ellison syndrome do not have evidence of peptic ulcer disease [17•,19]. Diarrhea and weight loss are common symptoms. In addition, dysphagia, esophagitis, and endoscopic abnormalities of the esophagus may be present in up to 60% of patients [20,21]. Elevated basal serum gastrin levels (> 100 pg/mL) combined with gastric acid hypersecretion (> 15 mEq/h) or elevation of gastrin levels (> 200 pg/mL) following a secretin stimulation test confirm the biochemical diagnosis. The results of testing fasting serum gastrin level and basal acid output are positive in 100% of patients, and the secretin stimulation test result is positive in 85% of patients [22]. Zollinger-Ellison syndrome must be excluded before performing any operation for duodenal ulcer disease. The symptoms and diagnostic criteria for the remaining less common pancreatic islet cell tumors are presented in Tables 1 and 2.

Medical management

After establishment of a firm biochemical diagnosis, adequate medical therapy is necessary to correct the abnormalities caused by excessive hormone secretion. Patients with insulinoma can be treated with frequent feedings as well as cornstarch, which slows the absorption of food and may prevent hypoglycemic troughs [23••]. Medications include diazoxide (helpful in about 60% of patients) [24], calcium channel blockers [25], and octreotide. The efficacy, as well as unresolved issues pertaining to the use of octreotide in controlling symptoms, are discussed in a paper by Maton [26•]. In general, the unpredictable nature of octreotide in inhibiting insulin release from insulinomas has limited its therapeutic usefulness in this disease [27].

An excellent study investigating the management of gastric acid hypersecretion in patients with Zollinger-Ellison syndrome is presented by Metz *et al.* [28••]. For successful long-term medical management of this disease, the acid secretion must be less than 10 mEq/h for the hour prior to the next dose of antisecretory medication. Patients may require two to five times the usual dose of H_2-receptor antagonists needed for idiopathic peptic ulcer disease. In addition, 10% to 25% of Zollinger-Ellison patients require omeprazole every 12 hours rather than once a day. Patients who have undergone previous partial gastrectomy require acid outputs of less than 5 mEq/h to heal mucosal disease and prevent ulcer recurrence [29]. Furthermore, the subset of Zollinger-Ellison patients who exhibit severe esophageal disease may require acid outputs of less than 1 mEq/h to heal strictures and reduce the need for frequent esophageal dilatation [21].

Octreotide is effective in reducing the secretory diarrhea and plasma concentrations of vasoactive intestinal peptide in more than 80% of patients with VIPoma. Octreotide has also been shown to decrease plasma concentrations of glucagon and cause resolution of the

Table 1. Signs and symptoms, hormone production, incidence, and pathology of less common pancreatic endocrine tumors

Tumor type	Signs or symptoms	Hormone	Incidence	Identification at surgery, %	Location, %: Pancreas	Location, %: Duodenum	Malignant, %	With MEN-1
Glucagonoma	Rash, weight loss, malnutrition, diabetes	Glucagon	Rare	98–100	>99	—	70	Rare
VIPoma	Watery diarrhea, hypokalemia, hypochlorhydria	VIP	Rare	100	85	15	40	Rare
Somatostatinoma	Diabetes, cholelithiasis, steatorrhea, weight loss	Somatostatin	Rare	100	50	50	70	—
GRFoma	Acromegaly	GRF	Rare	100	30	10	30	30%
ACTHoma	Cushing's syndrome	ACTH	Rare	100	100	—	100	—
Neurotensinoma	Tachycardia, hypotension, cyanosis, malabsorption, hypokalemia	Neurotensin	Rare	100	100	—	>80	—
PTH-like-oma	Hypercalcemia, bone pain	PTH-like factor	Rare	100	100	—	100	—
Nonfunctioning	Abdominal pain, gastrointestinal bleeding, mass	Pancreatic polypeptide, neuron-specific enolase	1 in 5 million	100	>99	—	60	Common

ACTH—adrenocorticotropic hormone; GRF—growth hormone releasing factor; MEN-1—multiple endocrine neoplasia type 1; PTH—parathyroid hormone; VIP—vasoactive intestinal polypeptide.

Table 2. Diagnostic criteria for less common endocrine tumors of the pancreas

Tumor type	Diagnostic study	Results
Glucagonoma	Fasting plasma glucagon	Increased (>500 pg/mL)
VIPoma	Fasting plasma VIP	Increased (>250 pg/mL)
GRFoma	Fasting plasma GRF	Increased
Somatostatinoma	Fasting plasma somatostatin	Increased
ACTHoma	Urinary free cortisol	Increased
	Plasma ACTH	Increased
	Dexamethasone	Failure to suppress
	CRH	Failure to suppress
Neurotensinoma	Fasting plasma neurotensin	Increased
PTH-like-oma	Serum calcium	Increased
	Serum PTH	Undetectable
	Serum PTH-like factor	Increased

ACTH—ardrenocorticotropic hormone; CRH—corticotropin releasing hormone; GRF—hormone releasing factor; PTH—parathyroid hormone; VIP—vasoactive intestinal polypeptide.

rash associated with glucagonoma [26•]. Control of the diabetes mellitus and improvement of nutritional status using total parenteral nutrition if necessary are also important in the medical management of glucagonomas. Octreotide has been successful in controlling the symptoms caused by excessive growth hormone secretion in GRFomas [26•] but not the elevated adrenocorticotropic hormone (ACTH) levels in ACTHoma. It should be noted that Cushing's syndrome associated with an ACTHoma usually occurs with an islet cell tumor that secretes another peptide and causes another syndrome, most commonly Zollinger-Ellison syndrome [30]. In patients with ACTH-producing islet cell tumor, the symptoms of Cushing's syndrome are severe and by the time the diagnosis is made, each of these patients has hepatic metastases and a poor prognosis [31].

Localization

Despite sophisticated technology, 50% of insulinomas and gastrinomas are not evident on preoperative imaging studies [32••], thus prompting a myriad of recent publications detailing the sensitivity and specificity of various imaging modalities. Table 3 lists the accuracy of a variety of localization studies found by different investigators. Insulinomas are located in the pancreas in 99% of cases, whereas gastrinomas are located in extrapancreatic sites in 28% to 44% of cases, most commonly in the duodenum or lymph nodes [33]. van Heerden *et al.* [34•] provide an overview of localization studies used in patients with insulinomas. Many insulinomas are 2 cm or smaller in diameter, and thus are not detected using noninvasive techniques such as ultrasonography, computed tomography (CT), or magnetic resonance (MR) imaging. Selective celiac axis angiography, which produces a hypervascular blush of the adenoma in the pancreas, had previously been considered the single best imaging study, with sensitivities up to 95% [35]. However, its accuracy has appeared to decrease, with only 50% of insulinomas imaged in recent reports [12]. Portal venous sampling has an average sensitivity of 82% (range, 70% to 95%), and this sensitivity is independent of tumor size [36]. While portal venous sampling does not provide precise imaging of the tumor, it can provide localization to the head, body, or tail of the pancreas in 80% of patients and is considered by some to be the most sensitive test for indicating evidence of small adenomas [37,38]. Some suggest that the diagnostic ability of portal venous sampling falls considerably when the tumor is localized in the pancreatic tail [39], but others have not had that problem [37]. Other disadvantages of this imaging modality include its considerable expense, as well as the complication rate of 3% and mortality rate of 0.4% [40,41]. Doppman *et al.* [42•] describe a new technique called the calcium angiogram in which pancreatic arteriography is performed to image the tumor and identify which arteries perfuse different areas of the pancreas. Calcium gluconate is then rapidly injected into each selectively catheterized artery and plasma samples are obtained from the hepatic veins for insulin concentrations. A twofold elevation of insulin levels is considered to be a positive localization. Preliminary results demonstrated insulin gradients in the hepatic vein in 9 (100%) of 9 patients and unequivocal localization of tumor in 6 (66%) of 9 patients.

Two recent papers discuss the advantages of endoscopic ultrasonography in localizing pancreatic endocrine tumors [43•,44•]. The high-frequency resolution of this technique can distinguish structures as small as 2 to 3 mm in diameter. Endocrine tumors generally appear as homogeneous hypoechoic masses with smooth margins. Endoscopic ultrasonography was found to have a sensitivity of 80% to 85% and a specificity of 95%. With preliminary results suggesting superiority to angiography, endoscopic ultrasonography may emerge as the most sensitive preoperative imaging modality for the detection of small endocrine tumors of the pancreas [43•]. Endoscopic ultrasonography does not resolve the problem of localization of extrapancreatic tumors, however, and thus may be less helpful in localizing gastrinomas than insulinomas. It can reliably exclude a tumor in the head of the pancreas in Zollinger-Ellison patients.

Lamberts has had extensive experience with the use of isotope-labeled somatostatin analogs such as ^{123}I-Tyr^{3}-octreotide and ^{111}In-octreotide in the visualization of islet cell tumors. These results are discussed in recent review articles [45•,46•]. Primary endocrine pancreatic tumors as well as previously unrecognized metastases could be visualized in 80% of patients. Insulinomas were somewhat more difficult to visualize with this technique than gastrinomas because octreotide receptors were not present on all tumors. Lamberts *et al.* [46•] also noted that a positive octreotide scan can predict patients who will have a favorable response in terms of clinical symptoms to octreotide treatment.

Table 3. Preoperative localization studies of pancreatic islet cell tumors

Study	Localization modality	Patients, *n*	True positive results, *n(%)*
	Imaging		
Doherty *et al.* [12], Wank *et al.* [70]	Computed tomography	60	26(43)
Doherty *et al.* [12], Frucht *et al.* [71]	Magnetic resonance imaging	35	9(26)
Doherty *et al.* [12], Norton *et al.* [33]	Ultrasonography	43	10(23)
van Eyck *et al.* [45•], Lamberts *et al.* [46•]	Octreotide isotope-labeling	21	18(86)
Rösch *et al.* [43•]	Endoscopic ultrasonography	38	31(82)
Doherty *et al.* [12], Maton *et al.* [72]	Selective angiography	70	39(56)
	Regional localization		
Doherty *et al.* [12]	Insulinoma PVS	22	17(77)
Doppman *et al.* [42•]	Calcium angiography	9	9(100)
Miller *et al.* [73]	Gastrinoma PVS	55	32(58)
Thom *et al.* [47•]	Secretin angiography	36	32(89)

PVS—portal venous sampling.

Localization studies are critical in the assessment of patients with Zollinger-Ellison syndrome, since 25% to 50% of cases will have metastatic disease at the time of diagnosis [47•]. CT scanning reliably detects tumors greater than 3 cm in diameter. For smaller lesions, MR imaging with fat suppression was found to be superior to dynamic contrast-enhanced CT [48]. Selective arterial secretin injection studies have a 90% to 100% positive predictability rate and are more sensitive than portal venous sampling in the localization of duodenal gastrinomas (Fig. 1) [47•,49•]. Recently, selective arterial secretin injection was used to identify the vessel feeding an occult gastrinoma. At the time of surgery, methylene blue was injected through the catheter to selectively stain the gastrinoma [50•].

The remaining endocrine tumors of the pancreas, such as glucagonomas and VIPomas, are usually greater than 5 cm in size at the time of diagnosis. They are therefore easily imaged by CT scan or MR imaging [51].

Surgical management

The operative goal in patients with insulinoma is to locate and remove all of the tumor while avoiding unnecessary resection of normal pancreatic tissue. Tumors measure less than 2 cm in the majority of cases and are equally distributed throughout the pancreas [38]. Eighty percent of patients have solitary, benign β islet cell tumors [52•]. Because of their small size, these tumors often cannot be directly visualized at the time of surgery. Palpation has a sensitivity of 75% to 95% [36], but may miss tumors in the head of the pancreas because of the increased thickness of the gland in this region. Intraoperative ultrasonography has emerged as the best method for operative detection of insulinomas. It is less useful for localizing gastrinomas because of their common extrapancreatic location. An excellent review discusses the experience with intraoperative ultrasonography to date [32••]. Several studies have shown intraoperative ultrasonography to be more sensitive than palpation in the operative detection of insulinomas. Because it allows precise localization of tumors, intraoperative ultrasonography has enabled simple enucleation of insulinomas rather than blind pancreatic resections or Whipple pancreaticoduodenectomies. In addition, intraoperative ultrasonography accurately documents the relationship of the tumor to pancreatic vascular and ductal structures (Fig. 2). A critical point in the use of intraoperative ultrasonography is the need for an extended Kocher maneuver and adequate mobilization of the entire pancreas. Insulinomas found in the head of the pancreas are generally enucleated. Lesions in the body or tail of the pancreas are either enucleated or resected by distal or subtotal pancreatectomy depending on their relationship to the pancreatic duct. Blind distal pancreatectomy in cases where no tumor is found is no longer advocated [37,52•]. The rates of surgical cure for benign insulinomas range from 77% to 98% [52•].

The introduction of powerful antisecretory medications that adequately control gastric acid hypersecretion has shifted the goal of surgical intervention in patients with Zollinger-Ellison syndrome away from total gastrectomy and towards resection of the gastrinoma itself for potential cure. The vast majority (>80%) of gastrinomas are found in the gastrinomas triangle, which includes the head of the pancreas and the duodenum [53], although gastrinomas occurring in the stomach, jejunum, liver, ovary, kidney, lymph nodes, and greater omentum have also been reported [54]. Careful palpation and intraoperative ultrasonography are initially used to locate the tumor (Fig. 1 *bottom*). The greater and lesser omenta as well as regional lymph nodes are also explored. Despite thorough exploration, no tumor can be found in 15% to 50% of cases [55]. It has recently emerged that between 30% to 40% of Zollinger-Ellison patients have gastrinomas located in the duodenum (Fig. 3). Since these tumors are typically sin-

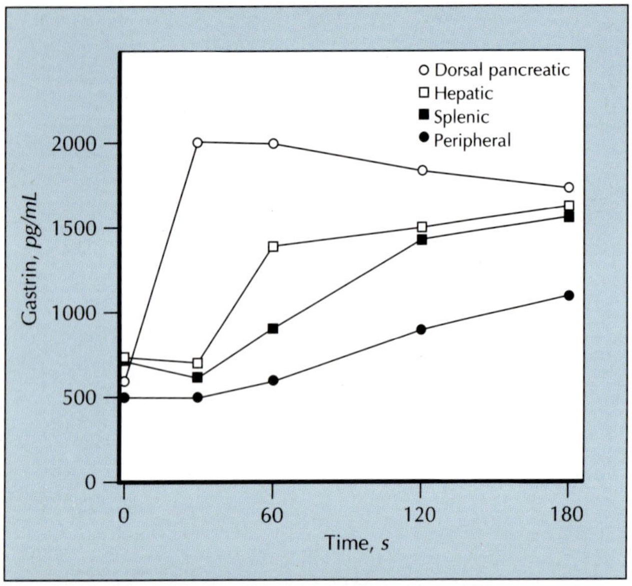

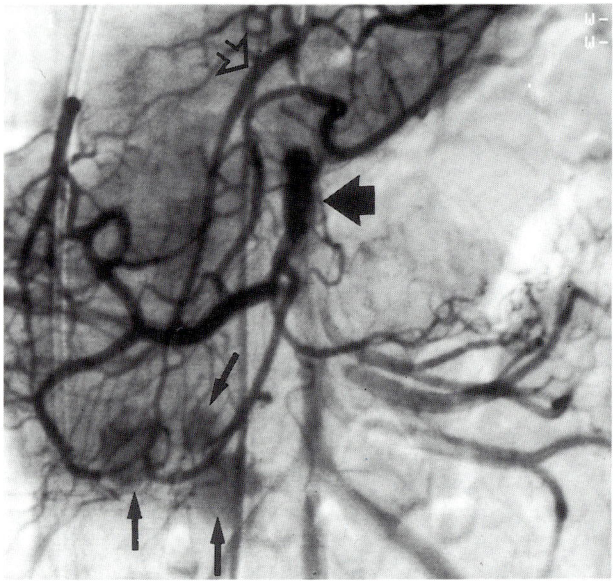

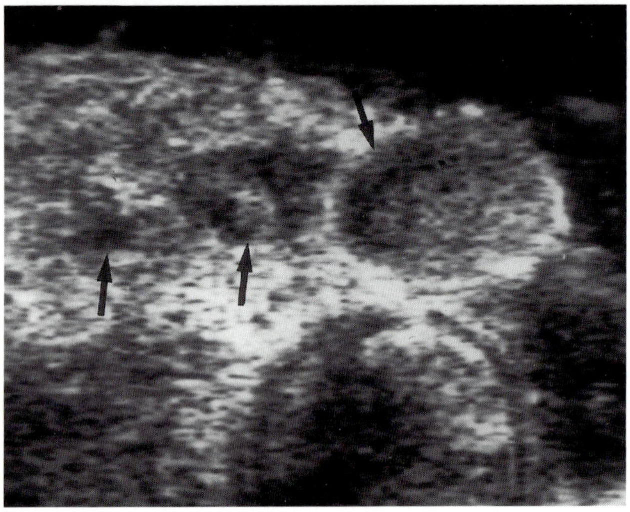

Fig. 1. Top left, Results of secretin angiogram in a patient with Zollinger-Ellison syndrome. Venous samples for gastrin measurement were obtained from the right hepatic vein following selective intra-arterial secretin injections. The elevated hepatic vein serum gastrin level found after injection of the dorsal pancreatic artery localizes the functioning gastrinoma to the head of the pancreas or duodenum. **Top right**, Selective angiogram in same patient. Radio-opaque contrast injected into the dorsal pancreatic artery (*open arrow*) reveals three round hypervascular lesions (*thin arrows*) in the head and uncinate process of the pancreas. These lesions proved to be islet cell neoplasms. Opacification of the superior mesenteric artery (*thick arrow*) is also seen. **Bottom,** Intraoperative ultrasonogram using a 7.5-MHz transducer. The three tumors visualized in *top right panel* appear sonolucent *(arrows)* compared with the surrounding pancreas.

gle, submucosal, and very small, they can easily be overlooked and thus be the cause of an unsuccessful surgical procedure [56]. Frucht *et al.* [55] reported that operative endoscopic transillumination had a greatly increased sensitivity (83%) over intraoperative ultrasonography and palpation (42%) in identifying duodenal gastrinomas and should therefore be performed routinely in all Zollinger-Ellison patients undergoing exploratory laparotomy for cure (Fig. 4). Thompson *et al.* [57••] discusses the importance of duodenotomy in the surgical treatment of these patients. Duodenotomy is especially important in identifying tumors on the medial wall of the duodenum, as these lesions are not transilluminated. Gastrinomas in the body or tail of the pancreas should be resected by distal or subtotal pancreatectomy-splenectomy [58]. Gastrinomas in the head of the pancreas are generally enucleated, although some centers perform pancreaticoduodenectomy in the majority of these patients [59•]. Duodenal tumors are removed with a full thickness elliptical excision of the duodenum. Delcore and Friesen [60•] advocate pancreaticoduodenectomy in the case of multiple metastases to pancreaticoduodenal lymph nodes, multiple duodenal wall gastrinomas, or involvement of the ampulla of Vater. If all tumor is removed in patients with Zollinger-Ellison syndrome, the immediate postoperative cure rate is 40% to 90%, although nearly 50% will recur at 6 years [17•].

Metastatic disease

Although malignant insulinomas are rare (5% to 10%), inspection of regional lymph nodes and the liver must be performed at the time of laparotomy. Limited metastatic disease can often be successfully resected.

Metastases occur in 25% to 90% of patients with gastrinomas, and the 5-year survival is only 20% to 38% [61•]. Duodenal primary gastrinomas were found to have a higher incidence of metastases (55%) than pancreatic gastrinomas (22%) in one study [17•]. In addition,

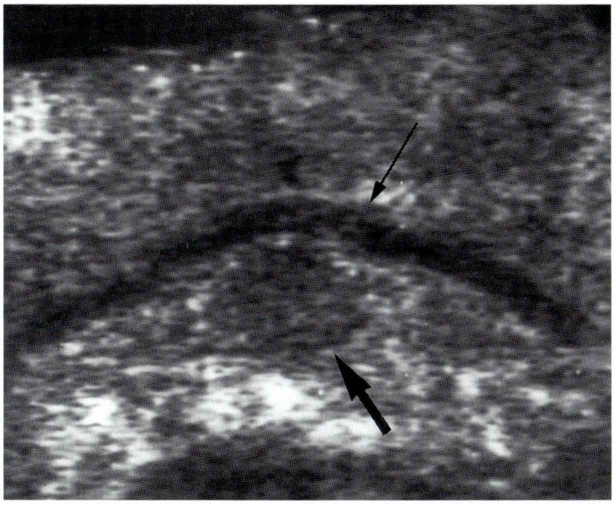

Fig. 2. Intraoperative ultrasonogram showing an 8-mm islet cell tumor (*thick arrow*) located just deep to the pancreatic duct (*thin arrow*). The lesion, which was not visualized by preoperative studies, also was not palpable at the time of surgery. Because of the close proximity of the tumor to the pancreatic duct, a distal pancreatectomy rather than enucleation of the lesion was performed.

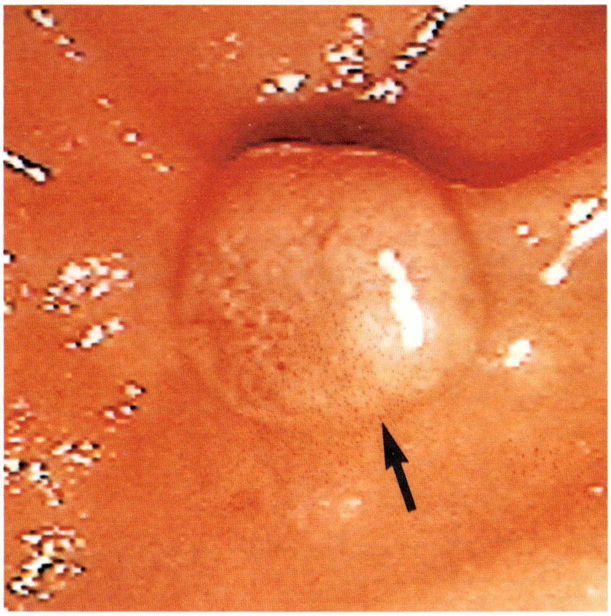

Fig. 3. Endoscopic view of a duodenal gastrinoma (*arrow*). The tumor, which is located on the anterior wall of the descending duodenum, measures less than 1 cm in size and is seen as a polypoid lesion through a side viewing endoscope. (*From* Norton [74]; with permission.)

duodenal gastrinomas as small as 2 mm have metastasized to regional lymph nodes [57••]. Miliary or extensive bilobar hepatic and distant metastatic disease are considered inoperable and are generally treated with chemotherapy including streptozotocin, doxorubicin hydrochloride, and/or 5-fluorouracil. Other treatments include hepatic artery embolization, chemoembolization [62], or recombinant interferon alfa-2b [63]. Patients with metastatic disease considered resectable by radiologic studies who underwent aggressive resection had a 5-year survival of 79% compared with 28% in patients who had inoperable metastatic disease [61•].

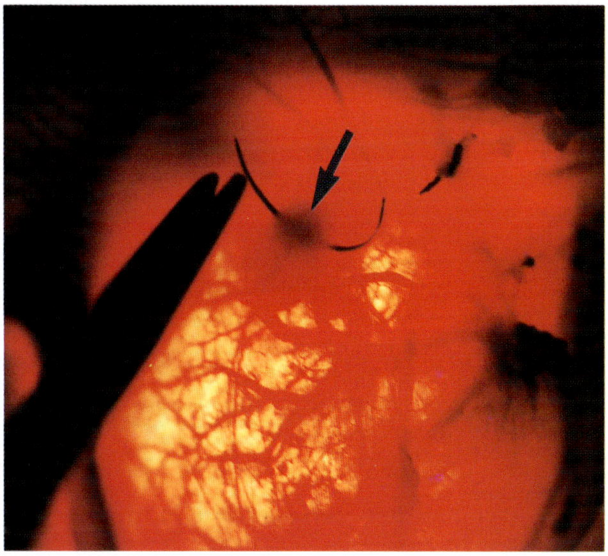

Fig. 4. Operative endoscopic transillumination of a duodenal gastrinoma. The lesion appears as a focal light defect (*arrow*) and measures only 2 mm in diameter. (*From* Sugg *et al.* [75]; with permission.)

The majority of the more rare neuroendocrine tumors of the pancreas have metastases at the time of diagnosis or surgery. However, aggressive surgical treatment such as pancreaticoduodenectomy, liver resection, or subtotal pancreatectomy-splenectomy may help ameliorate symptoms and extend survival if all tumors can be resected. In the case of somatostatinomas, glucagonomas, and PTH-like-omas, surgery to debulk the tumor may be important, as medical management is often not effective in controlling symptoms of hormone excess. Adrenalectomy is often required to control the hypercortisolism produced by ACTHomas [23••].

Multiple endocrine neoplasia type 1

Five percent to 25% of patients with islet cell tumors of the pancreas will have multiple endocrine neoplasia type 1 (MEN-1) syndrome. These patients always have multiple pancreatic islet cell tumors [64]. Gastrinomas occur in 54% of patients with MEN-1, and insulinomas occur in 20% [65]. Preoperative portal venous sampling or calcium angiogram is recommended in MEN-1 patients with insulinoma to better determine which of the multiple tumors found at exploration is responsible for excessive insulin production [52•]. Removal of the functionally dominant islet cell tumor is the most important step in the treatment of these patients.

The treatment of MEN-1 patients with Zollinger-Ellison syndrome is controversial. Previously it was thought that recurrence of acid hypersecretion was certain in these patients unless total gastrectomy or total pancreatectomy was performed. It was also thought that the malignant potential of islet cell neoplasms in patients with MEN-1 was relatively low. Currently, however, there is evidence that most gastrinomas in MEN-1 patients are malignant [65,66]. Thompson [67•] advocates performing transhepatic portal venous sampling for gastrin and exploring those patients showing regionalized secretion of gastrin. He also routinely performs duodenotomy as well as periduodenal and peripancreatic lymph node dissection whenever a duodenal gastrinoma is found. Palpable tumors in the head of the pancreas are enucleated and a distal pancreatic resection is generally performed even when no palpable tumors have been identified in this area. Using this aggressive surgical approach, 10 of 11 patients were rendered eugastrinemic [67•]. Others have not had similar results despite performing similar procedures [65,68]. It is important to surgically correct primary hyperparathyroidism as the initial procedure in MEN-1 patients with Zollinger-Ellison syndrome, as this usually results in a marked decrease in serum levels of gastrin [69].

References and recommended reading

Papers of particular interest, published within the annual period of review, have been highlighted as:
• Of special interest
•• Of outstanding interest

1. FRIESEN SR: **Tumors of the Endocrine Pancreas.** *N Engl J Med* 1982, **306**:580–590.

2. BUCHANAN KD, COLLINS JSA, VARGHESE A, JOHNSTON CF, SHAW C: **Sandostatin and the Belfast Experience.** *Digestion* 1990, **45 (suppl 1)**:11–16.

3. JENSEN RT, NORTON JA: **Pancreatic Endocrine Tumors.** In *Textbook of Gastroenterology*. Edited by Yamada T, Alpers DH, Owyang C, Powell DW, Silverstein FE. Philadelphia: Lippincott; 1991:1912–1936.

4. KLÖPPEL G, HEITZ PU: **Pancreatic Endocrine Tumors.** *Pathol Res Pract* 1988, **183**:155–168.

5. MUKAI K, GREIDER MH, GROTTING JC, ROSAI J: **Retrospective Study of 77 Pancreatic Endocrine Tumors Using the Immunoperoxidase Method.** *Am J Surg Pathol* 1982, **6**:387–399.

6. CREUTZFELDT W: **Endocrine Tumors of the Pancreas: Clinical and Morphological Patterns.** In *The Pancreas*. Edited by Fitzgerald PS, Morrison AB. Baltimore: Williams and Wilkins; 1980:208–230.

7. JENSEN RT, GARDNER JD: **Gastrinoma.** In *The Pancreas: Biology, Pathobiology, and Disease*, edn 2. Edited by Go VLW, Brooks FA, DiMagno EP, Gardner JD, Lebenthal E, Scheele GA. New York: Raven Press; 1993:936–986.

8. LARSSON LI, GRIMELIUS L, HÅKANSON R, REHFELD JF, STADIL F, HOLST J, ANGERVALL L, SUNDLER F: **Mixed Endocrine Pancreatic Tumors Producing Several Peptide Hormones.** *Am J Pathol* 1975, **79**:271–284.

9. CHIANG HCV, O'DORISIO TM, HUANG SC, MATON PN, GARDNER JD, JENSEN RT: **Multiple Hormone Elevations in Zollinger-Ellison Syndrome: Prospective Study of Clinical Significance and of the Development of a Second Symptomatic Pancreatic Endocrine Tumor Syndrome.** *Gastroenterology* 1990, **99**:1565–1575.

10. WYNICK D, WILLIAMS SJ, BLOOM SR: **Symptomatic Secondary Hormone Syndromes in Patients With Established Malignant Pancreatic Endocrine Tumors.** *N Engl J Med* 1988, **319**:605–607.

11. GRAMA D, ERIKSSON B, MÅRTENSSON H, CEDERMARK B, AHRÉN B,
• KRISTOFFERSSON A, RASTAD J, ÖBERG K, ÅKERSTRÖM G: **Clinical Characteristics, Treatment, and Survival in Patients With Pancreatic Tumors Causing Hormonal Syndromes.** *World J Surg* 1992, **16**:632–639.

Retrospective analysis of 85 patients with endocrine pancreatic tumors. Discusses symptoms, diagnosis, and treatment over follow-up period of 3 to 18 years.

12. DOHERTY GM, DOPPMAN JL, SHAWKER TH, MILLER DL, EASTMAN RC, GORDEN P, NORTON JA: **Results of a Prospective Strategy to Diagnose, Localize and Resect Insulinomas.** *Surgery* 1991, **110**:989–997.

13. SERVICE FJ, O'BRIEN PC, KAO PC, YOUNG WF: **C-Peptide Suppression Test: Effects of Gender, Age, and Body Mass Index; Implications for the Diagnosis of Insulinoma.** *J Clin Endocrinol Metab* 1992, 74:204–210.

14. GORDEN P, ROTH J, FREYCHET P, KAHN R: **The Circulating Proinsulin-like Components.** *Diabetes* 1972, **21**:673–677.

15. FRIESEN SR: **Treatment of the Zollinger-Ellison Syndrome: A 25-Year Assessment.** *Am J Surg* 1982, **143**:331–338.

16. THOMPSON JC, REEDER DD, VILLAR HV, FENDER HR: **Natural History and Experience With Diagnosis and Treatment of the Zollinger-Ellison Syndrome.** *Surg Gynecol Obstet* 1975, **140**:721–739.

17. NORTON JA, DOPPMAN JL, JENSEN RT: **Curative Resection in Zollinger-**
• **Ellison Syndrome: Results of a 10-Year Prospective Study.** *Ann Surg* 1992, **215**:8–18.

Prospective study of 73 patients, in 78% of whom gastrinomas were found and resected. Duodenal primary gastrinomas had a much greater incidence of malignancy and a shorter disease-free interval than pancreatic gastrinomas. Long-term disease-free survival in patients with localized sporadic Zollinger-Ellison syndrome was 30%. Patients who presented with metastatic disease had a 20% 5-year survival rate.

18. CAMERON AJ, HOFFMAN HN: **Zollinger-Ellison Syndrome: Clinical Features and Long-Term Follow-Up.** *Mayo Clin Proc* 1974, **49**:44–51.

19. ANDERSEN DK: **Current Diagnosis and Management of Zollinger-Ellison Syndrome.** *Ann Surg* 1989, **210**:685–703.

20. WAXSMAN I, GARDNER JD, JENSEN RT, MATON PN: **Peptic Ulcer Perforation as the Presentation of Zollinger-Ellison Syndrome.** *Dig Dis Sci* 1991, **36**:19–24.

21. MILLER LS, VINAYEK R, FRUCHT H, GARDNER JD, JENSEN RT, MATON PN: **Reflux Esophagitis in Patients With Zollinger-Ellison Syndrome.** *Gastroenterology* 1990, **98**:341–346.

22. SLAFF JI, HOWARD JM, MATON PN, VINAYEK R, WANK SA, MCCARTHY DM, GARDNER JD, JENSEN RT: **Prospective Assessment of Provocative Gastrin Tests in 81 Consecutive Patients With Zollinger-Ellison Syndrome.** *Gastroenterology* 1986, **90**:1637–1643.

23. NORTON JA: **Neuroendocrine Tumors of the Pancreas and Duodenum.**
•• *Curr Probl Surg* 1994, in press.

In-depth, comprehensive review covering all aspects of neuroendocrine tumors of the pancreas and duodenum.

24. COMI RJ, GORDEN P, DOPPMAN JL, NORTON JA: **Insulinoma.** In *The Exocrine Pancreas: Biology, Pathology and Disease*. Edited by Go VLW, Brooks FA, DiMagno EP, Gardner JD, Lebenthal E, Scheele GA. New York: Raven Press; 1986:745–761.

25. MURAKAMI K, TANIGUCHI H, KOBAYSHI T, SEKI M, OIMOMI M, BABA S: **Suppression of Insulin Release by Calcium Antagonist in Human Insulinoma *In Vivo* and *In Vitro*: Its Possible Role for Clinical Use.** *Kobe J Med Sci* 1979, **25**:237–247.

26. MATON PN: **Use of Octreotide Acetate for Control of Symptoms in**
• **Patients With Islet Cell Tumors.** *World J Surg* 1993, **17**:504–510.

Octreotide, a synthetic octapeptide analogue of somatostatin, has been effective in treating symptoms caused by VIPomas, glucagonomas, and GRFomas. Its effects on plasma insulin and glucose are inconsistent, but it can be useful in controlling hypoglycemia in some patients with unresectable insulinomas.

27. MATON PN, GARDNER JD, JENSEN RT: **Use of Long-Acting Somatostatin Analogue SMS 201-995 in Patients With Pancreatic Islet Cell Tumors.** *Dig Dis Sci* 1989, **34 (suppl)**:28S–39S.

28. METZ DC, PISEGNA JR, FISHBEYN VA, BENYA RV, JENSEN RT: **Control**
•• **of Gastric Acid Hypersecretion in the Management of Patients With Zollinger-Ellison Syndrome.** *World J Surg* 1993, **17**:468–480.

Excellent overview detailing the recent advances in the medical and surgical management of gastric acid hypersecretion in patients with Zollinger-Ellison syndrome.

29. MATON PN, FRUCHT H, VINAYEK R, WANK SA, GARDNER JD, JENSEN RT: **Medical Management of Patients With Zollinger-Ellison Syndrome Who Have Had Previous Gastric Surgery: A Prospective Study.** *Gastroenterology* 1988, **94**:294–299.

30. MATON PN, GARDNER JD, JENSEN RT: **Cushing's Syndrome in Patients With the Zollinger-Ellison Syndrome.** *N Engl J Med* 1986, **315**:1–5.

31. JENSEN RT, DOPPMAN JL, GARDNER JD: **Gastrinoma.** In *The Exocrine Pancreas: Biology, Pathobiology, and Disease*. Edited by Go VLW, Brooks FA, DiMagno EP, Gardner JD, Lebenthal E, Scheele GA. New York: Raven Press; 1986:727–744.

32. ZEIGER MA, SHAWKER TH, NORTON JA: **Use of Intraoperative Ul-**
•• **trasonography to Localize Islet Cell Tumors.** *World J Surg* 1993, **17**:448–454.

Presents comparative data in which the sensitivity of intraoperative ultrasonography exceeds all other preoperative and intraoperative imaging modalities in the detection of pancreatic islet cell tumors.

33. Norton JA, Doppman JL, Collen MJ, Harmon JW, Maton PN, Gardner JD, Jensen RT: **Prospective Study of Gastrinoma Localization and Resection in Patients With Zollinger-Ellison Syndrome.** *Ann Surg* 1986, 204:468–479.

34. van Heerden JA, Grant CS, Czako PF, Service FJ, Charboneau JW:
• **Occult Functioning Insulinomas: Which Localizing Studies Are Indicated?** *Surgery* 1992, 112:1010–1015.
Retrospective study in which 100% of occult, benign insulinomas were found and resected using intraoperative ultrasonography and palpation. Based on these results, the authors conclude that extensive preoperative studies are not cost-effective and are unnecessary.

35. van Heerden JA, Edis AJ, Service FJ: **The Surgical Aspects of Insulinomas.** *Ann Surg* 1979, 189:677–682.

36. Böttger TC, Junginger T: **Is Preoperative Radiographic Localization of Islet Cell Tumors in Patients With Insulinoma Necessary?** *World J Surg* 1993, 17:427–432.

37. Norton JA, Shawker TH, Doppman JL, Miller DL, Fraker DL, Cromack DT, Gorden P, Jensen RT: **Localization and Surgical Treatment of Occult Insulinomas.** *Ann Surg* 1990, 212:615–620.

38. Rothmund M, Angelini L, Brunt LM, Farndon JR, Geelhoed G, Grama D, Herfarth C, Kaplan EL, Largiader F, Morino F, Peiper H, Proye C, Röher H, Rückert K, Kümmerle F, Thompson NW, van Heerden JA: **Surgery for Benign Insulinoma: An International Review.** *World J Surg* 1990, 14:393–399.

39. Böttger TC, Weber W, Beyer J, Junginger T: **Value of Tumor Localization in Patients With Insulinoma.** *World J Surg* 1990, 14:107–114.

40. Gianello P, Gigot JF, Berthet F, Dardenne AN, Lambotte L, Rahier J, Otte JB, Kestens PJ: **Pre- and Intraoperative Localization of Insulinomas: Report of 22 Observations.** *World J Surg* 1988, 12:389–397.

41. Roche A, Raisonnier A, Gillon-Savouret MC: **Pancreatic Venous Sampling and Arteriography in Localizing Insulinomas and Gastrinomas: Procedure and Results in 55 Cases.** *Radiology* 1982, 145:621–627.

42. Doppman JL, Miller DL, Chang R, Gorden P, Eastman RC, Norton JA:
• **Intraarterial Calcium Stimulation Test for Detection of Insulinomas.** *World J Surg* 1993, 17:439–443.
Presents the calcium angiogram as a less morbid alternative to portal venous sampling in localizing occult insulinomas. Intra-arterial calcium stimulation provided unequivocal localization of tumor in 66% of patients.

43. Rösch T, Lightdale CJ, Botet JF, Boyce GA, Sivak MV, Yasuda K,
• Heyder N, Palazzo L, Dancygier H, Schusdziarra V, Classen M: **Localization of Pancreatic Endocrine Tumors by Endoscopic Ultrasonography.** *N Engl J Med* 1992, 326:1721–1726.
Study of 37 patients in which endoscopic ultrasonography was significantly more sensitive than angiography in localizing endocrine tumors of the pancreas (82% vs 27%, respectively).

44. Palazzo L, Roseau G, Salmeron M: **Endoscopic Ultrasonography in**
• **the Preoperative Localization of Pancreatic Endocrine Tumors.** *Endoscopy* 1992, 24 (suppl 1):350–353.
Study demonstrating the superior diagnostic accuracy rate (87.5%) of endoscopic ultrasonography versus ultrasonography (8.5%) and CT (17%) in the localization of pancreatic endocrine tumors. The problems posed by extrapancreatic tumors are also addressed.

45. van Eyck CHJ, Bruining HA, Reubi JC, Bakker WH, Oei HY,
• Krenning EP, Lamberts SWJ: **Use of Isotope-Labeled Somatostatin Analogs for Visualization of Islet Cell Tumors.** *World J Surg* 1993, 17:444–447.
Study showing that the higher density or higher affinity of somatostatin receptors in many of the islet cell tumors allowed visualization by radioactive isotope–labeled octreotide scanning in 80% of patients.

46. Lamberts SWJ, Reubi JC, Krenning EP: **Somatostatin Receptor Imag-**
• **ing in the Diagnosis and Treatment of Neuroendocrine Tumors.** *J Steroid Biochem Mol Biol* 1992, 43:185–188.
Good overview of the experience to date with isotope-labeled octreotide scanning in visualizing a variety of neuroendocrine tumors.

47. Thom AK, Norton JA, Doppman JL, Miller DL, Chang R, Jensen RT:
• **Prospective Study of the Use of Intraarterial Secretin Injection and Portal Venous Sampling to Localize Duodenal Gastrinomas.** *Surgery* 1992, 112:1002–1009.
Prospective study demonstrating that intra-arterial secretin injection was more sensitive (89%) than portal venous sampling (60%) in localizing gastrinomas. The intra-arterial secretin test was particularly sensitive in patients with duodenal gastrinomas, and the authors advocate using this test rather than portal venous sampling in patients with occult gastrinomas.

48. Semelka RC, Cumming MJ, Shoenut JP, Magro CM, Yaffe CS, Kroeker MA, Greenberg HM: **Islet Cell Tumors: Comparison of Dynamic Contrast-Enhanced CT and MR Imaging With Dynamic Gadolinium Enhancement and Fat Suppression.** *Radiology* 1993, 186:799–802.

49. Imamura M, Takahashi K: **Use of Selective Arterial Secretin Injection**
• **Test to Guide Surgery in Patients With Zollinger-Ellison Syndrome.** *World J Surg* 1993, 17:433–438.
Comprehensive overview of the use of the secretin angiogram in the preoperative and postoperative management of Zollinger-Ellison syndrome. The test is shown to have a 100% positive and a 100% negative predictability rate.

50. Ko TC, Flisak M, Prinz RA: **Selective Intra-arterial Methylene Blue In-**
• **jection: A Novel Method of Localizing Gastrinoma.** *Gastroenterology* 1992, 102:1062–1064.
Interesting case report of a 6-mm duodenal gastrinoma visualized and resected only after methylene blue was injected into the gastroduodenal artery feeding the tumor.

51. Norton JA, Levin B, Jensen RT: **Cancer of the Endocrine System.** In *Cancer: Principles and Practice of Oncology,* edn 4. Edited by DeVita VT, Hellman S, Rosenberg SA. Philadelphia: J.B. Lippincott; 1993:1333–1435.

52. Pasieka JL, McLeod MK, Thompson NW, Burney RE: **Surgical Ap-**
• **proach to Insulinomas: Assessing the Need for Preoperative Localization.** *Arch Surg* 1992, 127:442–447.
Retrospective study of 50 patients with hyperinsulinemia in which CT scanning localized 26% of tumors, angiography 44%, and transhepatic venous sampling 94%. The authors conclude that preoperative localization studies are essential in the surgical treatment of insulinomas.

53. Stabile BE, Morrow DJ, Passaro E: **The Gastrinoma Triangle: Operative Implications.** *Am J Surg* 1984, 147:25–31.

54. Pipeleers-Marichal M, Donow C, Heitz PU, Klöppel G: **Pathologic Aspects of Gastrinomas in Patients With Zollinger-Ellison Syndrome With and Without Multiple Endocrine Neoplasia Type 1.** *World J Surg* 1993, 17:481–488.

55. Frucht H, Norton JA, London JF, Vinayek R, Doppman JL, Gardner JD, Jensen RT, Maton PN: **Detection of Duodenal Gastrinomas by Operative Endoscopic Transillumination: A Prospective Study.** *Gastroenterology* 1990, 99:1622–1627.

56. Thompson NW, Vinik AL, Eckhauser FE: **Microgastrinomas of the Duodenum: A Cause of Failed Operations for the Zollinger-Ellison Syndrome.** *Ann Surg* 1989, 209:396–404.

57. Thompson NW, Pasieka J, Fukuuchi A: **Duodenal Gastrinomas, Duo-**
•• **denotomy, and Duodenal Exploration in the Surgical Management of Zollinger-Ellison Syndrome.** *World J Surg* 1993, 17:455–462.
Excellent article discussing the surgical management of duodenal gastrinomas.

58. Norton JA, Sugarbaker PH, Doppman JL, Wesley RA, Maton PN, Gardner JD, Jensen RT: **Aggressive Resection of Metastatic Disease in Selected Patients With Malignant Gastrinoma.** *Ann Surg* 1986, 203:352–359.

59. Stadil F, Bardram L, Gustafsen J, Efsen F: **Surgical Treatment of**
• **the Zollinger-Ellison Syndrome.** *World J Surg* 1993, 17:463–467.
Retrospective study of 53 patients with Zollinger-Ellison syndrome. Twenty-one patients underwent operation, and 21% were cured. The best results occurred when patients with gastrinomas localized to the head of the pancreas or duodenum by portal venous sampling underwent pancreaticoduodenectomy.

60. Delcore R, Friesen SR: **Role of Pancreatoduodenectomy in the Man-**
• **agement of Primary Duodenal Wall Gastrinomas in Patients With Zollinger-Ellison Syndrome.** *Surgery* 1992, 112:1016–1023.
Review of the increasing experience with duodenal gastrinomas and the indications for pancreaticoduodenectomy in selected patients. Addresses the controversial issue of "blind" pancreaticoduodenectomy in the treatment of Zollinger-Ellison syndrome.

61. Carty SE, Jensen RT, Norton JA: **Prospective Study of Aggressive**
• **Resection of Metastatic Pancreatic Endocrine Tumors.** *Surgery* 1992, 112:1024–1032.
Prospective study showing that patients with limited metastases who underwent aggressive surgery had improved survival over patients whose disease was determined to be inoperable. In contrast, patients with extensive metastatic disease who underwent aggressive surgery showed no survival advantage over patients with inoperable disease.

62. Neŭsović M, Ćirić J, Radojković S, Žarković M, Durović M: **Improvement of Metastatic Endocrine Tumors of the Pancreas by Hepatic Artery Chemoembolization.** *J Endocrinol Invest* 1992, 15:543–547.

63. Biesma B, Willemse PHB, Mulder NH, Verschueren RCJ, Kema IP, Debruijn HWA, Postmus PE, Sleijfer DT, Devries EGE: **Recombinant Interferon Alpha-2b in Patients With Metastatic Apudomas: Effect on Tumours and Tumour Markers.** *Br J Cancer* 1992, 66:850–855.

64. Thompson NW, Lloyd RV, Nishiyama RH, Vinik AI, Strodel WE, Allo MD, Eckhauser FE, Talpos G, Mervak T: **MEN-I Pancreas: A Histological and Immunohistochemical Study.** *World J Surg* 1984, 8:561–574.

65. Sheppard BC, Norton JA, Doppman JL, Maton PN, Gardner JD, Jensen RT: **Management of Islet Cell Tumors in Patients With**

Multiple Endocrine Neoplasia: A Prospective Study. *Surgery* 1989, **106**:1108–1118.

66. FRIESEN SR: **Treatment of the Zollinger-Ellison Syndrome: A 25-Year Assessment.** *Am J Surg* 1982, **143**:331–338.

67. • THOMPSON NW: **Surgical Treatment of the Endocrine Pancreas and Zollinger-Ellison Syndrome in the MEN-I Syndrome.** *Henry Ford Hosp Med J* 1992, **40**:195–198.

Study of 11 patients with MEN-1 and Zollinger-Ellison syndrome in which an aggressive surgical approach resulted in eugastrinemia in 10 of the patients. The frequency and often multiple nature of duodenal gastrinomas in MEN-1 patients are emphasized.

68. VAN HEERDEN JA, SMITH SL, MILLER LJ: **Management of the Zollinger-Ellison Syndrome in Patients With Multiple Endocrine Neoplasia Type 1.** *Surgery* 1986, **100**:971–977.

69. NORTON JA, CORNELIUS MJ, DOPPMAN JL, MATON PN, GARDNER JD, JENSEN RT: **Effect of Parathyroidectomy in Patients With Hyperparathyroidism, Zollinger-Ellison Syndrome, and Multiple Endocrine Neoplasia Type 1: A Prospective Study.** *Surgery* 1987, **102**:958–966.

70. WANK SA, DOPPMAN HL, MILLER DL, COLLEN MJ, MATON PN, VINAYEK R, SLAFF JI, NORTON JA, GARDNER JD, JENSEN RT: **Prospective Study of the Ability of Computed Axial Tomography to Localize Gastrinomas in Patients With Zollinger-Ellison Syndrome.** *Gastroenterology* 1987, **92**:905–912.

71. FRUCHT H, DOPPMAN JL, NORTON JA, MILLER DL, DWYER AJ, FRANK JA, VINAYEK R, MATON PN, JENSEN RT: **Gastrinomas: Comparison of Magnetic Resonance Imaging With Computed Tomography, Angiography, and Ultrasound.** *Radiology* 1989, **171**:713–717.

72. MATON PN, MILLER DL, DOPPMAN HL, COLLEN MJ, NORTON JA, VINAYEK R, SLAFF JI, WANK SA, GARDNER JD, JENSEN RT: **Role of Selective Angiography in the Management of Zollinger-Ellison Syndrome.** *Gastroenterology* 1987, **92**:913–918.

73. MILLER DL, DOPPMAN JL, METZ D, MATON PN, JENSEN RT: **Portal Venous Sampling in Zollinger-Ellison Syndrome: Technique, Results and Complications in 95 Procedures.** *Radiology* 1992, **182**:235–242.

74. NORTON JA: **Surgical Treatment of Islet Cell Tumors With Special Emphasis on Operative Ultrasound.** In *Frontiers of Gastrointestinal Research*. Edited by Jensen RT. Basel: S Karger AG; 1993: in press.

75. SUGG SL, NORTON JA, FRAKER DL, METZ DC, PISEGNA JR, FISHBEYN V, BENYA RV, SHAWKER TH, DOPPMAN JL, JENSEN RT: **A Prospective Study of Intraoperative Methods to Diagnose and Resect Duodenal Gastrinomas.** *Ann Surg* 1993, **218**:138–144.

Jennifer B. Meko, MD, and Jeffrey A. Norton, MD, Department of Surgery, Washington University School of Medicine, St. Louis, MO 63110, USA.

Laparoscopy and endoscopy

Editorial overview

Bruce V. MacFadyen, Jr, MD

University of Texas Medical School, Houston, Texas, USA

Current Opinion in General Surgery 1994:195–197

Laparoscopic inguinal herniorrhaphy

The papers in this section discuss three common surgical procedures that are performed laparoscopically. In the paper on laparoscopic inguinal herniorrhaphy, Moses Fallas and Edward Phillips (pp 198–202) report on their review of 1721 laparoscopic hernia repairs performed with various techniques including simple closure of the internal ring, the plug and patch technique, and the intraperitoneal and the extraperitoneal repair with mesh. It should be noted that in the 31 laparoscopic hernia repairs performed by simple closure of the internal ring, there was a 23% incidence of complications with two recurrences, one case of neuralgia, and four technical failures, whereas the 220 laparoscopic plug and patch hernia repairs had a complication rate of 12% and a hernia recurrence rate of 5.9%. The intraperitoneal placement of mesh was associated with a 1% recurrence rate and a complication rate of 15%.

These data, along with the series of MacFadyen *et al.* [1] and Fitzgibbons *et al.* [2], confirm that reinforcement of the entire inguinal region with a synthetic mesh is the preferred method, which is consistent with Stoppa's results using an anterior incision. Laparoscopically, the reinforcement can be performed as an intraperitoneal onlay mesh (IPOM), transabdominal preperitoneal prosthesis (TAPP), or totally extraperitoneal procedure. As noted by the authors, anterior hernia repairs do have low morbidity, mortality, and recurrence rates, although patients return to work later than those undergoing laparoscopic repair.

Several issues discussed by Fallas and Phillips should be noted. The first is whether the mesh should be placed intraperitoneally or retroperitoneally. From their data and those of others, it appears that the retroperitoneal mesh location is preferred. The second issue is whether to place the retroperitoneal mesh transabdominally or purely in an extraperitoneal approach. As noted in the review, the disadvantage of the TAPP and IPOM is the development of intra-abdominal adhesions and possible small bowel obstruction; this complication has been reported by Fitzgibbons *et al.* [2], although the incidence is low. It should be noted that the purely extraperitoneal method does not allow easy visualization of both inguinal regions, although the method described by Fallas and Phillips allows bilateral evaluation when the laparoscope is initially inserted transabdominally. It should also be noted that there is very little statistical difference in morbidity and recurrence rates for the IPOM, TAPP, and extraperitoneal approaches.

The third issue is hernia recurrence. Early recurrence, *ie*, recurrence in the first 6 to 12 months, is most likely related to technical failure, whereas recurrence after 2 to 5 years is related to tissue disintegration. It has been shown that 90% of the original hernia recurrences develop in the first 2 years, and Stoppa *et al.* [3] have observed that the large permanent mesh reinforces the entire inguinal region and significantly decreases the incidence of recurrence.

A fourth issue is the morbidity rate, which is relatively low with the TAPP or extraperitoneal repair. Neuralgia results from injury to the lateral femoral cutaneous nerve and the femoral branch of the genitofemoral nerve and has been shown to be related to lateral and posterior placement of staples on the mesh and vigorous dissection around the iliac vessels. Avoiding these technical pitfalls will significantly decrease the incidence of neuralgia.

In conclusion, the main benefits of laparoscopy lie in recurrent and bilateral inguinal hernia repairs and especially in improving return-to-work time. Although Fallas and Phillips emphasize the extraperitoneal technique, the data thus far do not suggest any significant

Abbreviations

ECRP—endoscopic retrograde cholangiopancreatography; **IPOM**—intraperitoneal onlay mesh; **TAPP**–transabdominal preperitoneal prosthesis.

 ISBN 1-85922-671-X ISSN 1065–6243

advantage of the extraperitoneal over the TAPP technique so long as the entire inguinal region is reinforced with synthetic mesh.

Common bile duct stones

In the paper discussing the laparoscopic and endoscopic management of common bile duct stones, David Pitcher, Daniel Martin, and Karl Zucker (pp 203–207) review the options that are currently available to the practicing surgeons. Endoscopic retrograde cholangiopancreatography (ERCP) has been the primary pre- and postoperative modality, and its use has increased with the introduction of laparoscopic cholecystectomy. The use of laparoscopic common bile duct exploration has developed slowly because it involves advanced laparoscopic techniques such as suturing and knot tying. The indications for preoperative ERCP include jaundice, cholangitis, pancreatitis, abnormal liver function, and an increase in bile duct diameter as determined by ultrasonography. As the authors point out, patients with jaundice, pancreatitis, and cholangitis were more likely to have common bile duct stones, whereas patients with abnormal liver function or a dilated common bile duct had a lower incidence ranging from 5% to 29%.

Intraoperatively, the laparoscopic approach to common bile duct stones includes exploration via the cystic duct and choledochotomy. Determining which method is better will depend on the size and location of the stone and the technical skill of the surgeons. In Petellin's [4] experience with choledochotomy, it was noted that complete ductal clearance was achieved in 90% of the cases. However, the incidence of retained stones after common bile duct exploration can be reduced to less than 1% if choledochoscopy is also used. Because laparoscopic common bile duct exploration is technically demanding, conversion to an open procedure may be required in up to 25% of the patients, or postoperative ERCP may need to be done. It should be noted that there is a 10% complication rate in laparoscopic common bile duct exploration and that the operative time is 146 minutes compared with 83 minutes for laparoscopic cholecystectomy alone. On the other hand, the transcystic approach is easier to perform, although it requires dilation of the cystic duct to 5 mm, and the surgeon is unable to explore the proximal bile duct 90% of the time.

Another unique option is the intraoperative antegrade sphincterotomy described by DePaulo [5]. In this technique, a standard ERCP papillotome is passed transcystically through the ampulla of Vater and visualized by an endoscope inserted into the duodenum, and a sphincterotomy is performed at the 12 o'clock position. The procedure eliminates the risk of pancreatic duct cannulation and postendoscopy pancreatitis and allows easy access to the proximal common bile duct and removal of stones 1 to 1.5 cm in diameter, while increasing operative time by only 17 minutes.

Mechanical, laser, and electrohydraulic lithotripsy, which can be used via the cystic or common bile ducts or via ERCP, are very useful in the treatment of large common bile duct stones. Laser and electrohydraulic lithotripsy must be delivered through a small fiber inserted into the common bile duct under direct vision with a flexible choledochoscope, which increases safety and reduces the risk of common bile duct perforation. Pitcher *et al.* emphasize that the success rate was 70.7% for laser lithotripsy, 81.7% for mechanical lithotripsy, and 91.8% for electrohydraulic lithotripsy.

Postoperative stone removal can be performed transhepatically or via ERCP. To increase the rate of common bile duct stone clearance to more than 95% via ERCP, a 7 French catheter is placed transabdominally through the cystic duct into the duodenum, which allows placement of a wire postoperatively and endoscopic transfer, so that the papillotomy can be done with few complications.

In conclusion, it is apparent that there are multiple options for managing common bile duct stones other than surgery, and the surgeon must be familiar with all of these options. However, the surgeon must keep in mind that conversion to an open operation is still an excellent option.

Laparoscopic colectomy

In their paper on controversies regarding laparoscopic colectomy for malignant disease, David Ota, Heidi Nelson, and Jane Weeks (pp 208–213) address several pertinent issues. Their first consideration regards cancer control and the adequacy of colon resection. The number of lymph nodes is an important predictor of survival, and as noted in this paper, laparoscopic colon resection can result in a lower number of recovered lymph nodes. This problem may be related to the learning curve in this technique; the number may increase with experience. This area of concern may indicate that the surgeon who does only an occasional colon resection should not be doing laparoscopic colon resection, but rather an open method. With the development and clinical use of laparoscopic ultrasonography, previously undetected lymph nodes will be localized more easily, thus increasing the accuracy of resection. How many lymph nodes constitute an adequate resection is debatable, but the number is probably 10 to 15.

The issue of tumor implantation in the surgical incision has always concerned the surgeon. It appears that the use of specimen bags and removal of the specimen through a small incision is the preferred method, as opposed to pulling the specimen though the distal bowel, which may result in its contamination.

Besides the concern of lymph node status, the "no touch technique" has previously been considered inviolable. Most surgeons now agree, however, that there is no statistical evidence that this technique has any advantage in a standard colon resection. Therefore, this should not be a significant issue in laparoscopic colon resection.

Morbidity and mortality rates are important concerns in any operative procedure. It has been observed, however, that as the technical skill of the surgeon increases, the overall incidence of complications decreases, and in larger series, morbidity is similar to that of a standard open operation.

Cost analysis and the quality of life will be major issues that surgeons must address in this decade. One should keep in mind that the total cost of the illness—not just the hospitalization cost—is the major concern. Hospitalization cost is only one aspect of the patient's care, and the cost-utility method is probably the best method for evaluating the overall treatment of illness. Heretofore, data on the total cost of illness have not been investigated carefully, but with the increased cost-consciousness of physicians, patients, and hospital administrators, this information will be obtained and will significantly influence surgical practice.

References

1. MacFadyen BV Jr, Arregui ME, Corbitt JD Jr, Filipi CJ, Fitzgibbons RJ Jr, Franklin ME, McKernan JB, Olsen DO, Phillips EH: **Complications of Laparoscopic Herniorrhaphy**. *Surg Endosc* 1993, 7: 155–158.
2. Fitzgibbons R, Annabale R, Litke B, *et al.*: **Nutritional Clinical Trial on Laparoscopic Inguinal Hernia Repair: Preliminary Results [Abstract]**. *Surg Endosc* 1993, 7:115.
3. Stoppa RE, Rivas JL, Warlaumont CR, *et al.*: **The Use of Dacron in the Repair of Hernias of the Groin**. *Surg Clin North Am* 1984, 64:269–285.
4. Petelin J: **Laparoscopic Approach to Common Duct Pathology**. *Surg Laprosc Endosc* 1991, 1:33–41.
5. DePaulo AL, Hashiba K, Bafutto M. *et al.*: **Laparoscopic Antegrade Sphincterotomy**. *Surg Laparosc Endosc* 1993 3:157–160.

Bruce V. MacFadyen, Jr, MD, University of Texas Medical School, 6431 Fannin, Houston, TX 77030, USA.

Laparoscopic inguinal herniorrhaphy

Moses J. Fallas, MD, and Edward H. Phillips, MD

Cedars-Sinai Medical Center, Los Angeles, California, USA

Traditional open hernia repairs are usually performed as outpatient procedures under local anesthesia, with minimal morbidity and low recurrence rates. To be widely accepted, any new procedure must at least match current standards of performance. This review summarizes the most widely used techniques for laparoscopic inguinal herniorrhaphy. Early results of over 1700 cases using these techniques are reported. Recurrence was lowest using the total extraperitoneal repair. In selected patients, laparoscopic inguinal herniorrhaphy is a safe and comparable alternative to standard open repairs.

Current Opinion in General Surgery 1994:198–202

More than 500,000 hernia procedures are performed annually in the United States alone. Traditional repairs are routinely completed as outpatient procedures under local anesthesia in less than 1 hour, with minimal postoperative pain. Recurrence rates are acceptable, in some series, as low as 1.6% [1]. Patients can return to work in 1 to 2 weeks, and patient acceptance of the procedure is very high. Therefore, it is easy to understand the slow acceptance of laparoscopic hernia repair. There is a potential for increased morbidity, as laparoscopy violates the peritoneal cavity. This can lead to bowel obstructions due to adhesions, or trocar site defects. Mesh is used in all repairs, and general anesthetic must be administered to safely perform the operation. In spite of these objections, the potential advantages of less postoperative pain and earlier return to work have prompted many surgeons to pursue clinical work in laparoscopic hernia repair. We review current techniques for laparoscopic inguinal herniorrhaphy and describe our own unique approach for this operation.

Types of repair

Closure of internal ring

In 1982, Ger *et al.* [2] performed laparoscopic closure of the internal ring for small indirect defects. The ring was simply closed with staples, without addressing the hernia sac. For larger herniae he inserted mesh into the preperitoneal portion of the sac and stapled it in place, thus closing the ring.

Plug and patch

In 1989, Schultz *et al.* (Paper presented at Third World Congress of Endoscopic Surgery, Bourdeaux France, 1992) described the transperitoneal plug and patch technique. Initially, they inserted rolled mesh to plug the defects, but this led to an unacceptable rate of recurrence. Schultz then modified the procedure by covering this plug with a small patch, which was then closed over with a flap of peritoneum and preperitoneal fat, holding it in place against the muscle wall. Herniae still recurred through the unrepaired inguinal tissue, so the technique was further modified by placing mesh over the entire inguinal floor and fixing it in place with staples.

Transabdominal preperitoneal prosthetic

The transabdominal preperitoneal prosthetic (TAPP) repair is the most commonly performed laparoscopic hernia operation. The peritoneum is incised, and a peritoneal flap is created. The hernia sac, Cooper's ligament, abdominal wall, and conjoined tendon are all dissected to clearly identify any defects. Mesh is then fixed to Cooper's ligament, the conjoined tendon, and transversalis fascia lateral to the internal ring, to cover the indirect, direct, and femoral areas. The peritoneal flap is then closed, covering the mesh (Arregui *et al.*, Paper presented Third World Congress of Endoscopic Surgery, Bordeaux, France, 1992).

Intraperitoneal

Fitzgibbons (Paper presented at SAGES Postgraduate Course, Washington, DC, 1992) developed a technique that leaves mesh fixed and exposed within the peritoneum. This procedure is quicker and easier to perform than a TAPP repair, because much of the dissection is avoided. Fitzgibbons began his work using intraperitoneal onlay mesh (IPOM) in the porcine model, and he found that adhesion formation was less when the mesh was placed laparoscopically, rather than via laparotomy. This worked well with indirect herniae, but failed with direct herniae [3]. Because of a case of

Abbreviations

IPOM—intraperitoneal onlay mesh; **TAPP**—transabdominal preperitoneal prosthetic.

 ISBN 1-85922-671-X ISSN 1065–6243

possible mesh erosion into bowel, he has discontinued performance of IPOM repairs.

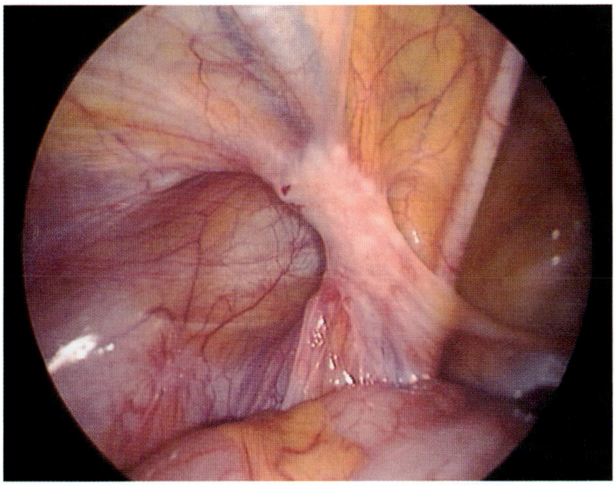

Fig. 1. Laparoscopic view of indirect left inguinal hernia.

Franklin (Personal communication) also uses an intraperitoneal mesh technique. He makes a small incision in the peritoneum overlying Cooper's ligament, and staples the mesh to the ligament. He then fixes the mesh with transfascial abdominal wall sutures. Keith needles are used to pass sutures inward through the abdominal wall, through the mesh, and then back out through the abdominal wall, where it is tied within a small incision.

Total extraperitoneal

Our team began total extraperitoneal hernia repairs in 1990. We use a modified Cheatle-Henry repair [4,5], using preperitoneal prosthetic mesh. Stoppa and Warlaumont [6] have reported excellent results using an abdominal wall incision to achieve a repair in this manner, with recurrence rates as low as 1.4%. In our technique the peritoneum is not incised, and the space between the abdominal wall and the peritoneum is developed with carbon dioxide and blunt dissection [7••]. This avoids the potential of bowel obstruction due to adhesions to the peritoneal closure.

The abdominal cavity is entered laparoscopically via an umbilical incision. A general exploration using a 30°angled laparoscope is performed, and herniae are identified (Fig. 1). With the patient in the reversed Trendelenburg position, a skin incision is made just superior to McBurney's point in the right and left sides of the abdomen. With a view from within the peritoneal cavity, a clamp is used to bluntly dissect down to the peritoneum, and then a 10- to 11-mm blunt-tip trocar is inserted between the peritoneum and the abdominal wall. Blunt dissectors or graspers are then used to separate the peritoneum from the underside of the abdominal wall. With carbon dioxide insufflation via the trocar, the peritoneum is dissected from the infraumbilical area down to Cooper's ligament and the femoral vessels. During the first part of this dissection vision is provided by the intra-abdominal laparoscope. When enough dissection is accomplished to allow the insertion of an 11-mm midline trocar into the preperitoneal space, a laparoscope is inserted in the preperitoneal space in the following manner.

An incision is made approximately 2 cm below the umbilical trocar. Blunt dissection with a clamp is again used to dissect through the abdominal wall until the peritoneum is reached. A disposable blunt-tip trocar is inserted through this incision between the peritoneum and the posterior abdominal wall. The laparoscope is then inserted through this trocar into the preperitoneal space. Under direct vision, the preperitoneal tissue and fat are dissected from the direct and indirect portions of the inguinal canal, and from Cooper's ligament. This allows excellent visualization of the aponeurotic sling, spermatic cord, femoral vessels, femoral canal, and iliopectineal line. Although we prefer to do so, the cord does not have to be mobilized in direct herniae. In indirect herniae the sac is reduced bluntly. In enlarged indirect or scrotal herniae it is occasionally transected using an endoscopic surgical loop to ligate it on the side of the abdominal cavity.

After both inguinal regions are completely dissected, a 12 by 11 cm sheath of mesh is rolled longitudinally, inserted into the preperitoneal space, and attached to Cooper's ligament, as previously described [7••]. Once both mesh rolls are attached to Cooper's ligament (Fig. 2, *top left*), the sutures holding the mesh are cut (Fig. 2, *top right*), and the mesh is unfurled superiorly (Fig. 2, *bottom*). Staples are then used to fix the mesh to the underside of the abdominal wall, near the conjoined tendon, to prevent the mesh from being pushed in to the defect. The slit in the mesh is then approximated around the cord in the preperitoneal space with tacking staples.

The trocar sites are injected with 0.5% bupivacaine hydrochloride. A laparoscope is replaced in the intraperitoneal space through the umbilical trocar, and carbon dioxide is evacuated from the preperitoneal space, allowing assessment for adequacy of the repair (Fig. 3) and identification of possible "reduction en masse." After inspection, the laparoscope and intraperitoneal trocars are removed, and the 11-mm trocar sites are closed with 0-Vicryl. The skin incisions are closed with subcuticular 4-0 Vicryl.

Total extraperitoneal repair without peritoneoscopy

McKernan (Paper presented at the Third World Congress of Endoscopic Surgery, Bordeaux, France, 1992) accomplishes the total extraperitoneal repair without entering the peritoneal cavity, even for a laparoscopic examination. The operation is begun by entering the preperitoneal space with the Hasson blunt-tip trocar, introduced in the infraumbilical hernia. After inserting an operating laparoscope, McKernan insufflates carbon dioxide to aid blunt dissection of the preperitoneal space in the lower abdomen until the rectus muscle is seen anteriorly and the peritoneum posteriorly. He then inserts two additional midline trocars

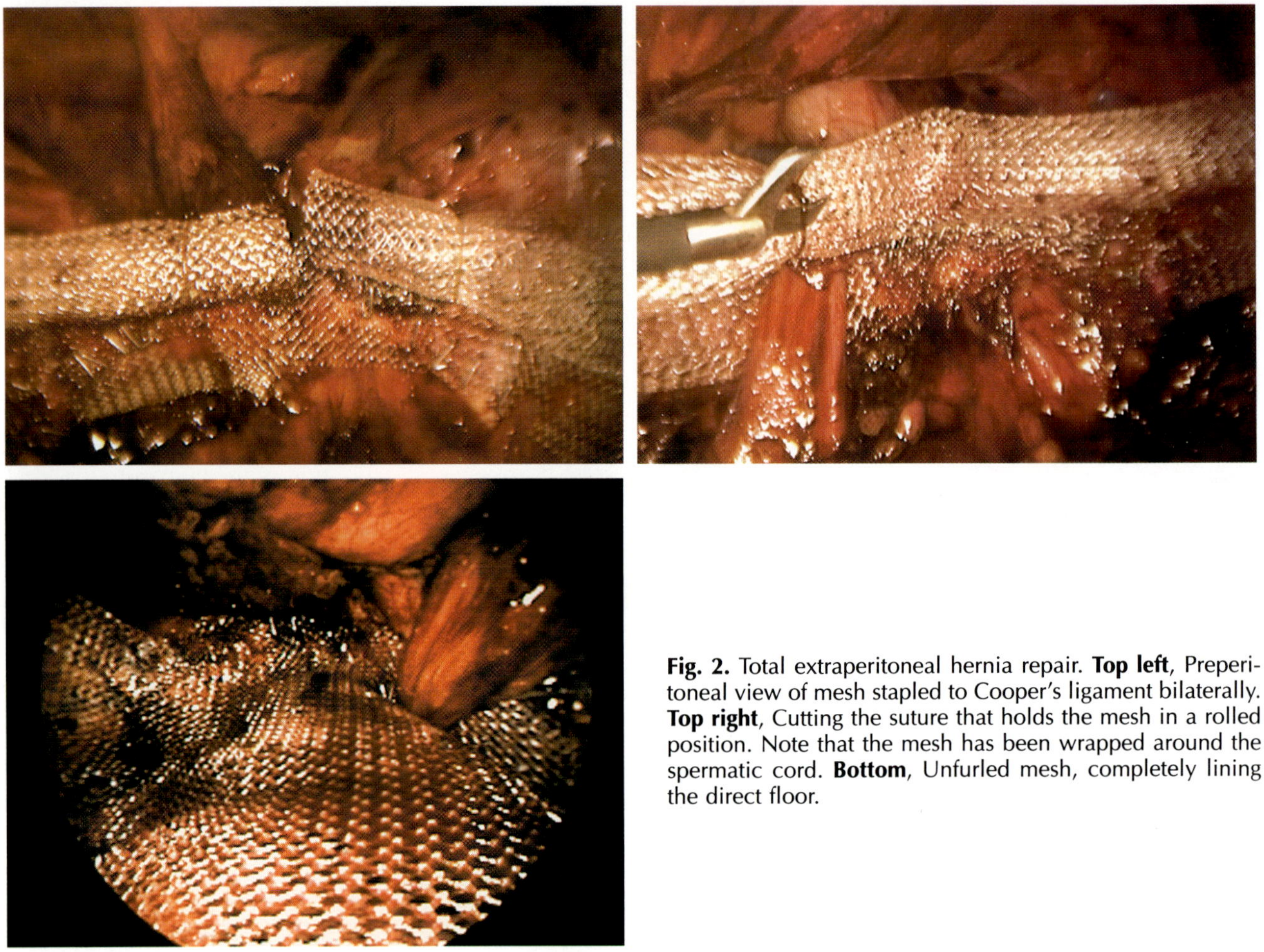

Fig. 2. Total extraperitoneal hernia repair. **Top left**, Preperitoneal view of mesh stapled to Cooper's ligament bilaterally. **Top right**, Cutting the suture that holds the mesh in a rolled position. Note that the mesh has been wrapped around the spermatic cord. **Bottom**, Unfurled mesh, completely lining the direct floor.

in the preperitoneal space and performs a modified Stoppa repair. In a direct inguinal hernia, the preperitoneal sac and contents are dissected from the fascial defect. In an indirect defect, the spermatic cord and vascular structures are dissected out in the preperitoneal area. A small indirect sac is dissected from the cord structures, while large indirect sacs are divided, leaving the distal sac, which may extend into the scrotum, in place. The mesh is then inserted and fixed to Cooper's ligament and the underside of the rectus muscle [8].

Results

We have previously reported the cumulative results of a total of 1721 laparoscopic hernia repairs [7••]. These comprised five groups, according to the operative technique employed. Total extraperitoneal repair was performed in 22% of cases. Transabdominal preperitoneal approach was used in the largest number of repairs, which accounted for 52% of the total repairs performed. The plug and patch, intraperitoneal, and simple closure of the internal ring techniques accounted for 13%, 11% and 2%, respectively, of the total number of repairs.

The recurrence rate was lowest for the 381 repairs performed using a total extraperitoneal technique. In this group there were 30 other complications (8%), 20 of which were small hematomas. Seromas occurred in five cases. There were two cases of neuralgia. Testicular pain, chronic pain, and urinary complications each were reported in one case.

Of 895 TAPP repairs, recurrence was reported in five cases (0.6%). Including recurrences, a total of 45 complications were reported (5%). These included seven neuralgias, 16 hematomas, one hemorrhage requiring transfusion, two trocar site infections, testicular pain in five cases, and chronic pain in one case. Hydrocele and ileus each occurred in one case.

The IPOM procedure was performed in 194 repairs. There were two recurrences (1%). Including recurrences, a total of 29 complications were reported (15%). There were seven neuralgias, four hematomas, and one hemorrhage requiring transfusion. Patients complained of testicular pain in four cases. There was one bladder injury, and four other urinary complications. Hydrocele occurred in four cases, and pubic osteitis in one case.

There were 220 plug and patch repairs performed, with a total of 27 complications (12%). There were 13 re-

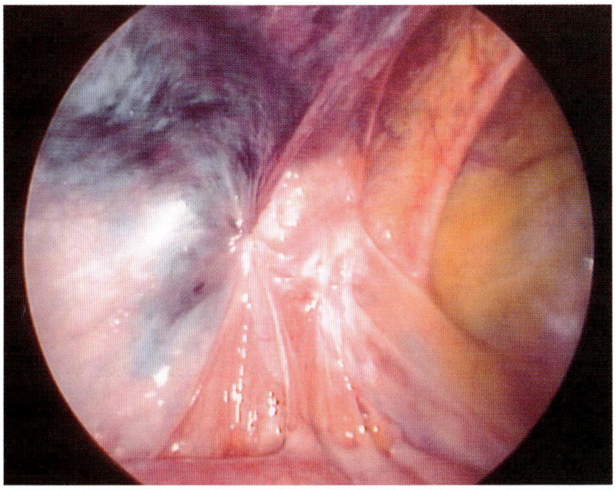

Fig. 3. Total extraperitoneal hernia repair. Laparoscopic intraperitoneal view after repair has been completed.

currences (5.9%). Other complications included three hematomas, four cases of testicular pain, and five urinary complications. There were two cases of small bowel obstruction.

Following 31 repairs performed by the method of simple closure of the internal ring, there were seven complications (23%), including two recurrences, one neuralgia, and four technical failures. This group had the highest rate of complications, although the sample size was relatively small, accounting for only 2% of the repairs reported in this series. This group also had the highest rate of recurrence, at 6.5%.

The overall complication rate was 8%, which includes recurrence complications. Hematoma was the most frequent complication, reported in 2.5% of the repairs. A small bowel obstruction occurred in two cases in the entire series; both followed the plug and patch technique.

Discussion

Although the available follow-up is short, the recurrence rate of 1.3% in this series compares quite favorably with recurrence rates associated with classic hernia repairs, which range from 0% to 7% for indirect, 1% to 10% for direct, and 5% to 35% for recurrent herniae. Most herniae recur within 1 year of repair; nearly 90% recur within 2 years [9].

Fitzgibbons *et al.* (Paper presented at SAGES Annual Meeting, Phoenix, AZ, 1993) and MacFadyen *et al.* [10•] reported the results of differing techniques of laparoscopic herniorrhaphy from several centers and concluded that laparoscopic hernioplasty was safe and effective. Fitzgibbons *et al.* reported 736 repairs in 597 patients. There were 25 (3.4%) recurrences (IPOM had a 4.6% incidence), and an additional 267 complications (36%), most of which were minor. There was one (0.2%) death due to a myocardial infarction. MacFadyen (Paper presented at SAGES 1992 Postgraduate Course, Washington, DC, 1992) reported 635 repairs in 563 patients (some of the same cases). There were nine (1.4%) recurrences and 52 (8%) complications, only two of which were major.

Those who argue that the use of mesh is not justified in primary hernia repair are concerned about the possibility of mesh infection. However, in Amid *et al.*'s [11] total experience of 7133 mesh repairs, the infection rate was 0.028%. So far the total extraperitoneal and TAPP methods for prosthetic repair of herniae show promise in low rates of recurrence and complications. By placing the mesh in the preperitoneal space we achieve two theoretical advantages. One advantage is that clearance of bacteria may be greater than in the subcutaneous tissue. The second advantage is that contamination from either the skin or a superficial wound infection is less likely, because the mesh is inserted via a trocar. Furthermore, the prosthesis is not left in direct contact with the subcutaneous tissue, in contrast to nonlaparoscopic mesh repairs. Instead, it is kept isolated from the exterior by the relative remoteness of the trocar site from the mesh and the continued protective effect of intraperitoneal pressure, which seals the prosthesis between the intact peritoneum and abdominal wall.

The most frequently mentioned disadvantage of the IPOM and TAPP techniques is the potential for adhesion formation and the risk of small bowel obstruction associated with the use of exposed intraperitoneal prosthetic material. However, intra-abdominal adhesions have not yet been observed to be a major problem (Paper presented at SAGES Postgraduate Course, Washington, DC, 1992).

Not all inguinal herniae can be recognized on laparoscopic examination. Indirect herniae are the easiest to identify. In fact, small subclinical indirect herniae are sometimes incidentally found at laparoscopy. Direct defects are more commonly overlooked than indirect defects. It is also more difficult to identify a recurrent hernia where preperitoneal fat may be incarcerated and the peritoneum is not indented.

Extensive surgery or multiple prior surgeries in the lower abdomen or pelvis are a relative contraindication to laparoscopic herniorrhaphy. The conventional approach is preferable when laparoscopic operative time and risk would be unnecessarily increased by the need to take down adhesions. While prior appendectomy usually does not present a problem, the total extraperitoneal approach is difficult with a prior lower midline Pfannenstiel or paramedian incision.

Conclusions

Total extraperitoneal laparoscopic inguinal hernia repair provides the benefit of avoiding the peritoneal cavity while performing a repair that traditionally has a very low recurrence rate. This operation does not violate the peritoneal cavity, except at the umbilical trocar site, and should not create pelvic adhesions. While the complication rate of endoscopic techniques is unknown, early results justify the continued use of these repairs. Further technical improvements and prospective randomized studies with careful follow-up will determine the proper usage of laparoscopic methods among the many approaches to inguinal hernia repair.

References and recommended reading

Papers of particular interest, published within the annual period of review, have been highlighted as:

- • Of special interest
- •• Of outstanding interest

1. CORBITT JD: **Laparoscopic Herniorrhaphy**. *Surg Laparosc Endosc* 1991, **1**:23–25.
2. GER R, MONROE R, DUVIVIER R, *ET AL.*: **Management of indirect inguinal hernias by a laparoscopic closure of the neck of the sac**. *Am J Surg* 1990, **159**:370.
3. SALERNO GM, FITZGIBBONS RJ, FILIPI CJ: **Laparoscopic Inguinal Hernia Repair**. In *Surgical Laparoscopy*. Edited by Zucker KA. St. Louis: Quality Medical Publishing; 1991:281–293.
4. CHEATLE GL: **An Operation for the Radical Cure of Inguinal and Femoral Hernia**. *BMJ* 1920, **2**:68.
5. READ R: **The Cheatle-Henry Approach to the Groin**. *Surg Rounds* 1983, 50–57.
6. STOPPA RE, WARLAUMONT CR: **The Preperitoneal Approach and Prosthetic Repair of Groin Hernia**. In *Hernia*. Edited by Nyhus LM, Condon RE. Philadelphia: JP Lippincott; 1989:199–225.
7. •• PHILLIPS EH, CARROLL BJ: **Laparoscopic Inguinal Hernia Repair**. *Gastrointest Endosc Clin North Am* 1993, **3**:297–307.

Presents detailed description of our own approach to laparoscopic inguinal hernia repair.

8. MCKERNAN JB, LAWS H: **Laparoscopic Preperitoneal Prosthetic Repair of Inguinal Hernias**. *Surg Rounds* 1992, **15**:597–608.
9. CONDON RE, NYHUS LM: **Complications of Groin Hernias**. In *Hernia*. Edited by Nyhus LM, Condon RE. Philadelphia: JB Lippincott; 1989:106–118.
10. • MACFADYEN BV, ARREGUI M, CORBITT J, FILIPI CJ, FITZGIBBONS RJ JR, FRANKLIN ME, MCKERNAN JB, OLSEN DO, PHILLIPS EH, ROSENTHAL D:**Complications of Laparoscopic Herniorrhaphy**. *Surg Endosc* 1993, **7**:155–158.

The principle of laparoscopy was applied to anterior inguinal hernia repair in a series of 762 patients with 841 inguinal hernias. The early results indicate that the overall complication rates were low. It is concluded that laparoscopic inguinal herniorrhaphy is a safe and effective procedure.

11. AMID PK, SHULMAN AG, LICHTENSTEIN IL: **Selecting Prosthetic Mesh for the Repair of Groin Hernia**. *Postgrad Gen Surg* 1992, **4**:150–155.

Moses J. Fallas, MD, 8635 West Third Street, Suite 795W, Los Angeles, CA 90048, USA.

Laparoscopic and endoscopic management of common bile duct stones

David E. Pitcher, MD, Daniel T. Martin, MD, and Karl A. Zucker, MD

University of New Mexico School of Medicine and Veterans Administration Medical Center, Albuquerque, New Mexico, USA

The rapid evolution and acceptance of laparoscopic cholecystectomy for the management of symptomatic cholelithiasis and acute and chronic cholecystitis are unprecedented in modern surgical practice. With rapid advances in laparoscopic and endoscopic instrumentation and surgical skills, many surgeons are developing minimally invasive techniques and strategies for treating the patient with known, suspected, or unsuspected choledocholithiasis. Recent articles describing the current status, complications, results, and future directions of laparoscopic and endoscopic management of common bile duct stones are reviewed. The role of endoscopic retrograde cholangiopancreatography and sphincterotomy, laparoscopic exploration of the common bile duct, choledochoscopy, and percutaneous transhepatic extraction techniques are discussed.

Current Opinion in General Surgery 1994:203–207

Laparoscopic cholecystectomy has rapidly gained acceptance as the preferred method for treating patients with symptomatic cholelithiasis, chronic cholecystitis, and most patients with acute cholecystitis and gallstone pancreatitis. Of all patients with gallstones, an estimated 8% to 15% of individuals less than 60 years of age and 15% to 60% of those greater than 60 years of age will be found to have choledocholithiasis at the time of cholecystectomy [1]. In most centers with experienced biliary endoscopists, patients suspected of having common duct stones or other biliary pathology prior to planned operative intervention have been routinely advised to undergo preoperative endoscopic retrograde cholangiopancreatography (ERCP), with sphincterotomy and stone extraction if necessary. Until recently, most unsuspected choledocholithiasis discovered at the time of laparoscopic cholecystectomy was managed either by postoperative ERCP with sphincterotomy and stone extraction or by open cholecystectomy and common bile duct exploration. As laparoscopic surgical skills and instrumentation have improved, increasing numbers of surgeons are attempting intraoperative clearance of common duct stones with a variety of minimally invasive laparoscopic and endoscopic techniques [2,3].

Management strategies for patients with choledocholithiasis continue to evolve but depend in general on the local endoscopic and laparoscopic surgical skill level. Table 1 lists the currently described management options for patients with known, suspected, unsuspected, and retained common bile duct stones.

Biliary endoscopy

Preoperative biliary endoscopy has become a common method for evaluating and treating patients with suspected choledocholithiasis prior to laparoscopic cholecystectomy. This trend has been attributed to the lack of ability of most surgeons to clear the common duct laparoscopically and the subsequent need to convert to an open laparotomy and formal common bile duct exploration. ERCP has also been frequently used postoperatively for those patients found on intraoperative cholangiography, to have previously unsuspected common duct stones. Success rates for ERCP with stone extraction (if necessary) have ranged from 85% to 95% [3]. Occasionally, two or more attempts at biliary endoscopy are required to cannulate the common bile duct successfully and perform papillotomy and sphincterotomy. Although usually successful, this approach is not without risk. In several recently published collective review articles, the incidence of major complications has been reported to be as high as 10% with a procedure-related mortality of 1% or more [4–6]. In addition, 60% to 85% of preoperative ERCP will reveal no evidence for choledocholithiasis, despite a moderate to high degree of clinical suspicion [2,7]. This would suggest that many preoperative ERCPs are unnecessary and may place a significant number of patients at unnecessary additional risk in the attempt to avoid open surgery.

A recent article by Cotton [6] provides an excellent overview of the role of ERCP in the era of laparo-

Abbreviations

ERCP—endoscopic retrograde cholangiopancreatography; **LCBDE**—laparoscopic common bile duct exploration.

 ISBN 1-85922-671-X ISSN 1065–6243

Table 1. Management options for known or suspected choledocholithiasis

Preoperative
High suspicion: ERCP
Moderate suspicion: ERCP optional
Low suspicion: no ERCP
Intraoperative
Laparoscopic CBDE (transcystic or via choledochotomy)
Balloon catheter extraction
Fluoroscopically guided wire basket extraction
Choledochoscopy
Intraoperative ERCP
Laparoscopic antegrade sphincterotomy
Open conversion with CBDE
Expectant management (stones < 5 mm)
Percutaneous access to cystic or common duct via soft catheter, T tube, or guide wire for postoperative stone extraction
Postoperative
ERCP
Percutaneous extraction via T tube or equivalent access
Basket extraction
Mechanical lithotripsy
Laser lithotripsy
Percutaneous transhepatic extraction
Electrohydrolic lithotripsy
Oral dissolution therapy
Open CBDE
Biliary-enteric bypass

CBDE—common bile duct exploration; ERCP—endoscopic retrograde cholangiopancreatography.

scopic cholecystectomy. In this paper, the indications for preoperative ERCP are defined on the basis of the degree of suspicion of common duct pathology and the local endoscopic expertise. Patients can be divided into three groups based upon the predictive values of historic factors (recent jaundice, cholangitis, pancreatitis), abnormal liver function tests, and bile duct size as measured by ultrasonography. Patients with any past or present jaundice, cholangitis, or acute pancreatitis in conjunction with liver function abnormalities and a dilated common bile duct on ultrasonography are deemed very likely to have common bile calculi. This group of patients should generally undergo preoperative ERCP if the expertise is available and laparoscopic common bile duct exploration is not. The second group of patients consists of those without any historical or clinical indicators of common duct pathology. Most endoscopists agree that these patients do not need preoperative ERCP, because only 2% or fewer will be found to have choledocholithiasis at the time of surgery. The most controversial group of patients includes those who may have one or two abnormalities of liver functions and only mild clinical indications of common duct pathology. As Cotton points out, there are no controlled trials addressing this group of patients, and there is no agreement among endoscopic experts. The second major factor influencing the indications for preoperative ERCP is local endoscopic expertise. Cotton describes a paradoxical increase in the use of preoperative ERCP if the local expertise with biliary endoscopy is only moderate or low. This he attributes to a lack of confidence in the ability to clear the duct postoperatively if stones are found at the time of operation. Endoscopists with high expertise are more likely to be confident of and successful in clearing the duct postoperatively. Cotton's own data from the Duke University Medical Center reveal a 94% success rate in clearing the common bile duct of stones.

The indications for postoperative biliary endoscopy after laparoscopic cholecystectomy are more clear-cut and basically include any postoperative indication of ongoing ductal pathology (*eg*, retained stones, bile leak, ductal injury, and missed pathology). An algorithm for the use of ERCP in conjunction with laparoscopic cholecystectomy as proposed by Cotton is shown in Figure 1.

Laparoscopic exploration

Despite the success of ERCP and other nonsurgical methods of managing common duct stones, many surgeons have recognized the potential health-care and economic benefits of a single-stage minimally invasive approach. Surgeons are now developing the necessary laparoscopic surgical skills and borrowing techniques from both conventional methods of common bile duct exploration and flexible biliary endoscopy to perform increasing numbers of successful laparoscopic common bile duct explorations (LCBDEs).

Recent articles by Hunter and Soper [2] and Petelin [8••] provide an excellent overview of the methods and results of LCBDE. Techniques for bile duct access using either the transcystic duct approach or a laparoscopic choledochotomy are discussed. The transcystic approach has clearly become the preferred method of common bile duct access because it obviates the need for extensive common bile duct dissection, intracorporeal suturing of the choledochotomy, and in most cases laparoscopically guided T-tube placement. In Petelin's experience, more than 90% of LCBDEs were accomplished utilizing the transcystic approach. Recent dramatic improvements with portable C-arm fluoroscopic technology along with the development of smaller (≤ 3.0 mm in diameter) and more versatile flexible choledochoscopes have been primarily responsible for the increasing success of this approach.

After access to the common bile duct is gained, several methods of stone extraction can be used. Both reports describe the use of fluoroscopic transcystic fogarty catheters, wire baskets, and mechanical, electrohydrolic, and pulsed-dye laser lithotriptors. Techniques using laparoscopic transcystic choledochoscopy are described as well. Benefits and limitations of each of these LCBDE techniques are discussed. In general, Hunter and Soper and Petelin advocate using simpler techniques of common duct clearance prior to choledochoscopy or lithotriptor techniques. Hunter and Soper also describe various management techniques and strategies for common duct stones that

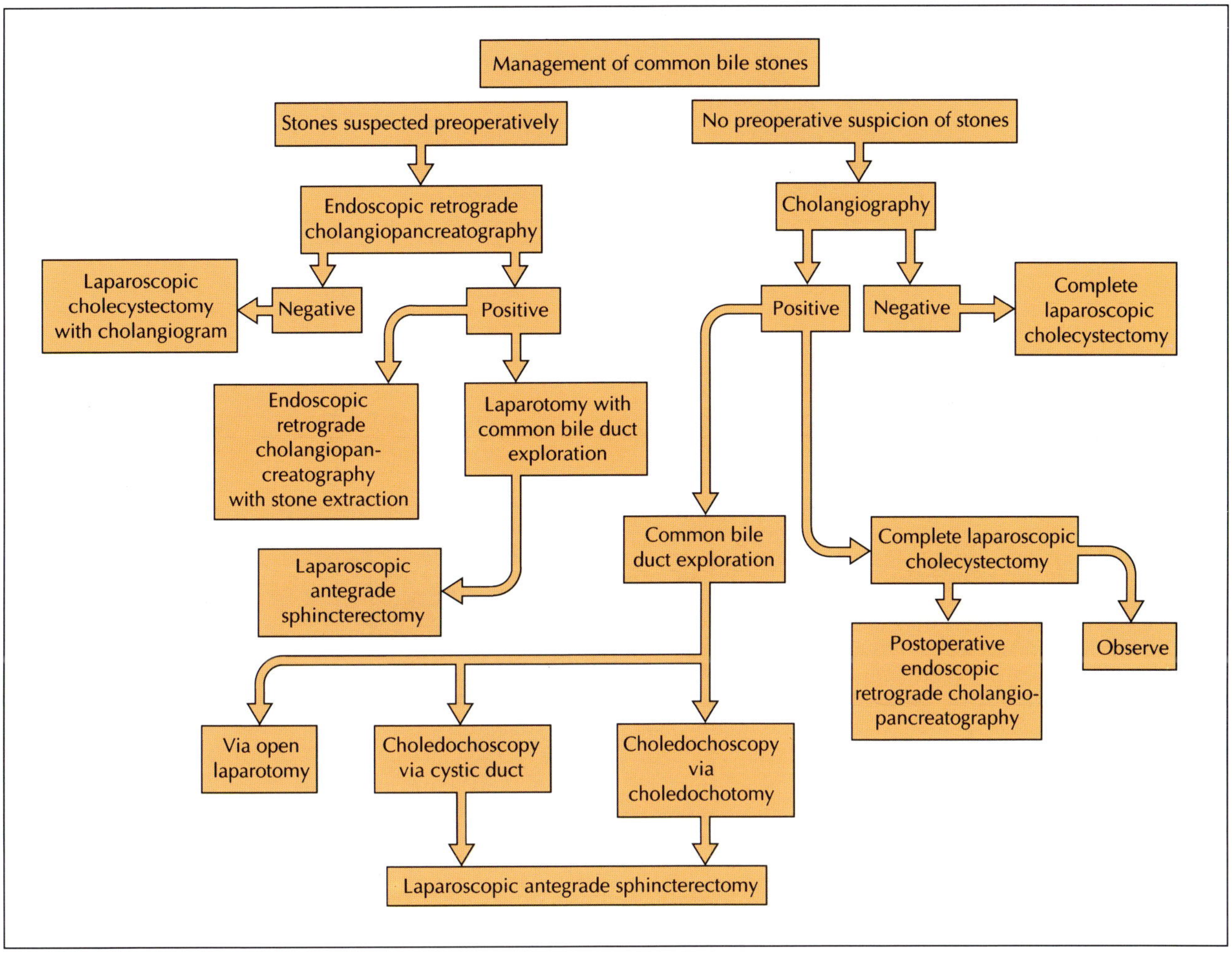

Fig. 1. Management of common bile duct stones. (*From* Cotton [6]; with permission.)

are refractory to laparoscopic extraction. Options described include open conversion, postoperative ERCP, or percutaneous access to the common duct with transcystic soft catheters or guide wires or placement of T tubes.

Petelin [8••] presents his own results as well as data from five other series reporting on experiences with LCBDE [9,10•,11–14]. Of 3365 laparoscopic cholecystectomies, 270 (8%) had cholangiograms interpreted as abnormal. The success rate for LCBDE from these combined series ranged from 57% to 98% (as a percent of attempted LCBDEs). The open conversion rate varied from none to 22%, and postoperative ERCP or other radiologic clearance was used in up to 55% of those patients with abnormal cholangiograms. Petelin's own data cover 77 attempted LCBDEs with a success rate of 96% (74 of 77 patients). The most useful method for common bile duct clearance was fluoroscopy with wire basket extraction in 2%, fogarty balloon extraction in 27%, and choledochoscopy in 62%. Petelin reports that multiple methods may be tried in each patient, beginning with the simplest and progressing to the most difficult. Of the three patients who underwent unsuccessful LCBDE, one was converted to open common bile duct exploration, and two underwent successful postoperative ERCP with stone extraction. Complications occurred in eight (10%) of those patients undergoing LCBDE, although only one complication, a minor bile leak, could be considered attributable to LCBDE directly. Mean operative time averaged 146 minutes for LCBDE compared with 83 minutes for laparoscopic cholecystectomy alone, although the mean length of stay was 46 hours for LCBDE compared with 26 hours for laparoscopic cholecystectomy alone.

Laparoscopic antegrade sphincterotomy, recently described by DePaulo *et al.* [15••], is another useful technique for clearing the common bile duct. This technique involves transcystic passage of a standard endoscopic papillotome through the ampulla (Fig. 2). A side-viewing endoscope is simultaneously passed through the mouth and into the duodenum and used to position the sphincterotome in the classic "12 o'clock" location (Fig. 3). The sphincterotomy is then performed, and stones are removed using previously described techniques or allowed to pass spontaneously. Because the sphincterotomy is passed forward through the common bile duct and ampulla, there is essentially no risk of pancreatic duct cannulation or postendoscopic pancreatitis. In addition, there would appear to be a greatly diminished likelihood of perforation by

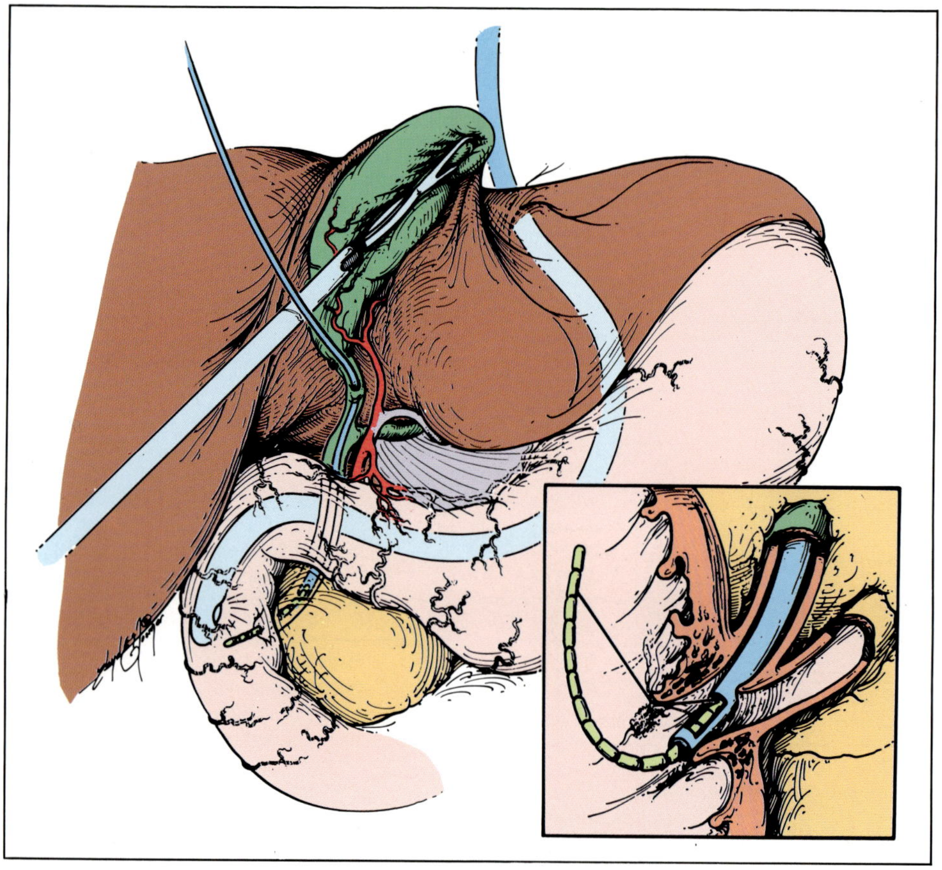

Fig. 2. The technique of antegrade sphincterotomy. (*Courtesy of* M. Curet, Albuquerque, NM.)

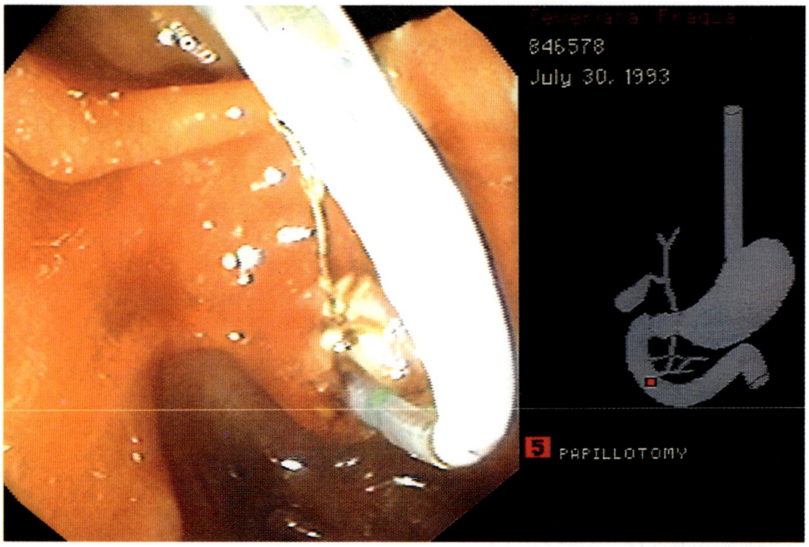

Fig. 3. Endoscopic view (via the side-viewing duodenoscope) of antegrade sphincterotomy. (*Courtesy of* M. Curet, Albuquerque, NM.)

the sphincterotome of the creation of false channels. In DePaulo's series, laparoscopic antegrade sphincterotomy was performed successfully in 21 patients with no related complications. The entire procedure added a mean of only 17 minutes to the total operative time. Although it is apparently a very safe and effective method of performing sphincterotomy, the indications for this procedure are still unclear.

Lithotripsy and cholangioscopy

Other methods for the management of common duct stones refractory to common surgical and endoscopic techniques are reviewed in articles by Ponsky [16] and Graham [17•]. Techniques discussed include the use of mechanical lithotriptors, electrohydrolic lithotriptors, pulsed dye laser lithotriptors, mother-daughter cholangioscopy, transhepatic cholangioscopy, and biliary stents. These techniques rely upon access to the biliary tree via a percutaneous route (T-tube tract, transhepatic) or via a peroral transpapillary route (*eg*, ERCP). In general, a transhepatic route is used only when endoscopic or trans–T-tube therapy has failed, or for intrahepatic stones. All of these techniques may require multiple sessions for stone clearance. Success rates for mechanical lithotripsy, electrohydrolic lithotripsy, and laser lithotripsy from multiple series are summarized in Graham's article. Mechanical lithotripsy was successful in 411 of 503 patients (81.7%) from six series, with a range of 48.7% to 93.5%. Electrohydrolic lithotripsy was successful in 158 of 172 patients (91.8%) from 12 series, with a range of 60% to 100%. Laser lithotripsy was successful in 63 of 89 patients (70.7%) from five series, with a range of 64.3% to 85.7%. In general, the electrohydrolic and laser lithotripsy techniques are more costly and run a higher risk of thermal injury to the common duct. If all efforts at percutaneous or transpapillary extraction fail, open common duct exploration or biliary bypass can still be considered. For those stones refractory to all extraction techniques in patients deemed poor operative risks, biliary stents, extracorporeal shock wave lithotripsy, and contact dissolution techniques remain viable alternatives.

Conclusions

Management strategies for common duct stones in the era of laparoscopic cholecystectomy continue to evolve. Increasing numbers of surgeons are exploring the common duct laparoscopically with a high degree of success. Multiple techniques are available for accomplishing LCBDE and for management of common duct stones refractory to conventional endoscopic and percutaneous extraction techniques. ERCP continues to play an important role in both the preoperative and postoperative management of common duct stones. The ultimate goal for common duct stone management should be a single-stage procedure with minimal morbidity and low cost.

References and recommended reading

Papers of particular interest, published within the annual period of review, have been highlighted as:

- • Of special interest
- •• Of outstanding interest

1. **NIH Consensus Conference Statement.** *Am J Surg* 1993, 165:390–396.
2. Hunter JG, Soper NJ: **Laparoscopic Management of Common Bile Duct Stones.** *Surg Clin North Am* 1992, 72:1077–1097.
3. Zucker KA, Bailey RW: **Laparoscopic Cholangiography and Management of Choledocholithiasis.** In *Surgical Laparoscopy Update.* Edited by Zucker KA. St. Louis: Quality Medical Publishing; 1993:145–193.
4. Reiter JJ, Bayer HP, Mennicken L: **Results of Endoscopic Papillotomy: A Collective Experience From Nine Endoscopic Centers in West Germany.** *World J Surg* 1978, 2:505–509.
5. Cotton PB, Lehman G, Vennes JA: **Endoscopic Sphincterotomy Complications and Their Management: An Attempt at Consensus.** *Gastrointest Endosc* 1991, 37:383–390.
6. Cotton PB: **Endoscopic Retrograde Cholangiopancreatography and Laparoscopic Cholecystectomy.** *Am J Surg* 1993, 165:474–478.
7. Scott TR, Zucker KA, Bailey RW: **Laparoscopic Cholecystectomy: A Review of 12,397 Patients.** *Surg Laparosc Endosc* 1992, 2:191–198.
8. Petelin JB: **Laparoscopic Approach to Common Duct Pathology.** *Am J Surg* 1993, 165:487–491.
•• This article provides an excellent description of the common methods of LCBDE and describes the author's results in over 90 patients. Data from five other series are also presented. The author stresses the importance of utilizing a variety of techniques as necessary for common duct clearance.
9. Jacobs M, Verdeja JC, Goldstein HS: **Laparoscopic Choledocholithotomy.** *J Laproendosc Surg* 1991, 1:79–82.
10. Hunter JG: **Laparoscopic Transcystic Common Bile Duct Exploration.** *Am J Surg* 1992, 163:53–58.
• This article provides an in-depth description of laparoscopic transcystic common bile duct exploration and reviews the results of five series on LCBDE. Useful technical tips and common technical problems are discussed.
11. Petelin J: **Laparoscopic Approach to Common Duct Pathology.** *Surg Laparosc Endosc* 1991, 1:33–41.
12. Spaw AT, Reddick EJ, Olsen DO: **Laparoscopic Laser Cholecystectomy: Analysis of 500 Procedures.** *Surg Laparosc Endosc* 1991, 1:2–7.
13. Sackier JM, Berci G, Phillips E, Carroll B, Shapiro S, Paz-Partlow M: **The Role of Cholangiography in Laparoscopic Cholecystectomy.** *Arch Surg* 1991, 5:111–115.
14. Carroll BJ, Phillips EH, Daykhovsky L, *et al.*: **Laparoscopic Choledochoscopy: An Effective Approach to the Common Duct.** *J Laproendosc Surg* 1992, 2:15–21.
15. DePaulo AL, Hashiba K, Bafutto M, Zago R, Machado MM: **Laparoscopic Antegrade Sphincterotomy.** *Surg Laparosc Endosc* 1993, 3:157–160.
•• The authors discuss their initial results with a novel technique for antegrade sphincterotomy for common duct clearance in 21 patients. This technique appears to avoid the potential complication of postendoscopic pancreatitis seen with retrograde pancreatic duct cannulation and retrograde sphincterotomy. Unlike ERCP, antegrade sphincterotomy can be performed intraoperatively with the patient in a supine position and can be completed as a single-stage procedure (obviating the need for postoperative ERCP). This technique appears to be another useful method for clearing the common duct.
16. Ponsky JL: **Alternative Methods in the Management of Bile Duct Stones.** *Surg Clin North Am* 1992, 72:1099–1107.
17. Graham SM, Flowers JL, Zucker KA: **Endoscopic Management of the Difficult Common Bile Duct Stones.** *Surg Laparosc Endosc* 1993, 3:54–59.
• This paper reviews the techniques and results of methods useful in managing "difficult" common bile duct stones. Techniques described and reviewed include mechanical lithotripsy, electrohydraulic lithotripsy, mother-daughter cholangioscopy, and the use of biliary stents.

David E. Pitcher, MD, Daniel T. Martin, MD, and Karl A. Zucker, MD, Division of Surgical Endoscopy, Department of Surgery, University of New Mexico School of Medicine, 2211 Lomas Boulevard NE, Albuquerque, NM 87131-5341, USA.

Controversies regarding laparoscopic colectomy for malignant diseases

David M. Ota, MD, Heidi Nelson, MD, and Jane C. Weeks, MD

University of Missouri–Ellis Fischel Cancer Center, Columbia, Missouri, Mayo Clinic, Rochester, Minnesota, and Dana-Farber Cancer Center Institute, Boston, Massachusetts, USA

Surgical investigators have shown that a hemicolectomy can be done laparoscopically. This minimally invasive approach to treat colon cancer potentially reduces hospitalization time, hastens return to normal activity, and reduces health care costs. Hopefully, all of these favorable outcomes can be achieved without compromising cancer control. At present, however, the issues regarding laparoscopic colectomy are not clear, and prospective studies are necessary to validate that this new procedure is superior to open colectomy. Because cancer control might be compromised by this new procedure, laparoscopic colectomy should not be accepted by the surgical community because of the allure of new technology or the hope that it is equivalent to open colectomy in controlling a curable disease. Rather, a randomized trial of laparoscopic colectomy compared with open colectomy is needed to prove that cancer control is not different and that laparoscopic colectomy is cost-effective.

Current Opinion in General Surgery 1994:208–213

During the past 5 years there has been tremendous interest in developing minimally invasive surgical techniques for inflammatory and neoplastic diseases of the abdominal cavity. The relatively rapid acceptance of laparoscopic cholecystectomy as the standard procedure for cholelithiasis has been remarkable. Laparoscopic appendectomy and Nissen fundoplication have been described and will soon become standard therapy as well. Soon after laparoscopic procedures for benign inflammatory diseases were developed, minimally invasive surgery was adapted for neoplastic diseases of the abdominal cavity. Initially these involved diagnostic and palliative procedures such as staging, enteric bypasses, colostomy, and feeding tubes. More recently, surgeons who believed that laparoscopic surgery could be adapted for treating intestinal tumors have performed colectomies with laparoscopic techniques. Although there have been several articles reporting the feasibility of laparoscopic colectomy for malignant disease [1–4, 5••], caution should be exercised before this procedure is considered equivalent to open colectomy. Issues such as compromised cancer control, complications, quality of life, and health care costs must be considered. A review of laparoscopic colectomy for treating potentially curable colon cancer is timely, and the need for a randomized trial of open compared with laparoscopic colectomy is now apparent.

Cancer control

Cancer control issues surrounding laparoscopic colectomy include extent of lymphadenectomy, wound implantation of malignant cells, adequacy of intraperitoneal staging, and no-touch technique. The extent of lymphadenectomy for treating colorectal carcinomas has been controversial since Miles [6] published his paper on the rationale for the abdominal perineal resection. Miles' theory was that a wider dissection removed more lymph nodes that contained metastatic disease and thereby increased the chance for cure. Gabriel *et al.* [7] observed that colorectal carcinoma spread in an orderly fashion from proximal to distal lymph nodes. However, it was observed that nodal disease could occur far from the primary tumor site without involvement of adjacent lymph nodes. This "skip lymph node metastasis" was attributed to unusual lymphatic drainage from partially obstructed lymphatic vessels producing a retrograde lymphatic flow, resulting in nodal metastases far from the primary tumor site [8]. This concept was used to support Miles's theory that a wide lymphadenectomy was necessary to maximize the chance of cure; the theory dominated surgical management of this disease for many decades.

In 1982 Sugarbaker and Corlew [9••] analyzed the results of lymphadenectomy from several studies that retrospectively compared extended regional hemicolectomy with a regional colectomy. An extended regional lymph node dissection involved removing the regional arterial blood supply with a periaortic node dissection. A regional lymph node dissection involved removing lymph nodes along a regional arterial blood supply The authors concluded that an extended regional lymphadenectomy could theoretically result in a 5% survival advantage over a regional lymph node dissection, and no statistical significance was found in the studies that were reviewed retrospectively. The current standard of therapy for a resectable colon carcinoma is to perform a colectomy with at least 5 cm of proximal and distal luminal margins and to take the regional arterial blood supply at its origin. A lesion in the right colon requires a colonic resection of the ileocolic and right arteries. A lesion in the transverse colon is treated with a transverse colectomy taking the middle colic artery. For left colonic carcinomas, resection should include the left colic artery, whereas a resection of a sigmoid tumor should include the superior rectal artery.

Although the extent of lymphadenectomy has not been shown to influence survival, there is important prognostic information in the regional lymph nodes of the resected mesentery. Cady [10] has argued that regional lymph nodes are not governors but rather indicators of survival. Removal of the regional lymph nodes for breast, prostatic, bladder, and cervical carcinoma provides important staging information and does not necessarily add to survival. In the past few years, systemic adjuvant chemotherapy has been shown to be effective in increasing survival of high-risk patients [11]. At present, high risk is defined as positive nodes in the resected mesentery. Thus, node-positive colon carcinoma patients should receive adjuvant chemotherapy whereas node-negative patients do not benefit from such postoperative therapy. If laparoscopic colectomy provides fewer lymph nodes in the resected specimen compared with open laparotomy and colectomy, then the potential exists for understaging this disease. This could lead to withholding adjuvant therapy from patients who might benefit from it, resulting in a lower survival rate.

Whereas operative techniques can influence the extent of nodal resection, there are many variables that contribute to the number of nodes found in a resected colon specimen. For example, Herrera-Ornelas *et al.* [12] reexamined the resected mesentery after it was dissected by the pathologist. They used a defatting solution to remove adipose tissue and found undetected positive lymph nodes in specimens that were otherwise node negative. Although this process is time-consuming, requires a vented hood to handle the organic solvent fumes, and is not widely practiced, it points out that gross pathologic identification of lymph nodes may be inaccurate.

The number of nodes in a resected specimen has been equated with adequacy of the node sampling. When 20 nodes are recorded in the final pathology report, the surgeon feels satisfied with his technique. However, in addition to the pathologist missing small nodes in the surgical specimen, a normal variation in node number is expected. What is most important is the influence of nodal count on survival. The number of lymph nodes in the resected colonic specimen has not been shown to influence survival. This would suggest that lymph node recovery in the resected specimen may not be important.

We recently reviewed the number of nodes reported in resected specimens from Dukes B and C colon tumors (Table 1). This database was assessed for the number of lymph nodes found in the resected colon mesentery and is one measure of the adequacy of the laparoscopic lymphadenectomy. Only those tumors in the right, left, and sigmoid colon were examined. There was a wide range in the number of nodes found in these cases and a similar wide variation was noted for left and sigmoid colons. For example, the standard deviation was greater than the mean number of nodes from left hemicolectomies. Another observation was the significantly higher nodal count in the right colon compared with the left and sigmoid colon. In comparing open colectomy with laparoscopic colectomy, these differences in nodal count should be considered.

Early reports have suggested that lymph node counts in laparoscopic colectomy specimens are similar to open colectomy specimens. However, most of these studies had a considerable mix of proximal and distal colorectal carcinomas. In a recent study of 14 laparoscopic right hemicolectomies at the MD Anderson Cancer Center, the author observed a mean of 8.8 ±5.45 nodes; this was significantly less than what was observed in the historical right hemicolectomies done by open laparotomy. Similar findings comparing open with laparoscopic colectomy during a similar time period were also reported (Vayer *et al.*, Paper presented at 92nd Annual Meeting of Colon/Rectal Surgeons, Phoenix, AZ, 1993). The mean node count was 6.6 for the laparoscopic group; this was significantly less than the 9.6 node count found in the open laparotomy group. At present it is unclear whether these differences are clinically meaningful, and the challenge will be to conduct a randomized study to resolve this issue.

Table 1. Lymph nodes in resected specimens from Astler-Coller Dukes B and C colon carcinomas*

Location†	Patients who underwent colectomy, *n*	Mean nodes ±SD (±SEM)
Right colon	101	18.8±11.2(±1.1)
Left colon	60	15.8±16.2(±2.1)‡
Sigmoid colon	43	11.0±8.6(±1.3)§

*Dukes A and D tumors were excluded. B1, 38 patients; B2, 104 patients; C1, 54 patients.
†Carcinomas of the hepatic flexure, transverse colon, and splenic flexure were excluded.
‡$P<0.002$ compared with right colon (Mann-Whitney test).
§$P<0.00001$ compared with right colon (Mann-Whitney test).

Another significant cancer control issue is the incidence of tumor implantation at either the port site or the specimen wound. Several reports have described carcinoma implantation after laparoscopic cholecystectomy for gallstone disease, and relatively early carcinoma was reported in the final pathologic assessment [13,14]. Similar case reports regarding tumor implantation at wound or port site after laparoscopic colectomy have now appeared in the literature [15,16,17••]. In one instance the implant was noted in a node-positive specimen (stage III) whereas in another case the tumor implant was found in a node-negative colon resection (stage II). At the time of the procedure there was no evidence of peritoneal carcinomatosis. Implantation was found at either the extraction wound or a port site. Such reports are disturbing because tumor recurrence in the incision site for an open laparotomy and colectomy is very uncommon. However, the denominator for these laparoscopic colectomies is unknown; thus, the true incidence will never be known until a large prospective study is done.

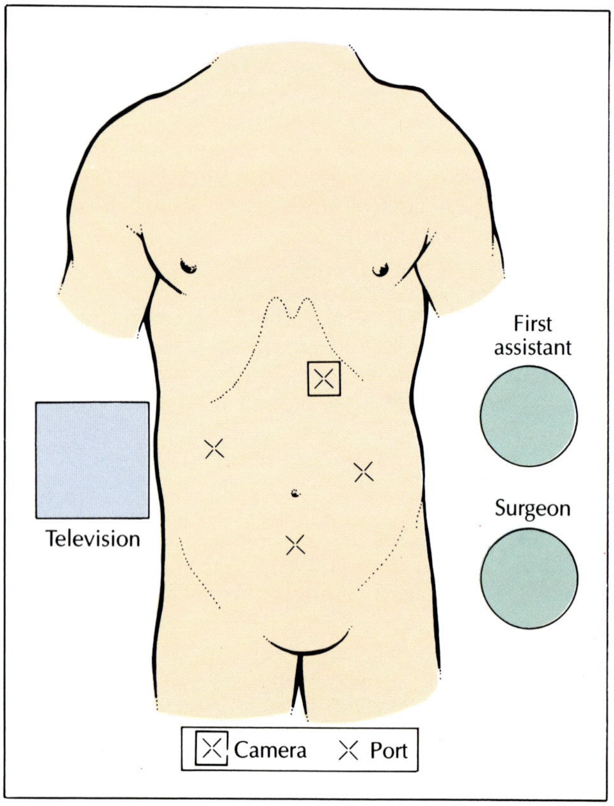

Fig. 1. Port site placement for laparoscopic right hemicolectomy. The patient is placed on a bean bag, which is then secured to the operating table with adhesive tape. This is done because the patient is placed in a deep Tendelenberg position. The camera is placed through the left upper quadrant 10-mm Hasson port and controlled by the assistant. The right 10-mm port is placed over the transverse colon. The assistant uses a Babcock clamp placed through the right port. Left and infraumbilical 10-mm ports are used by the surgeon. The right colon is exteriorized through a transverse 5-cm excision made around the right port.

The mechanism for tumor wound implantation after laparoscopic colectomy is related to operative technique. Tumors that have invaded the serosa can potentially shed malignant cells, and grasping the colonic wall for retraction during the laparoscopic procedure can dislodge these cells. Either the extraction wound or port site may be inoculated, and eventually the tumor will grow. From a technique standpoint the laparoscopic surgeon should avoid grasping the colonic wall near the tumor. Laparoscopic Babcock clamps are now widely available and should be used carefully (Figs. 1 and 2). Even with ideal technique, however, in laparoscopy the surgeon loses tactile sensation; what was once grasped with fingers for retraction is now held with redesigned operative instruments that offer no tactile feedback.

Intraperitoneal staging is another limitation of laparoscopic colectomy. The surgeon is no longer able to palpate the liver for metastases, although the surface of the liver can be seen and either external or intracorporeal liver ultrasound can be done. Intraperitoneal metastasis to ovaries, pelvic cul-de-sac, or paracolic gutters can be missed. The incidence of understaging is unknown and can best be determined in a randomized trial. Another potential disadvantage of laparoscopic colectomy is that the no-touch technique cannot be used. The rationale for the no-touch technique was that intraoperative manipulation of the primary tumor during dissection of the colon and mesentery could dislodge tumor cells in regional venules and veins, potentially disseminating disease to distant organs. For these reasons the initial step in the no-touch technique was ligating the regional arterial and venous blood supply before the colon and mesentery were mobilized [18]. In 1988 Wiggers *et al.* [19••] reported the results of a prospective randomized trial of the no-touch isolation technique versus a conventional resection technique. Patients were registered and randomly assigned preoperatively. Eligibility and exclusion criteria were given and were judged reasonable. There were 117 patients in the "no-touch" group and 119 patients in the control arm. All evaluable patients had resectable disease. Complications were equal in both groups and survival was not significantly different between the two treatment groups. Although the authors saw a trend toward improved survival with the no-touch technique, the final conclusion was that there was no statistical improvement in survival with this technique. Hence, early ligation of regional blood vessels during a laparoscopic procedure is not important.

The cancer control issues with laparoscopic colectomy are very important. Compromising cure for the sake of using new technology or 2 to 3 fewer days of hospitalization is not acceptable. Open laparotomy and colectomy can be done with minimal postoperative mortality, and it seems that until we have long-term prospective data demonstrating the efficacy of this procedure, we must proceed cautiously. The common bile duct injuries observed during a laparoscopic cholecystectomy should serve as a reminder that the laparoscopic colectomy procedure should be studied prospectively before it is accepted as standard technique.

Complications

Like the laparoscopic cholecystectomy, laparoscopic colectomy has resulted in unusual complications. Ureteral injury during either a right or left hemicolectomy is rare in open colectomy, but such injuries have

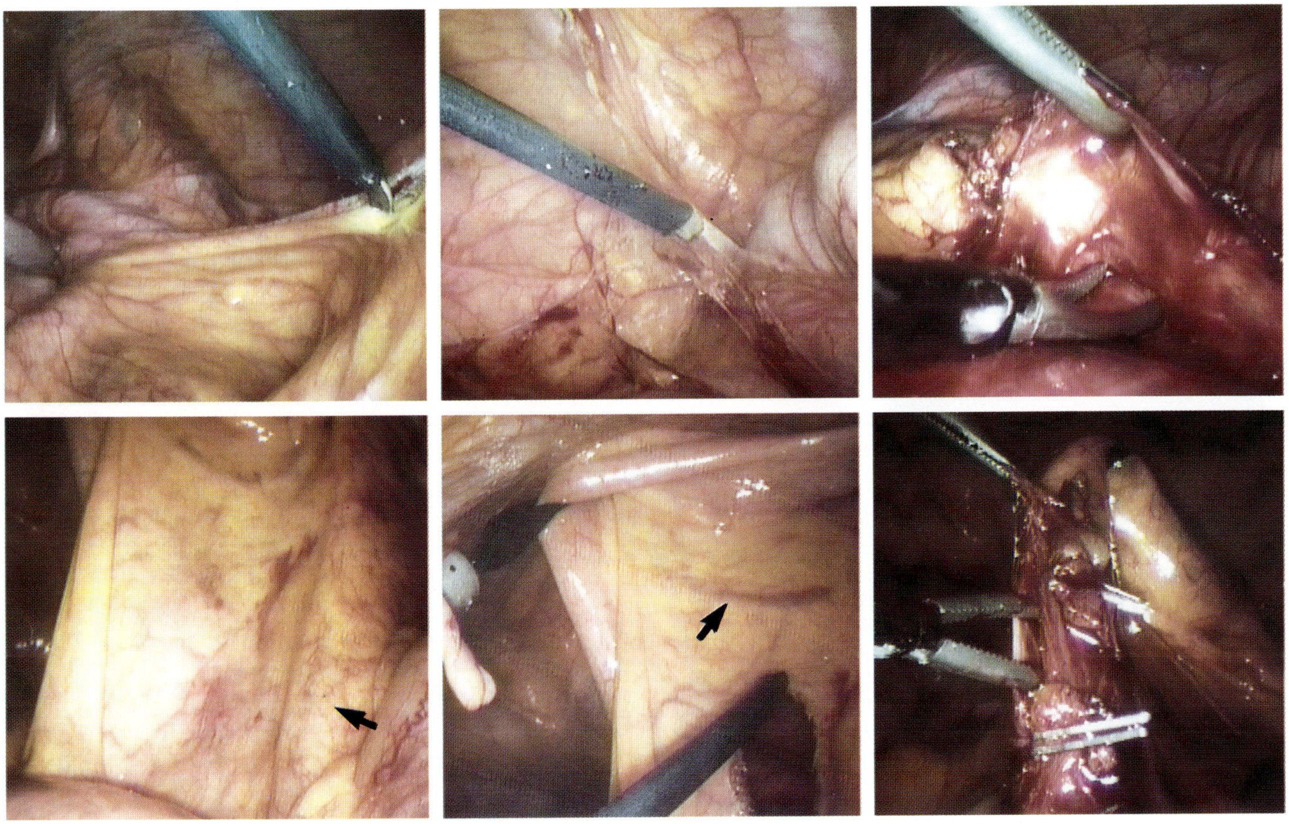

Fig. 2. Laparoscopic right hemicolectomy. **Top left,** View from the left upper quadrant Hasson port looking into the right lower quadrant. The terminal ileum and cecum have been retracted cephalad with laparoscopic Babcock clamps. The peritoneum on the underside of the ileal mesentery is being opened with a spatula. Blunt dissection with the spatula tip is used to find the bloodless plane between the mesentery and the retroperitoneal fat. The assistant is retracting the cecum cephalad with the Babcock retractor in the right port, and the surgeon is using another Babcock in the left port to retract the ileum. **Top center,** The laparoscope is in the left upper quadrant port looking at the white line of Toldt. The dissection has continued along the lateral aspect of the right colon. The attachment of the right colon to the abdominal wall is being taken down using the cautery and blunt dissection with the spatula placed through the infraumbilical port. The surgeon's right hand is retracting the cecum cephalad with the Babcock clamp in the left port. **Top right,** View from the left upper quadrant looking down into the right lower quadrant. The grasper is in the infraumbilical port lifting up the retroperitoneal fat, and the laparoscopic dissector is placed through the left port; with careful blunt dissection, the right ureter was identified. **Bottom left,** View from the left upper quadrant looking down into the right lower quadrant. The terminal ileum and right colon mesentery have been completely mobilized off the retroperitoneum and lateral abdominal wall. The surgeon is holding up the terminal ileum with a laparoscopic Babcock clamp, which is placed through the infraumbilical port, in his left hand. The assistant is lifting the cecum with a Babcock clamp in the right port. The scope is looking directly at the ileal mesentery. Bowing of the ileocolic artery (*arrow*) can be seen. **Bottom center,** An avascular window in the mesentery adjacent to the ileocolic artery. The terminal ileum is held up to the anterior abdominal wall with the mesentery placed on a stretch. With the spatula in the mesenteric opening, the spatula cautery is used to create the window. The mesentery is slowly opened up toward the ileal-cecal arcade vessel (*arrow*). The window is carried down to the base of the mesentery, where the ileocolic artery and vein are located. **Bottom right,** The ileocolic artery and vein are dissected from the surrounding tissues with blunt dissection. The vein has been doubly clipped—proximally and distally—and transected. The laparoscopic dissector is coming around the ileocolic artery, which is also doubly clipped and transected. A chromic loop is then placed around the artery, and the dissection is continued cephalad toward the transverse colon. The entire ileal and right colon mesentery have thus been mobilized and transected. The terminal ileum and colon will now come up through the 5-cm incision made over the right laparoscopic port. The specimen is then exteriorized, and the terminal ileum and transverse colon are transected with an intestinal stapler. The specimen is then removed. The two ends are approximated, and a side-to-side staple anastomosis is performed. The ileocolic anastomosis is then dropped into the abdominal cavity, and the 5-cm incision is closed.

been observed with the laparoscopic technique. Another significant injury is an inadvertent, undetected bowel perforation. The mechanism of such an injury may be instrument trauma from grasping and retracting or from an unnoticed cautery injury. Other complications include uncontrolled hemorrhage, bladder injury, and hypercapnia-induced cardiac arrhythmias or dysfunction. Such complications are avoidable as long as the surgeon can detect the injury and respond appropriately. Some injuries can obviously lead to higher costs.

Cost analysis and quality of life

The appeal of laparoscopic surgery is that patient recovery is faster and may therefore result in lower health care costs and better quality of life compared with open laparotomy. Shorter hospitalization time, less use of analgesia, and fewer complications should reduce costs. Less postoperative pain, earlier return of gastrointestinal function, and faster return to normal activity should lead to better quality of life. Although all surgeons would agree with these concepts, attempts to quantify these parameters sometimes take on the quality of the pursuit of the Holy Grail. Under the pressure of spiraling medical costs, new tools are emerging that make it possible to conduct rational analyses of the economic and quality-of-life effects of medical interventions [20••]. Recently, these tools have been applied to cancer treatment with intriguing results and conclusions [21••].

The primary goal of a randomized study of laparoscopic colectomy will be to evaluate whether it is equivalent to open colectomy measured in disease-free and overall survival. If it fails to meet that test, issues of cost and quality of life are irrelevant. However, if laparoscopic colectomy does not compromise survival, the choice between procedures should be guided by an assessment of their respective effects on the secondary endpoints of cost and quality of life.

Shortened length of hospital stay is certainly one indicator of improved quality of life. It is widely accepted that patient reports are an essential component of a meaningful assessment of quality of life. There are now a number of short, reliable questionnaires available that can assess patients' overall quality of life and their experiences in specific areas such as pain and functional status. It will be important to incorporate these measures into randomized trials of laparoscopic colectomy so that the necessary data will be available to make comparisons with respect to quality of life if the newer technology proves to offer comparable cancer control.

Similarly, an analysis of the costs and cost-effectiveness of laparoscopic colectomy is an integral part of evaluating this new technology. A consideration of the costs of medical interventions is necessary only if we are willing to acknowledge that there is some limit to what we as a society are willing to pay for health care. Although open discussion of these limits may not always be politically acceptable, the revolution now taking place in our health care system in response to rising health care costs (14% of gross national product and rising) suggests that there may be a *de facto* limit.

Economic analyses of health care may taken any of four forms. The simplest, a "cost minimization" study, assumes that the alternative approaches being considered are equally effective in all ways and simply compares the costs associated with each. The cheapest approach is assumed to be superior. In most circumstances, however, alternative approaches are not medically equivalent because of differences in their effects of length of life, quality of life, or both. Three approaches have been developed for assessing whether the additional benefit in length or quality of life resulting from a more expensive procedure justifies the extra cost [22].

In "cost-effectiveness" analysis, the extra cost of the more expensive procedure is compared to the extra benefit in years of life saved. For example, a cost-effectiveness analysis of laparoscopic colectomy would evaluate how much more it costs than open colectomy and whether it results in any gains in years of life compared with the standard approach. If laparoscopic colectomy produces better or equivalent survival and is less expensive than the standard approach, it would be considered "dominant," and no further analysis would be required to identify it as the superior option. However, if it costs more than colectomy but results in slightly improved survival, one could calculate how many dollars were required for each year of life gained to estimate the "cost-effectiveness ratio." A "cost-utility" analysis is similar to a cost-effectiveness analysis but also takes into account the effect of the procedure on quality of life. A "cost-benefit" analysis measures both the cost and the benefit of a health intervention in monetary terms. The cost-benefit ratio compares how much an intervention costs with how much patients might be willing to pay for the added benefit. Because of the difficulties inherent in assigning a dollar value to years of life saved, cost-benefit analyses are rarely used to evaluate medical interventions.

The most comprehensive economic analysis of laparoscopic colectomy would be a cost-utility analysis because that would take into account not only differences in cost between laparoscopic and open procedures but also any potential differences in clinical and quality-of-life outcomes. If a randomized trial shows equivalent survival and cancer control, then the cost-utility ratio will depend on differences in costs and quality-of-life outcomes. For example, the lower the operating costs and the better the quality of life in patients undergoing the laparoscopic procedure, the more favorable the cost-utility ratio. This analysis will also be influenced by length of stay, so that even if operating costs are higher for a laparoscopic procedure, shortened length of stay may result in lower costs overall [3,22]. If laparoscopic colectomy returns patients to work sooner, it may result in lower indirect costs and therefore lower total costs. And even if costs prove to be higher for laparoscopic colectomy, the cost-utility ratio may still be within generally accepted norms if the procedure is associated with significant quality-of-life benefits for patients. It is clear that like the more traditional clinical endpoints, the components of an economic analysis are best evaluated in a randomized trial so that one can be certain that any differences in costs and quality of life are attributable to differences between the procedures rather than differences in the types of patients who are selected for one procedure or the other.

Conclusions

There is no doubt that laparoscopic surgery has made a significant impact on abdominal surgery. Less postoperative abdominal pain, shorter hospitalization time, and reduced health care costs are strong arguments for minimally invasive surgery in the treatment of potentially curable colon carcinomas. However, these are assumptions and not proofs. Moreover, the potential for compromising cancer control and raising health care costs are serious drawbacks. Surgical investigators must prove that laparoscopic colectomy is superior and not just equivalent to open laparotomy colectomy. Equivalency means that 5-year survival and local or regional disease control are not compromised. The potential benefits include shorter hospitalization time, reduced health care costs, and earlier return to normal activities. Before laparoscopic colectomy can replace open laparotomy colectomy, a prospective randomized clinical trial comparing disease control, complications, health care costs, and quality of life must be done.

References and recommended reading

Papers of particular interest, published within the annual period of review, have been highlighted as:

- • Of special interest
- •• Of outstanding interest

1. Jacobs M, Verdeja JC, Goldstein HS: **Minimally Invasive Colon Resection (Laparoscopic Colectomy)**. *Surg Laparosc Endosc* 1991, **1**:144–150.
2. Fowler DL, White SA: **Laparoscopy-Assisted Sigmoid Resection**. *Surg Laparosc Endosc* 1991, **1**:183–188.
3. Schlinkert RT: **Laparoscopic-Assisted Right Hemicolectomy**. *Dis Colon Rectum* 1991, **34**:1030–1031.
4. Phillips EH, Franklin M, Carroll BJ, Fallas MJ, Ramos R, Rosenthal D: **Laparoscopic Colectomy**. *Ann Surg* 1992, **216**:703–707.
5. •• Falk PM, Beart RW, Wexner SD, Thorson AG, Jagelman DG, Lavery IC, Johansen OB, Fitzgibbons RJ Jr: **Laparoscopic Colectomy: A Critical Appraisal**. *Dis Colon Rectum* 1993, **36**:28–34.

Although most publications on laparoscopic colectomy express enthusiasm for the procedure, this article states that this new procedure is similar to open colectomy in terms of outcome and cost. The only potential difference is post-operative quality of life. A randomized trial is needed to see if significant cost-saving can be demonstrated.

6. Miles EE: **A Method of Performing Abdomino-perineal Excision for Carcinoma of the Rectum and of the Terminal Portion of the Pelvic Colon**. *Lancet* 1908, 1812–1813.
7. Gabriel WB, Dukes C, Bussy HJ: **Lymphatic Spread in Cancer of the Rectum**. *Br J Surg* 1935, **23**:395–413.
8. Grinnell RS: **Lymphatic Block With Atypical and Retrograde Lymphatic Metastasis and Spread in Carcinoma of the Colon and Rectum**. *Ann Surg* 1966, **163**:272–280.
9. •• Sugarbaker PH, Corlew S: **Influence of Surgical Techniques on Survival in Patients With Colorectal Cancer: A Review**. *Dis Colon Rectum* 1982, **25**:545–557.

This article critically reviews the role of wide lymphadenectomy in increasing colon cancer survival and concludes that extended lymphadenectomy is unlikely to increase survival compared with regional lymphadenectomy.

10. Cady B: **Lymph Node Metastasis: Indicators but Not Governors of Survival**. *Arch Surg* 1984, **119**:1067–1072.
11. Steele G: **Adjuvant Therapy for Patients With Colon and Rectal Cancer: Clinical Indications for Multimodality Therapy in High-Risk Groups and Specific Surgical Questions for Future Multimodality Trials**. *Surgery* 1992, **112**:847–849.
12. Herrera-Ornelas L, Justiniano J, Castillo N, Petrelli N, Stule JP, Mittelman A: **Metastases in Small Lymph Nodes From Colon Cancer**. *Arch Surg* 1987, **122**:1253–1256.
13. Clair DG, Lautz DB, Brooks DC: **Rapid Development of Umbilical Metastases After Laparoscopic Cholecystectomy for Unsuspected Gallbladder Carcinoma**. *Surgery* 1993, **113**:355–358.
14. Fong Y, Brennan MF, Turnbull A, Colt DG, Blumgart LH: **Gallbladder Cancer Discovered During Laparoscopic Surgery: Potential for Iatrogenic Tumor Dissemination**. *Arch Surg* 1993, **128**:1028–1032.
15. Walsh DCA, Wattchow DA, Wilson TG: **Subcutaneous Metastases After Laparoscopic Resection of Malignancy**. *Aust N Z J Surg* 1993, **63**:563–565.
16. O'Rourke N, Price PM, Kelly S, Sikora K: **Tumor Inoculation During Laparoscopy**. *Lancet* 1993, **342**:368.
17. •• Fusco MA, Paluzzi MW: **Abdominal Wall Recurrence After Laparoscopic-Assisted Colectomy for Adenocarcinoma of the Colon**. *Dis Colon Rectum* 1993, **36**:858–861.

Examines isolated reports of port site recurrences. The incidence appears to be low, but without a randomized prospective study, it will be difficult to assess the true incidence of these anecdotal cases.

18. Turnbill RB Jr, Kyle K, Watson FR, *et al.*: **Cancer of the Colon: The Influence of the No-Touch Isolation Technic on Survival Rates**. *Ann Surg* 1967, **166**:420–427.
19. •• Wiggers T, Jeekel J, Arends JW, *et al.*: **No-Touch Isolation Technique in Colon Cancer: A Controlled Prospective Trial**. *Br J Surg* 1988, **75**:409–415.

This definitive study shows that early arterial and venous legation do not contribute to survival.

20. •• Detsky AS, Naglie I: **A Clinician's Guide to Cost-Effective Analysis**. *Ann Intern Med* 1990, **113**:147–154.

This is an excellent review of cost-effective analysis and how it can be applied to assess the cost and actual benefits of new medical technology. The analytical tools for comparing effectiveness, quality of life, and benefits of new therapy with those of standard therapy are described.

21. •• Smith TJ, Hillner BE, Desch CE: **Efficacy and Cost-Effectiveness of Cancer Treatment: Rational Allocation of Resources Based on Decision Analysis**. *J Natl Cancer Inst* 1993, **85**:1460–1474.

In this era of managed care, new therapies will undergo rigorous analyses regarding outcome, quality of life, and cost. These studies will involve all areas of medicine that heretofore were accepted but now do not meet the criteria of cost-effectiveness.

22. Bass EB, Pitt HA, Lillemoe KD: **Cost-Effectiveness of Laparoscopic Cholecystectomy Versus Open Cholecystectomy**. *Am J Surg* 1993, **165**:466–471.

David M. Ota, MD, The University of Missouri–Ellis Fischel Cancer Center, 115 Business Loop 70 West, Columbia, MO 65203, USA.

Surgical oncology and tumor immunology

Editorial overview

Timothy J. Eberlein, MD

Brigham and Women's Hospital, Boston, Massachusetts, USA

Current Opinion in General Surgery 1994:215–216

The topics chosen this year for the section on surgical oncology concern issues in the arenas of both clinical and basic science. I have tried to choose common clinical areas of interest where controversy exists, and because it would be impossible and beyond the scope of the reviews to cover all aspects of basic science, I have concentrated on cellular immunology and molecular biology, two areas that are important to surgical scientists and that I hope will affect the future diagnosis and treatment of surgical patients with malignancy.

As Yvedt Matory (pp 217–223) points out in her review, genetic screening of breast cancer will become increasingly important. Identification of an inherited breast cancer gene will help clinicians and patients with strong familial histories and premalignant pathologies to consider hormonal manipulation or prophylactic surgical management. Other genetic markers, however, such as *HER2/neu*, *p53*, and angiogenesis factor will also play a role in the diagnosis and selection of patients for more aggressive therapies, which will subsequently affect overall prognosis.

Mammography and physical examination are still the mainstays in the diagnosis of breast cancer in women over 50 years of age [1,2]. Work is now being done with magnetic resonance imaging, and although results are promising, they are premature, and the technique remains too costly for routine screening. Breast-conserving surgery has proven to be effective in the treatment of primary breast cancers. Criteria for inclusion, the extent of resection, and the need and extent of axillary dissection will require further clarification, however. Ductal carcinoma *in situ*, lymphatic vessel invasion, and multifocality will have important implications in the recommendation of breast-conserving therapy. Randomized trials of adjuvant therapies, both chemical and hormonal, are in progress and will help to clarify the role of these modalities and to target appropriate patient populations. With the proposed changes in our health care system, selection of patients most likely to benefit from these adjuvant treatments will become increasingly important. For example, although patients receiving tamoxifen therapy might be expected to benefit from a reduction in opposite breast cancers or from a reduction in cardiovascular events, they may also have increases in endometrial, hepatocellular, and colorectal malignancies.

In an excellent review, Raphael Pollock (pp 224–229) discusses the management of soft tissue sarcomas and suggests that limb-saving surgery with or without radiation therapy is preferred over ablative radical surgery. Although adjuvant chemotherapy for soft tissue sarcomas has not been particularly effective, neoadjuvant treatment either administered locally (*ie*, extremity sarcoma) or systemically may hold great promise. Genetic changes or objective mitotic activity might again identify those patients who would benefit most from neoadjuvant and adjuvant treatment.

Radiotherapy continues to be an important adjuvant in the management of soft tissue sarcomas. Low grade tumors and tumors that are widely resected (compartmental resections) are often spared radiation therapy. Preoperative radiation therapy as discussed by Pollock can improve the chance for resectability but needs to be carefully planned and performed in a multimodality setting to decrease morbidity and optimize the result.

As with so many malignancies, surgery remains the standard of treatment for local tumor control, however, more conservative surgery with close margins may still be preferable to radical ablative procedures. Molecular, biochemical, and histologic properties currently under study may help target the appropriate patient populations to undergo wider excisions or receive adjuvant radiation therapy [3]. The use of free tissue transfer, bone graft, and other reconstructive modalities would not only improve the functional results but also allow a more standardized surgical resection.

In a thorough review, Alan Meagher and John Pemberton (pp 230–237) suggest that more conservative surgery—often accompanied by other adjuvant modalities—can be equally as efficacious in the treatment of rectal cancers. The extent of linear margins (which are becoming more conservative) and the extent of mesorectal resection remain controversial in the treatment of these patients. While Meagher and Pemberton have nicely summarized several studies that demonstrate inclusion and exclusion criteria for rectal-conserving surgery, answers to these biologic questions will be confirmed only as a result of randomized, prospective trials such as those currently underway by the Cancer and Leukemia Group B and the Eastern Cooperative Oncology Group. The use of molecular biology to identify oncogene products such as *ras* may facilitate the selection of those patients suitable for conservative rectal excision as well as those who may profit from adjuvant treatment.

 ISBN 1-85922-671-X ISSN 1065–6243

In summary, local excision of adenocarcinomas of the distal rectum may be feasible in tumors less than 4 cm in diameter or less than 30% of the rectal circumference. Tumors should be mobile, nonulcerated, and well to moderately differentiated without mucin production. These tumors may be excised by the peranal approach. Patients with cancers or villous adenomas greater than 4 cm and within 6 cm of the anal verge are candidates for coloanal anastomosis. Complications following peranal excisions are rare. Transsacral excisions have a high rate of continence and lack of nighttime soilage. Major complications of this procedure include wound infection and rectal fistula, and although they are often self-limiting, they necessitate a diverting colostomy. Complications such as pelvic abscess, infection, anastomotic disruption, fistula, and stricture formation are more frequent after a coloanal anastomosis than after rectum-conserving procedures. As experience with patient selection and conservative surgical techniques increase, the results and the surgeon's ease in recommending these procedures will improve [4].

The review of cellular therapy by James Yang (pp 238–244) is superb. Understanding the cellular immunologic mechanisms of tumor recognition, specifically the types of lymphocytes that are useful (CD8+–specific cytotoxic lymphocytes) as well as those cells that may not be as effective or may possibly hinder the immune response (CD4+, T-helper 2, and interleukin-4–producing helper cells), will lead to more effective adoptive immunotherapy protocols. A clear grasp of the interaction between the T-cell receptor and major histocompatibility complex and the identification of antigen systems in various tumors will be meaningful. This work has been done in melanoma by van der Bruggen *et al.* [5] and Traversari *et al.* [6], who have described the human gene in coding a nine-amino-acid peptide that is recognized by cytotoxic T cells. Similar approaches are being used in our laboratory and in others with such oncogene products as *HER2/neu*. Elucidation of tumor recognition as well as the biologic properties of tumors (*ie*, how they develop and escape recognition by the immune system) will result in the design of more effective and less toxic therapies for the treatment of various solid tumors.

In an elegant review, Michael Lotze (pp 245–254) has taken these basic biologic mechanisms to the molecular level. Through the use of quantitative polymerase chain reaction, more sophisticated answers to the questions surrounding cellular processes are possible. We have now begun to distinguish the cellular interaction of suppressor genes such as *p53* and oncogenes such as *HER2/neu* and *ras*. Further knowledge of the cellular intricacies driven by these genes and their products will not only open new frontiers in basic biology but will potentiate the development of novel therapeutic interventions for patients with cancer.

As Lotze states, several medical centers are utilizing protocols involving gene therapy. These therapies involve the use of tumors that are transfected with various cytokines to produce an effective tumor vaccine. Multiple methods for transfection have been optimized, and studies of animal models are currently underway to identify the mechanism of tumor eradication. Other gene therapies include transfection of fibroblasts and specific T lymphocytes. These newer means of gene transfer hold promise for eventual benefit of patients.

References

1. Shapiro S, Venet W, Strax P, Venet L: *Periodic Screening for Breast Cancer: The Health Insurance Plan Project and Its Sequelae, 1963–1986.* Baltimore: Johns Hopkins University Press; 1988.
2. Tabar L, Gad A: **Screening for Breast Cancer: The Swedish Trial.** *Radiology* 1981, **138**:219.
3. Singer S, Corson JM, Gonin R, Labow B, Eberlein TJ: **Prognostic Factors Predictive of Survival and Recurrence for Extremity Soft Tissue Sarcoma.** *Ann Surg* 1993, in press.
4. Steele G Jr, Busse P, Huberman MS, LeClair JM, Falchuk ZM, Mayer RJ, Bothe AP Jr, Ravikumar TS, Stone M, Jessup JM: **A Pilot Study of Sphincter-Sparing Management of Adenocarcinoma of the Rectum.** *Arch Surg* 1991, **126**:696–701.
5. van der Bruggen P, Traversari C, Chomez P, Lurquin C, De Plaen E, Van den Eynde B, Knuth A, Boon T: **A Gene Encoding an Antigen Recognized by Cytolytic T Lymphocytes on a Human Melanoma.** *Science* 1991, **254**:1643–1647.
6. Traversari C, van der Bruggen P, Luescher IF, Lurquin C, Chomez P, Van Pel A, De Plaen E, Amar-Costesec A, Boon T: **A Non-peptide Encoded by Human Gene MAGE-1 is Recognized on HLA-A1 by Cytolytic T Lymphocytes Directed Against Tumor Antigen MZ2-E.** *J Exp Med* 1992, **176**:1453–1457.

Timothy J. Eberlein, MD, Brigham and Women's Hospital, Division of Surgical Oncology, Department of Surgery, 75 Francis Street, Boston, MA 02115, USA.

The diagnosis and treatment of breast cancer

Yvedt L. Matory, MD

Brigham and Women's Hospital, Boston, Massachusetts, USA

There have been several new developments in breast cancer research. Investigators are closer to identifying the breast cancer gene, which may aid in the diagnosis and treatment of the disease. The more established routine of screening mammography has been questioned by the results of the Canadian National Breast Screening Study. Many authors challenge this study's validity. Largely because of screening mammography, noninvasive breast cancer is one of the most frequently diagnosed types of breast cancer. The treatment options for noninvasive breast cancers are discussed along with recent publications. The option of breast-conserving therapy for early stage cancers is also reviewed. Recent investigators have sought to identify the most appropriate patients for breast conservation. This overview also discusses treatment options for advanced cancers and the use of hormonal therapy for all patients with breast cancer.

Current Opinion in General Surgery 1994:217–223

Screening

Genetic

Human breast cancer is usually caused by genetic alteration of somatic cells of the breast, but on occasion, susceptibility to the disease is inherited. Mapping the genes responsible for inherited breast cancer could influence screening and treatment strategies for all women. King (*reviewed in* Roberts [1•]) and Hall *et al.* [2] have identified chromosome 17q21 as the locale of a gene for inherited susceptibility to breast cancer in families with early-onset disease. Among these families, the odds that the result was correct was 5.98; a score of 3 was then considered convincing. This work has narrowed the search to within 50 million base pairs. Further studies pooling patients from the European Linkage Consortium have narrowed the search to within 3 million base pairs [1•]. Efforts continue, with groups in Europe and in the United States aggressively seeking to identify the precise gene. Identification of this gene may help to provide guidance for patients with a strong family history of breast cancer and it may direct clinicians in the treatment of patients with premalignant lesions (Fig. 1).

Mammography

Over the past decade, several studies evaluating from 30,000 to 283,000 patients have found that screening mammography reduces breast cancer mortality [3]. The improvement in 5-year survival, noted in these series, ranges from 12% to 40%. The findings of improved survival with screening have been consistent in women over 50 years of age. Studies involving younger women were not randomized, or younger women were not clearly separated from the older patients [4] (American Cancer Society, Unpublished data). The Canadian National Breast Screening study [5••,6••] was designed to evaluate the benefit of screening mammography in patients aged less than 50 years. This study evaluated 50,430 patients between ages 40 and 49 (part 1) [5••] and 39,405 patients aged 50 to 69 years (part 2) [6••].

In part 1 [5••], patients were randomly assigned to receive either annual mammogram and physical examination (MP) or initial physical examination followed by the usual care (UC), which consists of follow-up by a self-administered questionnaire only. The mean follow-up time for both studies was 8.5 years. More patients (3.89/1000) were found to have breast cancer in the MP group at the time of initial presentation, compared with 2.46 per 1000 patients in the UC group. Seven years into the part I study, 191 women in the MP group had invasive breast cancer versus 157 women in the UC group. In the MP group, 102 had nodal involvement, and 66 patients in the UC group had positive nodes (38 and 49 patients respectively had unknown nodal status). The proportion of patients who died of breast cancer was similar in each group, with the greatest survival in patients whose cancer was diagnosed by mammography only. In young patients, MP detected more small node negative cancers than did UC. This result was not associated with improved survival.

In part 2 [6••], older women received either MP or yearly physical examination only (PO). At the time of

Abbreviations

DCIS—ductal carcinoma *in situ*; **EIC**—extensive intraductal component; **HDC/ABMT**—high-dose chemotherapy and autologous bone marrow transplant; **LCIS**—lobular carcinoma *in situ*; **MP**—annual mammogram and physical examination; **PO**—yearly physical examination only; **UC**—initial physical examination followed by usual care.

ISBN 1-85922-671-X ISSN 1065–6243

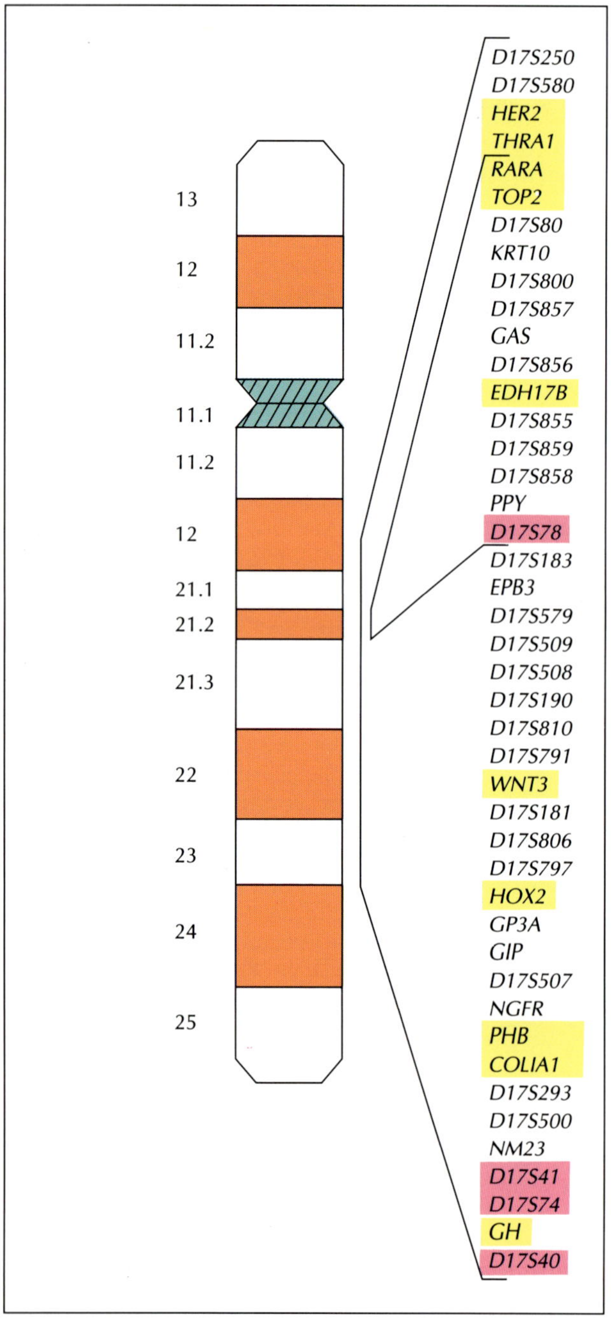

Fig. 1. The breast cancer susceptibility gene, *BRCA1*, was initially mapped to a 50-million base pair region of chromosome 17q (*large bracket*) with four DNA markers (*pink*). As more and more markers became available, investigators found 14 that narrow the region to 2 or 3 million base pairs (*small bracket*). Candidate genes, most of which have now been excluded, are in *yellow*. (*From* Roberts [1•]; with permission.)

initial presentation, women in the MP group were detected to have more cancers than those in the PO group (7.2/1000 vs 3.45/1000). In up to 7 years of follow-up, 217 cases of invasive cancer without node involvement were found in the MP group and 184 such cases were found in the PO group. In the MP group, 98 patients had node involvement, and there were 90 such patients in the PO group. Fifty-five and 46 patients, respectively, had unknown node status. The two groups had similar survival rates. Survival was slightly higher in women whose cancer was detected by mammogram alone. This portion of the study suggests that MP will detect more small node negative tumors than physical examination alone. However, in up to 7 years of follow-up, there was no difference in survival between the PO and MP groups.

Overall, several limitations to these studies have been noted [7–15]. Of most concern is the quality of the screening mammograms. Radiography was performed at many different centers, and neither radiologists nor technicians were given instructions on procedure or interpretation. An internal review by the project reference radiologist revealed that 42% of "interval" cancers could have been detected during the preceding screening rounds. In contrast, the physical examiners were instructed on how to perform a good breast examination. In addition, the follow-up of 7 years may be too short to reveal a significant difference in survival in either part of this study.

Noninvasive breast cancer

Lobular carcinoma *in situ*

There is little consensus on the treatment for lobular carcinoma *in situ* (LCIS), perhaps because few prospective randomized trials have been published that review treatment options for this disease. At Michigan State, 250 patients were evaluated prospectively as part of the National Cancer Institute's Surveillance, Epidemiology, and End Results (SEER) registry [16•]. The median follow-up was 93 months. Two hundred twelve women had a mastectomy, and 65 had less than a mastectomy. In the total group, one patient developed an ipsilateral cancer, and 37 developed contralateral cancers. Two of these 38 second cancers were invasive. There was one known death from breast cancer in the entire series. Although the authors do not clearly separate the results of patients who had mastectomy from those that did not, the overall findings support the conclusion that LCIS can be managed safely by local excision alone.

In light of the high association with contralateral breast cancer in LCIS, local excision alone is the treatment of choice. Unilateral total mastectomy is not appropriate because it does not address the increased risk of contralateral breast cancer. In the absence of a lesion detected by physical examination or mammogram, biopsy of the contralateral breast is not indicated [17].

Ductal carcinoma *in situ*

Two notable studies have been published recently that evaluate the role of radiation therapy and breast-conserving surgery in the treatment of ductal carcinoma *in situ* (DCIS).

The first of these is a retrospective review of 70 patients, 34 of whom had a modified radical mastectomy

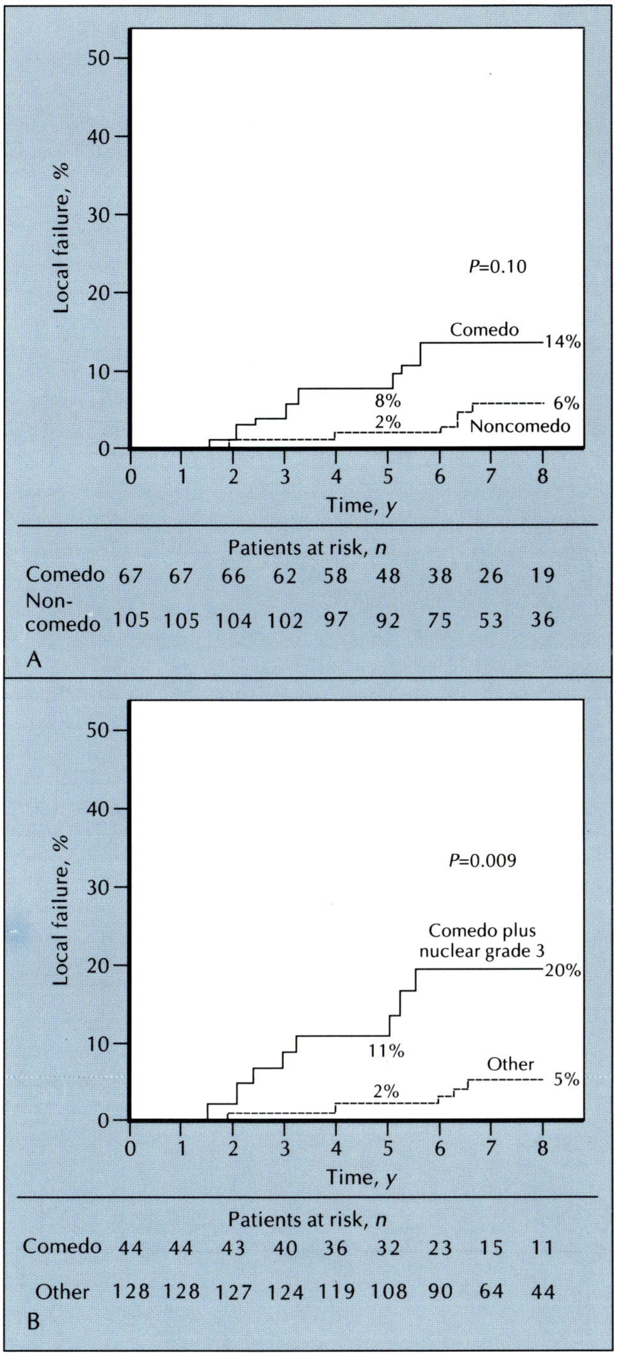

Fig. 2. Local recurrence of ductal carcinoma *in situ* of the breast. **A**, Comparison of the histologic subtype of comedo versus noncomedo intraductal carcinoma. **B**, Comparison of the presence (*solid line*) versus the absence (*dashed line*) of the combination of the histologic subtype of comedo carcinoma plus nuclear grade 3. (*From* Solin *et al.* [24•]; with permission.)

and 36 had local excision and radiation therapy [18]. One patient treated with radical surgery relapsed and three patients treated conservatively relapsed. The authors state that incomplete excision was the reason for failure in the patients treated conservatively. There was no difference in overall survival between the two treatment groups, but there were more relapses in the group treated with breast conservation. These authors appropriately conclude that randomized trials will be needed to confirm their results.

A larger study of 259 women from nine institutions in Europe and in the United States also evaluates the role of breast-conserving therapy in the treatment of breast cancer [19]. All patients underwent a complete gross excision of the primary cancer and definitive irradiation. The median follow-up time was 78 months. The 10-year overall survival was 94%, with a 16% local failure rate. Of the patients who had local recurrences, 86% remain without evidence of distant metastases.

This is one of the largest series published, and it helps to establish the validity of breast-conserving therapy for intraductal cancer. Indeed, there is a rising trend towards breast-conserving treatment of DCIS. Coleman *et al.* [20] reviewed studies that involved a total of 2336 women from across the United States over a 5-year period. This was the treatment option for 30% of patients in 1984 and 45% in 1988. Breast-conserving therapy was more likely to be performed for smaller lesions (< 2 cm) and in younger patients.

The treatment options for microscopic DCIS are total mastectomy, wide excision followed by breast irradiation, or wide excision alone. Total mastectomy should include removal of the nipple-areolar complex because of the risk of microscopic Paget's disease. Breast preservation with or without irradiation should include complete excision of the margins and removal of microcalifications. The ongoing National Surgical Adjuvant Breast Project Protocol 17 trial evaluates all of these treatment options; once published, it will provide guidance for the treatment of this disease entity.

Gross DCIS, with lesions frequently larger than 2.5 cm, is associated with a higher recurrence rate, a higher incidence of invasion, and a greater association with node metastases than smaller lesions [21]. It is best managed in a manner similar to invasive breast cancer either with total mastectomy and low axillary dissection or wide excision, low axillary dissection, and breast irradiation. There is evidence that the comedo subtype of DCIS is also associated with a high incidence of local recurrence compared with other subtypes (Fig. 2) [22,23•,24•]. This too should be managed either with breast-conserving therapy or total mastectomy and low axillary node dissection.

Early invasive breast cancer

Breast conservation has been compared with mastectomy in several early trials [25–29]. Recent studies have confirmed the validity of this treatment option. Several other studies have attempted to identify the patient population that will most benefit from this type of therapy.

Researchers from the National Cancer Institute recently reported a prospective randomized trial of 237 patients with stage I and II breast cancer who received either a modified radical mastectomy or lumpectomy and radiation therapy [30••]. All patients had an axillary node dissection. The median follow-up time was 68 months. No difference in overall survival or disease-free survival was observed. The estimated 5-year actuarial survival for modified radical mastectomy patients was 85%, and for patients undergoing lumpectomy, axillary node dissection, and radiation, the survival was 89%. The local regional control was also similar in both groups (Fig. 3).

Researchers for the European Organization for the Research and Treatment of Cancer (EORTC) Breast Cancer Cooperative Group [31•] published a comparable study in 1992. Modified radical mastectomy was compared to breast-conserving therapy in 10,801 patients with stage I and stage II breast cancer. The median follow-up was 6 years and actuarial survival was 73% after modified radical mastectomy and 71% after breast-conserving therapy. Local recurrence at 8 years was 9% and 15% respectively. In the breast-conserving therapy group local recurrence was higher for tumors 2 to 5 cm (16%) than for smaller tumors (7%) at 8 years.

Breast-conserving therapy continues to be supported as an excellent treatment option for stage I and II breast cancers. Use of this approach for larger lesions was addressed in a series published by Khanna *et al.* [32]. Sixty-eight patients with invasive cancers ranging from 4 to 12 cm were treated with wide excision, node dissection, and radiation therapy. The median follow-up was 46 months. The 5-year actuarial disease-free survival was 68%. The local recurrence rate was 8.5%. A good cosmetic result as determined by the physician was reported for 90% of patients. This report provides additional data to support the use of breast conservation for the treatment of patients with large tumors. The survival of patients in this study is similar to that of patients with large lesions treated with mastectomy.

The importance of margins of resection in achieving local control for patients undergoing breast-conserving therapy was also evaluated by Ghossein *et al.* [33]. A total of 521 patients with breast cancer were treated with varying degrees of resection. Fifty-six of these patients were treated with quadrantectomy and 142 with a wide excision; the remaining 323 were excised with a minimal rim of tissue. All groups had comparable tumor stage, size, and radiation therapy. Margin involvement for patients with minimal excision was 41%, with wide excision, 14%, and after quadrantectomy, 7%. Local failure for these patients, respectively, was 15%, 7%, and 5%. Local failures were inversely proportional to the amount of breast tissue excised. These data support a growing body of literature that suggests that excision of wider volumes of tissue are needed to achieve good local and regional control.

Investigators from the Harvard Medical School [34,35] also evaluated the importance of extent of resection in 507 patients with stage I and II breast cancer. All patients received breast-conserving surgery and radiation therapy, and the median follow-up time was 100 months. All patients had total removal of the primary tumor without confirmation of the pathologic margins. Patients were stratified by clinical tumor size (T stage) and the presence or absence of an extensive intraductal component (EIC). The patients were then divided into three groups based on the volume of excised tissue.

The largest resections were associated with a lower risk of recurrence than the smallest resections in EIC positive patients. The recurrence rates were 10% for the largest resections and 29% for the smallest resections in EIC positive T1 tumors; for those with T2 tumors, these rates were 9% and 36% respectively. The recurrence rates were significantly lower in EIC-negative patients:

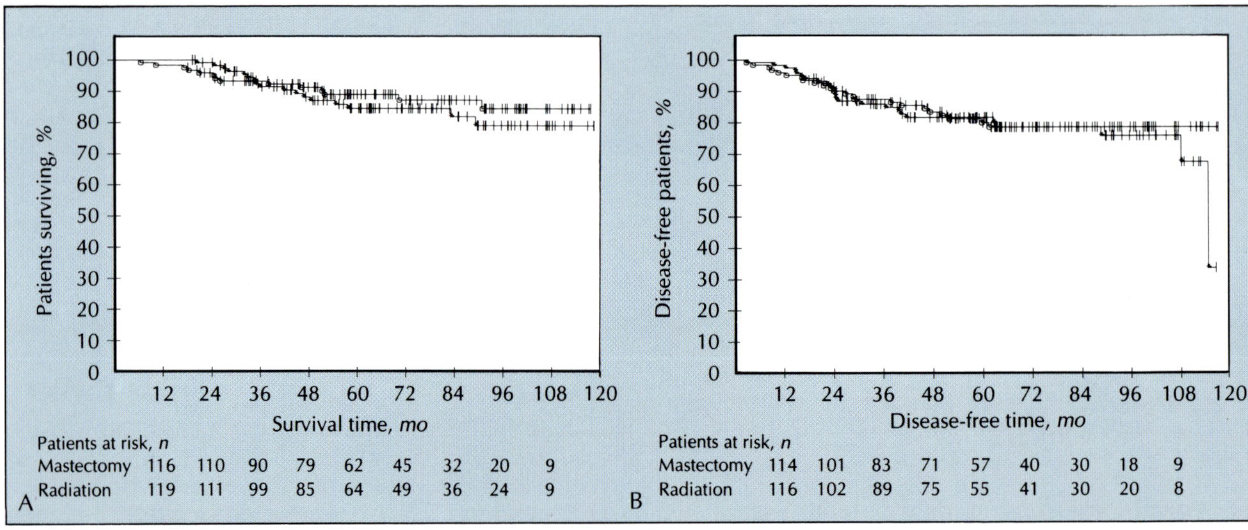

Fig. 3. A, Overall survival of the mastectomy and lumpectomy plus radiation treatment groups. **B**, Disease-free survival of both groups. Patients in the breast-conservation arm who failed only in the breast and were rendered disease-free with mastectomy do not appear as failures on this chart. *Crossed lines* indicate patients undergoing mastectomy. *Circles* indicate patients who received radiation therapy. (*From* Lichter *et al.* [30••]; with permission.)

0% for the largest resections and 9% for the smallest resections. The similar rates for T2 tumors were 3% and 6%. These authors concluded that for patients with early EIC-negative breast cancer, limited resection is acceptable. For patients with EIC-positive tumors, resection should be more extensive.

On the basis of these studies and others, breast conservation with adequate resection, axillary dissection, and breast irradiation is regarded as equal treatment to mastectomy in terms of survival. This was supported by the papers presented at the 1990 National Institutes of Health Consensus Development Conference (#81) on the treatment of early stage breast cancer. There is consensus that multicentric disease, pregnancy, radiation-induced cancer, or diffuse malignant microcalcifications are contraindications for breast conservation [3]. Further studies are needed to determine if the presence of an EIC-positive tumor and focal margin involvement are also contraindications to breast conservation.

Advanced breast cancer

For patients with advanced breast cancer, stage IIIB and IV, the greatest promise for disease stability lies with high-dose chemotherapy and autologous bone marrow transplant (HDC/ABMT). Eddy [36••] analyzed 15 studies published in the last 10 years evaluating the efficacy of this treatment. Most of these were nonrandomized trials. There was an overall response rate of 36% (range, 0% to 55%) and a complete response rate of 70% (range, 6% to 94%). The duration of response ranged from 3 to 13 months. These findings were compared to those of 45 randomized control trials of patients who received conventional doses of chemotherapy. The overall response rates averaged 39% (range, 13% to 81%) and the average complete response rate was 8% (range, 0% to 36%). It is important to note that high complete response rates have been observed with conventional high-dose chemotherapy and with induction therapy. However, complete and partial response rates tend to be even higher with HDC/ABMT. Median duration of response is generally shorter for HDC/ABMT than for conventional chemotherapy, 6.6 months versus 9.7 months. Overall 2-year survival for HDC/ABMT had a weighted average of 43%. In randomized trials of conventional chemotherapy, the weighted 2-year survival rate was 39%. The treatment-related mortality from HDC/ABMT averaged 12% versus 1% for conventional chemotherapy.

Ongoing research in the use of growth factors and peripheral blood stem cells might decrease the mortality associated with HDC/ABMT. The author of this study acknowledges the limitations of this review, such as trial selection, and variation in treatment and in evaluation of responses [36••]. He concludes that the superior response associated with HDC/ABMT may not be associated with a survival benefit and may be minimized by the associated high morbidity and mortality.

Hormonal therapy

The value of antiestrogen therapy in the treatment of breast cancer has been described since 1960 [37]. Subsequent trials have shown that the overall response to antiestrogen drugs is about 30%, and up to 50% in patients with estrogen-receptor–positive tumors. This figure is higher, up to 75%, in women with estrogen-receptor values greater than 100 fmol/mg of cytosol protein. The Early Breast Cancer Trialists' Collaborative Group 1992 [38••,39••] also found treatment with tamoxifen (the most frequently used antiestrogen) to be an effective regimen. The combined trials involve 15,000 women treated with tamoxifen and the same number in the untreated control group. During the first 5 years, there was an estimated 8.3% increase in recurrence-free survival. Beyond 5 years, tamoxifen was of no proven benefit in the prevention of breast cancer recurrence. In addition, tamoxifen was associated with an increase in the time between recurrence and death, with a 3.6% decrease in mortality at 5 years and 6.2% at 10 years. These data suggest that tamoxifen produces a survival advantage beyond the time at which it is no longer preventing recurrence.

If the women are separated on the basis of nodal status, the results are more impressive. For node-negative patients, a 6.2% increase in recurrence-free survival was observed compared with 10.1% for node-positive patients. Tamoxifen provides the greatest advantage to women with a poor prognosis and it provides an adjuvant benefit to all patients.

In a recent review, Catherino and Jordan [40] explored additional benefits of tamoxifen as well as associated toxicity. A summary of nine trials suggests that the rates of contralateral breast cancer were lower for tamoxifen-treated patients than were those of patients given placebo (a mean of 1.6% vs a mean of 2.4%, respectively). In addition, the incidence of both cardiovascular disease and osteoporosis also appears to be lower in patients who received tamoxifen. However, there is an increased incidence of some life-threatening diseases. They include thromboembolic events (1.5% in treated patients vs 0.2% in untreated patients), endometrial cancer (0.5% versus 0.1%, respectively) and hepatocellular cancer (0.04% versus 0.0%, respectively). Tamoxifen is clearly beneficial for short-term treatment of less than 5 years. Longer treatment may result in the onset of serious side effects.

Conclusions

There have been several advances over the past year in the diagnosis and treatment of breast cancer. We eagerly await the identification of the breast cancer gene to improve the treatment of high-risk patients. Although the role of screening mammography has been questioned, the overwhelming evidence is that it is beneficial. The ideal treatment for LCIS and DCIS has yet to be defined, but analysis of specific tumor characteristics may identify the best options. Early breast cancers can be safely treated with breast conservation in most cases, and high-dose chemotherapy with bone marrow transplantation holds great promise for patients with advanced disease. Tamoxifen has some benefit for all patients with invasive breast cancer.

References and recommended reading

Papers of particular interest, published within the annual period of review, have been highlighted as:

- • Of special interest
- •• Of outstanding interest

1. • ROBERTS L: **Zeroing in on a Breast Cancer Susceptibility Gene.** *Science* 1993, **259**:622–625.

The editors of *Science* have nicely chronicled the advances in the discovery of the breast cancer gene beginning with the efforts of Mary-Claire King.

2. HALL JM, LEE MK, NEWMAN B, MORROW JE, ANDERSON LA, HUEY B, KING M: **Linkage of Early-Onset Familial Breast Cancer to Chromosome 17q21.** *Science* 1990, **250**:1684–1689.

3. BORGEN PI, KINNE DW: **Breast Cancer: Strategies for the 1990's.** *Compr Ther* 1992, **18**:24–29.

4. SEIDMAN H, GELB S, SILVERBERG E, LAVERDA N, LUBERA JA: **Survival Experience in the Breast Cancer Detection Demonstration Project.** *CA Cancer J Clin* 1987, **37**:258.

5. •• MILLER AB, BAINES CJ, TO T, WALL C: **Diagnostic Imaging. Canadian National Breast Screening Study: 1. Breast Cancer Detection and Death Rates Among Women Aged 40 to 49 Years.** *Breast Diseases* 1993, **4**:20–21.

This study and part II (Miller *et al.*, *Breast Diseases* 1993, 4:21–22) are among the most controversial publications of the year in the field of breast cancer investigation. Younger patients were evaluated in part I of the study. Screening mammograms detected more node-negative tumors and small tumors, although no survival benefit was seen over 7 years of follow-up.

6. •• MILLER AB, BAINES CJ, TO T, WALL C: **Diagnostic Imaging. Canadian National Breast Screening Study: 2. Breast Cancer Detection and Death Rates Among Women Aged 50 to 69 Years.** *Breast Diseases* 1993, **4**:21–22.

This study and part I (Miller *et al.*, *Breast Diseases* 1993, 4:20–21) are among the most controversial publications of the year in the field of breast cancer investigation. Older patients were screened for breast cancer with yearly mammography in part II. As with part I, more node negative tumors and smaller tumors were identified by screening. Similarly, there was no survival advantage for the screened patients.

7. DODD GD: **Screening for Breast Cancer in Younger Women: A Continuing Dilemma.** *Breast Diseases* 1993, **4**:9–11.

8. BASHINKI SH: **The Canadian National Breast Screening Study: Opportunity for a Rethink.** *Can Med Assoc J* 1993, **148**:1670.

9. COURTEAU JP, BOUCHARD F: **Canadian National Breast Screening Study.** *Can Med Assoc J* 1993, **148**:875.

10. BURHENNE HJ: **Canadian National Breast Screening Study.** *Can Med Assoc J* 1993, **148**:875–876.

11. CARO JJ, O'BRIEN JA, HARTZ SC: **Canadian National Breast Screening Study.** *Can Med Assoc J* 1993, **148**:876.

12. WARREN L: **Canadian National Breast Screening Study.** *Can Med Assoc J* 1993, **148**:877.

13. OWEN G: **Canadian National Breast Screening Study.** *Can Med Assoc J* 1993, **148**:879–880.

14. HOWE D: **Canadian National Breast Screening Study.** *Can Med Assoc J* 1993, **148**:880.

15. MILLER AB, BAINES CJ, TO T, WALL C: **Canadian National Breast Screening Study.** *Can Med Assoc J* 1993, **148**:880–883.

16. • WALT AJ, SIMON M, SWANSON GM: **The Continuing Dilemma of Lobular Carcinoma In Situ.** *Arch Surg* 1992, **127**:904–909.

This article supports the assessment that LCIS can be treated safely with excision only.

17. SMITH BL, BERTAGNOLLI M, KLEIN BB, BATTER S, CHANG M, DOUVILLE L, EBERLEIN TJ: **Evaluation of the Contralateral Breast.** *Ann Surg* 1992, **216**:17–21.

18. TEISSIER CB, PIAT JM, JANSER JC, RENAUD R, RODIER JF, JUNG GM: **Radical Surgery and Conservative Treatment of Ductal Carcinoma In Situ of the Breast.** *Eur J Cancer* 1992, **28**:649–654.

19. SOLIN LJ, RECHT A, FOURQUET A, KURTZ J, *ET AL.*: **Ten-Year Results of Breast-Conserving Surgery and Definitive Irradiation for Intraductal Carcinoma (Ductal Carcinoma In Situ) of the Breast.** *Cancer* 1991, **68**:2337–2344.

20. COLEMAN EA, KESSLER LG, WUN LM, FEUER E: **Trends in the Surgical Treatment of Ductal Carcinoma In Situ of the Breast.** *Am J Surg* 1992, **164**:74–76.

21. LAGIOS MD, MARGOLIN FR, WESTDAHL PR, ROSE MR: **Mammographically Detected Duct Carcinoma In Situ: Frequency of Local Recurrence Following Tylectomy and Prognostic Effect of Nuclear Grade on Local Recurrence.** *Cancer* 1989, **63**:618–624.

22. BELLAMY CO, MCDONALD C, SALTER DM, CHETTY U, ANDERSON TJ: **Noninvasive Ductal Carcinoma of the Breast: The Relevance of Histologic Categorization.** *Hum Pathol* 1993, **24**:16–23.

23. • SCHWARTZ GF, FINKEL GC, GARCIA JC, PATCHEFSKY AS: **Subclinical Ductal Carcinoma In Situ of the Breast: Treatment by Local Excision and Surveillance Alone.** *Cancer* 1992, **70**:2468–2474.

In some cases, small-size DCIS can be treated with local excision alone. However, in most cases, more extensive surgery is optimal with or without irradiation.

24. • SOLIN LJ, YEH IT, KURTZ J, FOURQUET A, RECHT A, KUSKE R, MCCORMICK B, CROSS MA, SCHULTZ DJ, AMALRIC R, *ET AL.*: **Ductal Carcinoma In Situ (Intraductal Carcinoma) of the Breast Treated with Breast-Conserving Surgery and Definitive Irradiation: Correlation of Pathologic Parameters With Outcome of Treatment.** *Cancer* 1993, **71**:2532–2542.

The rate of local recurrence varies with pathologic characteristics of the primary tumor. Comedo carcinoma and nuclear grade 3 are associated with the highest recurrence.

25. VERONESI U, SACCOZZI R, DEL VECCHIO M, BANFI A, CLEMENTE C, DELENA M, GALLUS G, GRECO M, LUINI A, MARUBINI E, *ET AL.*: **Comparing Radical Mastectomy with Quadrantectomy, Axillary Dissection, and Radiotherapy in Patients With Small Cancers of the Breast.** *Cancer* 1958, **1**:238–241.

26. VERONESI U, BANFI A, DEL VECCHIO M, SACCOZZI R, CLEMENNNTE C, GRECO M, LUINI A, MARUBINI E, MUSCOLINO G, RILKE F: **Comparison of Halsted Mastectomy With Quadrantectomy, Axillary Dissection, and Radiotherapy in Early Breast Cancer: Long Term Results.** *Eur J Cancer Clin Oncol* 1986, **22**:1085–1089.

27. VERONESI U, SALVADORI B, LUINI A, BANFI A, ZUCALI R, DELVECCHIO M, SACCOZZI R, BERETTA E, BORACCHI P, FARANTE G: **Conservative Treatment of Early Breast Cancer: Long-Term Results of 1,232 Cases Treated With Quadrantectomy, Axillary Dissection, and Radiotherapy.** *Ann Surg* 1990, **211**:250–259.

28. FISHER B, BAUER M, MARGOLESE R, POISSON R, PILCH Y, REDMOND C, FISHER E, WOLMARK N, DEUTSCH M, MONTAGUE E: **Five-Year Results of a Randomized Clinical Trial Comparing Total Mastectomy and Segmental Mastectomy With or Without Radiation in the Treatment of Breast Cancer.** *N Engl J Med* 1985, **312**:665–673.

29. FISHER B, REDMOND C, POISSON R, MARGOLESE R, WOLMARK N, WICHERHAM L, FISHER E, DEUTSCH M, CAPLAN R, PILCH Y: **Eight-Year Results of a Randomized Clinical Trial Comparing Total Mastectomy and Lumpectomy With or Without Irradiation in the Treatment of Breast Cancer.** *N Engl J Med* 1989, **320**:822–828.

30. •• LICHTER AS, LIPPMAN ME, DANFORTH DN, D'ANGELO T, STEINBERG SM, DEMOSS E, MACDONALD HD, REICHERT CM, MERINO M, SWAIN SM, *ET AL.*: **Mastectomy vs Breast-Conserving Therapy in the Treatment of Stage I and II Carcinoma of the Breast: A Randomized Trial at the National Cancer Institute.** *J Clin Oncol* 1992, **10**:976–983.

These data add further weight to the conclusion that breast conservation has equivalent survival to mastectomy for early stage breast cancer.

31. • VAN DONGEN JA, BARTELINK H, FENTIMAN IS, LERUT T, MIGNOLET F, OLTHUIS G, VAN DER SCHUEREN E, SYLVASTER R, TONG D, WINTER J, *ET AL.*: **Factors Influencing Local Relapse and Survival and Results of Salvage Treatment After Breast-Conserving Therapy in Operable Breast Cancer: EORTC Trial 10801, Breast Conservation Compared With Mastectomy in TNM Stage I and II Breast Cancer.** *Eur J Cancer* 1992, **28A**:49–50.

This is a multi-institution trial that also finds an equivalent survival for early stage breast cancers treated with mastectomy or breast conservation. They found an exceptionally high recurrence rate in patients with midsize lesions.

32. KHANNA MM, MARK RJ, SILVERSTEIN MJ, JUILLARD G, LEWINSKY B, GIULIANO AE: **Breast Conservation Management of Breast Tumors 4 cm or Larger.** *Arch Surg* 1992, **127**:1038–1043.

33. GHOSSEIN NA, BARBA AS, PRESSMAN P, STACEY P, LORENZ E, SHULMAN M, SADARANGANI GJ: **Breast Cancer: Importance of Adequate Surgical Excision Prior to Radiotherapy in the Local Control of Breast Can-**

cer in Patients Treated Conservatively. *Surg Gynecol Obstet* 1992, 174:189–194.

34. Recht A: **Patient Selection for Treatment With Conservative Surgery and Radiation Therapy.** *Cancer Invest* 1992, 10:471–476.

35. Vicini FA, Eberlein TJ, Connolly JL, Recht A, Abner A, Schnitt S, Silen W, Harris J: **The Optimal Extent of Resection for Patients With Stage I or II Breast Cancer Treated With Conservative Surgery and Radiotherapy.** *Ann Surg* 1991, 214:200–205.

36. •• Eddy DM: **High-Dose Chemotherapy With Autologous Bone Marrow Transplantation for the Treatment of Metastatic Breast Cancer.** *J Clin Oncol* 1992, 10:657–670.

This is a very thorough analysis of one of the most promising adjuvant treatments for advanced breast cancer. At this early stage of investigation, the side effects may outweigh the benefits.

37. DiSaia PJ: **Hormone-Replacement Therapy in Patients With Breast Cancer.** *Cancer Supplement* 1993, 71:1490–1500.

38. •• Early Breast Cancer Trialists' Collaborative Group: **Systemic Treatment of Early Breast Cancer by Hormonal, Cytotoxic, or Immune Therapy: 133 Randomized Trials Involving 31,000 Recurrences and 24,000 Deaths Among 75,000 Women.** *Lancet* 1992, 339:71–85.

This article and another by the same group (*Lancet* 1992, 339:1–15) comprise a multinational analysis of 133 randomized trials evaluating the adjuvant therapy of early breast cancer.

39. •• Early Breast Cancer Trialists' Collaborative Group: **Systemic Treatment of Early Breast Cancer by Hormonal, Cytotoxic, or Immune Therapy: 133 Randomized Trials Involving 31,000 Recurrences and 24,000 Deaths Among 75,000 Women.** *Lancet* 1992, 339:1–15.

This article and another by the same group (*Lancet* 1992, 339:71–85) comprise a multinational analysis of 133 randomized trials evaluating the adjuvant therapy of early breast cancer.

40. Catherino WH, Jordan VC: **A Risk-Benefit Assessment of Tamoxifen Therapy.** *Drug Saf* 1993, 8:381–397.

Yvedt L. Matory, MD, Brigham and Women's Hospital, Surgical Oncology Division, 75 Francis Street, Boston, MA 02115, USA.

Limb-sparing therapy for soft tissue sarcomas

Raphael E. Pollock, MD, PhD

The University of Texas MD Anderson Cancer Center, Houston, Texas, USA

Effective therapy for soft tissue sarcoma of the extremities continues in its lengthy evolution from mandatory amputation or radical compartment resection to multimodality limb salvage procedures. This current approach typically includes preoperative neoadjuvant systemic chemotherapy, followed by negative margin surgical resection in conjunction with radiotherapy. The scope and functional outcome of these resections has been markedly enhanced by the application of microvascular-dependent free tissue transfer techniques. Because of the rarity of this tumor system, problems in soft tissue sarcoma receive proportionally less attention. Nonetheless, the past year has witnessed several important advances in this field, as is discussed.

Current Opinion in General Surgery 1994:224–229

Soft tissue sarcoma is an extremely rare clinical entity that comprises only 0.7% of the new adult malignancies diagnosed annually in the United States. The therapy for this disease has undergone remarkable evolution over the past 30 years. Local recurrence rates of 90% were typical in the earlier era when these tumors were simply enucleated. Up to 70% of extremity soft-tissue sarcoma patients treated by amputation died of pulmonary metastases that were clinically undetectable at the time of resection.

This disheartening clinical spectrum began to improve with the introduction of external beam radiotherapy in the 1960s, leading to a less mutilating 2-cm margin wide local excision of the primary tumor. However, questions about the efficacy of preoperative versus postoperative versus interstitial radiotherapy are yet to be resolved. The introduction of systemic chemotherapy in the mid-1970s provided an approach to disseminated disease. However, the useful drugs are markedly toxic, and achievable response rates hover at the 50% level in most studies. The question of adjuvant versus neoadjuvant chemotherapy is still open, as are the potentially beneficial effects of myeloprotective strategies such as concomitant growth factor administration or stem cell rescue. Much work remains to be done; however, progress is hampered by the relative rarity of the sarcoma tumor system. Nonetheless, important advances have been made over the recent past in the chemotherapy, radiotherapy, and surgical components of the limb sparing multimodality treatment for this disease.

Chemotherapy

Azzarelli *et al.* [1•] prospectively considered the role of preoperative chemotherapy in primary soft tissue sarcomas of the extremities. From 1987 to 1991, 51 patients with grade 3 soft tissue sarcomas at least 5 cm in diameter (including 18 recurrences) received intra-arterial doxorubicin (80 mg/m^2) as an 8-day slow infusion along with ifosfamide (6 mg/m^2 on days 1 and 2) and mesna (500 mg/m^2 three times a day on days 1 and 2). Negative margin surgery was then performed, followed by three cycles of postoperative chemotherapy. Some patients received concomitant radiotherapy. Clinical response was determined preoperatively and defined as improvement in clinical parameters (size, mobility, consistency, decreased symptoms). Pathologic response was defined as necrosis in greater than 75% of the tumor, based on at least eight different pathological tumor samplings.

The conclusions of this study can be criticized because of the nonrandomized design, the small number of patients studied, the inclusion of recurrent lesions, the use of radiotherapy in some, but not all, patients, and the short follow-up time. However, it is interesting that 47% of patients demonstrated a clinical response and 45% a pathological response. The responding patients had an 85% 4-year metastasis-free actuarial survival, whereas the nonresponders had a markedly inferior 59% 4-year metastasis-free actuarial survival (P= 0.10). Definitive proof of the neoadjuvant approach will require a prospective randomized design with a no-treatment arm. However, as circumstantial

Abbreviation

EORTC—European Organization for Research and Treatment of Cancer.

© 1994 Current Science ISBN 1-85922-671-X ISSN 1065–6243

evidence accumulates suggesting a survival advantage for patients treated with neoadjuvant chemotherapy, a no-treatment prospective randomized design will be increasingly untenable on an ethical basis alone.

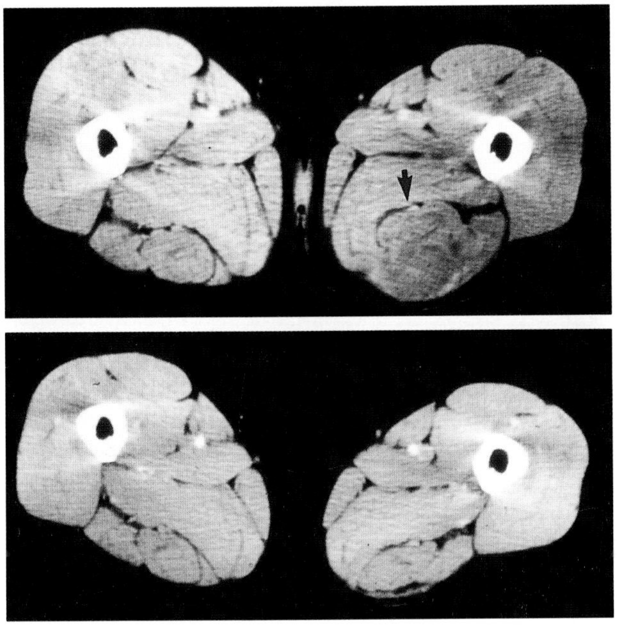

Fig. 1. Patient with large posterior thigh malignant fibrous histiocytoma before (*top panel*) and after (*bottom panel*) three courses of systemic chemotherapy (doxorubicin and DTIC [5-(3.3-dimethyl-1-triazino)-imidazole-4-carboxamide]).

This second report by Azzarelli *et al.* [2] incorporates a larger series of patients. In this larger study, 101 patients with large extremity soft tissue sarcomas, 45% of which were recurrent, were treated with neoadjuvant intra-arterial doxorubicin. At the conclusion of the study, 78 patients could be evaluated. These included all patients with histologically confirmed soft tissue sarcoma of the extremity that could be resected with adequate margins, excluding hemipelvectomy. (Patients requiring hemipelvectomy were studied on an advanced disease protocol.) Patients with recurrent lesions were eligible for inclusion provided that they had not received chemotherapy or radiation as part of their initial treatment.

Four different sequential treatments were used at different times during the study, although all regimens included intra-arterial doxorubicin as the salient feature of treatment. Response was evaluated on the basis of clinical and radiologic examination to determine changes in tumor size, consistency, improved demarcation of margins, mobility, and relationship to deeper structures. On the basis of these ratings, a lesion was classified as demonstrating 1) progressive disease, 2) stable disease, 3) objective response, or 4) complete regression. Pathologic response was scored as per a variety of standard criteria the application of which were admittedly subjective. For purposes of analysis, classifications 1 and 2 and classifications 3 and 4 were pooled. Of the 78 evaluable patients, clinical response could be documented in 38% and pathologic response in 45%. However, these responding subsets of patients were not coincident. On the basis of clinical response, the 5-year actuarial survival was 63% in the 31 clinically responsive patients versus 36% for the 46 nonresponders ($P = 0.01$). Disease in approximately 10% of patients was sufficiently downstaged by neoadjuvant chemotherapy such that limb salvage could be performed rather than amputation.

A review by Verweij *et al.* [3] examined the historical development of chemotherapy as part of a multimodality approach for the therapy of soft tissue sarcoma. The focus of this review was to document the important role of the 28 multicenter studies conducted since 1976 under the aegis of the European Organization for Research and Treatment of Cancer (EORTC) Soft Tissue and Bone Sarcoma Group.

Beginning with single-agent chemotherapy trials, the review demonstrates the superiority of multiagent protocols in achieving measurable tumor regression. Because of problems with rate-limiting myelosuppressive toxicity and low response rates, it has been difficult to justify long-term adjuvant chemotherapy programs that might confer survival advantages for patients treated in the postoperative setting. The induction neoadjuvant chemotherapy approach has allowed the intact tumor to serve as an *in vivo* chemosensitivity test, as has been demonstrated by Pezzi *et al.* [4]; for this reason, the neoadjuvant approach is now being incorporated into prospective randomized chemotherapy trials (Fig. 1). EORTC protocol 62874 uses three cycles of preoperative doxorubicin plus ifosfamide in patients with locally advanced but still operable extremity soft tissue sarcoma, and it is currently accruing patients. As Verweij *et al.* [3] correctly assert, this large multicenter EORTC trial may provide the first prospectively randomized evidence that multiagent neoadjuvant chemotherapy has survival benefit for patients with soft tissue sarcoma.

Ravaud *et al.* [5•] contend that difficulties in comparing different chemotherapy trial results stem from differences in the prognostic variables used to select maximum-risk patients for trial participation. Given that most patients who die from soft tissue sarcoma succumb to uncontrolled metastatic disease, the authors in this study wanted to derive a uniform set of unfavorable parameters that would justify enrollment in adjuvant chemotherapy trials.

To achieve these purposes, the authors retrospectively analyzed their results for 141 patients with extremity soft tissue sarcoma who were untreated prior to study. These patients were treated without chemotherapy; their treatment consisted of surgery alone ($n = 13$) or surgery with radiotherapy ($n = 110$). Univariate analysis of multiple clinical parameters were performed as a function of overall, disease-free, local disease-free, and metastatic disease-free survival.

Age and sex did not affect survival. Extremity rather than truncal location led to improved overall survival, although other measures of survival were not affected by tumor location. This seeming paradox is explained

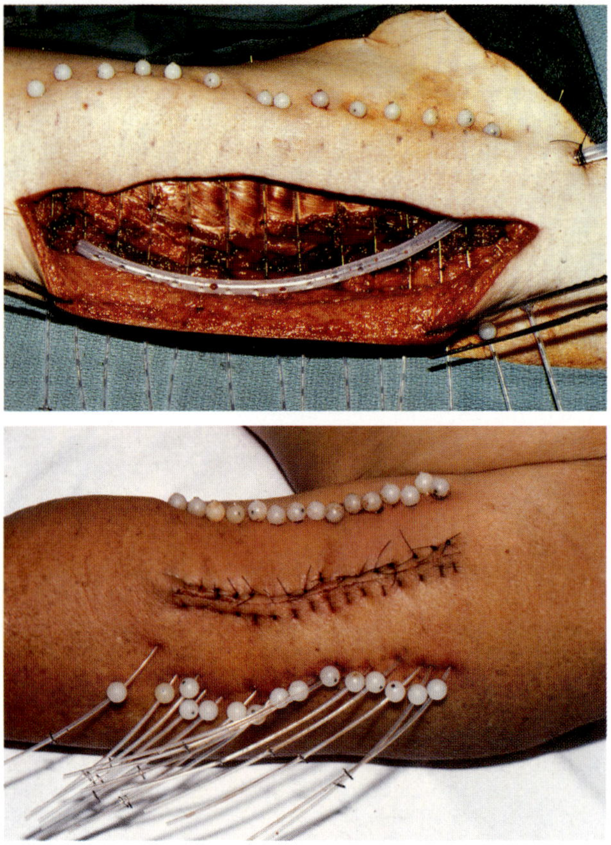

Fig. 2. Placement of brachytherapy catheters intraoperatively (*top panel*). After 5 days of wound healing, the catheters are loaded with ^{192}Ir wires (*bottom panel*). Five days later, wires and catheters are removed.

by improved overall survival in the subset of patients who had successful rescue treatment of an extremity relapse, which in turn is perhaps a reflection of lead-time bias. Tumor size of 5 cm or more conferred worse overall survival but did not affect other measures of survival. Invasion of neurovascular structures or bone impacted negatively on all survival parameters, as did tumor depth where superficially based tumors were more favorable than deep-seated lesions. Tumor histopathology was difficult to interpret reliably, whereas tumor grade was more consistently assessable. High tumor grade negatively impacted on all measures of survival. Macroscopic tumor margins likewise negatively affected all survival parameters. The relative contribution of the significant univariate survival correlates was assessed in a step-wise multivariate regression analysis. Tumor grade and tumor depth were most predictive of overall and metastatic disease-free survival; the authors concluded that any grade 3 tumor, any deep-seated grade 2 tumor, or any tumor with neurovascular or bone involvement has a high metastatic risk. This subset of sarcoma patients has such poor survival that their inclusion in postoperative adjuvant chemotherapy trials is warranted, notwithstanding the mediocre response rates, the cumulative chemotoxicity, and the lack of measurable tumor response in the adjuvant setting.

Radiotherapy

Tanabe *et al.* [6] of the University of Texas M.D. Anderson Sarcoma Service examined the influence of surgical margins on survival outcomes in 95 consecutive patients with intermediate or high grade sarcomas who underwent preoperative radiotherapy prior to limb-salvage excision of an extremity sarcoma. The clinical outcome of 24 patients who had microscopically positive final pathologic surgical margins was compared with the outcome for the 71 patients with negative margins. The microscopically positive margins were occasionally due to preoperatively unsuspected tumor involvement with critical neurovascular structures. Alternatively (and more commonly) the final pathology report was simply at a variance with the intraoperative frozen section analyses.

Patients with microscopically positive margins had an increased rate of local recurrence where there was a 62% 5-year local recurrence-free survival, versus a 91% 5-year local recurrence-free survival in the margin-negative patients. However, overall survival was equivalent in both groups (65% 5-year overall survival in margin-negative patients versus 70% 5-year overall survival in those with positive margins). While the impact of a local recurrence in extremity soft tissue sarcoma may not be trivial, disease outcome clearly is determined by disseminated rather than locally recurrent disease. It is also pertinent that nearly two thirds of the microscopically positive patients did not fail locally. Consequently, a policy of watchful waiting is appropriate for these preoperatively irradiated individuals and suggests that microscopic positivity does not invariably imply sarcoma viability in the preoperatively radiated tumor bed (Fig. 2).

Robinson *et al.* [7] reported the Royal Marsden Hospital Sarcoma Unit experience with preoperative radiotherapy for initially inoperable soft tissue sarcomas of the extremities. Preoperative radiotherapy is particularly useful in these patients because it may cause sufficient cytoreduction to permit limb salvage rather than amputation. This study sought to clarify the selection factors entering the decision to use preoperative radiotherapy and also identify the determinants of successful clinical outcome. The study population included 70 patients who received preoperative radiotherapy and surgery. Forty-two patients (60%) responded to the radiotherapy on the basis of serial physical examinations or computed tomographic scans, or both. This radiotherapy response was dose related. Eighty percent response rates were observed in patients receiving 60 Gy or more radiotherapy. In contrast, only 50% of patients had a demonstrable response to less than 60-Gy treatment. Pathologic response was scored as the presence of specimen necrosis, which was present in only 23 (33%) of 69 evaluable preradiotherapy biopsy specimens but 39 (72%) of 54 postradiotherapy biopsies, the usual caveats about sampling error using needle biopsy specimens notwithstanding. However, incidence of necrosis did not correlate with clinical response.

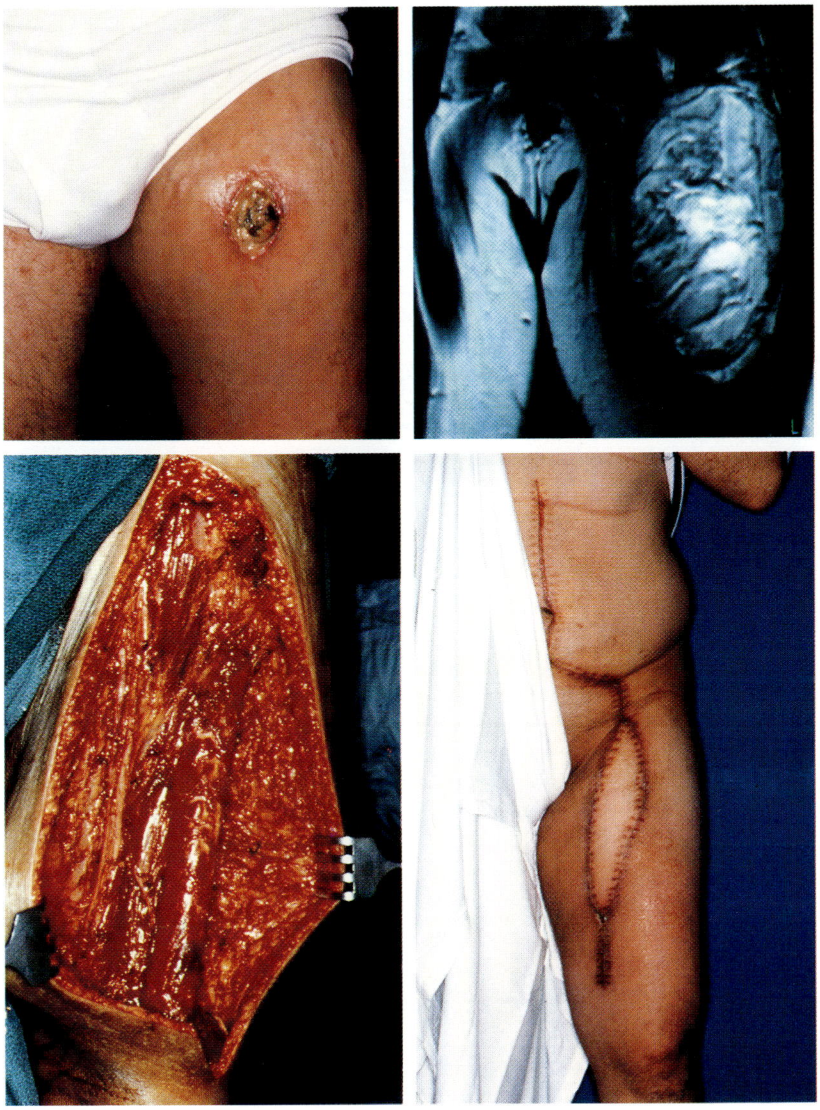

Fig. 3. Patient with a massive thigh sarcoma requiring preoperative chemotherapy and radiotherapy. **Top left**, Patient on presentation at MD Anderson Cancer Center. **Top right**, Magnetic resonance imaging scan of lesions. **Bottom left**, Tumor bed after resection. Note exposed bone and neurovascular structures. **Bottom right**, Reconstruction using rectus abdominis myocutaneous flap.

Neither response to preoperative radiotherapy nor amount of preoperative radiotherapy delivered correlated with local tumor control. Problems with wound healing and infection predominated among the various radiotherapy-related surgical complications (27 of 42 complications, which included eight wound breakdowns among the 10 major complications). The only factor that was associated with an increased incidence of wound complications was increased patient age; higher radiotherapy doses did not correlate with wound problems. Six patients had severely decreased range of motion in one or more joints, and eight patients had a morbid decrease in muscle power. However, 80% of patients had normal or excellent functional extremity results.

Surgery

Pignatti and Campanacci [8] briefly reviewed the basic surgical philosophy of Mario Companacci and colleagues at the Instituto Orthopedico Rizzoli, Bologna, Italy. The role of conservative surgery as part of a multimodality treatment program was defined, as was intraoperative management of sarcoma when critical neurovascular and osseous structures are involved with tumor.

Geer *et al.* [9••] examined the Memorial Sloan-Kettering Cancer Center experience with high-grade but small (less than 5 cm in diameter) extremity soft tissue sarcomas to determine the acceptable extent of resection and possible role (if any) for postoperative adjuvant nonsurgical treatments. Between 1982 and 1990, 174 patients were identified who had presented at the Memorial Hospital for primary treatment of small sarcomas of the extremities. After resection, local recurrence was observed in 11% of high-grade and 7% of low-grade tumors (no significant difference). No differences were observed between patients with high-grade and low-grade lesions regarding local recurrence-free survival. Depth, location, sex, or type of operation did not impact on local recurrence-free survival, whereas age of more than 50 years or positive surgical margins were associated with a significantly poorer local disease-free survival. Use of adjuvant radiotherapy did not have any apparent impact on local versus distant disease-free survival. Distant disease was observed in 7% of high-grade and 0% of low-grade lesions. However, there were no significant differences in disease-free survival between high- and low-grade patients. Distant disease-free survival was not affected by use of adjuvant chemotherapy. In summary, no factor correlated with a difference in overall survival for small sarcomas, and only age and positive margins adversely impacted on local disease-free survival. If these small sarcomas are adequately excised initially, no additional treatments are needed because there will be no increment in the extremely good survival for these patients.

Williard *et al.* [10] examined the Memorial Sloan Kettering Cancer Center experience regarding the decreasing role of amputation in the contemporary era of multimodality limb salvage. This retrospective review focused on patients who underwent amputation between 1982 and 1990 ($n=92$). As might be anticipated, significantly more amputation patients had high-grade tumors that were at least 5 cm in diameter, or tumors that invaded major neurovascular structures as compared with limb-salvage patients of the same time frame.

Overall survival in the amputation group was significantly worse than limb-salvage patients, attributable to the less favorable tumor characteristics. In fact, survival was better in limb-salvage patients who subsequently developed a local recurrence than those amputation patients who had never failed locally. These results support the conclusion that the most critical determinant of survival in soft tissue sarcoma is the capacity of a given primary tumor to distantly disseminate rather than the efficacy of local therapies.

Moseley [11•] reported the results of a prospective evaluation that compared preoperative intra-arterial doxorubicin followed sequentially by surgery and radiation ($n=18$) to regional limb perfusion with cisplatin followed by surgery and radiation ($n=20$). The trial was prospective but not randomized. Moreover, because perfusion does not provide reliable blood distribution to the buttocks and shoulder girdle as compared with infusion, patients with tumors in these areas were assigned to the infusion arm of study. In contrast, because doxorubicin is damaging to small vessels and can cause severe tissue toxicity if extravasated, patients with distal tumors preferentially received the perfusion arm of study.

Excellent local control was achieved in both groups. Response to chemotherapy did not correlate with degree of tumor necrosis. Length of hospitalization was 4 to 5 days in both groups. Complications were slightly increased in the perfusion group; however, excellent functional results were achieved for most patients in both groups. On the basis of this study, it is difficult to conclude that one form of regional drug delivery is superior to the other because of selection biases and lack of prospective randomization. Indeed, comparable results might have been achieved without the use of regional chemotherapy at all. Nonetheless, the authors demonstrate that these approaches are not particularly morbid in experienced hands and may salvage the occasional extremity that might otherwise require amputation.

Paz *et al.* [12•] examined the use of complex reconstruction (tissue transfer in conjunction with vascular synthetic grafts and bone prostheses as indicated) in 29 patients with extremity sarcomas who would have otherwise required amputation. Limb salvage was achieved in 96.6% of the patients; only 10.3% suffered a major wound complication. Long-term functional results were rated as good to excellent in 22 of the 29 patients. These excellent clinical outcomes were not achieved at the expense of tumor control in that disease-free and overall survival rates were comparable to those achieved in other series. However, the strength of this conclusion requires more time given the extremely short 2- and 3-year time intervals of follow-up for disease-free and overall survival.

Reece *et al.* [13] examined the University of Texas M.D. Anderson Cancer Center experience using free tissue transfer in extremity reconstructions after soft tissue sarcoma resection (Fig. 3). Eleven patients underwent immediate reconstruction, whereas eight patients had delayed reconstructions necessitated by complications of tumor treatment that otherwise would have required amputation. Limb salvage and postreconstruction ambulatory rates were both 95%. As might be anticipated, the immediate reconstruction group had shorter hospital stays and fewer postreconstruction complications.

References and recommended reading

Papers of particular interest, published within the annual period of review, have been highlighted as:
- • Of special interest
- •• Of outstanding interest

1. • Azzarelli A, Quagliuolo V, Casali P, Fissi S, Montalto F, Santoro A: **Preoperative Doxorubicin Plus Ifosfamide in Primary Soft-Tissue Sarcomas of the Extremities.** *Cancer Chemother Pharmacol* 1993, **31**(suppl 2):S210–S212.

This report prospectively demonstrates that documented clinical response to preoperative chemotherapy correlates with improved measures of survival.

2. Azzarelli A, Quagliuolo V, Fissi S, Casali P, Garbuglia A, Bignami P, Santoro A, Andreola S, Gennari L: **Intra-Arterial Induction Chemotherapy for Soft Tissue Sarcomas.** *Ann Oncol* 1992, **3**(suppl 2):S67–S70.

3. Verweij J, van Oosterom AT, Somers R, Santoro A, Roüessé J, Keizer J, Tursz T, Woll P, Steward W, Buesa J, Kerbrat P, Wagener D, Bramwell V, Thomas D, van Glabbeke M, Mouridsen HT: **Chemotherapy in the Multidisciplinary Approach to Soft Tissue Sarcomas: EORTC Soft Tissue and Bone Sarcoma Group Studies in Perspective.** *Ann Oncol* 1992, **3**(suppl 2):S75–S80.

4. Pezzi CM, Pollock RE, Evans HL, Lorigan JG, Pezzi TA, Benjamin RSS, Romsdahl MM: **Preoperative Chemotherapy for Soft-Tissue Sarcomas of the Extremities.** *Ann Surg* 1990, **211**:476–481.

5. • Ravaud A, Bui NB, Coindre JM, Lagarde P, Tramond P, Bonichon F, Stöckle E, Kahntor G, Trojani M, Chauvergne J, Marée D: **Prognostic Variables for the Selection of Patients With Operable Soft Tissue Sarcomas to be Considered in Adjuvant Chemotherapy Trials.** *Br J Cancer* 1992, **66**:961–969.

This report identifies key parameters of poor prognosis as a rationale for entry into adjuvant chemotherapy trials.

6. TANABE KK, POLLOCK RE, ELLIS LM, MURPHY A, SHERMAN N, ROMSDAHL MM: **Influence of Surgical Margins on Outcome in Patients With Preoperatively Irradiated Extremity Sarcomas.** *Cancer*, in press.

7. ROBINSON MH, BALL ABS, SCHOFIELD J, FISHER C, HARMER CL, THOMAS JM: **Preoperative Radiotherapy for Initially Inoperative Extremity Soft Tissue Sarcomas.** *Clin Oncol (R Coll Radiol)* 1992, 4:36–43.

8. PIGNATTI G, CAMPANACCI M: **Surgical Approach to Soft Tissue Sarcomas of the Extremities.** *Ann Oncol* 1992, **3**(suppl 2):S59–S61.

9. •• GEER RJ, WOODRUFF J, CASPER ES, BRENNAN MF: **Management of Small Soft-Tissue Sarcoma of the Extremity in Adults.** *Arch Surg* 1992, **127**:1285–1289.

This is the first report to establish the extremely favorable survival outcome for high-grade small sarcomas treated by adequate surgical excision alone.

10. WILLIARD WC, HAJDU SI, CASPER ES, BRENNAN MF: **Comparison of Amputation With Limb-Sparing Operations for Adult Soft Tissue Sarcoma of the Extremity.** *Ann Surg* 1992, **215**:271–275.

11. • MOSELEY H: **An Evaluation of Two Methods of Limb Salvage in Extremity Soft-Tissue Sarcomas.** *Arch Surg* 1992, **127**:1169–1174.

The role of regional chemotherapy remains unresolved in soft tissue sarcoma, as demonstrated in this single institution series.

12. • PAZ IB, WAGMAN LD, TERZ J, CHANDRASEKHAR B, LORANT JA, MOSCARELLO GM, ODOM-MARYON T: **Extended Indications for Functional Limb-Sparing Surgery in Extremity Sarcoma Using Complex Reconstruction.** *Arch Surg* 1992, **127**:1278–1281.

Complex reconstructive procedures after extirpative sarcoma resections have excellent functional results that do not compromise survival.

13. REECE GP, SCHUSTERMAN MA, POLLOCK RE, KROLL S, MILLER MJ, BALDWIN BJ, ROMSDAHL MM, JANJAN NA: **Immediate Versus Delayed Free-Tissue Transfer Salvage of the Lower Extremity in Soft-Tissue Sarcoma Patients.** *Ann Surg Oncol*, in press.

Raphael E. Pollock, MD, PhD, Chairman, Department of Surgical Oncology, The University of Texas MD Anderson Cancer Center, 1515 Holcombe Boulevard, Houston, TX 77030, USA.

Alternative surgical procedures for primary rectal carcinoma

Alan P. Meagher, FRACS, and John H. Pemberton, MD

Mayo Clinic, Rochester, Minnesota, USA

This review summarizes the recent literature on alternative surgical procedures for treating rectal carcinoma. After a brief examination of publications on preoperative staging, current reports on alternative surgical procedures, from local excision to anterior resection and extended resection, are discussed. Although radiotherapy and chemotherapy are assuming increasingly prominent roles in the management of rectal carcinoma, detailed examination of these therapies is beyond the scope of this review.

Current Opinion in General Surgery 1994:230–237

Preoperative staging

Selection of appropriate treatment modalities in patients with rectal carcinoma would most likely be facilitated by accurate preoperative staging. The current rage in preoperative studies is ultrasonography. In 118 patients with rectal cancer, Herzog *et al.* [1•] compared the results of preoperative endorectal ultrasonography with the pathologic findings. The overall accuracy in staging the depth of invasion was 89%. In 10% of patients the disease was understaged, and in 1% it was overstaged. The depth of invasion of tumors of the upper and middle rectum was assessed with significantly better accuracy than was that of tumors of the lower rectum ($P<0.001$). The accuracy of staging of lymph node involvement was 80% (false-positive rate, 15%; false-negative rate, 5%). Beynon *et al.* [2] studied 63 patients with primary rectal adenocarcinoma by endorectal ultrasonography. These investigators compared the depth of the carcinoma measured on ultrasonography (in centimeters) with the depth measured in the excised specimen. A significant correlation occurred between the ultrasonic depth and the depth on paraffin section ($P=0.001$; $r=0.46$), although there were a number of widely scattered results. Lymph nodes were not studied.

The evaluation of stenotic rectal tumors is not possible with conventional endorectal ultrasonography. Nielsen *et al.* [3] evaluated such lesions with a forward-looking endoprobe. The accuracy of assessing the depth of invasion was 82%. However, the detection of lymph nodes, whether involved by metastatic cancer or not, was poor: in only 16 or 22 patients undergoing radical surgery were lymph nodes detected at all, and no real attempt was made to predict which nodes were metastatic, because all appeared hypoechoic. Recognizing the limitations of ultrasonography in detecting lymph node involvement, Nielsen *et al.* [4] studied 20 excised specimens of colorectal cancer in an attempt to evaluate the lymph nodes under artificial but optimal conditions. Results were accurate in only 56% of all malignant nodes and 25% of benign nodes. Review articles by Durdey and Williams [5] and Feifel and Hildebrandt [6] stated that the accuracy of endorectal ultrasonography in detecting the stage of invasion through the bowel wall is more than 80% in most studies. However, the accuracy in staging lymph node metastases, which is of greatest clinical importance, is generally less than 80%. Ultrasonography is, nonetheless, an impressive tool for determining the depth of invasion reached by a rectal carcinoma; whether it has metastasized to the lymph nodes is another story. Overall, ultrasonography remains an intensely user-dependent diagnostic modality.

Other methods of staging are also under investigation. Okizuka *et al.* [7] studied 33 patients with magnetic resonance imaging. Invasion of the muscularis propria, perirectal fat, and adjacent organs was accurately predicted in 88%, 79%, and 100% of cases, respectively. Perirectal and distal lymph node metastases were accurately detected in 87% and 100% of cases, respectively, although the sensitivity of this method for detecting perirectal nodes was only 57% (four of seven cases). Gupta *et al.* [8] published a pilot study of positron emission tomography in staging colorectal carcinoma. Their results are promising, and further investigation may prove interesting. The positive predictive value of this modality for detecting tumor sites was 87%. Feifel and Hildebrandt [6] injected anti–carcinoembryonic antigen monoclonal antibody into the rectal submucosa of eight patients. However, in all patients there was nonspecific uptake by involved *and* noninvolved nodes.

Local excision

Whereas selection of patients suitable for local excision may be improved by preoperative staging, Brodsky *et al.* [9••] have also demonstrated the importance of careful pathologic examination of the specimen when rectal carcinoma has been locally excised. The specimens of 154 patients who had stage T1 or T2 rectal carcinomas within 11 cm of the anal verge, which were removed by anterior resection or abdominoperineal resection, were reexamined. The risk of lymph node metastasis with T1 and T2 tumors was 12% and 22%, respectively. Overall,

 ISBN 1-85922-671-X ISSN 1065–6243

the risk of lymph node metastasis with well-differentiated tumors was 0%. The risk of metastasis with tumors that had no lymphatic or blood vessel invasion was 17%, and it was 31% if evidence of either of these was present (*P*=0.04). No T1 tumors without lymphatic or blood vessel invasion had lymph node involvement. The authors concluded that local excision alone is adequate for well-differentiated or moderately differentiated T1 rectal cancers in the absence of lymphatic or blood vessel invasion, and for well-differentiated T2 tumors. Radical resection or local excision with radiation therapy may be more appropriate for the remainder.

In an attempt to address the effect of tumor grade on outcome after local excision, Lock *et al.* [10•] reviewed the cases of 152 patients who were treated by local excision of rectal carcinoma at St. Mark's Hospital between 1948 and 1984. Fifty-six patients had low-grade tumors, and only one of these patients subsequently died of carcinoma. Of the 81 patients with average-grade tumors, 10 died of carcinoma. Six of the 15 patients who had high-grade tumors underwent early reoperation, and three of them died of carcinoma. In the nine patients who did not undergo early reoperation, there were three related deaths (two from carcinoma and one after rectal excision for recurrence). The authors concluded that local excision was safe in low-grade tumors but not in average-grade tumors. Interestingly, the authors gave no definite advice about high-grade tumors, as six of nine patients who did not undergo reoperation survived more than 5 years.

Bailey *et al.* [11•] demonstrated that good results can be achieved with local excision when careful selection criteria are used. Local excision was attempted in well-differentiated or moderately well differentiated nonmucinous, mobile tumors, which ideally were on the posterior or posterolateral wall and involved less than 40% of the circumference of the rectum. Sixty-three patients underwent local excision, but abdominoperineal excision was subsequently advised in 10 because the pathologic findings revealed invasion beyond the muscularis propria. Of the remaining 53 patients, 23 underwent postoperative radiotherapy, which was introduced as a routine in the latter years of the study. Four of the 53 patients (8%) had a recurrence, but reexcision appears to have been successful in two. The median follow-up was 44 months. The 5-year disease-free survival rate was 90%. These authors and Nivatvongs and Wolff [12] emphasized the importance of meticulous surgical technique in treating such patients (Fig. 1).

Good results were also reported by Coco *et al.* [13•], who studied 36 patients who underwent local excision for rectal carcinomas. The selection criteria were similar to those used by Bailey *et al.* [11•]. Adjuvant radiotherapy was used in T2 lesions. The corrected 5-year survival rate was 90%. In a further study by Heimann *et al.* [14], of 15 patients with T1 or T2 lesions initially treated by local excision, only one died of metastatic carcinoma.

However, in a series of 40 patients treated with local excision between 1969 and 1985, Killingback [15•] re-

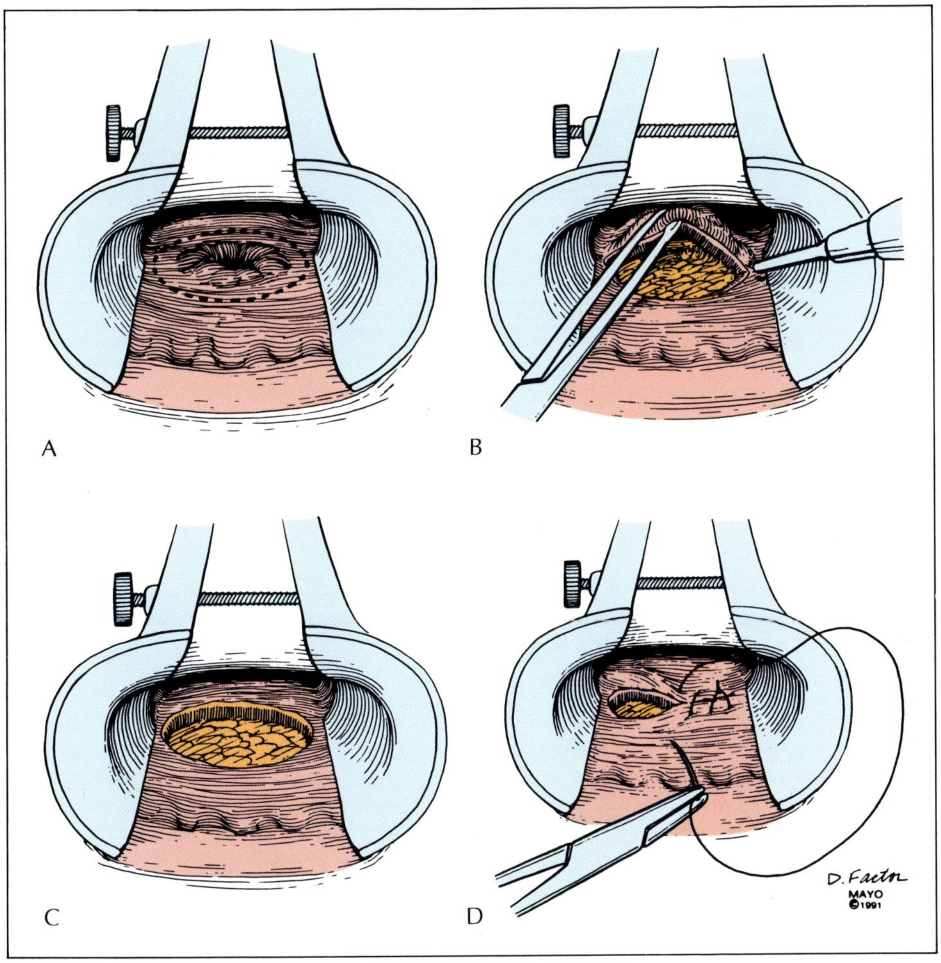

Fig. 1. Perianal excision for carcinoma of the low rectum. **A**, The line of excision, with a 1.5- to 2-cm margin, is marked with electrocautery. **B**, The incision is made while the inferior margin is grasped with an Allis clamp. **C**, A full-thickness disk of the lesion is removed, exposing the perirectal fat. **D**, The defect is closed transversely with a running absorbable suture. (*From* Nivatvongs and Wolff [12]; with permission.)

ported that invasion of the tumor was limited to the submucosa in only two patients, whereas 32 patients had invasion of the muscularis propria, and six had extrarectal invasion. After a minimum of 5 years, the cancer-specific mortality was 28%. In discussing the results, the author recognized that the poor outcomes were due largely to compromised patient selection. (Patients were sick and tumors were advanced.) Likewise, Wong *et al.* [16] reported a recurrence rate of 24% in 25 patients who underwent local excision of rectal carcinoma with postoperative radiotherapy. In 10 of these patients, local excision was performed because abdominoperineal excision was refused or the patients were too sick to undergo conventional surgery.

In a review of local excision and postoperative radiotherapy, Minsky [17] concluded that local excision and postoperative radiotherapy had a place in T1 and T2 tumors but not in T3 tumors; the local failure rate in these tumors is 24%. In contrast, Rosenthal *et al.* [18] reported on a phase I and II trial in which extensive low-lying rectal carcinomas were treated with local excision combined with preoperative and postoperative radiotherapy. Entry into the study was restricted to tumors that encompassed at least one third of the rectal circumference, and five of the 16 patients had T3 lesions. The actuarial 3-year relapse rate was 47%, although the actuarial 3-year survival rate was 94%.

At present, it is not possible to state confidently which criteria can be used in selecting patients for curative local excision of rectal carcinoma. The pathologic criteria of Brodsky *et al.* [9••] and the clinical criteria of Bailey *et al.* [11•] appear to be the best available. If good-quality ultrasonography is accessible, it can be helpful. As always, the patient's medical condition and wishes must be taken into account. Although postoperative radiotherapy is being increasingly used, no convincing data support its role. It is worth noting that local *surgical* alternatives are not the only alternatives: Papillon and Berard [19•] reported on 312 patients with well-differentiated or moderately well differentiated rectal carcinoma judged clinically to be stage T1 or T2 who were treated with endocavity irradiation with or without ^{192}Ir implants. The 5-year disease-free survival rate was 74%, and the cancer-specific mortality was only 7.7%.

Electrocoagulation

An alternative form of local treatment for rectal carcinoma, electrocoagulation, has some proponents. One disadvantage of this technique is that there is no pathologic specimen to assess the extent of invasion. In a study of 114 patients treated with electrocoagulation, Eisenstat and Oliver [20] reported that 81 were treated for cure and 33 for palliation. Of those treated for cure, 38% later required abdominoperineal excisions, and the 5-year survival rate for these 81 patients was 47%. This modality may have a role in palliation, as only one of the 33 patients treated for palliation required a colostomy before dying. Clearly, however, it has no role as a curative modality. Stahl *et al.* [21] reported on 33 patients who were treated with electrocoagulation, with curative intent. Nine (27%) died of recurrent or metastatic disease.

Transanal endoscopic microsurgery

In an attempt to extend the role of local excision to lesions higher in the rectum, the technique of transanal endoscopic microsurgery has been developed. However, only a minority of patients treated to date have had cancer. Moreover, because the technique was first introduced in 1983, there is insufficient follow-up to assess this method fully. The resectoscope used has a diameter of 40 mm and is made in two lengths, 12 and 20 cm. After introduction of the resectoscope, the field is extended by insufflation with carbon dioxide. An angled stereoscopic telescope is used, and specially designed scissors, forceps, needle holders, and suction devices are available (Fig. 2). Buess *et al.* [22•] reported the results of this technique in 274 patients, 74 of whom had carcinomas. Operative complications in the carcinoma group included two suture line dehiscences and two rectovaginal fistulas. Approximately one third of the patients underwent more radical surgical procedures after review of the pathologic specimens. In the 29 patients with T1 lesions followed up for up to 6 years, there was only one recurrence. Said *et al.* [23•] reported their experience with 233 patients, 51 of whom were treated for carcinoma. Follow-up ranged from 1 month to 6 years. Of the 22 patients with T1 lesions, one suffered a local recurrence. Twenty-nine patients had more advanced lesions; in 11 of these patients, treatment was only palliative. One of these patients had tumor progression requiring sigmoidectomy. It should be noted that this technique is designed specifically for lesions for which the alternative treatment is anterior resection rather than abdominoperineal resection.

Rectal excision

MacFarlane *et al.* [24••] updated the Basingstoke series of surgical treatment for rectal cancer. The actuarial local recurrence rate 5 years after curative anterior resection was 4% (95% CI, 0% to 7.5%), and the overall recurrence rate was 18% (95% CI, 10% to 25%). Even if cases judged by the surgeon at the time of resection to be locally noncurative were included, these rates only increased to 6% (95% CI, 0% to 11%) and 22% (95% CI, 13% to 29%). The operation was defined as curative if at the end of the procedure, the surgeon believed that all grossly detectable cancer was removed. Ten-year data for curative anterior resection demonstrated a local recurrence rate of 4% (95% CI, 0% to 11%) and an overall recurrence rate of 19% (95% CI, 7% to 32%).

It is the issue of total mesorectal excision, an issue brought forward by the group at Basingstoke, that is the most controversial because it contradicts a number of older and current clinical and pathologic studies suggesting that transection of the rectum 2 cm below a rectal carcinoma is sufficient. For example, in a recent study by Vernava *et al.* [25], 243 patients who had undergone anterior resection were divided into 1-cm groups based on the length of the distal resection margin (*eg*, 0 to 1-cm margin, 1- to 2-cm margin, etc.). No significant difference was found in local or distant recurrence when each interval was studied, down to 1 cm. Those with margins of less than 0.8 cm had more frequent anasto-

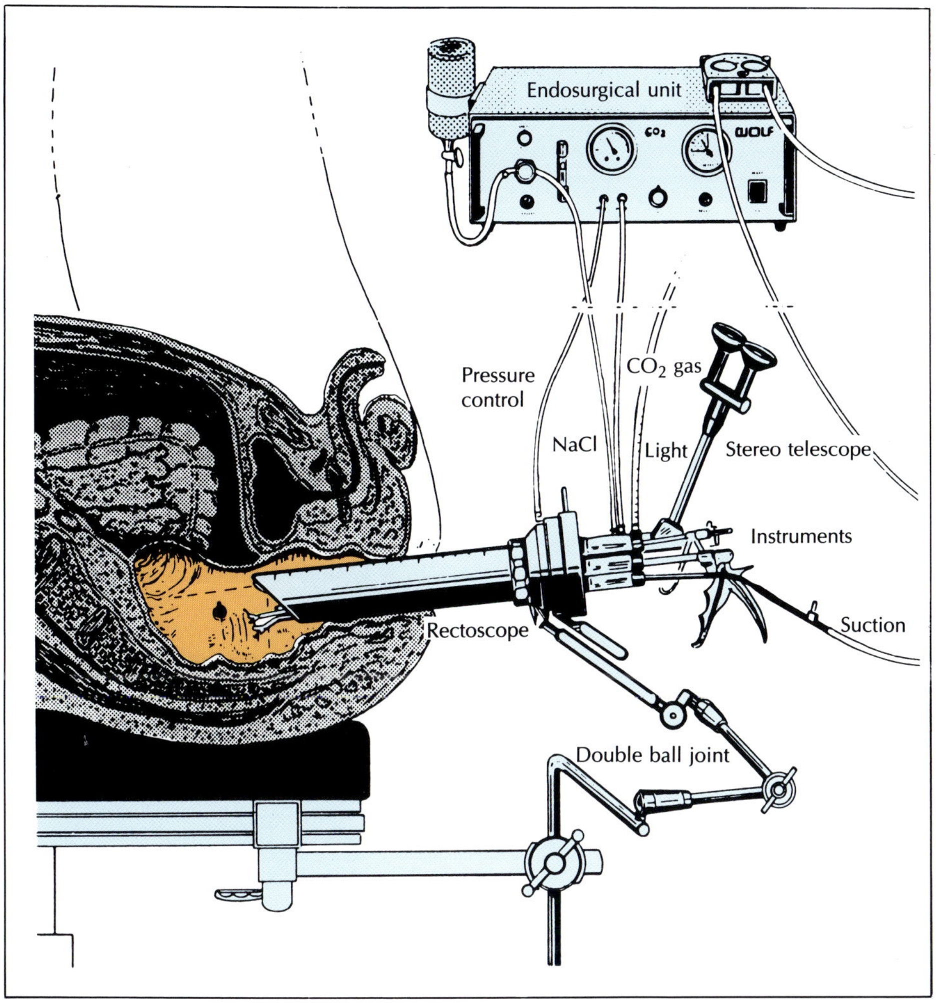

Fig. 2. Technique for transanal endoscopic microsurgery. (*From* Said *et al.* [23•]; with permission.)

motic recurrences than those with greater margins (30% vs 10.5%; P=0.01), and the former group also had a lower 5-year survival rate (49.3% vs 67.5%; P=0.01). Both groups were well matched for clinical and pathologic factors and for the use of adjuvant radiotherapy. In addition, MacFarlane *et al.* [24••] noted that the cost of total mesorectal excision is not inconsequential, and there is a 17.4% anastomotic leak rate (11% clinical and 6.4% radiologic), so that temporary protective colostomies are now employed routinely.

MacFarlane *et al.* [24••] compared their results of surgical treatment alone in high-risk patients with Dukes B and C carcinomas with the results of Krook *et al.* [26]. Krook *et al.*'s large, prospective, randomized study demonstrated that recurrence and survival rates in a similar high-risk group (here, patients with at least T1 or N1 tumors, which are equivalent to Dukes B or C tumors) were better in patients treated postoperatively with chemotherapy and radiotherapy than in those treated with radiotherapy alone; the local and overall recurrence rates were 25% and 62.5% in the group receiving surgery plus radiotherapy and 13.5% and 41.5% in the group receiving surgery plus chemotherapy and radiotherapy. In the Basingstoke high-risk group, the figures for local recurrence and overall recurrence were 5% and 22%, respectively. Importantly, in an accompanying editorial, Fielding [27] pointed out that one must be very cautious in making such comparisons because the two studies involve distinct patient populations and distinct pathologic and surgical evaluations. Fielding noted that although the findings are inconclusive, confounding factors alone are unlikely to be responsible for the differences. Controversy over the role of total mesorectal excision is likely to continue for some time.

In a paper by Ng *et al.* [28•], the prognostic importance of lateral surgical margins was reexamined. Sixteen of the 80 specimens studied had microscopic involvement of the lateral resection margin. Local recurrence occurred in 53% of these patients, compared with 28% of patients who had no involvement. Multivariate analysis showed involvement of the lateral resection margin to be of independent prognostic significance. In a review of previous papers on lateral resection margins, Wolff [29] concluded that the prognostic significance of this variable should be recognized, although the role of adjuvant therapy in patients with involved margins should be addressed in future studies.

Practical techniques of anterior resection

Gertsch *et al.* [30•] addressed the role of lavage of the rectal stump before a stapled anastomosis is performed. Ten patients underwent anterior resection with a circular stapler in which no cytotoxic lavage was used. After the anastomosis, the stapler and donuts were washed with saline, which was collected for cytologic examination. In nine of the 10 cases, malignant cells were identified. Although it is impossible to prove using the results of this study, these cells could implant and cause recurrence, which prompted the authors to conclude that rectal lavage has a place in the management of rectal carcinoma.

Mealy *et al.* [31] reviewed the cases of 114 consecutive patients who underwent anterior resection for rectal cancer. The authors had a policy of not using defunctioning stomas. The anastomosis was below the peritoneal reflection in 74 patients, and the six clinically significant leaks occurred in this group. All six underwent conversion to end colostomies, and one died. The interpretation of these results is extremely difficult. The authors concluded that the *routine* use of a defunctioning colostomy at anterior resection should be questioned. However, issues raised in subsequent correspondence regarding this paper included questions about the extent of mesorectal excision [32] and the treatment of all leaks with an end stoma [33] and a suggestion that the results may have been improved if all the low anastomoses were defunctioned [34]. Clearly, current opinions on the role of defunctioning low anterior resections are disparate. The decision to divert must be based on the patient's build, the type of pathology, the level of the anastomosis, and technical operative details, such as incomplete donuts.

With respect to donuts, the results of four large studies of the double-staple technique have been reported (Table 1). Redmond *et al.* [35•] reported on a prospective, consecutive series of 111 patients in whom all anastomoses were less than 10 cm from the anal verge. Ninety-six of the operations were for carcinoma. Although 9% of patients developed strictures, all were managed satisfactorily with dilatation alone. The local recurrence rate was 7%, with a mean follow-up of 40 months during which three-monthly sigmoidoscopic examinations were done. Baran *et al.* [36•] reported on 104 patients, 35 of whom had preoperative radiotherapy. It appears, from the studies listed in Table 1, that the double-staple technique is associated with results equal to those of other techniques.

There is increasing interest in constructing a colonic J pouch when anastomoses to the anal canal or anorectal junction are performed because the increased capacity of the pouch may result in improved function. Berger *et al.* [39••] reported on the results of colonic pouch–anal anastomosis in 162 patients who had carcinoma. A J pouch approximately 7 cm long was sutured to the dentate line, and a defunctioning stoma was routinely fashioned. Five patients developed anastomotic leakage, pelvic sepsis, or both. All drained spontaneously without the need for laparotomy. After 1 year, continence was perfect in 52% of cases, leakage of gas or mucus or occasional minor fecal soiling occurred in 44%, and major fecal soiling occurred in 4%. The mean number of stools per day was two. A pad was never used by 71% of patients. Four percent suffered fecal urgency, and 21% needed to evacuate a second time soon after a bowel motion. Although these results can be compared only with those in historical controls, they do appear to be better than those achieved with straight coloanal anastomoses.

Pelissier *et al.* [40•,41] reported on 33 colonic pouch–anal anastomoses in which the double-staple technique was used. A defunctioning colostomy was performed in all patients. There were two clinical anastomotic leaks, which did not require laparotomy. Function was compared with that in a group of matched, nonsurgically treated, normal control subjects. Surprisingly, there was no significant difference between the two groups in bowel frequency, urge to defecate, continence, urgency, or the need to wear a pad, although the surgically treated group tended to have more incontinence and an increased need to wear a pad. The only significant difference was that the ability to evacuate was better in controls, with satisfactory evacuation being achieved in one sitting in 97% of control subjects, compared with 48% of patients. Cohen [42•] reported on a series of 23 patients who had this procedure, in 14 of whom a double-staple technique was used (Fig. 3). Two patients had diverting stomas. There were no clinical anastomotic leaks, and the functional outcome was similar to that in the previously mentioned studies.

Abdominoperineal resection

Abdominoperineal resection is often thought to be associated with formidable morbidity and mortality. It is thus worth noting the results of a series of 155 abdominoperineal resections reported by Rothenberger and Wong [43•]. The mortality rate was 2.6%. The perineal wound was closed primarily in 92%, and there was only one pelvic abscess. There were three wound infections, two cases of pulmonary embolism, and one case of pneumonia. Urinary tract infections or urinary retention occurred in 15 patients, and seven patients developed small bowel obstruction. With modern surgical management, excellent results such as these can be achieved.

Table 1. Results of the double-staple technique for low anterior resection

Study	Patients, *n*	Patients with defunctioning stomas, %	Clinical leaks, %	Local recurrence, %	Stricture rate, %
Redmond *et al.* [35•]	111	29	2.7	7	9
Baran *et al.* [36•]	104	25	2.8	—	0
Griffen *et al.* [37•]	91	0	3.3	9	3.3
Moran *et al.* [38•]	55	9	9.1	7	5.5

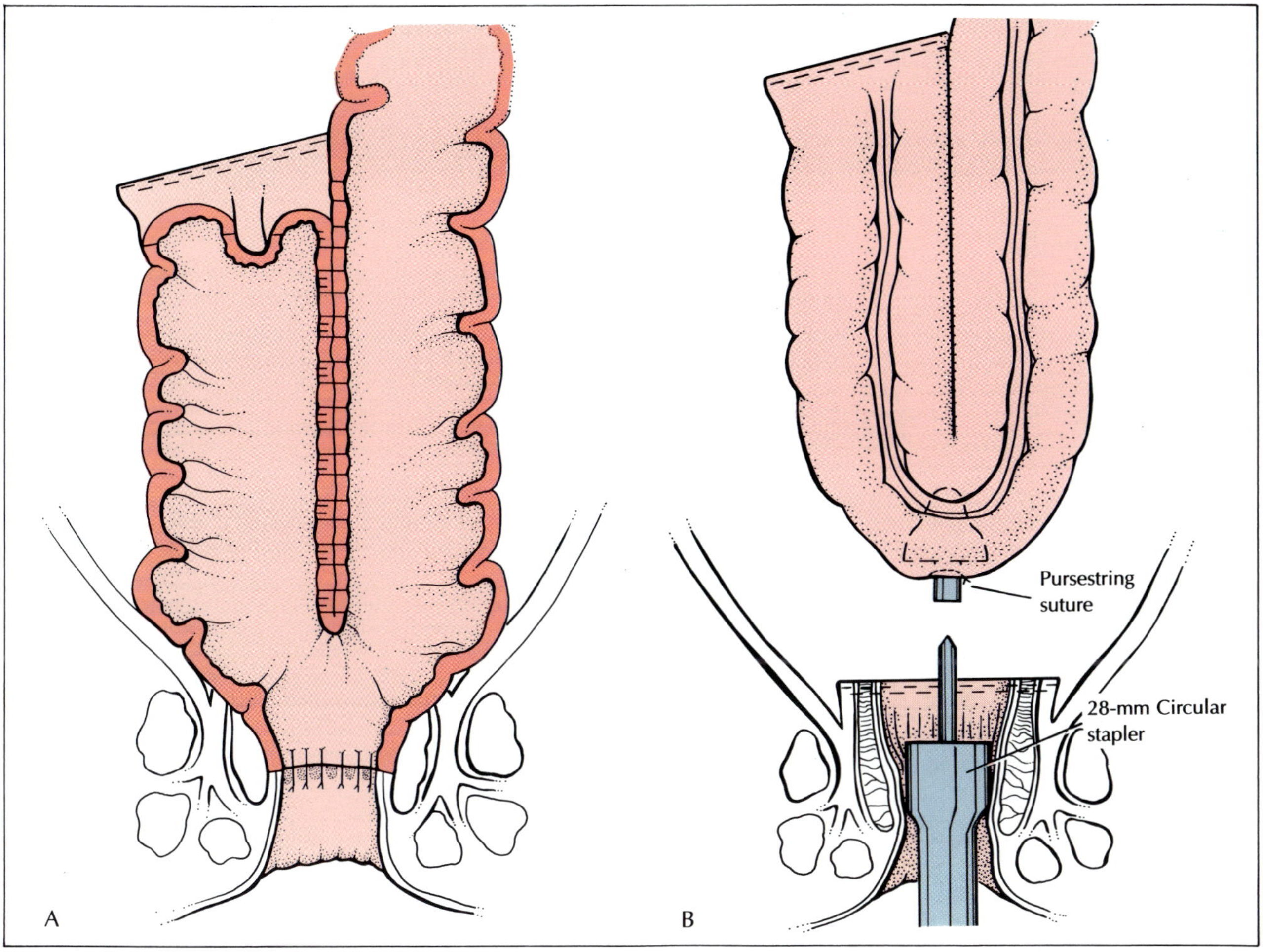

Fig. 3. A, Per anal sutured coloanal J-pouch reconstruction. **B**, Double-staple technique for low colorectal or high coloanal J-pouch reconstruction. (*From* Cohen [42•]; with permission.)

In a prospective, nonrandomized trial of three types of perineal wound management by Campos *et al.* [44•], 102 patients had either 1) packing of the presacral space after closure of the pelvic peritoneum, 2) closure of the pelvic peritoneum and the perineum with two perineal drains, or 3) closure of the perineal wound but no peritoneal closure, with two abdominal drains. Primary healing of the perineum was better with the third method (85%) than with the second (53%). Infection was also lower with the third (15%) than with the second (47%), and hospital stay was shortest with the third method.

The increasing use of postoperative radiotherapy has prompted the evaluation of different methods of excluding the small bowel from the pelvis. Thom *et al.* [45•] used a sling of polyglycolic acid mesh in 43 patients who then underwent postoperative radiotherapy. After a mean follow-up of 2 years, no associated small bowel injuries were noted. Lechner and Cesnik [46•] used the greater omentum to keep the small bowel above the sacral promontory. There have been no small bowel complications with a mean follow-up of 3 years. Chen *et al.* [47•] reported on 18 cases in which the posterior rectus sheath and peritoneum were mobilized and sutured to the posterior abdominal wall. The mean follow-up was 18 months, and there were two episodes of significant radiation enteritis.

In an important paper, Willett *et al.* [48•] reviewed the results of abdominoperineal resection in 64 patients with carcinomas confined to the muscularis propria (TNM stage I). None of 12 patients who had tumor confined to the submucosa had recurrence. However, of the 52 patients with muscularis propria involvement, the actuarial 6-year disease-free survival and freedom from metastasis rates were only 80% and 88%, respectively. The authors argue that adjuvant therapy may have a role in patients with penetration of tumor into the wall of the rectum. Furthermore, it is worth comparing these figures with those achieved with local excision because the figures for recurrence and survival are very similar.

Laparoscopic rectal excision

Laparoscopic colon and rectal surgery is being assessed in a number of centers; its advantages remain undefined. Of 63 patients who underwent laparoscopic colorectal procedures reported on by Falk *et al.* [49•], nine had rectal procedures (six had low anterior resections and three had abdominoperineal resections). The overall (n=63) major morbidity and mortality rates were 24% and 0%. Forty-one percent were converted to open procedures. Hospital stays appeared to be shorter than usual. Subcutaneous metastases in trocar sites following laparoscopic resection of malignancies, such as the two reported by Walsh *et al.* [50], are of some concern.

Extended resection

In a review article, Devine and Dozois [51] noted that in approximately 5% of primary rectal cancers, there is adherence to adjacent structures. In about half of such cases, the adherence is inflammatory, and in the other half, it is malignant. If en bloc removal can be performed with tumor-free margins, then 5-year survival rates of more than 50% have been reported. In most cases adherence is to the vagina, uterus, or dome of the bladder, and en bloc excision does not increase morbidity greatly in such cases. However, adherence to the bladder trigone or to the prostate may require pelvic exenteration. Ideally, these cases should be diagnosed preoperatively, so that treatment options can be discussed with the patient and preoperative radiotherapy can be used if it is considered appropriate. Curley *et al.* [52•], in a retrospective review of 101 patients who underwent extended excisions for colorectal carcinoma, noted that preoperative symptoms related to the genitourinary tract were present in 46 patients, and 43 (93%) had malignant invasion of these structures. However, 51% of patients without symptoms also had invasion of genitourinary structures, so that the finding of unanticipated invasion of adjacent structures will continue to be encountered. Preoperative investigation of patients *with* genitourinary symptoms appears to be warranted, and Curley *et al.* found that intravenous pyelography, computed tomography, and cystoscopy were accurate in diagnosing invasion of adjacent structures in 89%, 83%, and 87% of cases, respectively. However, invasion of adjacent organs is a relatively uncommon occurrence, and routine investigation does not appear to be warranted in patients in whom there is no suspicion of local invasion.

References and recommended reading

Papers of particular interest, published within the annual period of review, have been highlighted as:

- • Of special interest
- •• Of outstanding interest

1. • Herzog U, von Flue M, Tondelli P, Schuppisser JP: **How Accurate Is Endorectal Ultrasound in Preoperative Staging of Rectal Cancer?** *Dis Colon Rectum* 1993, **36**:127–134.

This article demonstrates that assessment of the depth of tumor invasion can be accurate in almost 90% of cases, although assessment of lymph node involvement is less accurate.

2. Beynon J, Mortensen NJMcC, Channer JL, Rigby H: **Rectal Endosonography Accurately Predicts Depth of Penetration in Rectal Cancer.** *Int J Colorectal Dis* 1992, 7:4–7.

3. Nielsen MB, Pedersen JF, Christiansen J: **Rectal Endosonography in the Evaluation of Stenotic Rectal Tumors.** *Dis Colon Rectum* 1993, 36:275–279.

4. Nielsen MB, Qvitzau S, Pedersen JF: **Detection of Pericolonic Lymph Nodes in Patients With Colorectal Cancer: An In Vitro and In Vivo Study of the Efficacy of Endosonography.** *AJR Am J Roentgenol* 1993, **161**:57–60.

5. Durdey P, Williams NS: **Pre-operative Evaluation of Patients With Low Rectal Carcinoma.** *World J Surg* 1992, 16:430–436.

6. Feifel G, Hildebrandt U: **New Diagnostic Imaging in Rectal Cancer: Endosonography and Immunoscintigraphy.** *World J Surg* 1992, **16**:841–847.

7. Okizuka H, Sugimura K, Ishida T: **Preoperative Local Staging of Rectal Carcinoma With MR Imaging and a Rectal Balloon.** *J Magn Reson Imaging* 1993, 3:329–335.

8. Gupta NC, Falk PM, Frank AL, Thorson AM, Frick MP, Bowman B: **Pre-operative Staging of Colorectal Carcinoma Using Positron Emission Tomography.** *Nebr Med J* 1993, **78**:30–35.

9. •• Brodsky JT, Richard GK, Cohen AM, Minsky BD: **Variables Correlated With the Risk of Lymph Node Metastasis in Early Rectal Cancer.** *Cancer* 1992, 69:322–326.

This important paper demonstrates that close pathologic examination of the excised specimen after local excision of rectal carcinoma for depth of invasion, differentiation, and lymphatic or blood vessel invasion can be of predictive value in estimating the risk of lymph node metastasis.

10. • Lock MR, Ritchie JK, Hawley PR: **Reappraisal of Radical Local Excision for Carcinoma of the Rectum.** *Br J Surg* 1993, **80**:928–929.

The authors demonstrate that tumor grade is a determinant of outcome after local excision of rectal carcinoma.

11. • Bailey HR, Huval WV, Max E, Smith KW, Butts DR, Zamora LF: **Local Excision of Carcinoma of the Rectum for Cure.** *Surgery* 1992, **111**:555–561.

In this large series, well-defined operative criteria are used. The results of local excision, often combined with radiotherapy, are excellent. Only four of 52 patients suffered recurrence, and two of these appear to have been successfully treated.

12. Nivatvongs S, Wolff BG: **Technique of Per Anal Excision for Carcinoma of the Low Rectum.** *World J Surg* 1992, **16**:447–450.

13. • Coco C, Magistrelli P, Granone P, Roncolini G, Picciocchi A: **Conservative Surgery for Early Cancer of the Distal Rectum.** *Dis Colon Rectum* 1992, **35**:131–136.

A corrected 5-year survival rate of 90% was achieved following local excision of rectal carcinoma. Patients who did not meet pathologic criteria after examination of the specimen were advised to undergo radical resections.

14. Heimann TM, Oh C, Steinhagen RM, Greenstein AJ, Perez C, Aufses AH: **Surgical Treatment of Tumors of the Distal Rectum With Sphincter Preservation.** *Ann Surg* 1992, **216**:432–436.

15. • Killingback M: **Local Excision of Carcinoma of the Rectum: Indications.** *World J Surg* 1992, **16**:437–446.

This important paper demonstrates that when local excision is attempted in unfavorable tumors, often because of the patient's general condition, recurrence rates are high.

16. Wong SC, Stern H, Cummings BJ: **Local Excision and Post-operative Radiation Therapy for Rectal Carcinoma.** *Int J Radiat Oncol Biol Phys* 1993, **25**:669–675.

17. Minsky BD: **Clinical Experience With Local Excision and Postoperative Radiation Therapy for Rectal Cancer.** *Dis Colon Rectum* 1993, 36:405–409.

18. Rosenthal SA, Yeung RS, Weese JL, Eisenberg BL, Hoffman JP, Coia LR, Hanks GE: **Conservative Management of Extensive Low-Lying Rectal Carcinomas With Transanal Local Excision and Combined Preoperative and Postoperative Radiation Therapy.** *Cancer* 1992, 69:335–341.

19. • Papillon J, Berard P: **Endocavity Irradiation in the Conservative Treatment of Adenocarcinoma of the Low Rectum.** *World J Surg* 1992, **16**:451–457.

This paper, from the center that has led the world in this technique, outlines the long-term results of endocavity irradiation when used as primary curative treatment for rectal cancer.

20. Eisenstat TE, Oliver GC: **Electrocoagulation for Adenocarcinoma of the Low Rectum.** *World J Surg* 1992, **16**:458–462.

21. Stahl TJ, Murray JJ, Coller JA, Schoetz DJ, Roberts PL, Veidenheimer MC: **Sphincter-Saving Alternatives in the Management of Adenocarcinoma Involving the Distal Rectum.** *Arch Surg* 1993, **128**:545–550.

22. • Buess G, Mentges B, Manncke K, Starlinger M, Becker HD: **Technique and Results of Transanal Endoscopic Microsurgery in Early Rectal Cancer.** *Am J Surg* 1992, **163**:63–70.

The results of this new technique for rectal adenomas and carcinomas are presented. Early results suggest that the technique may have a place in colorectal surgical practice.

23. • Said S, Huber P, Pichlmaier H: **Technique and Clinical Results of Endorectal Surgery.** *Surgery* 1993, **113**:65–75.

The authors operated for indications similar to those used by Buess *et al.* (*Am J Surg* 1992, 163:63–70) and have also been able to achieve promising results.

24. MacFarlane JK, Ryall RDH, Heald RJ: **Mesorectal Excision for Rectal**
•• **Cancer.** *Lancet* 1993, **341**:457–460.
The long-term results of total mesorectal excision are analyzed by an independent assessor. The very low local and distant recurrence rates indicate that meticulous operative technique performed by an experienced colorectal surgeon is worthwhile.

25. Vernava AM, Moran M, Rothenberger DA, Wong WD: **A Prospective Evaluation of Distal Margins in Carcinoma of the Rectum.** *Surg Gynecol Obstet* 1992, **175**:333–336.

26. Krook JE, Moertel CG, Gunderson LL, Wieand HS, Collins RT, Beart RW, Kubista TP, Poon MA, Meyers WC, Mailliard JA, *et al.*: **Effective Surgical Adjuvant Therapy for High-Risk Rectal Carcinoma.** *N Engl J Med* 1991, **324**:709–715.

27. Fielding LP: **Colorectal Carcinoma: Mesorectal Excision for Rectal Cancer.** *Lancet* 1993, **341**:471–472.

28. Ng IOL, Luk ISC, Yuen ST, Lau PWK, Pritchett CJ, Ng M, Poon
• GP, Ho J: **Surgical Lateral Clearance in Resected Rectal Carcinomas: A Multivariant Analysis of Clinicopathological Features.** *Cancer* 1993, 71:1972–1976.
This is the third publication to date that demonstrates the prognostic significance of lateral resection margin involvement. The role of adjuvant therapy in such patients has yet to be addressed.

29. Wolff BG: **Lateral Margins of Resection in Adenocarcinoma of the Rectum.** *World J Surg* 1992, **16**:467–469.

30. Gertsch P, Baer HU, Kraft R, Maddern GJ, Altermatt JH: **Malig-**
• **nant Cells Are Collected on Circular Staplers.** *Dis Colon Rectum* 1992, **35**:238–241.
This report demonstrates that clumps of malignant cells are collected on circular staplers. Lavage of the rectum before stapling is probably warranted.

31. Mealy K, Burke P, Hyland J: **Anterior Resection Without a Defunctioning Colostomy: Questions of Safety.** *Br J Surg* 1992, 79:305–307.

32. Thomas JM: **Letter.** *Br J Surg* 1992, 79:1109.

33. Cunliff WJ: **Letter.** *Br J Surg* 1992, 79:1109.

34. Karanjia ND, Heald RJ: **Letter.** *Br J Surg* 1992, **79**:1109.

35. Redmond HP, Austin OMB, Clery AP, Deasy JM: **Safety of Double-**
• **Stapled Anastomosis in Low Anterior Resection.** *Br J Surg* 1993, **80**:924–927.
In this consecutive series of 111 patients undergoing low anterior resection with the double-staple technique, 29% of whom had defunctioning stomas, the clinically significant leak rate was only 2.7%.

36. Baran JJ, Goldstein SD, Resnik AM: **The Double-Staple Technique in**
• **Colorectal Anastomoses: A Critical Review.** *Am Surg* 1992, **58**:270–272.
In a series similar to that of Redmond *et al.* (*Br J Surg* 1993, 80:924–927), 25% of patients had defunctioning stomas and there was a 2.8% clinically significant leak rate.

37. Griffen FD, Knight CD, Knight CD: **Results of the Double Stapling**
• **Procedure in Pelvic Surgery.** *World J Surg* 1992, **16**:866–871.
In this study, in contrast to those of Redmond *et al.* (*Br J Surg* 1993, 80:924–927) and Baran *et al.* (*Am J Surg* 1992, 58:270–272), none of the 91 patients had defunctioning stomas, and the clinically significant leak rate was still only 3.3%.

38. Moran BJ, Blenkinsop J, Finnis D: **Local Recurrence After Anterior Re-**
• **section for Rectal Cancer Using a Double Stapling Technique.** *Br J Surg* 1992, 79:836–838.
Of 55 patients who underwent anterior resection using the double-staple technique, 9% had defunctioning stomas and the clinical leak rate was 9.1%.

39. Berger A, Tiret E, Parc R, Frileux P, Hannoun L, Nordlinger B,
•• Ratelle R, Simon R: **Excision of the Rectum With Colonic J Pouch-Anal Anastomosis for Adenocarcinoma of the Low and Mid Rectum.** *World J Surg* 1992, 16:470–477.
This important paper very closely analyzes the outcome in 162 patients who underwent colonic J pouch–anal anastomoses. The use of this technique appears to result in superior functional outcome and does not adversely affect operative morbidity.

40. Pelissier EP, Blum D, Bachour A, Bosset JF: **Functional Results**
• **of Coloanal Anastomosis With Reservoir.** *Dis Colon Rectum* 1992, 35:843–846.
This paper, like that of Berger *et al.* (*World J Surg* 1992, 16:470–477), demonstrates the safety of this operation and the good functional results.

41. Pelissier EP, Blum D, Bachour A, Bosset JF: **Stapled Coloanal Anastomosis With Reservoir Procedure.** *Am J Surg* 1992, **163**:435–436.

42. Cohen AM: **Colon J-Pouch Rectal Reconstruction After Total or Subtotal**
• **Proctectomy.** *World J Surg* 1993, **17**:267–270.
This paper demonstrates the safety of this procedure: only two of the 23 patients had covering stomas, and there were no clinically significant leaks.

43. Rothenberger DA, Wong WD: **Abdominoperineal Resection for Ade-**
• **nocarcinoma of the Low Rectum.** *World J Surg* 1992, **16**:478–485.
This paper reveals the low morbidity and mortality rates that can be achieved with modern surgical management.

44. Campos RR, Ayllon JG, Paricio PP, Tebar JC, Mompean JAL, Ruiz RL,
• Martinez JAT, Martinez JM: **Management of the Perineal Wound Following Abdominoperineal Resection: Prospective Study of Three Methods.** *Br J Surg* 1992, 79:29–31.
Although this is not a randomized study, the findings suggest that leaving the pelvic peritoneum open and closing the perineal wound may be the optimal form of treatment for most of these patients.

45. Thom A, Baumann J, Chandler JJ, Devereux DF: **Experience With High-**
• **Dose Radiation Therapy and the Intestinal Sling Procedure in Patients With Rectal Carcinoma.** *Cancer* 1992, **70**:581–584.
This paper demonstrates the safety and efficacy of this method of protecting the small bowel from damage by postoperative radiotherapy.

46. Lechner P, Cesnik H: **Abdominopelvic Omentopexy: Preparatory Pro-**
• **cedure for Radiotherapy in Rectal Cancer.** *Dis Colon Rectum* 1992, **35**:1157–1160.
Like the study by Thom *et al.* (*Cancer* 1992, 70:581–584), this article describes a method of protecting the small bowel from postoperative radiotherapy and demonstrates the method to be effective.

47. Chen JS, ChangChien CR, Wang JY, Fan HA: **Pelvic Peritoneal Recon-**
• **struction to Prevent Radiation Enteritis in Rectal Carcinoma.** *Dis Colon Rectum* 1992, **35**:897–901.
Although the number of patients studied in this paper and in the papers by Thom *et al.* (*Cancer* 1992, 70:581–584) and Lechner and Cesnik (*Dis Colon Rectum* 1992, 35:1157–1160) is small, it appears that this method may not offer equally effective protection to the small bowel because two patients are shown to develop radiation enteritis.

48. Willett CG, Lewandrowski K, Donnelly S, Shellito PC, Convery K,
• Eliseo R, Compton CC: **Are There Patients With Stage I Rectal Carcinoma at Risk for Failure After Abdominoperineal Resection?** *Cancer* 1992, **69**:1651–1655.
This paper makes the important point that patients with stage I rectal carcinoma are still at significant risk for local recurrence, even after abdominoperineal resection.

49. Falk PM, Beart RW, Wexner SD, Thorson AG, Jagelman DG, Lavery
• IC, Johansen OB, Fitzgibbons RJ: **Laparoscopic Colectomy: A Critical Appraisal.** *Dis Colon Rectum* 1993, **36**:28–34.
An early, multicenter experience with laparoscopic colectomy is described.

50. Walsh DCA, Wattchow DA, Wilson TG: **Subcutaneous Metastases After Laparoscopic Resection of Malignancy.** *Aust N Z J Surg* 1993, 63:563–565.

51. Devine RM, Dozois RD: **Surgical Management of Locally Advanced Adenocarcinoma of the Rectum.** *World J Surg* 1992, **16**:486–489.

52. Curley SA, Carlson GW, Shumate CR, Wishnow KI, Ames FC: **Extended**
• **Resection for Locally Advanced Colorectal Carcinoma.** *Am J Surg* 1992, **163**:553–559.
This paper stresses the importance of investigating patients who have genitourinary symptoms and colorectal carcinoma, because these symptoms often indicate invasion of adjacent structures.

Alan P. Meagher, FRACS, and John H. Pemberton, MD, Department of Surgery, Section of Colon and Rectal Surgery, Mayo Clinic, 200 First Street SW, Rochester, MN 55905, USA.

Cellular immunotherapy of cancer

James C. Yang, MD

Surgery Branch, National Cancer Institute, Bethesda, Maryland, USA

Recent developments in the understanding of antigen processing and presentation and T-cell receptor recognition of antigens have immediate applications to the cellular immunotherapy of cancer. The specific antigens and processed peptide sequences responsible for T-cell recognition of some human melanomas have recently been identified. T cells with antitumor activity are undergoing genetic modification to improve their function and clinical efficacy. In addition, novel T-cell constructs are being created with chimeric T-cell receptors that confer new tumor reactivities to these lymphocytes. Current understanding of the basic processes involved in the immune recognition and destruction of tumors is allowing the manipulation of these processes to enhance experimental clinical therapies.

Current Opinion in General Surgery 1994:238–244

Recent advances in our understanding of T-cell biology have had direct consequences on the cellular immunotherapy of cancer. The mechanisms by which antigens are processed and presented to T cells, and the ways in which they stimulate these cells have only recently been clarified. In this review, a basic overview of T-cell physiology is given, and several critical discoveries with respect to tumor immunology are described. Furthermore, the application of these findings to therapeutic modalities and currently unresolved problems is discussed. An update on therapy with lymphokine-activated killer cells is also presented.

T-cell biology

T cells bearing the CD8 marker are known to interact with major histocompatibility complex (MHC) class I–restricted target cells and CD4-positive T cells with cells bearing MHC class II (primarily "professional" antigen presenting cells such as macrophages, dendritic cells, and B cells). Antigens are processed and presented in the context of class I MHC by an "intrinsic pathway," and an "extrinsic pathway" is utilized for CD4 restricted interactions [1,2•,3] (Fig. 1).

The class-I–targeted intrinsic pathway processes antigens primarily derived from the intrinsic proteins of the target cell itself. These proteins include not only those made after viral infection (such as viral nucleoprotein from influenza-infected cells) but also the normal structural proteins of the cell. Because of antigen processing that occurs in this pathway, it is now clear that such antigens do not have to be expressed on the cell surface in order to be recognized by T cells. Instead, they are cleaved intracytoplasmically to minimal determinants of eight or nine amino acids, which are transported into the endoplasmic reticulum, where they are assembled with the two component proteins of the MHC class I molecule. This complex is then exported to the cell surface, displayed, and recognized by T cells [4,5]. An eight- or nine-amino-acid minimal determinant within any single protein is highly specific for a particular MHC allele, but a protein could have other minimal determinants allowing it to be processed and presented by the different MHC molecules of different patients.

The extrinsic or class II–restricted antigen pathway pertains primarily to protein antigens from the extracellular environment. These antigens are ingested by pinocytosis, degraded in the endosome to peptides of 12 to 24 amino acids, and then mounted onto class II MHC molecules in a post-Golgi compartment as the MHC is being exported for display on the cell surface [6,7]. This process occurs in cells with antigen-presenting capability and is directed at stimulating the CD4-positive T-cell population. Once the correct peptide minimal determinant is bound onto the correct MHC molecule and displayed on the cell membrane, it can be recognized by the T-cell receptor.

The T-cell receptor complex has been reviewed elsewhere [8,9]. Fundamentally, it consists of an antigen–MHC binding heterodimer (typically an α and β chain or a γ and β chain) coupled with signal transduction elements used to activate T-cell effector func-

Abbreviations

LAK—lymphokine-activated killer; **MHC**—major histocompatibility complex;
MoAb—monoclonal antibody; **TIL**—tumor-infiltrating lymphocyte; **TNF**—tumor necrosis factor.

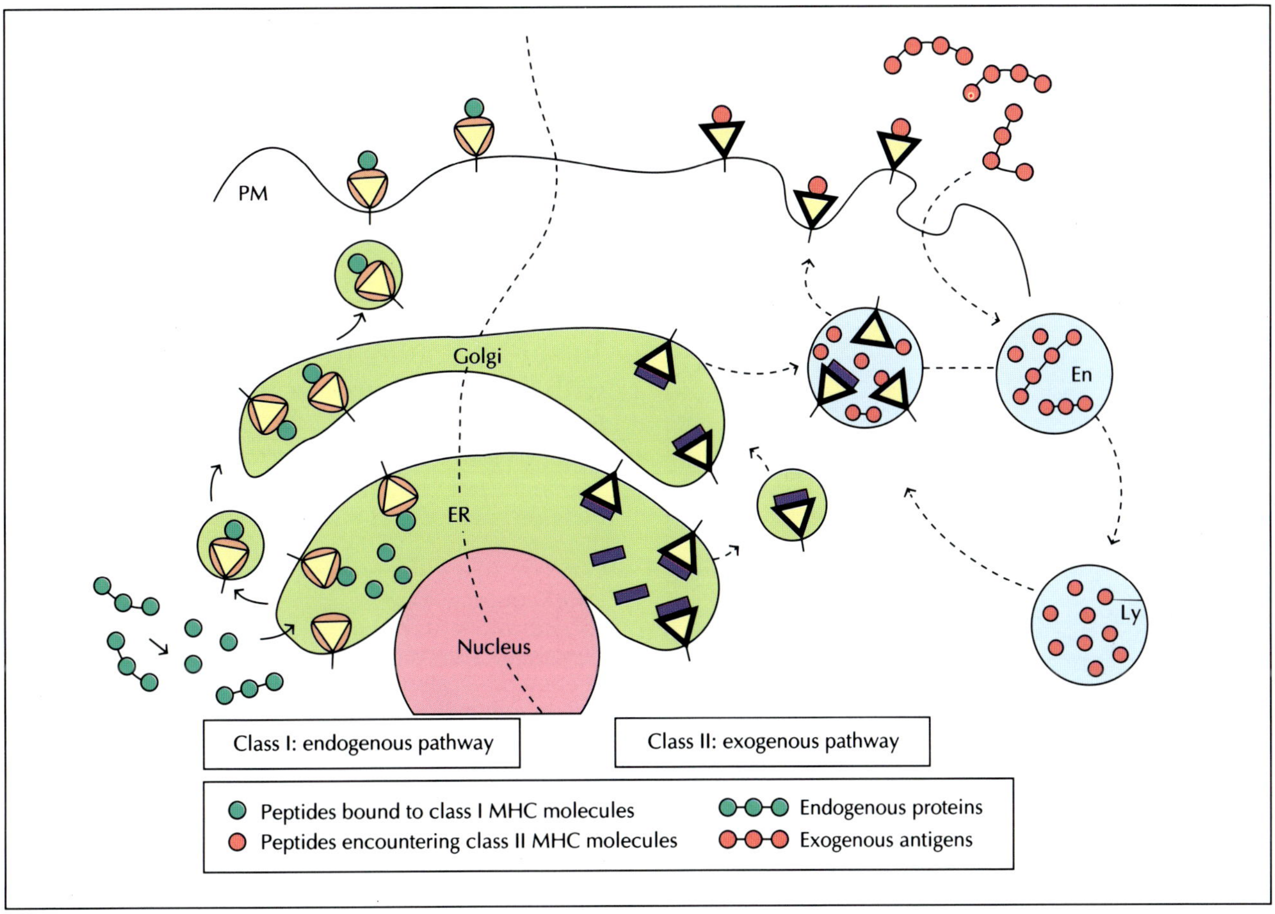

Fig. 1. The cellular processing and presentation of antigens. Endogenous proteins are degraded into peptides, which are bound by class I major histocompatibility complex (MHC) molecules (*open triangles*) in the endoplasmic reticulum (ER) and thus transported through the Golgi to the plasma membrane (PM). Exogenous antigens enter the cell by endocytosis and are degraded in endosomal (En) and lysosomal compartments (Ly). Peptides encounter class II MHC molecules (*dark triangles*) in a poorly defined cellular compartment before transport to the plasma membrane. The invariant chain (*open rectangle*) transiently associates with class II MHC molecules during exocytosis. (*From* Bjorkman and Parham [3]; with permission.)

tions. It interacts with either the CD4 or CD8 T-cell surface markers, which bind to constant, nonpolymorphic regions of the class II or class I MHC molecules, respectively. The ζ chain is a primary component of signal transduction by the CD3 complex leading to activation of phosphokinase C and cytoplasmic Ca^{2+} influx [10].

Tumor-specific T-cell antigens

Within the last year, exciting advances have been made in the area of identification of common antigens in melanomas, recognized by T cells, culminating in the cloning of the genes for a series of these antigens by van der Bruggen *et al.* [11••] at the Ludwig Institute in Brussels. Preliminary work by Darrow *et al.* [12], Topalian *et al.* [13•], O'Neil *et al.* [14••], and van der Bruggen *et al.* [11••] demonstrated that T cells obtained from melanoma patients (either by bulk culture of tumor-infiltrating lymphocytes [TILs] or by cloning of tumor and peripheral blood lymphocyte cocultures) not only recognized the patient's tumor in a specific MHC-restricted fashion, but also recognized most other melanomas from patients matched at the correct restricting MHC locus. This discovery implied (especially the work with cloned T-cell lines) that these melanomas shared a common antigen presented in the context of a specific MHC class I molecule. Using an HLA-A1–restricted T-cell clone from a patient immunized with a melanoma preparation, van der Bruggen *et al.* [11••] screened a genomic DNA library from the patient's melanoma line designated *MZ-2*. They identified a family of genes called *MAGE* that, when introduced into HLA-A1–positive cells, could make them susceptible to lysis by the antimelanoma T cells. Furthermore, by multiple truncations of the *MAGE-1* gene, Traversari *et al.* [15•] identified the specific nine-amino-acid peptide that the T cells recognized, EADPTGHSY. This peptide, when synthesized and externally pulsed onto cells expressing HLA-A1, where it would exchange with other peptides being presented by HLA-A1, also conferred lysability by the melanoma-reactive T-cell clone (Fig. 2).

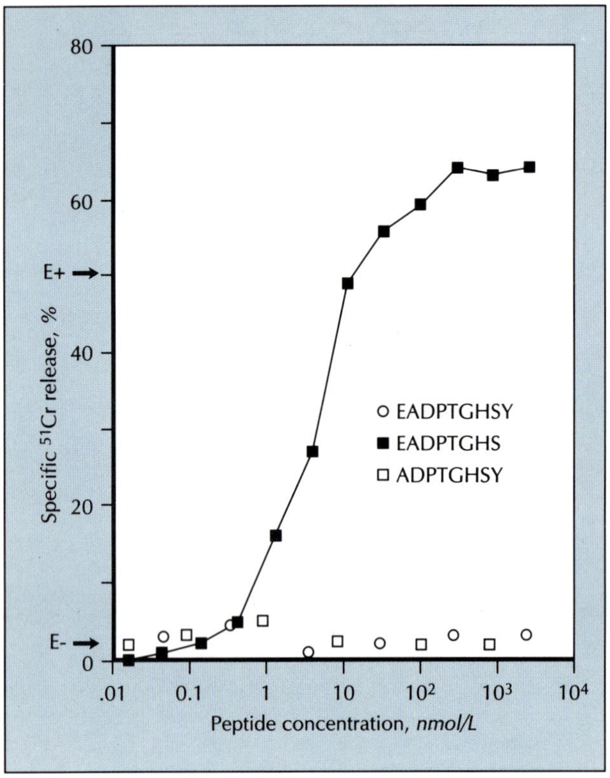

Fig. 2. Lysis of melanoma tumor lines by anti–melanoma-specific cytotoxic T lymphocytes (CTLs) from a patient designated MZ-2. *Arrows* indicate CTL lysis of an antigen-bearing tumor line (E+) and an antigen-deficient tumor line (E-) from patient MZ-2 in the absence of added peptide. The figure shows levels of lysis of the E- tumor line after preincubation with different concentrations of three peptides (EADPTGHSY, EADPTGHS, and ADPTGHSY) derived from the *MAGE-1* gene product. The correct nonapeptide, EADPTGHSY, is able to bind to the antigen groove of the HLA-A1 molecule and mediate the lysis of the antigen-deficient tumor line by specific cytotoxic T lymphocytes. Lysis is in a 4-hour ^{51}Cr-release assay at an effector/target ratio of 50. (*From* Traversari *et al.* [15•]; with permission.)

This elegant delineation of the precise nature of one T-cell recognition of a melanoma antigen was quickly followed by the cloning of another antigen from melanoma restricted by the more common HLA-A2 locus [16•]. This antigen proved to be tyrosinase, an enzyme in the synthetic pathway of melanin pigment. For both *MAGE-1* and tyrosinase, the genetic sequence of the tumor antigen was identical to that in normal tissues, contradicting the hypothesis that tumor antigens are likely to be mutated versions of normal proteins.

Apart from obvious benefits regarding prophylactic vaccination, the value of these discoveries to the therapy of melanoma are multiple. Vaccination may play a role in generating T cells for expansion and adoptive transfer therapy. The T cells and T-cell receptors involved in tumor recognition will soon be known and cloned for patients with certain MHC types. Transferring these receptors to autologous lymphocytes or stem cells to create effective T cells is possible if a patient cannot produce an adequate autologous TIL culture. Additionally, purified peptides could be used to antigen stimulate T-cell cultures, an intervention shown to enhance TIL efficacy in mice [17], but previously impractical in patients.

In the future, these antigens may prove instrumental in the generation of more effective T-cells with which to treat advanced disease.

Tumor-infiltrating lymphocyte therapy with native and genetically modified lymphocytes

Within the last year, the use of TILs from melanoma has demonstrated several findings. Patients with metastatic disease receiving TILs and high-dose interleukin-2 (720,000 IU/kg intravenously every 8 hours to tolerance) continue to show a 35% partial and complete response rate with no significant difference if they had previously received and failed therapy with high-dose interleukin-2 alone (Rosenberg, Unpublished data). Continued in vivo traffic studies with ^{111}In-labeled TILs during these therapeutic trials have shown that successful localization of ^{111}In-labeled TILs to tumor sites during therapy (as measured by scintigraphic visualization) was significantly associated with clinical tumor regression [18]. In addition, pretreatment with cyclophosphamide (25 mg/kg; intravenous bolus) 24 to 36 hours prior to TIL transfer augmented the ability to image tumor and significantly increased ^{111}In uptake in tumor deposits as measured by biopsy. With small numbers, a statistically significant association was not demonstrated between cyclophosphamide administration and clinical response. Currently, it is believed that cyclophosphamide does increase TIL localization to tumor by an as yet unidentified mechanism, but other factors may contribute substantially to clinical responses.

Other efforts have concentrated on genetically modifying TILs to augment their efficacy. Ongoing clinical trials using a retroviral transduction system have attempted to confer constitutive tumor necrosis factor (TNF) secretion on TILs, which could then localize to tumor and deliver a high concentration of TNF to the tumor microenvironment. These efforts have been slowed by unexpectedly low levels of expression of the products of introduced genes by lymphocytes. Using a retroviral vector with the Moloney leukemia virus LTR promoting the TNF gene and the SV40 promotor driving the neomycin resistance gene, transduced, selected tumor cells produce 1 to 2 logs more TNF than transduced, selected TILs [18]. Some improvement occurred using a modified TNF gene where the 17-kD secreted portion of TNF was coupled to the interferon gamma signal peptide, providing a cleavage site and mandatory secretion of TNF. This change produced an approximate fivefold increase in the amount of TNF secreted by transduced TILs [19] (Table 1). The concept of high local concentrations of TNF having major antitumor effects in patients with cancer has recently been substantiated by Lienard *et al.* [20]. Using total isolation and perfusion of extremities to avoid the dose-limiting toxicity of systemic TNF, they have reported 100% responses in patients with sarcoma and in transit melanoma when perfused with high-dose TNF, melphalan and interferon gamma. Because no TNF-related toxicities have been seen thus far in the administration of TILs genetically modified to secrete TNF, continued improvements in the expression levels of these retroviral vectors may result in the secretion of enough TNF by TILs to result in similar anti-tumor activity.

Efforts to introduce the gene for interleukin-2 have thus far failed to produce any meaningful interleukin-2 secretion or evidence of autonomous TIL growth, despite previous reports of success using the CTLL cell line [21]. A variety of other promotor constructs are being tried to overcome this expression block in TIL. Transient vector delivery systems using vaccinia, adenovirus, and other variant viral systems are also being tried.

Another approach with a great deal of promise has been to genetically modify components of the T-cell receptor to redirect T-cell recognition and reactivity. One recently described approach utilized a "single-chain" monoclonal antibody (MoAb) to ovarian carcinoma as the binding site of a neo–T-cell receptor, coupled to the intracellular domain of the signal-transducing FcRγ protein. FcRγ is closely related to the ζ chain of the T-cell receptor, and the single chain MoAb consisted of the V_H and V_L portions of the antiovarian cancer MoAb, MoV18, connected by a short peptide linker. Thus the antigen recognition site of the MoAb could be reconstructed by a single continuous peptide coded for by a single gene. When ligated to FcRγ and introduced into a TIL with reactivity to melanoma, this chimeric receptor could redirect these TILs to recognize the IGROV-1 ovarian cancer line, but not other nonovarian human tumors [22•] (Fig. 3). This approach could allow the creation of tumor-reactive T cells for the majority of tumors which do not currently generate tumor-specific TILs, but for which MoAbs exist. A variant of this approach using bispecific antibodies that cross-link a tumor antigen and the CD3 complex of the T cell has been tested and some clinical responses have been seen [23]. One drawback of this approach is the development of human antimouse Ig antibodies in nearly all patients.

Lymphokine-activated killer cells

Although interesting scientific work continues on the tumor-recognition elements of natural killer and lymphokine-activated killer (LAK) cells, clinical efforts have been less emphasized in the past year. Previous reports of randomized trials showing no benefit of the addition of LAK cells to interleukin-2 therapy in the treatment of metastatic cancer were limited by low response rates and short follow-up time. This past year Rosenberg *et al.* [24•] published the results of their randomized trial; follow-up time was greater than 5 years, and the overall response rates for patients with melanoma and renal cell cancer were 24% and 29%, respectively. With multiple-tumor histologies included, patient numbers for any specific tumor type were low.

Table 1. TNF production by TILs and tumor cells transduced with a retroviral vector containing a 17-kD TNF γ-signal peptide gene*

		TNF, *pg/mL/10⁶cells/d*†		
Cell line‡	Days after transduction	No transduction	Wild-type TNF vector§	17-kD TNF vector§
TIL patient A	49	33	189	825
	56	39	73	599
TIL patient B	34	5	380	2806
	45	10	119	899
	52	8	554	676
TIL patient C	18	97	77	271
	34	104	104	657
	73	89	72	188
TIL patient D	27	40	185	983
888 MEL	18	0	28,280	132,100
	97	0	31,170	193,750

**Adapted from* Hwu *et al.* [19]; with permission.
†TNF levels were determined by enzyme-linked immunosorbent assay. Supernatant collections (24 hours) were performed in the presence of 100 ng/mL soluble dimeric TNF receptor.
‡All are TIL cultures except 888 MEL, which represents a melanoma cell line.
§TILs were transduced and selected in G418, 0.3 mg/mL, for 5 days. Tumor control was transduced and selected continuously in G418, 0.6 mg/mL.
TIL—tumor-infiltrating lymphocyte; TNF—tumor necrosis factor.

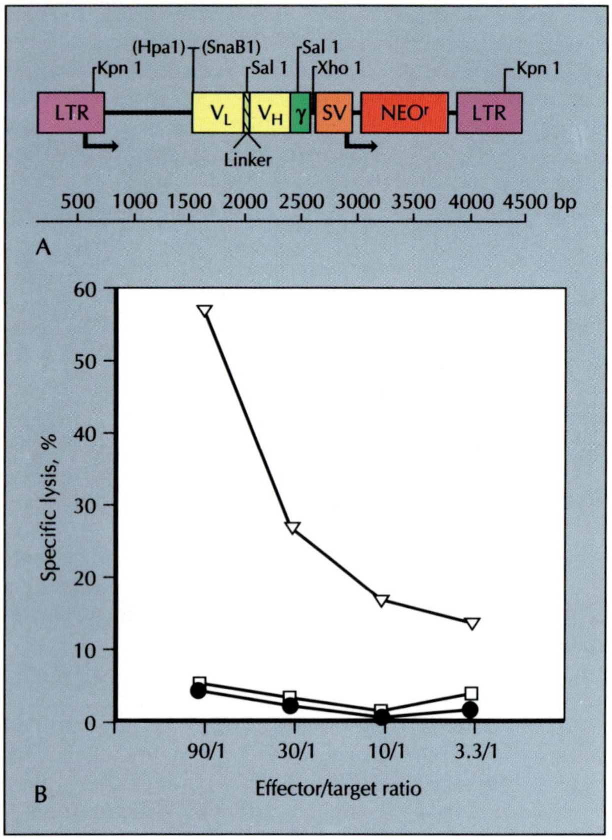

Fig. 3. **A**, Schematic of the retroviral vector used to insert a chimeric T-cell receptor into an antimelanoma tumor-infiltrating lymphocyte (TIL). The Moloney murine leukemia virus long terminal repeat (LTR) promotes a chimeric T-cell receptor consisting of the variable regions of the heavy (V_H) and light (V_L) chains of the antiovarian cancer antibody MoV18 (joined by a peptide linker), fused to the FcRγ signal transduction protein (γ). The neomycin resistance (Neo^r) selectable marker is promoted by the SV40 promoter (SV). **B**, Lysis of the human ovarian carcinoma cell line IGROV-1 by control antimelanoma TILs, (*circles*), the same TILs transduced with an irrelevant antitrinitrophenyl chimeric receptor construct (*squares*), and these TILs transduced with the construct shown in *panel A* (MoV-γ, *triangles*). Only the MoV-γ TIL lyses IGROV-1, and this lysis is specifically blocked by anti-idiotypic antibody against the MoV18 monoclonal antibody used to create this receptor (not shown). (*From* Hwu *et al.* [22••]; with permission.)

Nevertheless, they showed that for metastatic renal cell cancer, both treatment groups showed 4-year survival rates of approximately 25% without additional benefit from LAK cell administration (Fig. 4). For patients with metastatic melanoma, five of 27 patients treated with interleukin-2 and LAK cells survived beyond 4 years, and all patients receiving just interleukin-2 expired by 4.5 years (P_2 = 0.064) (Fig. 5). Although these results suggest that LAK cells could contribute to prolonged survival in patients with melanoma treated with interleukin-2, the numbers of patients is small, and the results will need to be confirmed.

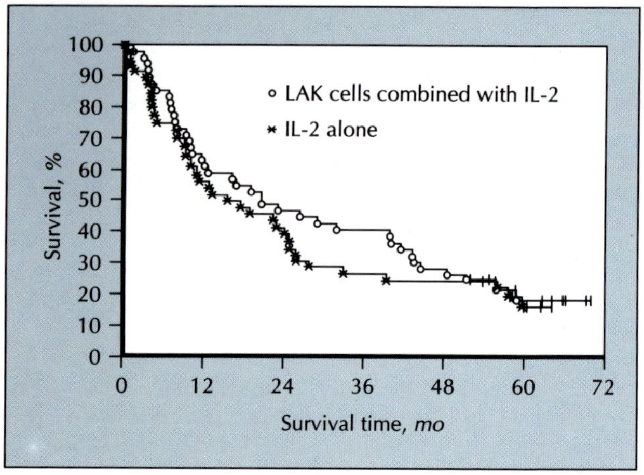

Fig. 4. Overall survival of patients with metastatic renal cell cancer randomly assigned to receive either interleukin-2 (IL-2) or lymphokine-activated killer (LAK) cells combined with IL-2 (P_2 = 0.52). (*From* Rosenberg *et al.* [24•]; with permission.)

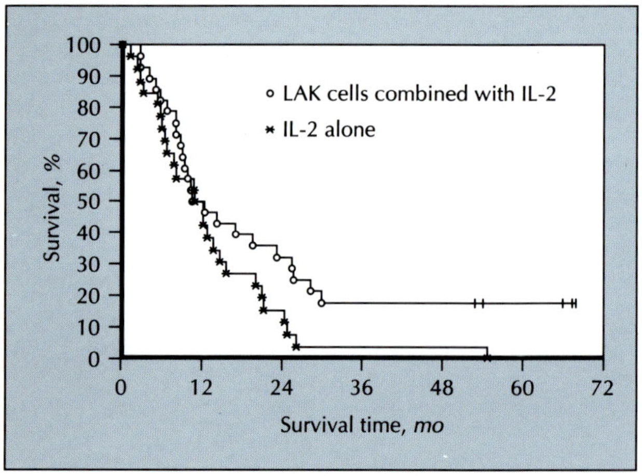

Fig. 5. Overall survival of patients with metastatic melanoma randomly assigned to receive either interleukin-2 (IL-2) or lymphokine-activated killer (LAK) cells combined with IL-2 (P_2 = 0.064 in favor of patients randomly assigned to receive LAK cells with IL-2). (*From* Rosenberg *et al.* [24•]; with permission).

Conclusions

Just 14 years ago, papers were published denying the existence of an antitumor immune response in patients with advanced cancer [25]. The past year has seen the documentation of such a response, elucidated down to the precise nine-amino-acid epitope of the tumor antigen recognized by a classic cytotoxic T lymphocyte in an MHC-restricted fashion. In parallel with this work, methods for utilizing T cells for therapy have been developed. The current challenge is to merge these disciplines and carry those immunologic advances into the therapy arena. Tumors engineered to secrete interleukin-2, TNF, interleukin-4 or interferonγ, or to express MHC or the B7 costimulatory T-cell signal have been shown to elicit enhanced local immune responses directed at parental or wild-type tumor antigens [26–31]. The exciting work of enhancing a weak immune response or correcting a deficient response must now make the leap from local immunity to systemic immunity capable of treating distant, disseminated bulk disease. Preclinical studies suggest that this development may not occur with simple vaccination with these constructs, and that a more powerful immune effector mechanism is required. The *ex vivo* expansion and adoptive cellular transfer of tumor-reactive T-cells may represent currently available technology capable of translating these discoveries into effective therapies.

Acknowledgment

I am indebted to Steven A. Rosenberg for his generous review of this manuscript and his many insightful comments.

References and recommended reading

Papers of particular interest, published within the annual period of review, have been highlighted as:

- • Of special interest
- •• Of outstanding interest

1. Yewdell JW, Bennink JR: **Cell Biology of Antigen Processing and Presentation to Major Histocompatibility Complex Class I Molecule-Restricted T Lymphocytes.** *Adv Immunol* 1992, **52**:1–123.

2. • Germain RN: **The Biochemistry and Cell Biology of Antigen Processing and Presentation.** *Annu Rev Immunol* 1993, **11**:403–450.

A review of the current understanding of MHC class I and class II antigen processing and presentation.

3. Bjorkman PJ, Parham P: **Structure, Function, and Diversity of Class I Major Histocompatibility Complex Molecules.** *Annu Rev Biochem* 1990, **59**:253–288.

4. Townsend A, Bodmer H: **Antigen Recognition by Class I-Restricted T Lymphocytes.** *Annu Rev Immunol* 1989, **7**:601–624.

5. Matsumura M, Fremont DH, Peterson PA, Wilson IA: **Emerging Principles for the Recognition of Peptide Antigens by MHC Class I Molecules.** *Science* 1992, **257**:927–934.

6. Chicz RM, Urban RG, Gorga JC, Lane WS, Stern LJ, Vignali DAA, Strominger JL: **The Predominant Naturally Processed Peptides Bound to HLA-DR1 Are Derived From MHC-Related Molecules and Are Heterogeneous in Size.** *Nature* 1992, **358**:764–769.

7. Brown JH, Jardetzky TS, Gorga JC, Stern LJ, Urban RG, Strominger JL, Wiley DC: **Three-Dimensional Structure of the Human Class II Histocompatibility Antigen HLA-DR1.** *Nature* 1993, **364**:33–39.

8. Weiss A: **Structure and Function of the T Cell Antigen Receptor.** *J Clin Invest* 1990, **86**:1015–1022.

9. Klausner RD, Lippincott-Schwartz J, Bonifacio JS: **The T Cell Antigen Receptor: Insights Into Organelle Biology.** *Annu Rev Cell Biol* 1990, **6**:403–431.

10. Irving BA, Weiss A: **The Cytoplasmic Domain of the T Cell Receptor Zeta Chain Is Sufficient to Couple to Receptor-Associated Signal Transduction Pathways.** *Cell* 1991, **64**:891–901.

11. •• van der Bruggen P, Traversari C, Chomez P, Lurquin C, De Plaen E, van den Eynde B, Knuth A, Boon T: **A Gene Encoding An Antigen Recognized by Cytolytic T Lymphocytes on a Human Melanoma.** *Science* 1991, **254**:1643–1647.

A landmark paper describing the cloning of a gene from a melanoma tumor line that confers HLA-Al– restricted recognition by a melanoma-specific cytotoxic T lymphocyte. This is the first identification in human tumors of a specific gene coding for a shared tumor antigen defined by T-cell recognition.

12. Darrow TL, Slingluff CL Jr, Seigler HF: **The Role of HLA Class I Antigens in Recognition of Melanoma Cells by Tumor-Specific Cytotoxic T Lymphocytes.** *J Immunol* 1989, **142**:3329–3335.

13. • Topalian SL, Hom SS, Kawakami Y, Mancini M, Schartzentruber DJ, Zakut R, Rosenberg SA: **Recognition of Shared Melanoma Antigens by Human Tumor-Infiltrating Lymphocytes.** *J Immunother* 1992, **12**:203–206.

A study of the cross-reactivity of antimelanoma TIL when specific MHC class I loci are matched or mismatched among a panel of autologous and nonautologous tumors.

14. •• O'Neil BH, Kawakami Y, Restifo NP, Bennick JR, Yewdell JW, Rosenberg SA: **Detection of Shared MHC-Restricted Human Melanoma Antigens After Vaccinia Virus-Mediated Transduction of Genes Coding for HLA.** *J Immunol* 1993, **151**:1410–1418.

A conclusive study demonstrating the existence of a widely shared melanoma antigen recognized by TIL in the context of HLA-A2. The study demonstrated that a panel of melanomas from patients without HLA-A2 can be recognized by HLA-A2–specific TIL when the HLA-A2 molecule is transiently introduced into these tumors using a vaccinia-based vector.

15. • Traversari C, van der Bruggen P, Luescher IF, Lurquin C, Chomez P, Van Pel A, De Plaen E, Amar-Costesec A, Boon T: **A Nonapeptide Encoded by Human Gene MAGE-1 Is Recognized on HLA-A1 by Cytolytic T Lymphocytes Directed Against Tumor Antigen MZ2-E.** *J Exp Med* 1992, **176**:1453–1457.

A follow-up to van der Bruggen *et al.* (*Science* 1991, 254:1643–1647). The specific 9-amino-acid sequence within the protein product of *MAGE-1* presented by HLA-A1 is defined.

16. • Brichard V Pel A, Wölfel T, Wölfel C, De Plaen E, Lethé B, Coulie P, Boon T: **The Tyrosinase Gene Codes for Antigen Recognized by Autologous Cytolytic T Lymphocytes on HLA-A2 Melanomas.** *J Exp Med* 1993, **178**:489–495.

This identifies another gene coding for a shared melanoma antigen, this time presented in the context of HLA-A2 (a class I allele of greater utility because it is present in nearly half of melanoma patients). This antigen was identified as tyrosinase, an enzyme uniquely expressed in adult pigmented tissue and a key component of the melanin synthetic pathway.

17. Yang JC, Perry-Lalley D, Rosenberg SA: **An Improved Method For Growing Murine Tumor Infiltrating Lymphocytes with *In Vivo* Antitumor Activity.** *J Biol Response Modifiers* 1990, 9:149–159.

18. Pockaj BA, Sherry R, Wei J, Yannelli JR, Carter CS, Leitman SF, Carrasquillo JR, White DE, Steinberg SM, Rosenberg SA, Yang JC: **Localization of ^{111} Indium-Labelled Tumor Infiltrating Lymphocytes to Tumor in Patients Receiving Immunotherapy: Augmentation With Cyclophosphamide and Association With Response.** *Cancer* 1993, in press.

19. Hwu P, Yannelli J, Kriegler M, Anderson WF, Perez C, Chiang Y, Schwarz S, Cowherd R, Delgado C, Mulé J, Rosenberg SA: **Characterization of Tumor Infiltrating Lymphocytes Transduced With the cDNA Encoding Tumor Necrosis Factor-Alpha.** *J Immunol* 1993, **150**:4104–4115.

20. Lienard D, Ewalenko P, Delmotte J-J, Renard N, Lejeune FJ: **High-Dose Recombinant Tumor Necrosis Factor Alpha in Combination With Interferon Gamma and Melphalan in Isolation Perfusion of the Limbs for Melanoma and Sarcoma.** *J Clin Oncol* 1992, **10**:52–60.

21. Karasuyama H, Tohyama N, Tada T: **Autocrine Growth and Tumorigenicity of Interleukin 2-Dependent Helper T Cells Transfected With IL-2 Gene.** *J Exp Med* 1989, **169**:13–25.

22. • Hwu P, Shafer GE, Treisman J, Schinkler DG, Gross G, Cowherd R, Rosenberg SA, Eshhar Z: **Lysis of Ovarian Cancer Cells By Human Lymphocytes Redirected With a Chimeric Gene Composed of an Antibody Variable Region and the Fc Receptor Gamma Chain.** *J Exp Med* 1993, **178**:361–366.

A novel approach to the generation of T cells with non-MHC restricted recognition of tumors based on the antigen-binding specificity of monoclonal antibodies. These T cells transduced with a chimeric T-cell receptor are capable of both lysis and cytokine release when they bind tumor targets *in vitro.*

23. Bolhuis RL, Lamers CH, Goey SH, Eggermont AM, Trimbos JB, Stoter G, Lanzavecchia A, De Re E, Miotti S, Rsapagliesi F: **Adoptive Immunotherapy of Ovarian Carcinoma With bs-MAb-Targeted Lymphocytes: A Multicenter Study.** *Int J Cancer* 1992, 7(suppl):78–81.

24. • Rosenberg SA, Lotze MT, Yang JC, Topalian SL, Chang AE, Schwartzentruber DJ, Aebersold P, Leitman S, Linehan WM, Seipp CA, White DE, Steinberg SM: **Prospective Randomized Trial of High-Dose Interleukin-2 Alone or in Conjunction With Lymphokine-Activated Killer Cells for the Treatment of Patients With Advanced Cancer.** *J Natl Cancer Inst* 1993, **85**: 622–632.

Long-term results of treatment of patients with metastatic cancer with interleukin-2 based immunotherapy. With median follow-up of more than 5 years, excellent overall survival and durable responses (including complete responses) are documented.

25. Hewitt HB: **A Critical Examination of the Foundations of Immunotherapy of Clinical Radiology.** *Clin Radiol* 1979, **30**:361–369.

26. CONNOR J, BANNERJI R, SAITO S, HESTON W, FAIR W, GILBOA E: **Regression of Bladder Tumors in Mice Treated With Interleukin 2 Gene-Modified Tumor Cells.** *J Exp Med* 1993, 177:1127–1134.

27. ASHER AL, MULÉ JJ, KASID A, RESTIFO NP, SALO JC, REICHERT CM, JAFFE G, FENDLY B, KRIEGLER M, ROSENBERG SA: **Murine Tumor Cells Transduced With the Gene for Tumor Necrosis Factor-Alpha.** *J Immunol* 1991, 146:3227–3234.

28. GOLUMBEK PT, LAZENBY AJ, LEVITSKY HI, JAFFEE LM, KARASUYAMA H, BAKER M, PARDOLL DM: **Treatment of Established Renal Cancer By Tumor Cells Engineered to Secrete Interleukin-4.** *Science* 1991, 254:713–716.

29. RESTIFO NP, SPIESS PJ, KARP SE, MULÉ JJ, ROSENBERG SA: **A Nonimmunogenic Sarcoma Transduced With the cDNA for Interferon Gamma Elicits CD8+ T Cells Against the Wild-Type Tumor: Correlation With Antigen Presentation Capability.** *J Exp Med* 1992, 175:1423–1431.

30. WEBER JS, JAY G, TANAKA K, ROSENBERG SA: **Immunotherapy of a Murine Tumor With Interleukin 2: Increased Sensitivity After MHC Class I Gene Transfection.** *J Exp Med* 1987, 166:1716–1733.

31. CHEN L, ASHE S, BRADY WA, HELLSTRÖM I, HELLSTRÖM KE, LEDBETTER JA, MCGOWAN P, LINSLEY PS: **Costimulation of Antitumor Immunity by the B7 Counterreceptor for the T Lymphocyte Molecules CD28 and CTLA-4.** *Cell* 1992, 71:1093–1102.

James C. Yang, MD, Surgery Branch, National Cancer Institute, 9000 Rockville Pike, Bethesda, MD 10892, USA.

Molecular biology and clinical applications to cancer

Michael T. Lotze, MD

University of Pittsburgh Medical Center, Pittsburgh, Pennsylvania, USA

New insights into the genetic changes associated with cancer, the genetic control of programmed cell death, and the availability of new tools to study biologic problems including targeted gene disruption and quantitative polymerase chain reaction have defined new questions and allowed more sophisticated answers in studies of fundamental cellular processes. The development of new approaches in the clinic, including nascent gene therapies, is rapidly evolving.

Current Opinion in General Surgery 1994:245–254

The twin concepts that cancer is a genetic disorder and that immune responses are genetically determined have become so well accepted that they could be considered trite expressions of modern biology. This review is quite clearly idiosyncratic and personal, reflecting twin interests in these two general areas. Much of what follows represents a synthesis of developments in these areas during the past year. The notion that a greater understanding of cancer would fundamentally lead to alterations in our approach to the disease has yet to be matched by major changes in cancer treatment outcome in any real sense in the clinic. Nevertheless, much of the exuberant activity in biotechnology and the modern academic medical center, as applied to cancer treatment, reflects the possibility of fundamentally altering the phenotypic expression of individual genes either through conventional chemotherapies and radiation therapy (about which we have a far more profound understanding) or through the application of nascent gene therapies.

Cancer-causing genes

Over 20 years ago it was demonstrated that only a single copy of chromosome 22 was found in meningiomas. Since then, many of the heritable genetic changes associated with familial cancers have been identified [1]. These are summarized in Table 1. Identification of these genetic alterations in individuals and their progeny represents not only a new opportunity for cancer screening, but also an important public health problem in terms of the required counseling of individuals with these inherited disorders. For example, the Wilms' tumor locus gene, *WT1* is associated with tumor suppressor functions and is clearly associated with the induction not only of the Wilms' tumor but potentially of some renal cell carcinomas as well. Targeted deletion of this gene in mice is associated with pulmonary dysfunction and a total failure to develop kidneys and gonads [2•]. Individuals having only a single functional copy of the WT1 gene have cryptorchidism and hypospadias, suggesting that gene dosage is indeed important for adequate production of this particular gene product.

Such so-called suppressor oncogenes appear to function in part by regulating the cell cycle. Traversion of the cell cycle in somatic cells during normal mitosis is increasingly understood from studies performed initially in yeast and more recently in mammalian cells [3••,4]. The resting G0 cell moves into G1-S with replication of chromosomal DNA and subsequent segregation of the replicated chromosomes at G2-M. So-called cell cycle checkpoints exist at each of these transitions (G1-S and G2-M). A complex set of cell proteins regulates traversion of the cell cycle. These include members of the p34 family and cyclins—the mitotic cyclins (cyclin B), S-phase cyclins (cyclin A) and G1 cyclins (cyclins C,D,E, and F). The complex of cyclin B and $p34^{cdc2}$ serves as a maturation-promoting factor allowing the initiation of the cell cycle. Understanding the cell cycle and development of therapeutic agents that can effectively induce arrest in cancer cells appears increasingly to be an attainable goal.

In human malignancy, *p53* is well recognized as the most frequently mutated oncogene. This molecule functions as a "negative brake" on the transition through G1-S and indeed as a cell cycle checkpoint following DNA damage induced by mutagens or ionizing radiation. Other mechanisms (Table 2) associated with genomic instability include decreases in DNA repair, problems with chromosomal segregation [4], and most recently a "mutator mutation" that allows accumulation of multiple mutations to numbers "greater than 100,000" in tumor cells [5••]. This process has recently been demonstrated [5••] in a group of colorectal carcinomas that had ubiquitous somatic deletion mutations. Interestingly, these tumors did not usually have *p53* mutations, suggesting that these cells could escape the normal censoring role of *p53*.

Initially, p53 was identified as a ubiquitous protein that appeared to be preferentially expressed in murine methylcholanthrene–induced sarcomas as studied by Deleo *et al.* [6]. Subsequently much has been learned

 ISBN 1-85922-671-X ISSN 1065–6243

Table 1. Dominantly inherited genetic predispositions to tumors*

Syndrome	Predominant tumor types	Chromosome	Gene	Location	Function
Alport	Smooth muscle tumors	x	*Collagen α5, α6*	Components of basement membranes	
Early-onset familial breast cancer	Breast carcinoma	17q	?	?	?
Familial adenomatous polyposis	Multiple colorectal adenomas	5q	*APC*	Cytoplasmic	?
Familial melanoma	Cutaneous malignant melanoma	9q	?	?	?
Gorlin	Basal cell carcinomas of the skin	9q	?	?	?
Hereditary nonpolyposis colorectal cancer	Colon and uterine carcinomas	2p	?	?	Replication fidelity?
Li-Fraumeni	Leukemia, soft-tissue sarcoma, osteosarcoma, brain tumor, breast and adrenal cortical carcinomas	17p	*p53*	Nuclear	Transcriptional regulation
Multiple endocrine neoplasia type 1	Parathyroid, endocrine pancreas, and pituitary tumors	11q	?	?	?
Multiple endocrine neoplasia type 2A	Medullary thyroid carcinoma, pheochromocytoma	10	*RET*	?	?
Neurofibromatosis type 1	Multiple peripheral neurofibromas	17q	*NF1*	Cytoplasmic	GTPase-activating protein
Neurofibromatosis type 2	Central schwannomas and meningiomas	22q	*NF2*	Cytoskeletal-membrane link	
Retinoblastoma	Retinoblastomas, osteosarcomas	13q	*Rb*	Nuclear	Transcriptional regulation
von Hippel-Lindau	Renal-cell carcinoma	3p	?	?	?
Wilms tumor	Nephroblastoma	11p	*WT1*	Nuclear	Transcriptional regulation

*Adapted from Kinzler and Vogelstein [1]; with permission.

Table 2. Mechanisms defective in genomic fidelity and associated with cancer

Cell cycle control check points
Machinery for DNA replication ("mutator mutations") and chromosome segregation
DNA repair processes

about this protein. Perhaps most surprising was the observation that *p53*-null mice (mice with the gene eliminated through targeted disruption) developed perfectly normally but then were susceptible to early malignancies occurring in the first several months following birth. Cells with wild type expression of *p53* arrest in G1 following mild gamma radiation, presumably to allow breaks in DNA to be repaired; in cells from *p53*-null mice, only a G2 checkpoint is noted. Studies in Chinese hamster ovary cells indicate that there are at least five GADD (growth arrest and DNA damage–inducible) genes induced following treatment with a wide variety of different DNA altering agents. The *GADD45* gene appears to be one of the first to be induced following DNA damage and has an intronic region that binds *p53*. The gene which causes increases in p53 protein (and presumed subsequent induction of *GADD45*) appears to be altered in ataxia telangiectasia [7•].

Normally, *p53* exists as a homotetramer and is bound by defective or mutant *p53* gene products, thus causing *p53* mutations to serve as a so-called "dominant negative" mutation. In addition, other genes and gene products will bind *p53*, including the MDM2 gene product, which binds the activation domain of *p53* [8••], as well as SV40T and the papilloma virus E6 gene product. It has been demonstrated recently that *p53* is required for apoptosis induced by irradiation but is not required for other forms of apoptosis (Fig. 1) induced in thymocytes by either crosslinking the T-cell receptor or treatment with glucocorticoids [9,10••,11]. Recently, overexpression of *p53* (using immunohistochemical techniques) was shown to be an independent marker for relapse-free and overall survival in node negative patients with resectable breast cancers [12••]. What does all this mean for the cancer clinician? Ways to increase normal *p53* expression either by effective inducible agents or binding factors that inhibit intracellular p53 binding proteins such as MDM2 would seem to be reasonable targets. In addition, wild type gene delivery using retroviral vectors would be testable in the clinic as has recently been proposed by Jack Roth at MD Anderson Hospital and approved by the Recombinant DNA Advisory Committee of the National Institutes of Health. The ability to target all cells may not be required, as was originally thought, because of a so-called "bystander effect" in which death of transfected cells induces other local cells to also die.

Apoptosis

Any individual somatic cell has a series of limited options at any one time which include mitosis, apoptosis, quiescence, or differentiation [13]. Apoptosis is now recognized as a genetically programmable cell death that is associated morphologically with plasma membrane blebbing, cell volume loss, condensation of the nuclear material, and a characteristic ladder of DNA degradation with nucleosomal intervals of approximately 200 base pairs. Just as mitosis is critically regulated, the notion that cell death induction could be a goal of cancer therapy (and its prevention a form of tumor escape) are now widely appreciated and accepted. Much of the current excitement in the area of apoptosis is defining the role of several genetic elements that regulate this important process. To date these include the *bcl*-2 family of proteins including *bcl*-x and *bax*, and others including Fas/APO-1, *myc*, *ras*, and *p53* [14–17,18••]. The protooncogene *bcl*-2 was isolated from the breakpoint of the chromosomal translocation t[14;18] that is found in over 60% of human follicular B-cell lymphomas. This translocation transposes the *bcl*-2 gene to the heavy chain locus of immunoglobulins. Subsequently it has been demonstrated that *bcl*-2 expression allows accumulation of B cells, permitting their enhanced survival rather than inducing their proliferation. Nothing is ever quite that simple and it now appears that there are two additional factors, perhaps forming a family of molecules, which are capable of binding to *bcl*-2 and regulating its function. These include bax and *bcl*-xs, which bind the *bcl*-2 gene product and allow apoptosis to proceed. A larger transcript that contains an additional 63 amino acids, *bcl*-x_L, appears to act like *bcl*-2 in preventing apoptotic cell death. The precise mechanism of *bcl*-2 action is unclear. Various studies initially localized the protein to the mitochondrial cell membrane but recently as well to the nucleus and to the endoplasmic reticulum where it may bind proteins required for apoptosis. Apoptosis can also be induced by crosslinking the APO-1/Fas molecule present on the cell surface of many mammalian cells. Crosslinking this receptor induces characteristic DNA fragmentation associated with apoptosis. Stimulation of chronic lymphocytic leukemia cell lines with mitogens such as *Staphylococcus aureus* Cowen 1 (Sac) or treatment with interleukin-2 causes both upregulation of the APO-1/Fas molecule as well as decreased expression of *bcl*-2 [17]. These two molecules appear to be functionally linked and the decreased expression of *bcl*-2 is thus associated with increased ability of APO-1/Fas to induce nuclear degradation. Likewise *bcl*-2 is expressed [17] in mature T cells but in only a small subset of double positive (CD4+, CD8+) thymocytes. Enhanced expression is observed during certain phases of fetal thymocyte development between days 15 and 16. This suggests that those thymocytes most likely to be induced to undergo apoptotic cell death may be protected from this during transient expression of *bcl*-2 both early and late in T-cell development.

Two very recent and surprising findings suggest the importance of *bcl*-2 expression. First, hematopoietic precursors transfected with *bcl*-2 are no longer growth factor dependent and continue to differentiate along different pathways in the total absence of lineage specific factors [18••]. In addition, although targeted disruption of *bcl*-2 is associated with apparently normal initial differentiation of immune cells, total disappearance of these cells occurs at about 4 weeks of age [19••]. This suggests not only the major importance of this molecule in normal hematopoietic development but also that means of targeting *bcl*-2 gene expression may be useful in the treatment of leukemias and lymphomas, using a variety of antisense strategies with phosphorothioate oligonucleotides or with antisense gene therapy. Such approaches are currently under-

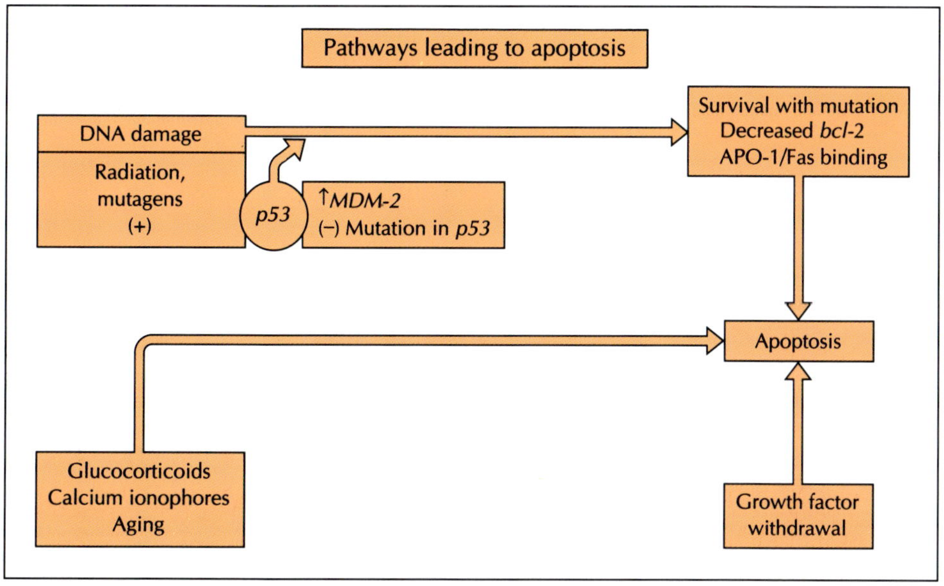

Fig. 1. Pathways leading to apoptosis. The characteristic changes of membrane blebbing and DNA fragmentation are observed with apoptotic cell death. Agents that increase p53 (*plus sign*) or are associated with a decrease in p53 (*minus sign*) are shown. (*Adapted from* Oliner *et al.* [8••]; with permission.)

going evaluation at a variety of centers. Expression of *bcl*-2 has also recently been described in 12% to 25% of non–small cell lung cancers [20••]. Interestingly, *bcl*-2 expression was positively correlated with survival, suggesting that patients with tumors that express *bcl*-2 have a better prognosis. This particular study demonstrated that *bcl*-2 status was more highly correlated (P= 0.010) with prognosis than sex, age, tumor differentiation, T stage, or N stage [21]. Thus, just like follicular lymphomas where it is associated with a more indolent course, expression of this oncogene probably identifies less virulent tumors.

The Fas antigen, a member of the tumor necrosis factor receptor family, is defective in *lpr* mice and associated with lymphoproliferation. The Fas ligand has yet to be identified but it has been suggested that a cell surface ligand exists on T cells. Presumably interaction of these T cells with cells expressing APO-1/Fas makes targets susceptible to its apoptotic signalling, potentially through decreased expression of *bcl*-2 products. Many groups are now attempting to identify the normal ligand for Fas. Northern blot tests show positive results for Fas in preparations of thymus, liver, heart, lung, and ovary [21]. Intravenous injection of this antibody in mice kills wild type mice but not the Fas deficient *lpr* mice. Severe damage of the liver with apoptotic cell changes suggest that this molecule is important in regulating hepatocyte growth and thus potentially in fulminant hepatitis. This limits the ability of agents crosslinking Fas to be used as systemic therapeutic agents for cancer. Potentially, antisense constructs to *bcl*-2, *myc* or Fas may allow targeted therapy in patients [22].

Targeted gene disruption

The control of immune responses by a variety of different gene products is becoming better understood. Using embryonic stem cells and targeting vectors that disrupt individual gene expression, it is possible to create chimeric and then, subsequently, homozygous animals lacking expression of individual genes (as was noted for the *p53* deletion mutants). This has become a very interesting area in modern immunology as individual cytokines and important signalling molecules are selectively eliminated. Some are found to have only minimal effects, demonstrating the immense redundancy that occurs within the immune system. Others have quite profound effects, potentially identifying better targets for therapeutic strategies to either enhance or decrease immune function. An excellent review of the current status of gene knock-outs in immunology is provided by Fung-Leung and Mak [23••] and is updated here in Table 3. One of the first of these knock-outs to be created was the β2 microglobulin molecule [37,38], which is necessary for delivery of class I molecules to the cell surface and is also associated with binding of other proteins such as CD1, thymocyte glycoproteins, and the intestinal IgG receptor. Even though CD8+ T cells are eliminated from such mice, the mice appear to be immunologically quite functionally intact. In fact, this initial observation of unexpected findings based on the expected biologic effects has been replicated throughout many of the knock-outs that have been developed. Among some of the more interesting recent findings is the absolute requirement for $p56^{lck}$ required for T-cell development and a lack of N-region diversity [36•] in T-cell receptors on T cells from animals without terminal deoxynucleotidal transferase. Profound inflammation is associated with knock-out of the transforming growth factor-β1 gene as would have been predicted [24••]. Extravasation of neutrophils is limited in P selection–deficient mice, and the ability of leukocytes to roll along the endothelial cells in blood vessels is severely compromised [51••]. Natural deletions also continue to be reported in patients. These include the p53 mutations noted above associated with Li-Fraumeni syndrome, and more recently, disruption of the collagen α5 and α6 genes associated with inherited smooth muscle tumors in patients with Alport's syndrome [52]. As noted, targeted disruption of *bcl*-2 causes loss of the immune system at about 4 weeks of age [19••]. Not only do these studies provide a richer understanding of the basic biology but they also suggest means by which inherited disorders might be rectified by gene therapies.

Quantitative polymerase chain reaction

Detecting small numbers of messenger RNA transcripts was made possible by the development of reverse transcription–polymerase chain reaction techniques. One of the fundamental difficulties in these approaches is the lack of true quantitation since small changes in template number, annealing capacity of individual primer pairs, and even position in the heating block of a thermal cycler can all profoundly affect the ultimate amount of amplified complementary DNA. These assay systems are extremely important for identifying transcripts in tumors as well as in immune effectors. Critically examining the total number of messenger molecules has been difficult at best. In the usual scenario, oligomers hybridizing to the 5′ and 3′ stretch of complementary DNA are used. The three cycles following reverse transcription of message traditionally performed during polymerase chain reaction include 1) the annealing phase, in which primers find template, followed by 2) an extension phase in which complimentary nucleotides find their partners in the growing double stranded DNA, followed by 3) melting to separate the two strands. The process is then repeated. Such amplification of usually a few hundred to several hundred bases can easily be accomplished using 25 to 30 cycles of amplification. We have been able to detect as few as one in 100,000 cells using this approach with gene-marked lymphocytes. More problematic has been the absolute quantification of message species. Based on studies initially developed in the late 1980s by Wang *et al.* [53], a competitor of known quantity can serve as an internal control, allowing precise delineation of the average number of message molecules per cell. The target messenger RNA and the internal standard are coamplified, which allows quantification of specific

Table 3. Genes involved in immune response and hematopoiesis that have been disrupted in the mouse germ line

Study	Gene	Effect of gene knockout
Kulkarni *et al.* [24••]	TGF-β	Excessive inflammation, early death
Fung-Leung and Mak [23••], Schorle *et al.* [25]	IL-2	T-cell development intact, late development of lymphadenopathy, splenomegaly, normal B-cell development
Paul [26], Kohn *et al.* [27]	IL-4	Marked decrease of IgG1, no IgE; not essential for ontogeny of thymocytes, B cells
Paul [26]	IL-10	Normal serum IgM, no increase of IFN-γ; animals smaller
Dalton *et al.* [28]	IFN-γ	Impaired production of antimicrobial products, decreased MHC class II antigens, decreased natural killer cell activity
Fung-Leung and Mak [23••]	IL-2Rβ	Not reported
Kamuo *et al.* [29]	IFN-γR	Decreased resistance to infections, MHC class II and NO production by macrophages
Rahemtulla *et al.* [30]	CD4	Decreased helper cell activity
Fung-Leung *et al.* [31]	CD8	Lack of cytotoxic cells
Schilham *et al.* [32•]	CD4, CD8	Have alloreactive but not viral reactive cells
Fung-Leung and Mak [23••]	CD5	Not reported
Nakayama *et al.* [19••]	*bcl*-2	Disappearance of lymphoid system at 4 weeks of age
Molina *et al.* [33], Killeen and Littman [34]	$p56^{lck}$	Pround block in thymocyte development, few peripheral T cells
Fung-Leung and Mak [23••]	*fyn*	Defective in signaling through TCRs, no change in peripheral T-cell function
Love *et al.* [35]	TCR ζ	Few TCRs and little CD5 on peripheral T cells
Komori *et al.* [36•]	Terminal deoxy-nucleotidal transferase	Lack of TCR N regions, increase in some variable region genes
Zijlstra *et al.* [37], Koller *et al.* [38]	β-2 Microglobulin	No CD8+ T cells, no class I MHC molecules
Cosgrove *et al.* [39], Grusby *et al.* [40]	MHC class II (I-A β chain)	Depletion of CD4+ T cells
Fung-Leung and Mak [23••]	Invariant chain	Lower level of MHC class II expression
Mombaerts *et al.* [41]	*RAG-1*	SCID, block in B and T cells
Shinkai *et al.* [42]	*RAG-2*	SCID, block in B cells, thymocyte differentiation
Tybulewicz *et al.* [43], Schwartzberg *et al.* [44]	c-*abl*	Neonatal lethality, lymphopenia (T and B), splenic atrophy
Kitamura *et al.* [45]	IgM μ chain	No serum IgM or mature B cells
Fung-Leung and Mak [23••]	Light chain λ5	Small population of B cells
Roes and Rajewsky [46]	IgD	Conventional B cells are found
Mucensky *et al.* [47]	c-*myb*	Severe anemia
Pevny *et al.* [48]	*GATA-1*	Failure of erythroid development
Mombaerts *et al.* [49]	TCR-α	Absence of α and β T cells, no decrease in number of thymocytes
Mombaerts *et al.* [49]	TCR-β	Absence of α and β T cells, decrease number of thymocytes
Itohara *et al.* [50]	TCR-δ	No γ or δ T cells, normal cells, α or β T cells
Mayadas *et al.* [51••]	P-selectin	Lack of leukocyte rolling and extravasation

**Adapted from* Fung-Leung and Mak [23••]; with permission.
IFN-γ—gamma interferon; IL—interleukin; MHC—major histocompatibility complex; SCID—severe combined immunodeficiency; TCR—T-cell receptor.

messenger RNA samples of less than 0.1 nanograms of total RNA or as few as 200 cells [54]. This has recently been applied in the setting of interleukin-4 transgenic mice (Fig. 2) with detection of as little as twofold differences [55••]. The critical problem with this technique, however, is the differential ability of complementary DNAs to be created at the reverse transcriptase phase from messenger RNA. This has recently been done by making cyclic RNAs from the plasmid internal controls, to allow subsequent complementary DNA formation of both the test messenger RNA as well as the control complementary RNA to go on in parallel. In addition, multiple messages can be simultaneously quantitated in such a fashion [56••].

Gene therapy for cancer

Gene therapy has indeed come of age [57••]. As of June 8, 1993, a total of 52 clinical protocols involving gene therapy have been approved by the Recombinant DNA Advisory Committee to the National Institutes of Health. A variety of approaches to introduce genes into human cells have been approved, including the use of incompetent murine retroviral vectors (which are most commonly employed) but also others, including adenoviral vectors, poxvirus vectors, liposomes used to directly introduce genes, and direct transfer of retrovirus producing cells *in vivo*. It is anticipated that the general approach used for cytokine gene therapy and other

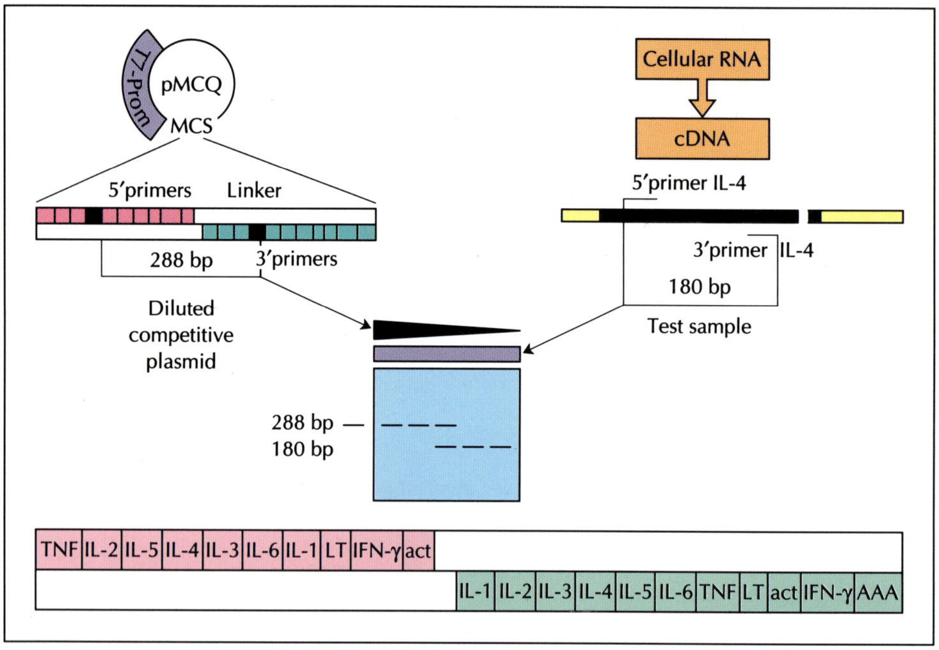

Fig. 2. Cytokine messenger RNA quantification by competitive polymerase chain reaction (PCR). The amount of PCR product is proportional to the amount of input DNA, as demonstrated by coamplification of constant amounts of target complementary DNA (cDNA) and serially diluted control plasmid pMQ. At *bottom,* the order of 5′ and 3′ primer-specific sequences in plasmid pMCQ is given. AAA—polyadenylation site; act—alpha chymotrypsin; IFN-γ—gamma interferon; IL—interleukin; LT—lymphotoxin; MCS—multiple cloning site; TNF—tumor necrosis factor. (*From* Platzer *et al.* [55••]; with permission.)

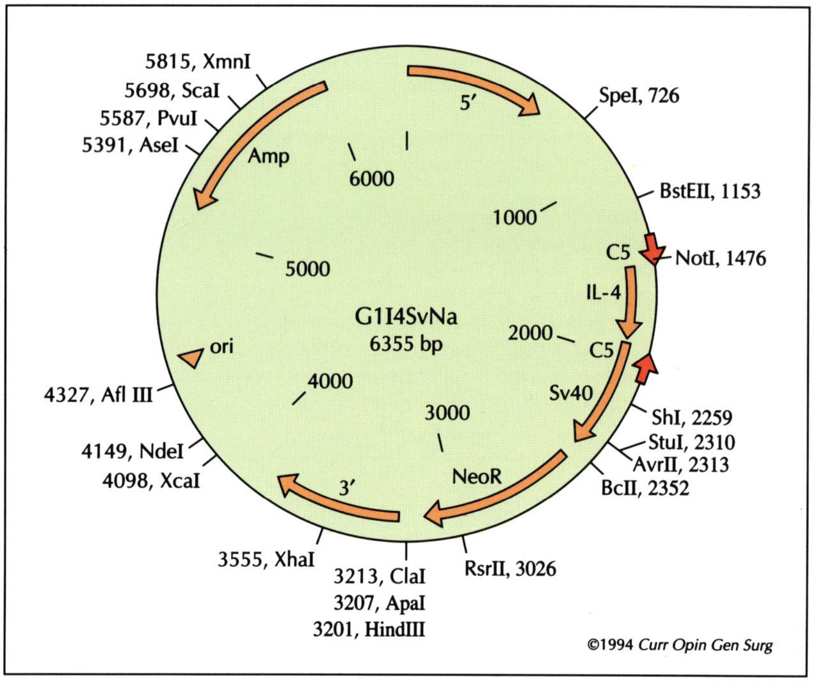

Fig. 3. Viral construct used for interleukin-4 (IL-4) gene therapy at the University of Pittsburgh, Pittsburgh, PA. The introduction of the virus requires the use of a "packaging cell line" that encapsidates the defective virus. (*Constructed by* W. Jacob, Genetic Therapy, Gaithersburg, MD.)

transferred genes, such as those used as part of marking studies that we performed at the National Cancer Institute [58] and at St. Jude's [59•], and more recently to introduce functional genes to subserve a variety of purposes, is growing at a logarithmic rate. Delivery of cytokines including interleukin-2, tumor necrosis factor α, interferon-γ, and interleukin-4 have already begun to be tested at a variety of institutions. These will soon include granulocyte-macrophage colony-stimulating factor gene therapy study to be initiated by Simons, Jaffee, Pardoll, and colleagues at Johns Hopkins. All of these approaches involve the delivery of an individual cytokine at the site of a tumor vaccine to elicit immunologic antitumor effects. These represent early phase I studies and, although based on substantive murine results, will require a prolonged period of evaluation [60]. In addition, it is unclear whether other means of local cytokine generation, including

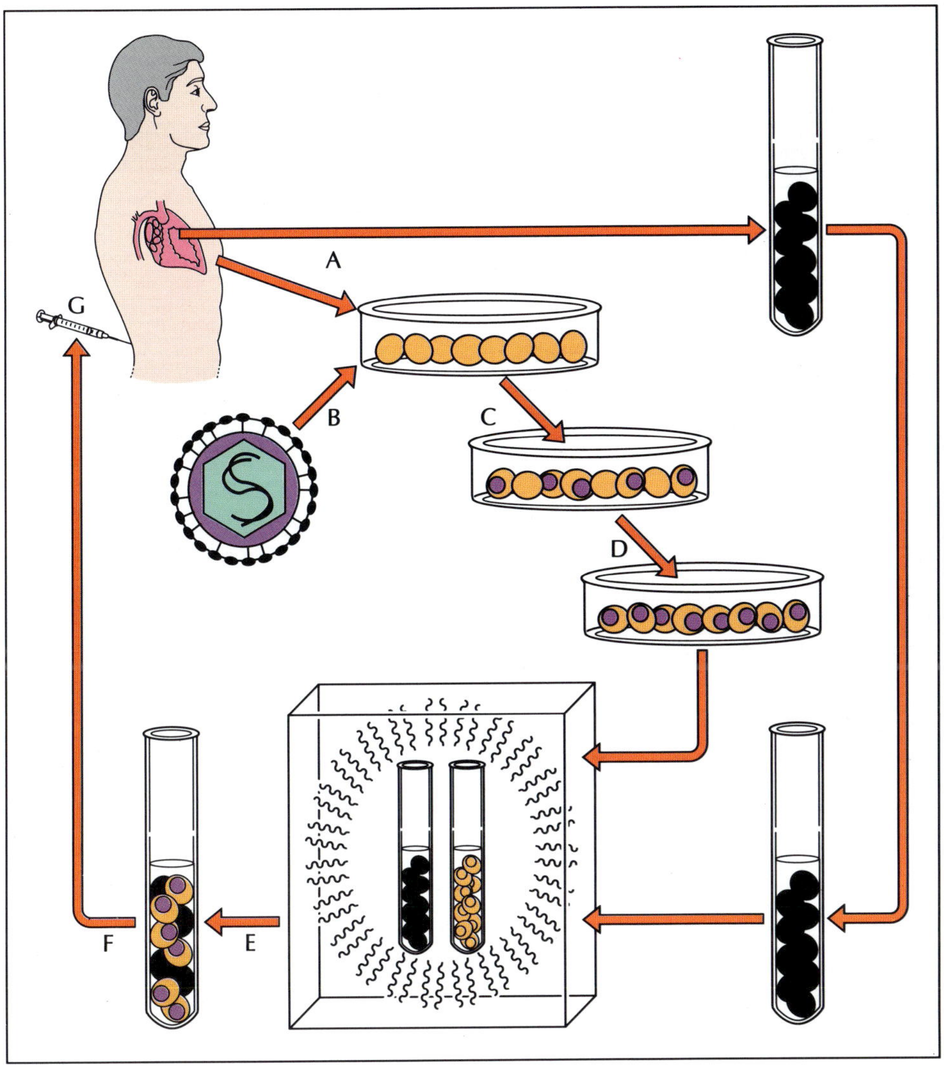

Fig. 4. Interleukin-4 (IL-4) gene therapy. **A**, Tumor cells and skin tissue are removed from patient. Tumor cells are frozen. Connective tissue cells (fibroblasts) are cultured. **B**, Retrovirus with gene for IL-4 is added to fibroblast cultures. **C**, IL-4 gene is incorporated into some of the fibroblasts. **D**, Researchers select fibroblasts that produce IL-4 protein and grow them in culture. **E**, Radiation is delivered to selected genetically altered fibroblasts and to thawed tumor cells. **F**, Altered fibroblasts and tumor cells are mixed to form a vaccine. **G**, Vaccine injected into patient's back at five locations. (*Courtesy of* University of Pittsburgh Medical Center, Pittsburgh, PA.)

traditional bacterial adjuvants, may not be more efficient than these gene transfer technologies [61••]. Our own interleukin-4 gene therapy protocol (and a proposed interleukin-12 gene therapy protocol) involves the production of interleukin-4 by transfected autologous fibroblasts (Figs. 3 and 4) and has recently been started in patients. Local production of cytokine at the site of a tumor vaccine is thought to activate the local endothelium, causing emigration of lymphocytes, macrophages, and eosinophils, and the late subsequent expansion of tumor specific T cells capable of migrating throughout the host. These approaches are now being coupled with systemic cytokine administration including interleukin-2 and interleukin-12 in attempts to enhance the antitumor effects in these murine models. Direct transfer of retroviral vectors to treat brain tumors has begun at the National Institutes of Health based on successful animal models [62••]. New means of gene transfer including particle bombardment [63••,64] with gold beads coated with DNA or even direct injection of DNA into muscle are being tested [65••]. Use of novel vectors, such as the adenoassociated virus [66], papillomavirus, and poxviruses, are being proposed as means to transfer genes of interest. The cost of developing the new therapies [67] is being borne by a variety of academic, federal, and commercial institutions. It is clear that much will be learned in these early steps [68•,69,70] of gene transfer and that the potential of targeting certain genes, in particular to cancer cells, will lead to rich insights into basic cellular biology and, ultimately, to patient benefit.

References and recommended reading

Papers of particular interest, published within the annual period of review, have been highlighted as:

- • Of special interest
- •• Of outstanding interest

1. KINZLER KW, VOGELSTEIN B: **A Gene for Neurofibromatosis 2.** *Nature* 1993, **363**:495.

2. • KREIDBERG JA, SARIOLA H, LORING JM, MAEDA M, PELLETIER J, HOUSMAN D, JAENISCH R: **WT-1 is Required for Early Kidney Development.** *Cell* 1993, 74:679–691.

This paper describes the use of targeted disruption to determine the function of the *WT1* locus in mice. At day 11 of gestation, cells from the anlage of the kidney and gonads undergo apoptotic cell death and fail to develop, creating an embryo lacking these organs.

3. MURRAY AW: **Creative Blocks: Cell-Cycle Checkpoints and Feedback**
•• **Controls.** *Nature* 1993, **359**:559–605.

This is an excellent overview of recent insights on how cells ensure that "copy editing" occurs before completion of the mitotic cycle. Failure to do this is responsible in part for the development of cancer.

4. HARTWELL L: **Defects in a Cell Cycle Checkpoint May Be Responsible for the Genomic Instability of Cancer Cells.** *Cell* 1992, **71**:543–546.

5. IONOV Y, PEINADO MA, MALKHOSYAN S, SHIBATA D, PERUCHO M: **Ubiqui-**
•• **tous Somatic Mutations in Simple Repeated Sequences Reveal a New Mechanism for Colonic Carcinogenesis.** *Nature* 1993, **363**:558–562.

Decreased fidelity of replication of somatic-cell DNA would lead to multiple mutations. Evidence for this has now been found in up to 12% of colon carcinomas, suggesting that this potentially hereditable alteration may be associated with the development of neoplastic transformation.

6. DELEO AB, JAY G, APPELLA E, DUBOIS GC, LAW LW, OLD LJ: **Detection of a Transformation-Related Antigen in Chemically Induced Sarcomas and Other Transformed Cells of the Mouse.** *Proc Natl Acad Sci U S A* 1979, **76**:2420–2424.

7. KASTAN MB, ZHAN Q, EL-DEIRY WS, CARRIER F, JACKS T, WALSH WV,
• PLUNKETT BS, VOGELSTEIN B, FORNACE AJ: **A Mammalian Cell Cycle Checkpoint Pathway Utilizing p53 and GADD45 is Defective in Ataxia-Telangiectasia.** *Cell* 1993, **71**:587–597.

Patients with ataxia-telangiectasis are susceptible to developing cancer. Irradiation of cells from these patients is not associated with the induction of normal *p53*, allowing failure to arrest in G1-S and accumulation of mutations that ultimately could contribute to neoplastic transformation.

8. OLINER JD, PIETENPOL JA, THIAGALINGAM S, GYURIS J, KINZLER KW,
•• VOGELSTEIN B: **Oncoprotein MDM2 Conceals the Activation Domain of Tumour Suppressor p53.** *Nature* 1993, **362**:857–860.

Inactivation of p53 can come about not only by mutation but also by its binding to proteins that inhibit its ability to activate the transcription of other genes presumably associated with inducing growth arrest. Inactivation of p53 in human sarcomas is associated with amplification of the oncogene *MDM2*, the product of which can bind p53.

9. LANE DP: **A Death in the Life of p53.** *Nature* 1993, **362**:786–788.

10. LOWE SC, SCHMITT EM, SMITH SW, OSBORNE BA, JACKS T: **p53 Is Re-**
•• **quired for Radiation-Induced Apoptosis in Mouse Thymocytes.** *Nature* 1993, **362**:847–858.

In this paper, the role of *p53* in inducing apoptotic cell death associated with irradiation and chemotherapeutic agents is established. Loss of *p53*-regulated events may be central to its role in tumor progression and its responsiveness to conventional chemotherapeutic agents and radiation therapy.

11. CLARKE AR, PURDIE CA, HARRISON DJ, MORRIS RG, BIRD CC, HOOPER ML, WYLIE AH: **Thymocyte Apoptosis Induced by p53-Dependent and Independent Pathways.** *Nature* 1993, **362**:849–852.

12. SILVESTRINI R, BENINI E, DAIDONE MG, BENERONI S, BORACCHI P,
•• CAPPELLETTI V, DI FRONZO G, VERONESI U: **p53 as an Independent Prognostic Marker in Lymph Node-Negative Breast Cancer Patients.** *J Natl Cancer Inst* 1993, **85**:965–970.

Overexpression of the p53 protein was detected in 44% of lymph node–negative breast cancer patients. Odds ratio of relapse was 3.24 compared with p53-negative tumors, and p53 overexpression appeared to be the most relevant indicator of relapse, even more than tumor size and estrogen receptor status.

13. WILLIAMS GT, SMITH CA: **Molecular Regulation of Apoptosis: Genetic Controls on Cell Death.** *Cell* 1993, **74**:777–779.

14. OLTVAI ZN, MILLIMAN CL, KORSMEYER SJ: **Bcl-2 Heterodimerizes In Vivo With a Conserved Homolog, Bax, That Accelerates Programmed Cell Death.** *Cell* 1993, **74**:609–619.

15. BOISE LH, GONZALEZ-GARCIA M, POSTEMA CE, DING L, LINDSTEIN T, TURKA LA, MAO X, NUNEZ G, THOMPSON CB: **Bcl-x, a bcl-2-Related Gene That Functions as a Dominant Regulator of Apoptotic Death.** *Cell* 1993, **74**:597–608.

16. MAPARA MY, BARGOU R, ZUGCK C, DOHNER H, USTAOGLU F, JONKER RR, KRAMMER PH, DORKEN B: **APO-1 Mediated Apoptosis or Proliferation in Human Chronic B Lymphocytic Leukemia: Correlation With bcl-2 Oncogene Expression.** *Eur J Immunol* 1993, **23**:702–708.

17. VEIS DJ, SENTMAN CL, BACH EA, KORSMEYER SJ: **Expression of the Bcl-2 Protein in Murine and Human Thymocytes and in Peripheral T Lymphocytes.** *J Immunol* 1993, **151**:2346–2354.

18. FAIRBAIRN LJ, COWLING GJ, REIPERT BM, DEXTER TM: **Suppression of**
•• **Apoptosis Allows Differentiation and Development of a Multipotent Hemopoietic Cell Line in the Absence of Added Growth Factors.** *Cell* 1993, **74**:823–832.

Transfection of the human *bcl-2* gene into an interleukin-3–dependent multipotent hematopoietic cell line allowed them to fully differentiate along various maturational pathways. This suggests that the role of growth factors is primarily to enable rather than induce differentiation along individual pathways.

19. NAKAYAMA KI, NAKAYAMA K, NEGISHI I, KUIDA K, SHINKAI Y, LOUIE M,
•• FIELDS LE, LUCAS PJ, STEWART V, ALT FW, LOH DY: **Disappearance of the Lymphoid System in *bcl-2* Homozygous Mutant Chimeric Mice.** *Science* 1993, **261**:1584–1588.

Targeted disruption of the *bcl-2* gene allows full and apparently normal development of an immune system that "disappears" at about 4 weeks of age. The failure to suppress apoptotic cell death, which occurs in normal cells, is presumably responsible for this lemming-like loss of B cells and T cells.

20. PEZELLA F, TURLEY H, KUZU I, TUNGEKAR MF, DUNNILL MS, PIERCE CB,
•• HARRIS A, GATTER KC, MASON DY: **bcl-2 Protein in Non-Small-cell Lung Carcinoma.** *N Engl J Med* 1993, **329**:690–694.

Twenty-five percent of squamous-cell carcinomas and 12% of adenocarcinomas of the lung express *bcl-2* by immunohistochemistry. These tumors appear to be associated with a more indolent course, just like lymphomas, compared with those tumors not expressing *bcl-2*.

21. OGASAWARA J, WATANABE-FUKUNAGA R, ADACHI M, MATSUZAWA A, KASUGAL T, KITAMURA Y, ITOH N, SUDA T, NAGATA S: **Lethal Effect of the Anti-Fas Antibody in Mice.** *Nature* 1993, **364**:805–810.

22. REED JC, CUDDY M, HALDAR S, CROCE C, HOWELL P, MAKOVER D, BRADLEY K: **Bcl-2 Mediates Tumorigenicity of a Human T-Lymphoid Cell Line: Synergy With myc and Inhibition by *bcl-2* Antisense.** *Proc Natl Acad Sci U S A* 1990, **87**:3660–3664.

23. FUNG-LEUNG WP, MAK TW: **Embryonic Stem Cells and Homologous**
•• **Recombination.** *Curr Opin Immunol* 1992, **4**:189–194.

The development of techniques to disrupt the function of genes in mice primarily is nicely presented here. Multiple "knockouts" have already been created and have led to unexpected insights regarding the function of individual genes.

24. KULKARNI AB, HUH CG, BECKER D, GEISER A, LYGHT M, FLANDERS KC,
•• ROBERTS AB, SPORN MB, WARD JM, KARLSON S: **Transforming Growth Factor β1 Null Mutation in Mice Causes Excessive Inflammatory Response and Early Death.** *Proc Natl Acad Sci U S A* 1993, **90**:770–774.

Transforming growth factor-β_1 is a homodimeric 25-kD protein that is involved in many cellular processes including proliferation and differentiation of many cell types, but especially those involving immunity. It is also involved in embryonic development, extracellular matrix formation, wound healing, bone development, hematopoiesis, and regulation of macrophage function. Targeted disruption of this gene allowed one third of fetuses to develop to term, but they developed massive inflammation 2 weeks after birth and died in the following 1 to 2 weeks. Tissue-specific gene therapy (perhaps targeted to the heart and lungs, where most of the inflammation occurred), with the transforming growth factor-βgene would seem reasonable next steps.

25. SCHORLE H, HOLTSCHKE T, HUNIG T, SCHIMPL A, HORAK I: **Development and Function of T Cells in Mice Rendered Interleukin-2 Deficient by Gene Targeting.** *Nature* 1991, **352**:621–624.

26. PAUL WE: **Poking Holes in the Network.** *Nature* 1992, **357**:16–17.

27. KOHN R, RAJEWSKY K, MULLER W: **Generation and Analysis of Interleukin-4 Deficient Mice.** *Science* 1991, **254**:707–710.

28. DALTON DK, PITTS-MEEK S, KESHAV S, FIGARI IS, BRADLEY A, STEWART TA: **Multiple Defects of Immune Cell Function in Mice With Disrupted Interferon-γ Genes.** *Science* 1993, **259**:1739–1744.

29. KAMUO R, SHAPIRO D, LE J, HUANG S, AGUET M, VILCEK ?: **Generation of Nitric Oxide and Induction of Major Histocompatibility Complex Class II Antigen in Macrophages From Mice Lacking the Interferon γ Receptor.** *Proc Natl Acad Sci U S A* 1993, **90**:6626–6630.

30. RAHEMTULLA A, FUNG-LEUNG WP, SCHILHAM MW, KUNDIG TM, SAMBHARA SR, NARENDRAN A, ARABIAN A, WAKEHAM A, PAIGE CJ, ZINKERNAGEL RM, MILLER RG, MAK TW: **Normal Development and Function of CD8+ Cells but Markedly Decreased Helper Cell Activity in Mice Lacking CD4.** *Nature* 1991, **353**:180–184.

31. FUNG-LEUNG WP, SCHILAM MW, RAHEMTULLA A, KUNDIG TM, VOLLENWEIDER M, POTTER J, VAN EWIJK W, MAK TW: **CD8 Is Needed for Development of Cytotoxic T Cells but Not Helper T Cells.** *Cell* 1991, **65**:443–449.

32. SCHILHAM MW, FUNG-LEUNG WP, RAHEMTULLA LA, KUENDIG T, ZHANG L,
• POTTER J, MILLER RG, HENGARTNER H, MAK TW: **Alloreactive Cytotoxic T Cells Can Develop and Function in Mice Lacking Both CD4 and CD8.** *Eur J Immunol* 1993, **23**:1299–1304.

Somewhat surprisingly, animals lacking the molecules CD4 and CD8 have sufficient numbers of α/β T cells, which are capable of generating alloreactive cytotoxic T cells, unlike the CD4+, CD8 – mice; mice lacking CD4 and CD8 were able to reject a skin graft expressing major histocompatibility molecules but not minor antigens only.

33. MOLINA TJ, KISHARA K, SIDEROVSKI P, VAN EWIJK W, NARENDRAN A, TIMMS E, WAKEHAM A, PAIGE CJ, HARTMANN KU, VELLETTE A, DAVIDSON

D, MAK TW: **Profound Block in Thymocyte Development in Mice Lacking p53 lck.** *Nature* 1992, **357**:161–164.

34. KILLEEN N, LITTMANN DR: **Helper T-cell Development in the Absence of CD4-p56lck Association.** *Nature* 1993, **364**:729–732.

35. LOVE PE, SHORES EW, JOHNSON MD, TREMBLAY ML, LEE EJ, GRINBERG A, HUANG SP, SINGER A, WESTPHAL H: **T Cell Development in Mice that Lack the Zeta Chain of the T Cell Antigen Receptor Complex.** *Science* 1993, **261**:918.

36. KOMORI T, OKADA A, STEWART V, FREDERICK W: **Lack of N Regions in**
• **Antigen Receptor Variable Region Genes of TdT-Deficient Lymphocytes.** *Science* 1993, **261**:1171–1178.

Terminal deoxynucleotidal transferase is required for addition of deoxynucleotides to available 3′ ends of encoded germline sequences for the T-cell receptor. Some of the diversity that characterizes the T-cell receptor is provided by so called *N regions*, which are lost in these animals.

37. ZIJLSTRA M, BIX M, SIMISTER NE, LORING JM, RAULET D, JAENISCH R: **β2-Microbglobulin Deficient Mice Lack CD4-8+ Cytotoxic T Cells.** *Nature* 1990, **344**:742–746.

38. KOLLER BH, MARRACK P, KAPPLER JW, SMITHIES O: **Normal Development of Mice Deficient in β2M, MHC Class I Proteins, and CD8+ T Cells.** *Science* 1990, **248**:1227–1230.

39. COSGROVE D, GRAY D, DIERICH A, KAUFMAN J, LEMEUR M, BENOIST C, MATHIS C: **Mice Lacking MHC Class II Molecules.** *Cell* 1991, **66**:1051–1066.

40. GRUSBY MK, JOHNSON RS, PAPAIOANNOU VE, GLIMCHER LH: **Depletion of CD4+ T Cells in Major Histocompatibility Complex Class II-Deficient Mice.** *Science* 1991, **253**:1417–1419.

41. MOMBAERTS P, IACOMINI J, JOHNSON RS, HERRUP K, TONEGAWA S, PAPAIOANNOU VE: **Rag-1-Deficient Mice Have No Mature B and T Lymphocytes Owing to Inability to Initiate V(D) Rearrangement.** *Cell* 1992, **68**:869–877.

42. SHINKAI Y, RATHBUN G, LAM KP, OLTZ EM, STEWART V, MENDELSOHN M, CHARRON J, DATTA M, YOUNG F, STALL AM, ALT FW: **RAG-2-Deficient Mice Lack Mature Lymphocytes Owing to Inability to Initiate V(D) Rearrangement.** *Cell* 1992, **68**:855–867.

43. TYBULEWICZ VLJ, CRAWFORD CE, JACKSON PK, BRONSON RT, MULLIGAN RC: **Neonatal Lethality and Lymphopenia in Mice With a Homozygous Disruption of the c-abl Proto-oncogene.** *Cell* 1993, **65**:693–702.

44. SCHWARTZBERG PL, STALL AM, HARDIN JD, BOWDISH KS, HUMARAN T, BOAST S, HARRISON ML, ROBERTSON EJ, GOGG SP: **Mice Homozygous for the abl-m1 Mutation Show Poor Viability and Depletion of Selected B and T Cell Populations.** *Cell* 1991, **65**:1165–1175.

45. KITAMURA D, ROES J, KUHN R, RAJEWSKY K: **A B Cell-Deficient Mouse by Targeted Disruption of the Membrane Exon of the Immunoglobulin μ Chain Gene.** *Nature* 1991, **350**:423–426.

46. ROES J, RAJEWSKY K: **Autonomous Expression of IgD Is Not Essential for the Maturation of Conventional B Cells.** *Int Immunol* 1991, **3**:1367–1371.

47. MUCENSKI ML, MCLAIN K, KIER AB, SWERDLOW SH, SCHREINER CM, MILLER TA, PIETRYGA DW, SCOTT WJ, POTTER SS: **Functional c-myb Gene Is Required for Normal Murine Fetal Hepatic Hematopoiesis.** *Cell* 1991, **65**:677–689.

48. PEVNY L, SIMON MC, ROBERTSON E, KLEIN WH, TSAI SF, D'AGATI V, ORKIN SH, COSTATINI F: **Erythroid Differentiation in Chimaeric Mice Blocked by a Targeted Mutation in the Gene for Transcription Factor GATA-1.** *Nature* 1991, **349**:257–260.

49. MOMBAERTS P, CLARKE AR, RUDNICKI MA, IACOMINI J, ITOHARA S, LAFAILLE JJ, WANG L, ICHIKAWA Y, JAENISCH R, HOOPER ML, TONEGAWA S: **Mutations in T-Cell Antigen Receptor Genes α and β Block Thymocyte Development at Different Stages.** *Nature* 1992, **360**:225–239.

50. ITOHARA S, MOMBAERTS P, LAFAILLE J, IACOMINI J, NELSON A, CLARKE AR, HOOPOER ML, FARR A, TONEGAWA S: **T Cell Receptor δ Gene Mutant Mice: Independent Generation of αβ T Cells and Programmed Rearrangements of γδ TCR Genes.** *Cell* 1993, **72**:337–348.

51. MAYADAS TN, JOHNSON RC, RAYBURN H, HYNES RO, WAGNER DD:
•• **Leukocyte Rolling and Extravasation Are Severely Compromised in P Selectin-Deficient Mice.** *Cell* 1993, **74**:541–554.

An increase in the number of circulating neutrophils presumably occurs because of this defect in the ability to roll along the endothelium, presumably decreasing the specific adherence at sites of inflammation and egress from the circulation.

52. ZHOU J, MOCHIZUKI T, SMEETS H, ANTIGNANC C, LAURILA P, DE PAEPE A, THYGGVASON K, REEDERS ST: **Deletion of the Paired α5 (IV) and α6 (IV) Collagen Genes in Inherited Smooth Muscle Tumors.** *Science* 1993, **261**:1167–1170.

53. WANG AM, DOYLE MV, MARK DF: **Quantitation of mRNA by the Polymerase Chain Reaction.** *Proc Natl Acad Sci U S A* 1989, **86**:9717–9721.

54. GILLILAND G, PERRIN S, BLANCHARD K, BUNN HF: **Analysis of Cytokine mRNA and DNA: Detection and Quantitation by Competitive Polymerase Chain Reaction.** *Proc Natl Acad Sci U S A* 1990, **87**:2725–2729.

55. PLATZER C, RICHTER G, UBERLA K, MULLER W, BLOCKER H, DIAMANTSTEIN
•• T, BLANKENSTEIN T: **Analysis of Cytokine mRNA Levels in Interleukin-4-Transgenic Mice By Quantitative Polymerase Chain Reaction.** *Eur J Immunol* 1992, **22**:1179–1184.

The ability to measure specific cytokine message concentrations within cells was very limited until techniques were developed to measure them with an internal competitor allowing precise quantitation of mRNA in tissues or cultured cells. In this application, increased expression of interleukin-5, interleukin-6, gamma interferon, and interleukin-4R was found in interleukin-4–transgenic mice.

56. LEGOUX P, MINTY C, DELPECH B, MINTY AJ, SHIRE D: **Simultane-**
•• **ous Quantitation of Cytokine mRNAs in Interleukin-1β Stimulated U373 Human Astrocytoma Cells by a Polymerization Chain Reaction Method Involving Co-Amplification With an Internal Multi-Specific Control.** *Eur Cytokine Netw* 1992, **3**:553–563.

This paper provides details of two separate plasmids encoding primer sequences from multiple cytokines and receptors and should be generally usable for investigators in the field.

57. MILLER AD: **Human Gene Therapy Comes of Age.** *Nature* 1992,
•• **357**:455–460.

A timely review of the gene therapy efforts now in progress at various institutions.

58. ROSENBERG SA, AEBERSOLD P, CORNETTA K, KASID A, MORGAN RA, MOEN R, KARSON EM, LOTZE MT, YANG JC, TOPALIAN SL, MERINO MJ, CULVER K, MILLER AD, BLAESE M, ANDERSON WF: **Gene Transfer Into Human Immunotherapy of Patients With Advanced Melanoma, Using Tumor-Infiltrating Lymphocytes Modified by Retroviral Gene transduction.** *N Engl J Med* 1990, **323**:570–578.

59. BRENNER MK, RILLER DR, MOEN RC, KRANCE RA, MIRRO J, ANDERSON
• WF, IHLE JN: **Gene-Marking to Trace Origin of Relapse After Autologous Bone-Marrow Transplantation.** *Lancet* 1993, **341**:85–86.

Study of two patients whose neuroblastoma recurred after they had received gene-marked bone marrow cells that had been "purged" prior to reinfusion. Evidence for relapse from the infused marrow was observed in both individuals. These techniques may be useful for identifying the adequacy of current tumor-purging strategies.

60. ROSENBERG S: **Gene Therapy for Cancer.** *JAMA* 1992, **268**:2416–2419.

61. HOCK H, DORSCH M, KUNZENDORF U, UBERLA, QIN Z, DIAMANSTEIN
•• T, BLANKENSTEIN T: **Vaccinations With Tumor Cells Genetically Engineered to Produce Different Cytokines. Effectivity Not Superior to Classical Adjuvant.** *Cancer Res* 1991, **53**:714–716.

Much effort has gone into creating vectors to target tumor cells and allow them to start producing a proinflammatory cytokine of choice. Although clinical protocols with interleukin-2, interleukin-4, gamma interferon, and tumor necrosis factor are currently going on. The experimental model presented suggests that none of them is better than conventional bacterial adjuvants.

62. CULVER KW, RAM Z, WALLBRIDGE S, ISHII H, OLDFIELD ED, BLAESE
•• RM: ***In Vivo* Gene Transfer With Retroviral Vector-Producer Cells for Treatment of Experimental Brain Tumors.** *Science* 1992, **256**:1550–1553.

This novel approach to gene therapy—direct injection of a cell line making retroviruses—has already gone into clinical trials. Promising initial results were presented at a Scandinavian Neurosurgery meeting although they have not yet been published. Targeting cells that are dividing is emphasized in this protocol, in which presumably only the dividing tumor cells are eliminated after treatment with the drug ganciclovir.

63. CHENG L, ZIEGELHOFFER PR, YANG NS: ***In Vivo* Promoter Activity**
•• **and Transgene Expression in Mammalian Somatic Tissues Evaluated by Using Particle Bombardment.** *Proc Natl Acad U S A* 1993, **90**:4455–4459.

Getting genes into cells is sometimes not an easy matter. The same general approach that was used to get genes across the hard outer cell wall of plants has now been shown to be useful in "bioballistically" introducing genes into a number of mammalian cell lines. This method represents an interesting opportunity for direct gene transfer for immunization approaches.

64. BURKHOLDER JK, DECKER J, YANG NS: **Rapid Transgene Expression in Lymphocyte and Macrophage Primary Cultures After Particle Bombardment-Mediated Gene Transfer.** *J Immunol Methods* 1993, in press.

65. ULMER JB, DONNELLY JJ, PARKER SE, RHODES GH, FEIGNER PL, DWARKI
•• VJ, GROMKOWSKI SH, DECK RR, DEWITT CM, FRIEDMAN A, HAWE LA, LEANDER KR, MARTINEZ D, PERRY HC, SHIVER JW, MONTGOMERY DL, LIU MA: **Heterologous Protection Against Influenzae by Injection of DNA Encoding a Viral Protein.** *Science* 1993, **249**:1745–1749.

Gene delivery, which has been a major goal of every gene therapist, was shown to be easy with direct transfer of DNA into muscle. The major problem with this approach is the large amount of genetic material required to get low levels of expression. Still, in this model it was possible to get an immune response to a viral protein using such techniques.

66. SAMULSKI RJ: **Adeno-Associated Virus: Integration At a Specific Chromosomal Locus.** *Curr Opin Genet Devel* 1993, 3:74–80.

67. LOTZE MT: **Trials and Tribulations: The Cost of Developing Gene Therapies.** *FASEB J* 1991, 5:3013–3014.

68. • TAHARA H, ZEH H, STORKUS WJ, PAPPO I, WATKINS S, GATELY MK, GUBLER U, WOLF SF, ROBBINS PD, LOTZE MT: **Fibroblasts Genetically Engineered to Secrete Interleukin-12 Can Suppress Tumor Growth In Vivo and Induce Antitumor Immunity To A Murine Melanoma.** *Cancer Res* 1994, in press.

The use of one of the most recently defined T-cell growth factors to obtain tumor rejection is described here. Interleukin-12 has the additional potential advantage that it appears to direct the development of primarily a T_{H1} type response, thought to be critical in antitumor immune responses.

69. LOTZE MT: **Clinical Protocol: The Treatment of Patients With Melanoma Using Interleukin-2, Interleukin-4, and Tumor Infiltrating Lymphocytes.** *Hum Gene Ther* 1992, 3:167–177.

70. HWU P, YANNELLI J, KRIEGLER M, ANDERSON WF, PEREZ C, CHIANG Y, SCHWARZ S, COWHERD R, DELGADO C, MULE J, ROSENBERG ?: **Functional and Molecular Characterization of Tumor-Infiltrating Lymphocytes Transduced With Tumor Necrosis Factor-α cDNA for the Gene Therapy of Cancer in Humans.** *J Immunol* 1993, 150:4104–4115.

Michael T. Lotze, MD, Section of Surgical Oncology, W1450 Biomedical Science Tower, University of Pittsburgh Medical Center, Pittsburgh, PA 15261, USA.

Vascular surgery

Editorial overview

Robert W. Hobson II, MD

University of Medicine and Dentistry of New Jersey,
New Jersey Medical School, Newark, New Jersey, USA

Current Opinion in General Surgery 1994:255–256

Vascular surgery continues to be a dynamic and challenging field. Consistent with the goals of this publication, three topics of current interest and evolving application have been selected for review. The authors of each section possess interest in and specialized knowledge of their topics, which should be of interest to all general and vascular surgeons.

In the first section, Kenneth Ouriel (pp 257–264) presents a concise and authoritative review on the use of thrombolytic therapy for acute arterial occlusion. Although lytic agents were introduced in the 1950s, their general use and clinical application became more widespread during the 1980s with the publication of retrospective as well as prospective clinical experiences. Although urokinase has emerged as the most commonly used member of the family of "plasminogen activators," advantages and disadvantages of streptokinase, recombinant tissue plasminogen activator, and acylated plasminogen streptokinase activator complex are discussed here. Ouriel reviews the classification of acute limb ischemia and presents cogent arguments in favor of lytic therapy, particularly in patients with class II disease who demonstrate elements of reversibility. He emphasizes that the goal of lytic therapy is not to replace operative intervention, but rather to diminish the operative requirement and thereby decrease the frequency of limb loss and mortality in a subset of patients with acknowledged high incidence of cardiovascular factors. The importance of delivering the lytic agent via direct catheter placement into the area of thrombosis within a native artery, autologous graft, or synthetic bypass is emphasized. Thrombosed vein grafts were less likely to undergo successful lysis as compared with prosthetic bypasses and native arteries. Furthermore, better results were observed in nondiabetic as compared with diabetic subjects. When the controversial issue of operative intervention versus thrombolytic therapy is discussed, the two should be considered complementary. However, a rationale for the use of lytic therapy in all patients with acute limb ischemia, as well as additional comparisons and contrasts between operative intervention and pharmacologic management, await larger prospective analyses. It is possible that subsets of patients will be identified who may receive greater benefit from this important adjunct to conventional surgical revascularization.

The next contribution (pp 265–271) reviews data on the efficacy of carotid endarterectomy in clinical practices. During the early 1980s, concern for the performance of carotid endarterectomy became heightened for several reasons. First, a perception existed that morbidity and mortality was unacceptably high; second, a lack of prospective randomized clinical trial data undermined confidence among our medical colleagues that the incidence of neurologic events was reduced significantly when compared with optimal medical management; and third, prospective analysis of the extracranial-intracranial bypass procedure demonstrated a lack of clinical efficacy, which was generalized by some clinicians to include the use of carotid endarterectomy in patients with extracranial carotid occlusive disease. The planning and execution of randomized clinical trials constituted the most responsible response to these growing concerns. Publication during 1991 of the results of three such trials concerning the management of patients with recent transient ischemic attack or nondisabling stroke in the presence of high-grade (≥70%) carotid stenosis has unequivocally defined the importance of carotid endarterectomy in symptomatic patients. The North American Carotid Endarterectomy Trial (NASCET), the European Carotid Surgery Trial (ECST), and the Veterans Administration symptomatic trial have confirmed clinical recommendations favoring operative intervention in symptomatic patients. It is no longer acceptable for clinicians to await symptomatic breakthrough on antiplatelet therapy and then warfarin sodium therapy before referring patients with high-grade stenosis for endarterectomy. The NASCET and ECST trialists continue to randomize patients with intermediate degrees of stenosis (30% to 69%). Surgical opinion suggests that these evaluations will confirm the 50% diameter-reducing stenosis as the minimally significant lesion for selecting operative management in these symptomatic patients.

Care of patients with asymptomatic carotid stenosis has been more controversial. The results of one

Abbreviations

ECST—European Carotid Surgery Trial; **NASCET**—North American Carotid Endarterectomy Trial.

 ISBN 1-85922-671-X ISSN 1065–6243

trial conducted in the Federal Republic of Germany (CASANOVA) were unable to demonstrate any differences between medical and surgical management; however, these trialists excluded patients with high-grade stenoses and lesions rapidly progressing to high-grade stenosis, thereby rendering the trial's results inconclusive. Clearly, the subset of patients who appear to benefit from operation in the Veterans Administration asymptomatic stenosis trial are patients with high-grade stenoses (area reducing stenosis ≥ 75%). In this group of patients, neurologic events (transient ischemic attack plus stroke) were reduced significantly when optimal medical management including antiplatelet therapy and carotid endarterectomy was compared with optimal medical management alone. Although the trial and its sample size were designed to address the influence of carotid endarterectomy on combined neurologic outcome, clinicians have emphasized the importance of analyzing data on stroke alone and stroke plus death. These topics will require analysis of a prospective randomized trial with a larger sample size, the results of which should be published within the next year or two. Consequently, the recently published results from the Veterans Administration asymptomatic trial have not entirely answered the question, and the topic remains controversial.

Patients are being managed operatively on an individual basis in centers after an audit-confirmed low incidence of operative complications among patients who have been cleared of increased risk factors for coronary artery disease. Nevertheless, the results of these randomized clinical trials have influenced indications for carotid endarterectomy in symptomatic and asymptomatic patients. Clearly, these trials have not defined all subsets of patients who might benefit from operation. The challenge of this decade is to define the importance of carotid plaque morphology, the incidence of silent computed tomography–confirmed cerebral infarction, the role and adequacy of collateral cerebral circulation, particularly in patients with asymptomatic carotid disease, and an analysis of combined risk factors that influence patient longevity, such as diabetes, coronary artery disease, and symptomatic peripheral vascular disease.

Finally, Virginia Newman and Richard Dean (pp 272–276) present a valuable discussion on the role of renal revascularization in patients with ischemic nephropathy. Traditionally, the importance of renovascular occlusive disease has centered around the management of potentially correctable hypertension. Clearly, renal revascularization under selected circumstances constitutes a major contribution to a group of patients with surgically remediable and usually severe hypertension. However, during recent years, the recognition that retrieval of excretory renal function could be accomplished has received additional emphasis under the heading of *ischemic nephropathy*. This term denotes the presence of anatomically severe occlusive disease of the extraparenchymal renal artery in patients with compromised excretory renal function. The authors have defined three patient groups for whom a rationale exists for renal revascularization. In the nonazotemic patient, the more traditional indications for revascularization continue; however, the authors report predictors of success in this population that include presence of collateral circulation to the chronically occluded kidney, at least 10% of total renal function coming from the functioning kidney on isotope renography, and the presence of a normal vascular bed distal to the stenotic lesion.

The use of renal vein renins, split renal function studies, and analysis of renal excretion have assumed lesser importance because of the difficulties involved with interpreting these physiological studies. In the azotemic patients with nearly end-stage renal disease and dialysis dependency, the risks of operation increase, and the goal of retrieving renal excretory function is considered. Based on the improvement in function in many patients, particularly the group with recent dialysis dependency, the authors recommend screening of adult patients over 50 years of age who have newly recognized renal insufficiency. Duplex ultrasonography has become the primary screening tool because of its reported accuracy of 96% in these patients.

The third group includes patients with acute vascular occlusion in the presence of chronic occlusive disease whose onset of renal failure is usually a consequence of thrombosis of a stenotic artery to a solitary kidney or to the only kidney with residual function. Performance of a single "one-shot" arteriogram has not aggravated renal failure in this population, and the presence or absence of a nephrogram does not necessarily imply success or failure with revascularization. Rather than immediate operation and attempted revascularization, a more carefully planned approach is recommended. Patients may require several days of dialysis, and successful revascularization has been reported after as long as 30 to 45 days in patients experiencing acute occlusion and oliguric renal failure. Prospective randomized assessment of operative intervention, including cost analyses on the efficacy of renal revascularization, will be required. In light of the costs of dialysis, however, identifying the subset of patients who will benefit from operation becomes increasingly important in our management of renovascular occlusive disease.

These topics represent three among many in which the practicing general and vascular surgeon must maintain knowledge of evolving recommendations for pharmacologic control as well as operative management of vascular disease. Incorporating these new concepts into one's practice becomes an essential focus of ongoing surgical education.

Robert W. Hobson II, MD, Section of Vascular Surgery, Medical Science Building G-532, UMDNJ-New Jersey Medical School, 185 South Orange Avenue, Newark, NJ 07103-2714, USA.

Thrombolytic therapy for acute arterial occlusion

Kenneth Ouriel, MD

University of Rochester Medical Center, Rochester, New York, USA

The standard treatment of peripheral arterial occlusion has been operative, employing embolectomy, thrombectomy, or bypass grafting to restore blood flow to the compromised extremity. Intra-arterial thrombolysis has been advocated as an initial intervention designed to unmask the anatomic lesion responsible for the occlusive event, with a directed or endovascular modality thereafter. Four thrombolytic agents are in clinical use: streptokinase, urokinase, recombinant tissue plasminogen activator, and acylated plasminogen streptokinase activator complex. The agents differ with respect to efficacy of thrombolysis, fibrin specificity, and cost. At present, urokinase is the most widely used. Recent randomized clinical trials suggest a benefit of thrombolytic therapy in the initial management of acute peripheral arterial occlusion, with improved patient survival and similar amputation rates compared with immediate open intervention. Each modality has its place in specific patient subcategories; the determination of which patients are best served by a specific modality awaits the results of large clinical trials.

Current Opinion in General Surgery 1994:257–264

Thrombolytic agents have been utilized clinically since the late 1940s [1]. The early pharmacologic preparations were obtained from the *Streptococcus* bacterium and were impure, containing streptodornase and other foreign proteins in addition to the active agent streptokinase [2]. These contaminants were responsible for a variety of untoward systemic effects and forced Tillett and Sherry [1] to limit the use of thrombolytic agents to extravascular disease processes, specially loculated hemothorax. In 1955 Tillett *et al.* [3] at New York University reported the results of a clinical trial of intravenous streptokinase in 11 patients, designed to define the safety of the intravascular administration of the agent. Unfortunately, pyogenic reactions were common, with low-grade fever developing in all of the patients and profound hypotension in four.

In 1956, Cliffton and Grossi [4] reported successful preliminary results with what was assumed to be the direct thrombolytic agent plasmin. In truth, Cliffton's agent comprised a mixture of plasminogen and streptokinase, designed to generate free plasmin. However, it is likely that the observed lytic effects occurred as a result of the streptokinase rather than the free plasmin [5]. Nevertheless, 1 year later Cliffton [6] reported an experience with 40 patients and documented the beneficial effects of direct intra-arterial streptokinase-plasmin infusions in two patients with peripheral arterial occlusions. Whereas Dotter and Rosch [7] are generally credited with pioneering catheter-directed peripheral arterial thrombolysis in 1974, Cliffton [6] actually documented the use of this technique 17 years earlier.

Pharmacology of thrombolytic agents

All thrombolytic agents represent "plasminogen activators," converting fibrin-bound plasminogen to fibrin-bound plasmin, which subsequently degrades the fibrin thrombus [8]. The administration of exogenous plasmin has little if any thrombolytic activity [9]. *In vitro* studies confirmed that free plasmin was relatively ineffective in degrading fibrin, but did result in significant degradation of fibrinogen and factors V and VIII [10]. These studies led to the formulation of a scheme of thrombolysis wherein plasminogen exists in two phases: a gel (thrombus) phase, in which it is bound to fibrin, and a soluble (plasma) phase, in which it is free (Fig. 1) [11]. Activation of soluble-phase plasminogen to free plasmin leads to degradation of fibrinogen and other plasma proteins, but is ineffective in dissolving fibrin within a thrombus. Free plasmin is also rapidly inactivated by antiplasmins. Gel-phase plasminogen, however, when activated to fibrin-bound plasmin, results in selective fibrinolysis in an environment relatively protected from antiplasmins. This mechanism explains why the degradation of fibrin thrombus is dependent on the concentration of plasminogen activators, but not dependent on the concentration of exogenously administered plasmin [12].

There are four thrombolytic agents currently approved by the US Food and Drug Administration: streptokinase, urokinase, recombinant tissue plasminogen activator (rt-PA), and acylated plasminogen streptokinase activator complex (APSAC). Each agent produces fibrinolysis through an activation of fibrin-bound plasmino-

Abbreviations

APSAC—acylated plasminogen streptokinase activator complex; **rt-PA**—recombinant tissue plasminogen activator.

 ISBN 1-85922-671-X ISSN 1065–6243

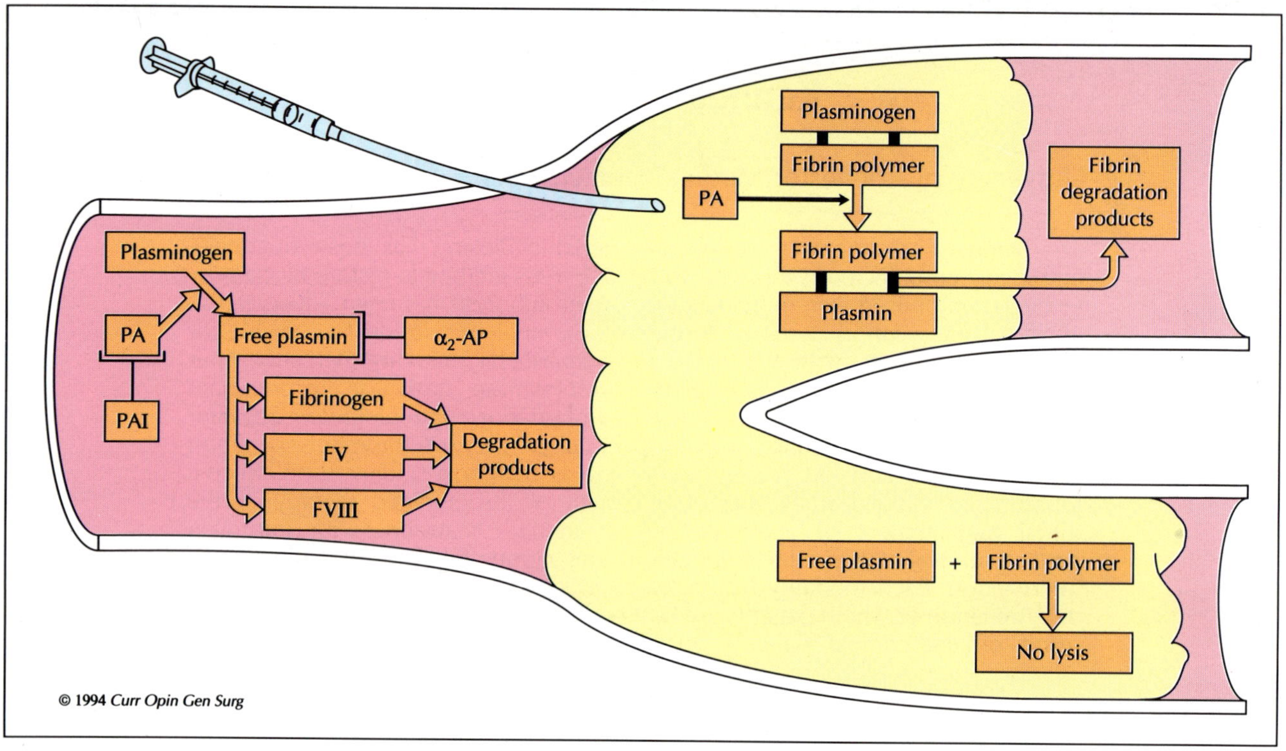

Fig. 1. Biomolecular interactions in the plasma and in the thrombus during pharmacologic thrombolysis. α_2-AP—α_2-antiplasmin; FV—factor V; FVIII—factor VIII; PA—plasminogen activator; PAI—plasminogen activator inhibitor.

Table 1. Properties of compenents of the thrombolytic system*

Component	Molecular weight, *kD*	Structure	Plasma half-life
Streptokinase	46	Single-chain	11 min
Urokinase	54	Two chains	10 min
rt-PA	70	One or two chains	5 min
APSAC	131	lys-plasminogen-streptokinase	70 min
Pro-urokinase	53	Single-chain	6 min
Plasminogen	88	Single-chain	2.2 d
Plasmin	88	Two chains	0.1 s
α_2-Antiplasmin	70	Single-chain	2.6 d
PAI	40	Single-chain	Unknown

**Data from* Marder [8].
APSAC—acylated plasminogen streptokinase activator complex; PAI—plasminogen activator inhibitor; rt-PA—recombinant tissue plasminogen activator.

gen to fibrin-bound plasmin (Table 1). The plasmin then hydrolyzes fibrin, leading to the dissolution of the thrombus and the restoration of blood flow. Streptokinase is a purified isolate from the *Streptococcus* bacterium and is an inactive single-chain 46,000 D protein. It forms a complex with plasminogen or plasmin, and this complex in turn activates additional plasminogen molecules. Urokinase, clinically employed in both high molecular weight (54,000 D) and low molecular weight (31,000 D) forms, is a two-chain compound present in urine. Unlike streptokinase, urokinase directly activates plasminogen without the need for initial binding to an additional plasminogen molecule. rt-PA is a single- or two-chain 70,000-D molecule and contains two kringle structures, one of which is important in the binding of rt-PA to fibrin [13]. Thus, rt-PA has been promoted as an agent with "fibrin specificity" and a low potential for systemic degradation. This contention has not been substantiated in the clinical setting, with similar decreases in plasma fibrinogen concentration following systemic administration of urokinase or rt-PA [14]. APSAC consists of an equimolar complex of streptokinase and plasminogen, originally developed to hasten fibrinolysis by eliminating the initial step of plasminogen binding. In practice, the benefits of APSAC may be related to its increased half-life rather than plasminogen supplementation.

The plasminogen activators differ in their relative rate of fibrin dissolution and in their fibrin-specificity [15]. An ideal agent would manifest a high degree of fibrinolytic activity with a low potential for systemic fibrinogen degradation. Reputedly streptokinase has the lowest activity and is not fibrin specific. Urokinase is intermediate, but rt-PA has been reported to be associated with the highest rate of fibrinolysis and the greatest degree of fibrin specificity. To date, however, few studies have actually documented clinical benefits of any one agent over another [8].

Pathophysiology

An arterial occlusive event occurs suddenly and without warning. A complex of six signs and symptoms are characteristically observed: pain, pallor, poikilothermia, pulselessness, paresthesia, and paralysis. Symptoms are usually of sufficient magnitude that the patient presents early, at a time when the thrombus is relatively susceptible to lytic dissolution. A useful classification of the severity of lower extremity ischemia is provided in a Society for Vascular Surgery/International Society for Cardiovascular Surgery report that places patients into one of three classes: viable and nonthreatened, viable but threatened, and nonviable [16]. In this schema, class II patients are generally the most appropriate candidates for thrombolysis; class I do not usually manifest sufficient symptoms to warrant the risks attendant thrombolytic therapy, and class III are, by definition, irretrievable with any treatment modality.

The cause of acute arterial occlusion can be divided into two categories: thrombosis and embolism. A thrombotic cause is observed more frequently than an embolic cause by a four-to-one ratio in most series of acutely compromised lower extremities [17]. Irrespective of cause, the original occlusive process is rapidly followed by prograde and retrograde propagation of thrombus to the next large collateral channel. The development of propagated thrombus attains significance in the setting of pharmacologic thrombolysis; the erythrocyte-rich, platelet-poor secondary thrombus is easy to lyse but the occluding head of platelet-rich thrombus or older embolus is relatively resistant [18].

Thrombotic arterial occlusion may be observed in native arteries or bypass conduits[19•,20••]. Thrombosis of native arteries usually develops in the setting of a preexisting stenosis, although acute thrombotic occlusion of near-normal arterial segments may develop with such entities as the antiphospholipid syndrome or the hypercoagulable state associated with malignancy. Thrombosis of a bypass conduit may occur with or without an anatomic lesion; failure of autogenous conduits is unlikely without a stenotic process but prosthetic conduits frequently fail in the absence of an identifiable lesion [21].

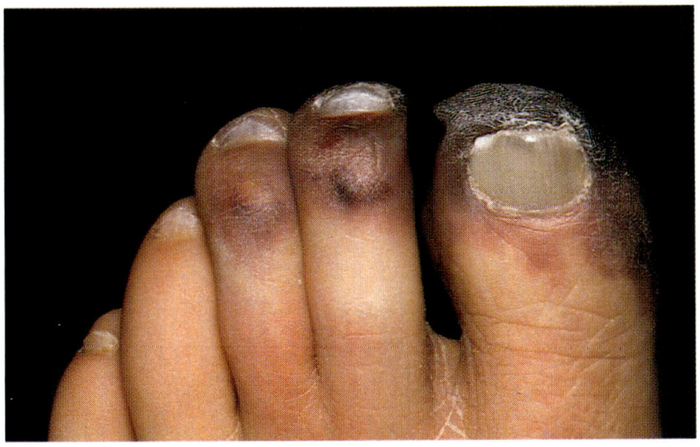

Fig. 2. The forefoot of a patient with atheroembolization from an aortic aneurysm shows ischemic changes in the first three digits.

Emboli characteristically originate in the heart, generally after an acute myocardial infarction or in the setting of atrial fibrillation. Arterioarterial emboli are also encountered, representing cholesterol or fibrin-platelet debris originating in a proximal aneurysm or ulcerated atherosclerotic plaque (Fig. 2). Cardiac emboli are typically large and associated with obstruction of the femoral or popliteal vessels, whereas arterioarterial emboli are smaller and usually associated with tibial or digital artery obstruction and such clinical entities as the "blue-toe syndrome."

Operation as the standard therapy

Operative therapy became the standard mode of intervention in acute arterial occlusion with the advent of surgical revascularization in the late 1940s [22,23]. The subsequent four decades witnessed an impressive improvement in technical advances, with the ability to operatively salvage the vast majority of acutely threatened limbs. The introduction of the balloon embolectomy catheter by Fogarty *et al.* [24] in 1963 offered an effective means of removing emboli and propagated thrombus through a single arteriotomy.

Operative interventions fall into two categories in acute limb ischemia: thromboembolectomy and bypass. Thrombectomy and thromboembolectomy are reserved for processes unassociated with preexisting anatomic defects, *eg*, in emboli to the common femoral artery or thrombosis of a prosthetic graft free of fixed narrowing. Alternatively, graft thrombectomy may be performed in conjunction with a patch angioplasty of an occluded native artery or bypass graft. Bypass is appropriate in all other circumstances, and it has been argued that all graft occlusions should be treated with the insertion of a new conduit.

Despite technical advances and decreases in the rate of amputation, limb salvage was achieved at the cost of an alarmingly high perioperative mortality rate, approaching 25% in the review of Blaisdell *et al.* [25] and approximately 20% in a later series by Jivegaard *et al.* [26]. More recently, Edwards *et al.* [27] replaced 111 occluded lower extremity bypass grafts with new autogenous vein conduits and documented a limb salvage rate of 90% at 5 years. However, these results were associated with a mortality rate of 26% at 6 months and only 12% of patients were alive at 5 years. The observations of these studies suggest that acute limb ischemia develops in a medically compromised subpopulation, a group that may be further jeopardized by invasive reconstructive procedures.

Technique of arterial thrombolysis

At the outset, the most important caveat of arterial thrombolysis relates to the goal of therapy. The aim of thrombolytic therapy in acute arterial occlusion is not to replace operation. Rather, thrombolysis merely uncovers the anatomic lesion responsible for the occlusive event in the majority of cases and operation or endovascular interventions must be subsequently employed to correct the unmasked lesion [28•,29•]. Thus, studies designed to document the effectiveness of thrombolysis are flawed when the primary outcome measure is avoidance of operation: indeed, the goal of arterial thrombolysis is to uncover and clearly define the etiologic mechanism and lessen the magnitude of a subsequent remedial intervention (Fig. 3).

Irrespective of the agent employed, arterial thrombolysis is best accomplished via a catheter-directed approach, with the delivery of activator agent directly into the substance of the thrombus [30••]. In contrast to the setting of acute coronary artery occlusion, intravenous routes of administration have been entirely unsatisfactory in the periphery. This difference is presumably a result of the larger size of peripheral thrombi and the resultant inability of activator agent to diffuse into the thrombus. Both antegrade and contralateral catheter insertion techniques have been successfully employed. The ipsilateral femoral artery is the insertion site in the antegrade approach, angling the needle in a distal direction. It is frequently difficult to pass the guidewire into an occluded bypass graft using an antegrade approach; the wire preferentially enters the profunda femoris artery and the close proximity of the graft orifice to the needle insertion site renders catheter manipulation arduous. The contralateral route is safest, especially in inexperienced hands, because failure to accomplish antegrade access may leave the patient with multiple needle-stick holes in the common femoral artery that can bleed during subsequent thrombolytic infusion through a contralateral approach. There is a tendency for thrombus to form on the wall of the catheter during any protracted intra-arterial procedure, and embolization of this "pericatheter thrombus" may occur as the thrombus is sheared off the catheter at the time of removal. The frequency of complications can be minimized by using small-bore catheters and concurrent heparin or aspirin therapy.

Several methods of infusion of thrombolytic agents are in routine use. A maximum duration of administration of 48 hours is recommended, because a prime correlate of complications appears to be the duration of infusion. Moreover, if successful lysis has not been accomplished after 48 hours, success is unlikely to be achieved with continued therapy. Continuous infusions are commonly employed, usually beginning with a large dose and tapering thereafter (Table 2). A "pulse-spray" technique has been used, bolusing the thrombolytic agent through a multiholed catheter along the length of the occlusive thrombus, potentially increasing the rate of dissolution. "Lacing" refers to the infusion of large amounts of agent along the length of the thrombus as the catheter is withdrawn, in an effort to attain even and complete distribution throughout the thrombus. To date, no consistent benefits have been documented with the use of one technique over another [31•].

It is important to follow the progress of thrombolysis with serial arteriographic studies. Catheter manipulation is necessary in the majority of instances, with frequent repositioning of the infusion holes to keep them within the substance of the unlysed thrombus. Distal

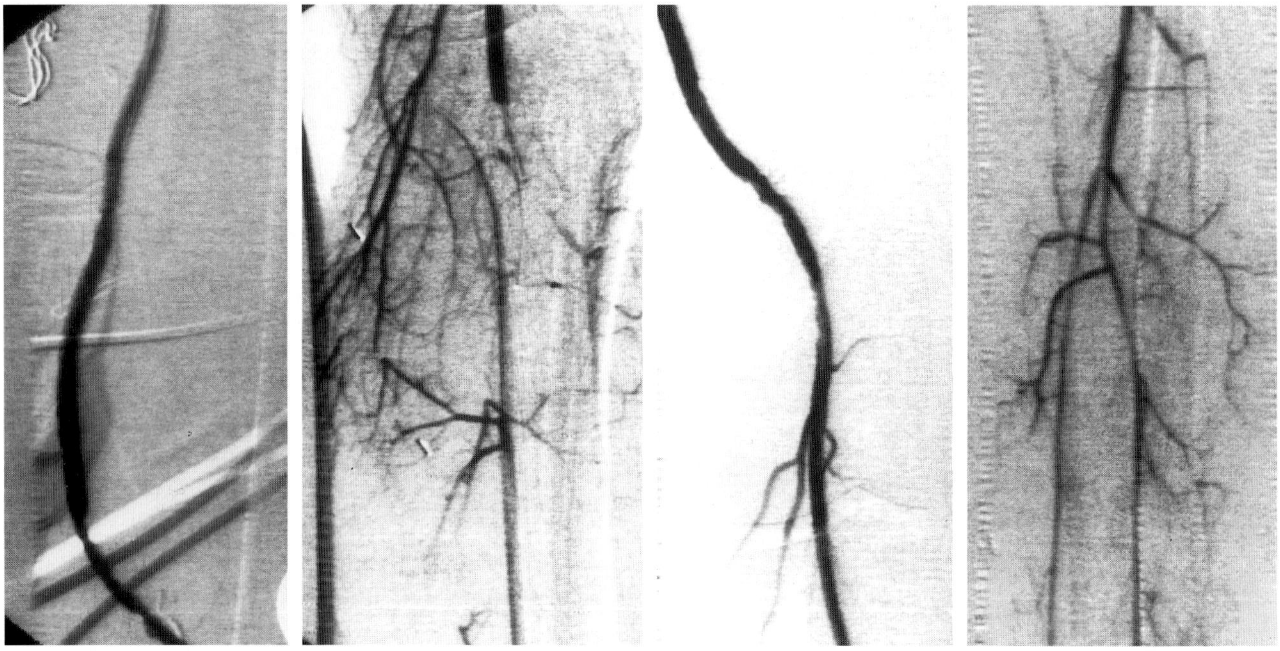

Fig. 3. Left, Arteriogram of a patient who presented with a severely ischemic foot and an occluded femoropopliteal vein graft. After 8 hours of urokinase infusion, the graft is open and stenotic lesions are unmasked in the distal graft. **Center left,** The popliteal artery abruptly occludes just below the level of the knee joint, with continuation of the thrombotic process into the crural arteries. **Center right,** The thrombus is completely lysed after positioning the catheter infusion holes into the distal popliteal thrombus and infusing urokinase for an additional 3 hours. **Right,** The popliteal trifurcation and posterior tibial and peroneal arteries are now patent.

Table 2. Urokinase treatment protocol for intra-arterial thrombolytic infusion

325 mg aspirin on presentation
Catheter positioned into substance of thrombus
Urokinase infusion, 4000 IU/min for 2 hours (concentration 5000 IU/mL, in normal saline)
Continue at 2000 IU/min for 2 hours
Decrease to 1000 IU/min, continue to a maximum of 48 hours of total therapy

embolization is a frequent complication of thrombolysis, but is fortunately treatable with an increase in the thrombolytic dose. Repositioning of the catheter into the distal emboli is not always necessary, as the material is usually sensitive to upstream administration of lytic agent.

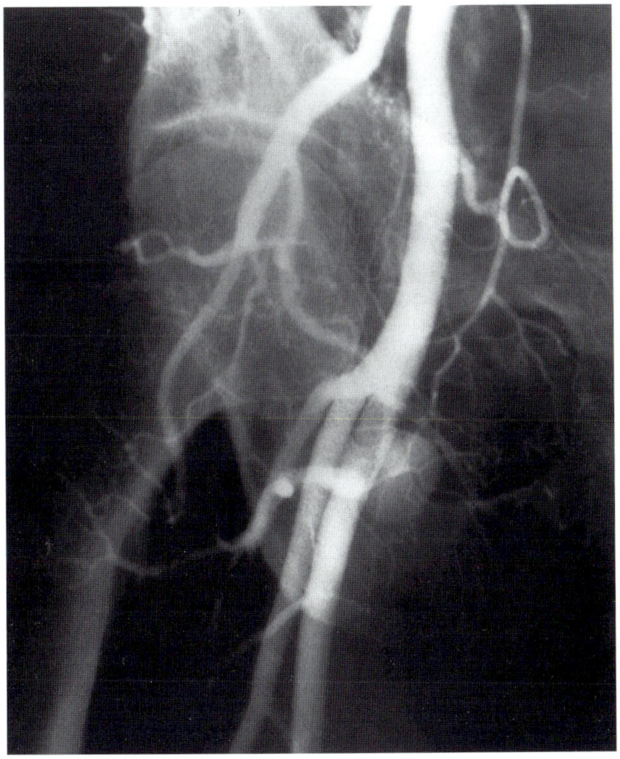

Fig. 4. An arteriogram of a false aneurysm at the site of a superficial femoral artery puncture for a thrombolytic infusion.

Monitoring of coagulation parameters during thrombolytic therapy remains controversial. Fibrinogen concentration, thrombin time, and other laboratory tests have been advocated as measures with which to gauge the risk of distant bleeding complications, but there do not exist conclusive evidence in this regard [8,32]. Bleeding complications almost always result from defects in vascular integrity, usually at the site of arterial cannulation (Fig. 4). These events bear little or no correlation with abnormalities in the coagulation tests, but accumulating evidence indicates that the duration of thrombolytic infusion may be an important predictor of hemorrhage.

Results of thrombolysis

Large, retrospective series of patients treated with intra-arterial thrombolytic therapy began to appear in the early 1980s [17,33–35]. Success was reported in over 90% of cases over a mean infusion duration of 6 to 12 hours. Amputation rates averaged less than 10%, with early mortality rates of less than 5% and bleeding complications in 5% to 10% of patients. Urokinase and rt-PA were argued to be safer and more efficacious than streptokinase. There were, however, severe limitations with these studies. Streptokinase was used early in the course of each series, usually at a time when the medical team had little experience in thrombolytic treatment. Patients with acute and chronic limb ischemia were included in many of the studies, precluding meaningful comparison with data on truly threatened extremities. Moreover, outcome measures were frequency subjective, bearing little clinical relevance to limb salvage or mortality.

These early series triggered several contradictory reports, all retrospective and somewhat anecdotal [36–38]. The data generated by these studies argued against the use of thrombolytic agents in acute arterial occlusion, principally on the basis of poor patency rates associated with sole therapy and the frequent need for concurrent operative intervention to achieve an acceptable result. The goal of thrombolysis, however, is not to replace or eliminate surgery. Rather ,thrombolytic therapy should be employed in an effort to diminish the magnitude of required interventions and thereby decrease the frequency of morbid and mortal events (Fig. 5). Studies that failed to tabulate long-term survival and limb salvage as primary endpoints predictably indicted thrombolysis as a useless therapeutic endeavor.

More recent trials have avoided these limitations by employing a randomized, prospective design and objective, clinically relevant endpoints [28]. In a randomized trial of intra-arterial urokinase compared with operative intervention in the initial treatment of acute limb ischemia, we documented a 62% reduction in 1-year mortality in the thrombolytic group [39]. This difference was attributed to a lower requirement for surgery concurrent with a decrease in the frequency of cardiopulmonary complications in the patients randomly assigned to thrombolysis. No increment in the requirement for amputation was observed, with 1-year limb salvage rates of approximately 20% in each treatment arm.

It is likely that different patient categories will benefit from one form of therapy over another (Fig. 6). In a multivariate analysis of patients treated with intra-arterial thrombolysis, five variables were found to be predictive of successful arteriographic dissolution (Table 3). Technical factors appeared most important. Successful lysis was seldom achieved if the infusion catheter could not be threaded into the thrombus or if a guidewire could not be passed through the occlu-

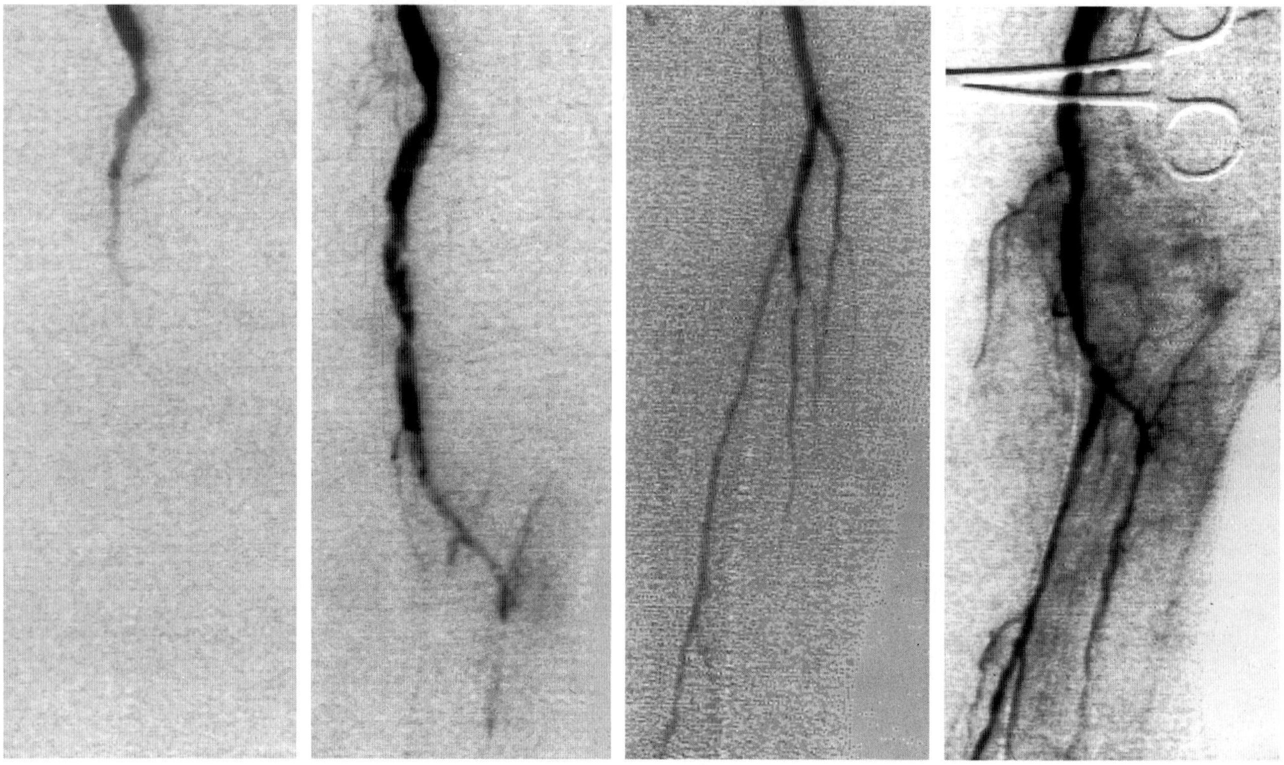

Fig. 5. The sequence of arteriograms obtained with urokinase infusion into a small, thrombosed popliteal aneurysm. **Left,** The initial film of the thrombosed aneurysm, without evidence of a tibial outflow vessel. **Center left,** Partial lysis of thrombus within the aneurysm and the proximal crural outflow tract after 6 hours of urokinase infusion. **Center right,** Complete lysis of the aneurysm thrombus and the posterior tibial and peroneal arteries after 11 hours of infusion. **Right,** Distal view at at 11 hours of patency of the posterior aneurysm with a bypass from the distal superficial femoral vein to the infragenicular popliteal saphenous vein, which ligated the superficial artery just beyond the proximal vein graft anastomosis.

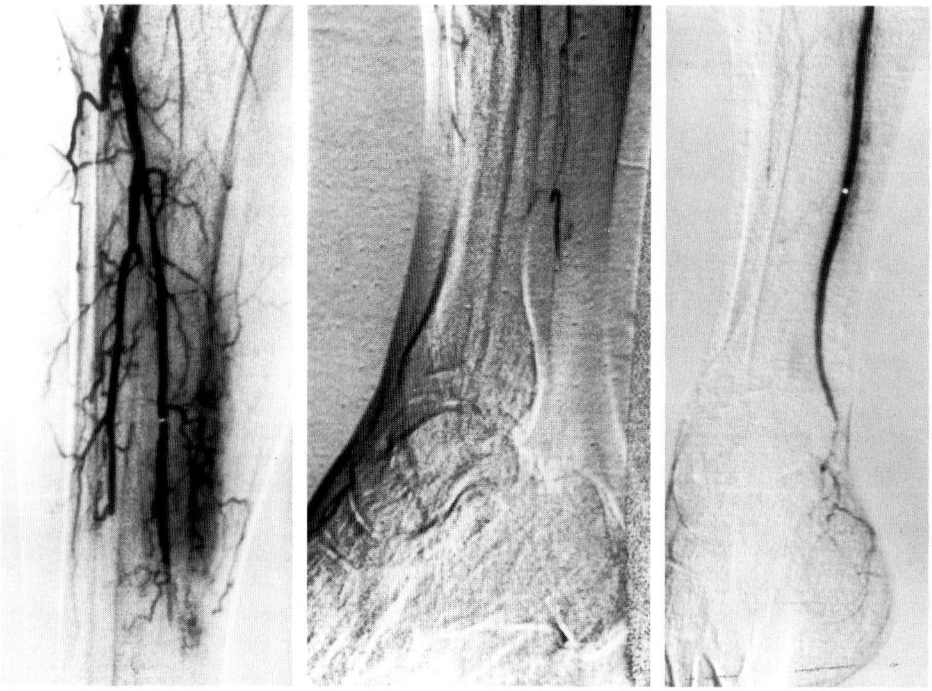

Fig. 6. Arteriograms of a patient with native arterial thrombosis on the basis of hypercoagulability (antiphospholipid syndrome). **Left,** Thrombolytic occlusion of all three crural vessels. **Center,** Absence of distal site appropriate for operative bypass. **Right,** Reconstruction of the posterior tibial artery after urokinase infusion directly into the artery for 6 hours. The patient was placed on chronic oral anticoagulation and maintained viability of the foot over 36 months of follow-up with a palpable posterior tibial pulse.

Table 3. Factors predictive of success in a multivariate analysis (stepwise linear regression) of 103 peripheral arterial and bypass graft occlusions treated with thrombolytic therapy*

Parameter	Patients, %	Success rate, %
Catheter into thrombus		
Yes	86	88
No	14	0
Guidewire traversed thrombus		
Possible	82	89
Impossible	18	16
Conduit involved		
Vein graft	18	55
Prosthetic graft	34	80
Native artery	48	78
Arterial segments involved		
One	51	88
Two	33	71
Three	16	40
Diabetes mellitus		
Present	29	49
Absent	71	80

*Data are univariate.

sive process. Several clinical factors also attained significance as independent predictors of arteriographic success. Vein grafts were less likely to undergo successful lysis than prosthetic grafts or native arteries. Lysis was more frequently achieved in nondiabetic patients than diabetic patients and in patients with fewer arterial segments involved.

The economics of thrombolysis have attained increased significance with the recent emphasis on the cost of health care. Thrombolysis appears to be associated with a similar length of hospital stay when compared with operative intervention [39]. The cost of hospitalization may be somewhat greater when thrombolytic therapy is employed, principally as a result of the cost of the lytic agent. When professional fees are considered, however, these differences vanish (Table 4). Clear advantages to the use of thrombolysis are realized when the cost data are expressed in relation to the dollars expended per life saved.

Table 4. Economic costs of thrombolytic versus operative intervention in the initial managment of acute peripheral arterial occlusion

	Thrombolysis (*n*=57)	Operation (*n*=57)
Hospital cost, $	22,171	19,775
Professional fees, $	2445	3517
Total costs, $	24,616	23,292
1-Year survival rate, %	58	84
Cost per life saved, $	29,305	40,158

It is likely that some patient subgroups will be most appropriately treated with thrombolytic interventions and other subgroups will be best treated with immediate operation. The definition of these distinct categories awaits the findings of large randomized studies. Presently, patients are best treated individually. Pending the availability of data on the results of thrombolysis in distinct subcategories of clinical presentation, appropriate therapy must be planned on the basis of reasonable clinical judgment and the experience of the angiographic and surgical teams.

References and recommended reading

Papers of particular interest, published within the annual period of review, have been highlighted as:
- • Of special interest
- •• Of outstanding interest

1. TILLETT WS, SHERRY S: **The Effect in Patients of Streptococcal Fibrinolysin (Streptokinase) and Streptococcal Deoxyribonuclease on Fibrinous, Purulent, and Sanguinous Pleural Exudations.** *J Clin Invest* 1949, **28**:173–190.
2. TILLETT WS, SHERRY S, CHRISTENSEN LR: **Streptococcal Deoxyribonuclease: Significance in Lysis of Purulent Exudates and Production by Strains of Hemolytic Streptococci.** *Proc Soc Exp Biol Med* 1948, **68**:184–188.
3. TILLETT WS, JOHNSON AJ, MCCARTY WR: **The Intravenous Infusion of the Streptococcal Fibrinolytic Principle (Streptokinase) Into Patients.** *J Clin Invest* 1955, **34**:169–185.
4. CLIFFTON EE, GROSSI CE: **Investigations of Intravenous Plasmin (Fibrinolysin) in Humans; Physiologic and Clinical Effects [Abstract].** *Circulation* 1956, **14**:919.
5. SHERRY S, FLETCHER AP, ALKJAERSIG N: **Developments in Fibrinolytic Therapy for Thromboembolic Disease.** *Ann Intern Med* 1959, **50**:560–570.
6. CLIFFTON EE: **The Use of Plasmin in Humans.** *Ann N Y Acad Sci* 1957, **68**:209–229.
7. DOTTER CT, ROSCH J, SEAMAN AJ: **Selective Clot Lysis With Low-Dose Streptokinase.** *Radiology* 1974, **111**:31–37.
8. MARDER VJ: **The Use of Thrombolytic Agents: Choice of Patient, Drug Administration, Laboratory Monitoring.** *Ann Intern Med* 1979, **90**:802–812.
9. ALKJAERSIG N, FLETCHER AP, SHERRY S: **The Mechanism of Clot Dissolution by Plasmin.** *J Clin Invest* 1959, **38**:1086.
10. MARDER VJ, SHERRY S: **Thrombolytic Therapy: Current Status, I.** *N Engl J Med* 1988, **318**:1512–1520.
11. SHERRY S, FLETCHER AP, ALKJAERSIG N: **Fibrinolysis and Fibrinolytic Activity in Man.** *Physiol Rev* 1959, **39**:343–382.
12. SHERRY S, LINDEMEYER RI, FLETCHER AP: **Studies on Enhanced Fibrinolytic Activity in Man.** *J Clin Invest* 1959, **38**:810–822.
13. AGNELLI G, BUCHANAN MR, FERNANDEZ F, HIRSH J: **The Thrombolytic and Hemorrhagic Effects of Tissue Type Plasminogen Activator: Influence of Dosage Regimens in Rabbits.** *Thromb Res* 1985, **40**:769–777.
14. GOLDHABER SZ, KESSLER CM, HEIT J, MARKIS J, SHARMA GVRK, DAWLEY D, NAGEL JS, MEYEROVITZ M, KIM D, VAUGHAN DE, *ET AL.*: **Randomized Controlled Trial of Recombinant Tissue Plasminogen Activator Versus Urokinase in the Treatment of Acute Pulmonary Embolism.** *Lancet* 1988, **ii**:293–298.
15. KANE KK: **Fibrinolysis: A Review.** *Ann Clin Lab Sci* 1984, **14**:443–449.
16. RUTHERFORD RB, FLANIGAN DP, GUPTA SK, JOHNSTON KW, KARMODY A, WHITTEMORE AD, BAKER JD, ERNST CB: **Suggested Standards for Reports Dealing With Lower Extremity Ischemia.** *J Vasc Surg* 1986, **4**:80–94.
17. MCNAMARA TO, FISCHER JR: **Thrombolysis of Peripheral Arterial and Graft Occlusions: Improved Results Using High-Dose Urokinase.** *AJR Am J Roentgenol* 1985, **144**:769–775.
18. JANG IK, GOLD HK, ZISKIND AA, FALLON JT, HOLT RE, LEINBACH RC, MAY JW, COLLEN D: **Differential Sensitivity of Erythrocyte-Rich and Platelet-Rich Arterial Thrombi to Lysis With Recombinant Tissue-Type Plasminogen Activator: A Possible Explanation for Resistance to Coronary Thrombolysis.** *Circulation* 1989, **79**:920–928.
19. • GARDINER GA JR, SULLIVAN KL: **Catheter-Directed Thrombolysis for the Failed Lower Extremity Bypass Graft.** *Semin Vasc Surg* 1992, **5**:99–103.

An excellent review of methods and results associated with thrombolysis of peripheral arterial bypass grafts.

20. •• McNamara TO: **Thrombolysis as an Alternative Initial Therapy for the Acutely Ischemic Lower Limb.** *Semin Vasc Surg* 1992, 5:89-98.

This article stresses the adjuvant nature of peripheral arterial thrombolysis, and the clinical predictors of patient subgroups that we may expect to associate with a high rate of success.

21. Ouriel K: **Differential Mechanism of Failure of Autogenous and Nonautogenous Bypass Conduits.** *J Cardiovasc Surg* 1994, in press.

22. Kunlin J. **Le Traitement de L'Arterite obliterante par la Greffe veineuse.** *Arch Mal Coeur Vaiss* 1949, **42**:371–372.

23. Dos Santos JC: **Sur la Desobstruction des Thrombus arterielles anciennes.** *Mem Acad Chir* 1947, **73**:409–411.

24. Fogarty TJ, Cranley JJ, Drause RJ, Strasser ES, Hafner CD: **A Method for Extraction of Arterial Emboli and Thrombi.** *Surg Gynecol Obstet* 1963, **116**:241–244.

25. Blaisdell FW, Steele M, Allen RE: **Management of Acute Lower Extremity Arterial Ischemia Due to Embolism and Thrombosis.** *Surgery* 1978, **84**:822–834.

26. Jivegard L, Holm J, Schersten T: **Acute Limb Ischemia Due to Arterial Embolism or Thrombosis: Influence of Limb Ischemia Versus Pre-existing Cardiac Disease on Postoperative Mortality Rate.** *J Cardiovasc Surg* 1988, **29**:32–36.

27. Edwards JE, Taylor LM Jr, Porter JM: **Treatment of Failed Lower Extremity Bypass Grafts With New Autogenous Vein Bypass Grafting.** *J Vasc Surg* 1990, **11**:136–145.

28. • Nilsson L, Albrechtsson U, Jonung T, Ribbe E, Thorvinger B, Thorne J, Astedt B, Norgren L: **Surgical Treatment Versus Thrombolysis in Acute Arterial Occlusion: A Randomized Controlled Study.** *Eur J Vasc Surg* 1992, **6**:189–193.

The first randomized, prospective comparison of operation and thrombolysis; its weakness is its small size.

29. • Allen DR, Smallwood J, Johnson CD: **Intra-arterial Thrombolysis Should be the Initial Treatment of the Acutely Ischemic Lower Limb.** *Ann R Coll Surg Engl* 1992, **74**:106–108.

This paper is a pro/con discussion of the theoretical and practical merits of thrombolysis and operation in acute limb ischemia.

30. •• McNamara TO, Bomberger RA, Merchant RF: **Intra-arterial Urokinase as the Initial Therapy for Acutely Ischemic Lower Limbs.** *Circulation* 1991, **83**(suppl I):I106–I119.

Methods and results of peripheral arterial thrombolysis.

31. • Kandarpa K, Chopra PS, Aruny JE, Polak JF, Donaldson MC, Whittemore AD, Mannic JA, Goldhaber SZ, Meyerovitz MF: **Prospective, Randomized Comparison of Forced Periodic Infusion and Conventional Slow Continuous Infusion.** *Radiology* 1993, **188**:861–867.

This is a carefully performed study of alternative methods of interarterial, catheter-directed thrombolysis.

32. Marder VJ, Sherry S: **Thrombolytic Therapy: Current Status (II).** *N Engl J Med* 1988, **318**:1585–1595.

33. Graor RA, Risius B, Young JR, Geisinger MA, Zelch MG, Smith JA, Ruschhaupt WF: **Low-Dose Streptokinase for Selective Thrombolysis: Systemic Effects and Complications.** *Radiology* 1984, **152**:35–39.

34. Krings W, Roth FJ, Cappius G, Schmidtke I: **Catheter-Lysis: Indications and Primary Results.** *Int Angiol* 1985, **4**:117–123.

35. Graor RA, Risius B, Lucas FV, Young JR, Ruschhaupt WF, Beven EG, Grossbard EB: **Thrombolysis With Recombinant Human Tissue-Type Plasminogen Activator in Patients With Peripheral Artery and Bypass Graft Occlusions.** *Circulation* 1986, **74**:I15–I20.

36. Sicard GA, Schier JJ, Totty WG, Gilula LA, Walker WB, Etheredge EE, Anderson CB: **Thrombolytic Therapy for Acute Arterial Occlusion.** *J Vasc Surg* 1985, **2**:65–78.

37. Ricotta J: **Intra-arterial Thrombolysis: A Surgical View [Comment].** *Circulation* 1991, **83**:I120–I121.

38. Lacombe M: **Surgical Versus Medical Treatment of Renal Artery Embolism.** *J Cardiovasc Surg* 1977, **18**:281–290.

39. Ouriel K, Shortell CK, DeWeese J, Green RM, Francis CW, Azodo M, Gutierrez O, Manzione J, Cox C, Marder VJ: **A Comparison of Thrombolytic Therapy With Operative Revascularization in the Initial Treatment of Acute Peripheral Arterial Ischemia.** *J Vasc Surg*, in press.

Kenneth Ouriel, MD, Department of Surgery, University of Rochester Medical Center, 601 Elmwood Avenue, Rochester, NY 14642-8410, USA.

Randomized clinical trial results define operative indications in symptomatic and asymptomatic carotid endarterectomy patients

Robert W. Hobson II, MD

University of Medicine and Dentistry of New Jersey,
New Jersey Medical School, Newark, New Jersey, USA

Randomized clinical trials on the efficacy of carotid endarterectomy have assisted in the selection of patients for operative intervention. Three such trials involving symptomatic carotid stenosis have confirmed the value of endarterectomy in patients with stenoses 70% or greater. Patients with recent transient ischemic attack or nondisabling stroke should be referred for noninvasive testing. If the patient's stenosis exceeds a threshold level (50% to 70% diameter-reducing lesion), arteriography should be performed and prompt endarterectomy scheduled , rather than antiplatelet therapy, as the primary means of treatment. Furthermore, the results of one clinical trial on asymptomatic stenosis have demonstrated benefits for operative intervention in reducing neurologic events (transient ischemic attack plus stroke). These data require additional confirmation in the analysis of stroke alone, which should be available within the next year from another clinical trial. These trials help to define indications for operation, and the thorough knowledge of their results has become essential to our practices.

Current Opinion in General Surgery 1994:265–271

The efficacy of carotid endarterectomy in patients with symptomatic and asymptomatic carotid stenosis has been defined by recently published randomized clinical trials [1••–4••]. Percentage of stenosis has emerged as the currently most accurate predictor of neurologic event rates. Clearly, the subset of patients who should be considered for operation include those with high-grade stenotic lesions, those with 70% diameter-reducing stenoses or greater in the symptomatic group [1••–3••], and those with 75% or more area stenoses in the asymptomatic group [4••]. The impetus for the emergence of randomized clinical trials on the efficacy of carotid endarterectomy was stimulated by several authors who emphasized the high risk of operation [5,6], the growth in number of operative procedures performed [7], and the lack of randomized clinical trials supporting surgery's efficacy [8]. In addition, publication of data from the extracranial-intracranial bypass trial, which demonstrated no benefit from surgical bypass, indirectly cast some doubt on the effectiveness of carotid endarterectomy for extracranial carotid occlusive disease [9]. Although planning for the Veterans Administration trial on asymptomatic carotid stenosis antedated these concerns [10], these various influences contributed to the funding of clinical trials on symptomatic disease [1••] (North American Symptomatic Carotid Endarterectomy Trial [NASCET]) and asymptomatic disease [11] (ACAS [Asymptomatic Carotid Atherosclerosis Study]) as sponsored by the National Institutes of Health as well as the recently published trial on asymptomatic carotid stenosis as sponsored by the Veterans Administration [4••]. These trials have assisted in defining primary operative candidates for symptomatic as well as asymptomatic extracranial carotid disease. The purpose of this chapter is to review the results of these trials and to highlight the application of these data in surgical practice.

Symptomatic carotid stenosis

Selection of patients for surgery was based on successful endarterectomy in patients with transient ischemic attack and nondisabling stroke and comparison of the natural history of similar patients. Because the incidence of stroke after transient ischemic attack has been reported to be about 30% over 5 years [12,13], accomplishing carotid endarterectomy with modest risk (≤ 3%

Abbreviation

NASCET—North American Symptomatic Carotid Endarterectomy Trial.

 ISBN 1-85922-671-X ISSN 1065–6243

to 5%) suggested efficacy for the procedure. Two randomized prospective trials had been conducted previously, both during the 1960s and early 1970s [14,15]. However, both suffered from design flaws that made the results less definitive. In the case of the small study reported on by Shaw *et al.* [14], the trial was terminated after only 41 patients had been randomized because of a high surgical morbidity and mortality. The second, larger study, the Joint Study of Extracranial Carotid Occlusion [15] was criticized because of the inclusion of patients with lesser degrees of stenosis, a variable operative complication rate among participating institutions, and the inclusion of some patients with symptoms not characteristic of carotid territory disease. These factors also contributed to the development of larger prospective randomized trials, one conducted in North America (NASCET) [1••] and one conducted in Europe (ECST or European Carotid Surgery Trial) [2••] as well as a smaller trial on symptomatic disease conducted within the Veterans Administration [3••].

Table 1. Clinical trials of the efficacy of carotid endarterectomy for symptomatic and asymptomatic carotid stenosis

Symptomatic carotid stenosis
North American Symptomatic Carotid Endarterectomy Trial [1••]
European Carotid Surgery Trialists' collaborative group [2••]
Veterans Administration Cooperative Trial on Symptomatic Carotid Stenosis [3••]
Asymptomatic carotid stenosis
Veterans Administration Cooperative Trial on Asymptomatic Carotid Stenosis [4••]
National Institutes of Health Asymptomatic Carotid Atherosclerosis Study [11]
Carotid Artery Stenosis with Asymptomatic Narrowing: Operation Versus Aspirin [44•]

The most influential clinical trial in symptomatic disease (Table 1) has been NASCET [1••]. In an analysis of 659 patients who had had transient ischemic attack or nondisabling stroke within the previous 120 days and who had ipsilateral carotid stenosis of 70% to 99%, the cumulative risk of any ipsilateral stroke at 24 months of follow-up was 26% for the 331 medical patients and 9% for the 328 surgical patients, an absolute risk reduction of 17% ($P<0.001$). For major or fatal ipsilateral stroke, the corresponding incidences were 13.1% and 2.5% for the medical and surgical groups, respectively, an absolute risk reduction of 10.6% or a greater than 5:1 benefit in favor of operation ($P<0.001$). The NASCET investigators concluded that carotid endarterectomy was highly beneficial for patients with recent hemispheric or retinal transient ischemic attacks or nondisabling stroke in the presence of ipsilateral high-grade carotid stenosis. However, these investigators have also made a plea for continued randomization of symptomatic patients with stenoses of 30% to 69%, among whom the differences between medical and surgical management currently are not significant. Furthermore, the incidence of stroke in the medical group increased significantly for each decile of patients with 71% to 80%, 81% to 90%, and 91% to 99% stenoses.

The results of another clinical trial on symptomatic carotid occlusive disease also was published in 1991 and presented data from the European Carotid Surgery Trial [2••]. These investigators randomized patients in a uniform protocol; however, it was based on an individual center's preference regarding selection of patients considered eligible for randomization. Although some reviewers considered this a methodologic flaw, the results of the study essentially confirmed those of the NASCET trial. Among a cohort of 778 patients with stenoses in the 70% to 99% range, at 3 years of follow-up the risk of surgical stroke or death, ipsilateral ischemic stroke, or any other stroke was 12.3% for the surgical group and 21.9% for the medical group, an absolute risk reduction of 9.6% ($P<0.01$). For the more significant disabling or fatal stroke, the incidence was 6% in the surgical group and 11% in the medical group ($P<0.05$). These investigators also studied 374 patients with stenoses of 0% to 29% and concluded that no benefit for carotid endarterectomy was observed in these patients. The results of carotid endarterectomy in patients with 30% to 69% stenoses remain uncertain.

Finally, a third trial concerning symptomatic carotid stenosis was the Veterans Administration Symptomatic Trial, in which 189 patients with transient ischemic attack or nondisabling stroke and ipsilateral stenosis of 50% or greater were randomized. During a mean follow-up of 11.9 months, the incidence of stroke or crescendo transient ischemic attack was 7.7% in the surgical group and 19.4% in the medical group, with an absolute risk reduction of 11.7% ($P=0.028$). Although the differences between groups with regard to stroke alone were not significant, the smaller sample size and shorter period of follow-up were responsible for these results. However, these results are viewed as confirmatory, recognizing the high clinical risk of stroke in the crescendo transient ischemic attack patient. As in NASCET, an increased risk of stroke was observed in patients with stenoses of 70% or greater.

Results from these randomized clinical trials influence our management of patients with recent transient ischemic attack and nondisabling stroke. Referral of symptomatic patients for noninvasive vascular testing to establish the severity of stenosis is recommended. With confirmation of severe stenosis (≥70%), carotid endarterectomy is the treatment of choice in better-risk patients in those centers reporting low operative risk of permanent stroke and death. Primary treatment with antiplatelet agents or in some instances warfarin (Coumadin; Dupont Pharmaceuticals, Wilmington, DE) coupled with referral for carotid endarterectomy only after occurrence of breakthrough symptoms on medication is no longer an acceptable clinical option.

Asymptomatic carotid stenosis

The more significant debate concerning indications for carotid endarterectomy has focused on the efficacy of operative intervention in patients with asymptomatic carotid stenosis. Application of carotid endarterectomy as a primary means of prophylaxis for transient ischemic attacks and stroke in patients with high-grade asymptomatic carotid stenosis is based on several assumptions: 1) patients can be identified by accurate noninvasive studies [16], and progression from less severe to significant stenosis can be documented [17]; and 2) arteriographic confirmation can be obtained with virtually no mortality and low stroke risk [18,19]. Stroke occurs at relatively high annual rates in the subset of patients with high-grade carotid stenosis, perhaps 3% to 5% or more [20,21]; and 3) carotid endarterectomy can be performed with low combined stroke morbidity and operative mortality, preferably less than 2% to 5% (Table 2).

Magnitude of stenosis

The definition of asymptomatic but clinically significant carotid stenosis is usually related to the magnitude of stenosis present at the carotid bifurcation and the proximal internal carotid artery. By convention as well as in laboratory studies documenting reductions in distal pressure and flow, the definition of hemodynamic significance has generally included stenoses equal to or greater than a 50% reduction in the luminal diameter of the artery on biplanar arteriography or constituting a 75% reduction in the artery's cross-sectional area. These definitions identify the threshold levels of hemodynamic significance. The percentage of stenosis is determined by comparing the least transverse diameter at the stenosis with the diameter of the distal uninvolved internal carotid artery where the arterial walls become parallel. The percentage may then be expressed as the function of the diameter or the cross-sectional area (Fig. 1). Direct interrogation of the carotid bifurcation using spectral analysis [22,23] and ultrasonographic imaging of the cervical carotid artery

Table 2. Morbidity and mortality associated with carotid endarterectomy for asymptomatic carotid disease, by study

Study	Operations, *n*	Mortality, *n(%)*	Morbidity, *n(%)* Transient	Morbidity, *n(%)* Permanent
Thompson *et al.* [38]	167	0	2(1.2)	2(1.2)
Moore *et al.* [39]	78	0	2(2.6)	0
Hertzer *et al.* [48]	95	1(1.1)	—	4(4.2)
Whitney *et al.* [49]	279	3(1.1)	5(1.8)	6(2.2)
Javid *et al.* [50]	65	1(1.5)	1(1.5)	1(1.5)
Anderson *et al.* [40]	120	0	0	0
Veterans Administration Clinical Trial [4••]	211	4(1.9)	2(0.9)	5(2.4)

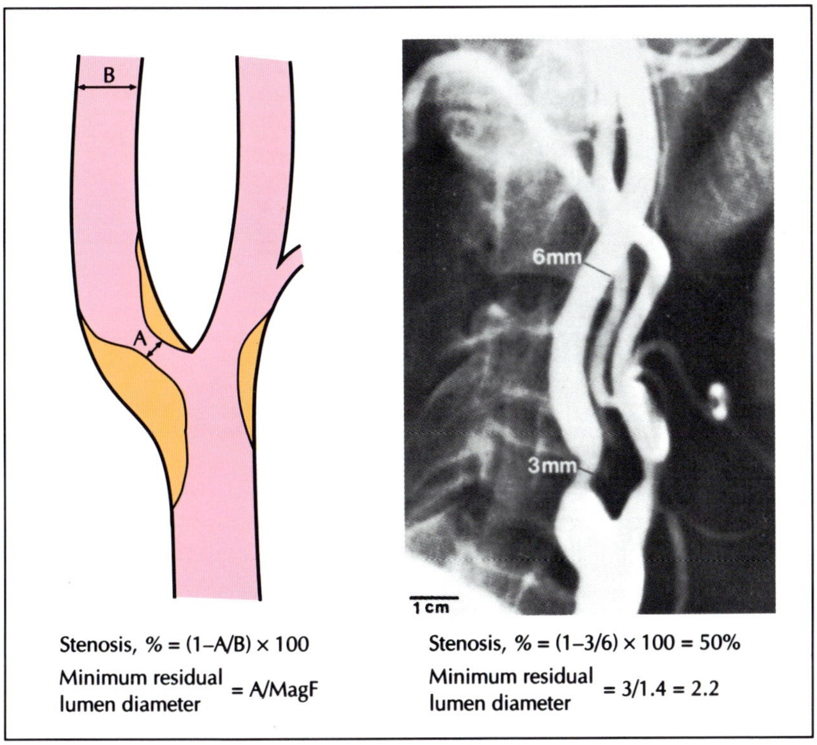

Fig. 1. Left, The percentage of stenosis is calculated by dividing the least transverse diameter of the internal carotid artery at the stenosis (*A*) by the diameter of the distal, uninvolved artery (*B*). The minimum residual lumen diameter is equivalent to the least transverse diameter (*A*) divided by the magnification factor (MagF) of the arteriogram. **Right,** An example illustrates a 50% stenosis by diameter and a minimum residual lumen diameter of 2.2 cm. (*From* Lynch and Hobson [16]; with permission.)

[24,25] have become increasingly important in the analysis of these cases. O'Leary *et al.* [26] assessed the impact of noninvasive testing on patient management and demonstrated an increase in the number of positive arteriogram results and a reduction in the incidence of less-significant findings directly related to the clinical application of duplex scanning.

The safety of arteriography has improved with the use of newer contrast media and the application of intra-arterial digital subtraction arteriographic techniques. One study on the complications of arteriography in six university medical centers involving patients presenting with transient ischemic attacks reported a stroke risk of less than 1% related to the procedure [19], generally involving a transfemoral route of catheterization. Recent analysis of data [18] from the Veterans Administration Cooperative Study on Asymptomatic Carotid Stenosis demonstrated a stroke rate of 0.4% without mortality in patients with asymptomatic stenoses and asymptomatic stenoses contralateral to a symptomatic lesion. Consequently, arteriography has been shown to be safe in asymptomatic patients, with a complication rate that can allow aggressive surgical management of patients with asymptomatic carotid stenosis. However, some clinicians rely on duplex scanning for characterization of carotid stenosis, thereby avoiding even this small risk [27].

Neurologic complications

Transient ischemic attacks accompanied by positive computed tomographic scan results or frank stroke occur at relatively high annual rates in patients with significant but asymptomatic carotid stenosis. Furthermore, the presumption that a clinical transient ischemic attack is innocuous awaits further clinical investigation. Some authors have reported a 30% to 40% incidence of positive computed tomographic scan results with transient neurologic events [28,29]. Consequently, the concept that a transient neurologic event has only minor or no clinical consequences [30] may be erroneous, because it also becomes the marker for patients at greatest risk of stroke during the first month after the initial transient ischemic attack [31].

Several authors have used noninvasive techniques to identify risk of subsequent stroke in the subset of patients with hemodynamically significant but asymptomatic stenoses. Kartchner and McRae [32] reported a 12% stroke rate after 2 years in a group of asymptomatic patients with hemodynamically significant stenoses identified by one oculoplethysmographic technique. Cullen *et al.* [33] used the measurement of ophthalmic artery pressure to identify 77 patients with hemodynamically insignificant stenosis and 29 with hemodynamically significant stenosis. Clinical follow-up at 18 months demonstrated that 11% of those without significant stenoses had become symptomatic, whereas 24% with significant stenoses had become symptomatic. Moneta *et al.* [34] reported on a group of 129 patients separated into those undergoing carotid endarterectomy and those receiving nonoperative treatment. Life table analysis at up to 24 months demonstrated a higher rate of transient ischemic attacks (28% vs 5%, P=0.008), internal carotid occlusion (29% vs 0%, P=0.003), and stroke (19% vs 4%, P=0.08) in the nonsurgical group. Of the strokes, none was preceded by transient ischemic attacks, eight of nine occurred within 9 months of the diagnosis of the high-grade lesion, and none occurred in the 10 patients who were refused operation because of coexisting medical problems. In the surgical group, one perioperative stroke (1.8%) occurred and no hospital deaths were reported. Moore *et al.* [35] reported similar data in a group of patients with asymptomatic stenoses of 50% or greater. In the unoperated group, the rate was 21% compared with 8% in the surgical group (P< 0.05). Chambers and Norris [20,21] reported data on 500 patients from their asymptomatic cervical bruit study. The ischemic cerebrovascular event rate in patients with area stenoses of greater than 75% was 18% (12% transient ischemic attack, 6% stroke rate, 3% ipsilateral to the stenosis) as compared with a neurologic event rate of less than 3% per year in those patients with stenoses of less than 75%. Their data and other reports have confirmed the association of high-grade stenosis with increased risk of transient ischemic attack and stroke. Although annualized stroke rates in patients with carotid bruit alone have been low [36,37], long-term studies on the incidence of stroke and transient neurologic events in an asymptomatic population with high-grade stenosis have not been well documented.

In the absence of data from multicenter prospectively randomized clinical trials on carotid endarterectomy in the asymptomatic population, justification for a prophylactic endarterectomy is based on the supposition that its associated complications are less than the expected morbidity and mortality of the nonoperated population. Consequently, surgical experience must be well documented by all practitioners who recommend prophylactic endarterectomy. Multiple reports in the literature have documented the relative safety of operation in these patients. Thompson *et al.* [38] reported a less than 2% incidence of perioperative morbidity and no operative deaths. Immediate and long-term results following carotid endarterectomy in the asymptomatic patient have also been evaluated by Moore *et al.* [39], who reported no operative deaths or perioperative strokes in a series of 78 operations and found a 95% stroke-free status in surviving patients.

Recently, our group [40] reported similar results, with the absence of perioperative stroke or death in the performance of 120 consecutive endarterectomies for high-grade asymptomatic carotid stenosis. Table 2 presents data from several clinical series on performance of carotid endarterectomy in asymptomatic patients. These data are generally consistent with the operative stroke and mortality rates recommended by Barnett *et al.* [41]. We agree with recent editorials that it is the responsibility of the operating surgeon to report local operative complication rates before carotid endarterectomy can be recommended in patients with asymptomatic stenosis [42,43].

Several trials have been conducted comparing medical and surgical management of asymptomatic carotid stenosis. Investigators from the CASANOVA (Carotid Artery Stenosis with Asymptomatic Narrowing: Operation Versus Aspirin) trial [44•] randomly assigned 410 patients to operative management or optimal medical management. After a mean follow-up of 3 years, these investigators were unable to demonstrate any significant difference in event rates between the medically and surgically treated patients. However, higher-risk patients were excluded from the study and referred preferentially for carotid endarterectomy. These patients included those with stenoses of 90% or greater as well as patients who demonstrated noninvasive evidence of significant progression of their stenoses. This fact, coupled with a qualitative flaw in the randomization protocol, cause the results of this trial to be generally regarded as inconclusive.

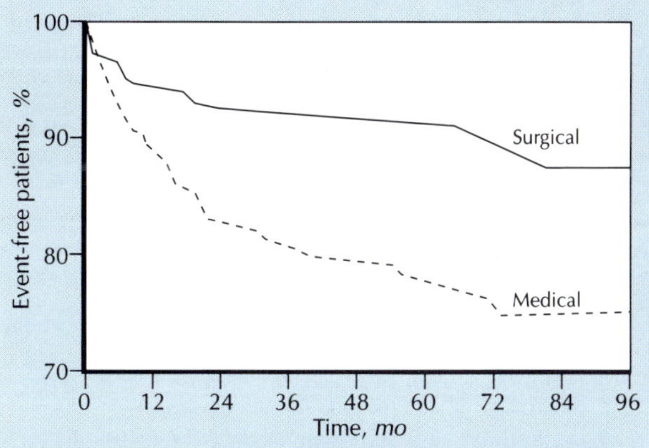

	0	12	24	36	48	60	72	84
Surgical patients, *n*	211	181	163	150	122	88	45	18
Medical patients, n	233	194	166	148	121	85	58	32

Fig. 2. Kaplan-Meier curves of an analysis of the time until the first neurologic event (ipsilateral stroke and transient ischemic attack, including transient monocular blindness) for patients treated surgically and medically for asymptomatic carotid stenosis. The number of patients remaining event-free and on-study at the beginning of each 12-month period is also provided. Treatment group comparisons by log-rank test demonstrated significant differences in favor of the surgical group ($P = 0.001$). The relative risk (surgical vs medical) was 0.38 (95% CI: 0.22, 0.67). (*From* Hobson *et al.* [4••]; with permission.)

A multicenter randomized clinical trial on asymptomatic carotid stenosis was conducted at 11 Veterans Affairs Medical Centers throughout the United States to determine the efficacy of carotid endarterectomy on the combined incidence of transient ischemic attack, transient monocular blindness, and stroke [4••]. The trial involved 444 adult male patients (mean age, 64.5 years) with asymptomatic carotid stenosis (minimal stenosis for randomization was 50% arterial lumen diameter reduction on arteriography in the presence of positive ocular plethysmography or duplex scan results or 75% area reduction). Patients were assigned randomly to optimal medical management, including antiplatelet medication (aspirin), plus carotid endarterectomy (211 patients) or optimal medical management alone (233 patients). All patients were followed up independently by a vascular surgeon and a neurologist at each center for a mean period of 47.9 months. The combined incidence of ipsilateral neurologic events was 8.0% in the surgical group and 20.6% in the medical group ($P < 0.001$), and the relative risk (surgical group vs medical group) was 0.38 (95% CI, range 0.22 to 0.67) (Fig. 2). Although the incidence of ipsilateral stroke alone was 4.7% in the surgical group and 9.4% in the medical group ($P = 0.056$), this two-to-one advantage in favor of the surgical group was diminished because of a combined 30-day operative mortality and stroke rate of 4.3%.

For those clinicians requiring significant reductions in stroke and death, the results of the Veterans Administration trial on asymptomatic carotid stenosis are not definitive and do not settle the controversy entirely [45•]. However, for the immediate future, it is the only randomized clinical trial to show efficacy for operation among this significant group of operative candidates. I continue to support the long-term follow-up of patients randomized to the other large clinical trial, the Asymptomatic Carotid Atherosclerosis Study, by the National Institutes of Health now that its acquisition of patients has been completed (effective November 1, 1993). Until outcome data are available from this trial, patients and referring physicians must define clinical recommendations based on currently available information.

For those patients with asymptomatic carotid stenosis, usually identified by noninvasive methodology, the threshold for considering prophylactic carotid endarterectomy is set at a 50% diameter-reducing stenosis or a 75% area-reducing stenosis. As an aside, it is acknowledged that this is a threshold at which to consider operative intervention; all arteriographically confirmed 50% diameter-reducing stenoses will not be accompanied by positive noninvasive study results (ocular plethysmography or duplex scan). Therefore, the area-reducing stenosis of 75% or greater should be considered as the minimal stenosis for operative intervention.

Based on the Veterans Administration clinical trial, operative complications were analyzed previously [46], and clinical audits [42] are recommended at individual centers to ensure an operative mortality and stroke morbidity of less than 3% [47]. It is my opinion that the 30-day perioperative stroke risk of 2.4% can be reduced by rigorous adherence to careful surgical technique and intraoperative evaluation of the technical adequacy of endarterectomy. Furthermore, the mortality (1.9%) was exclusively due to coronary artery disease. Randomization of patients occurred during an era (1983 to 1987) when identification of occult coronary artery disease with noninvasive stress testing or thallium scans was not readily available. Consequently, the patient with asymptomatic carotid stenosis who is undergoing initial consideration for prophylactic endarterectomy should have a thorough evaluation of cardiac risk factors and selective use of preoperative cardiac testing. In this manner, the patient with severe but occult coronary artery disease can be identified. At that point, consideration can be given for coronary angioplasty or aortocoronary bypass. In many patients, however, this process will be considered impractical due to the operative risk of coronary bypass in the elderly patient. This risk may assist clinicians in deciding to wait for neurologic events before proceeding to carotid endarterectomy. Conversely, the patient who is evaluated and cleared of coronary risk factors should then be considered for operative intervention. However, the option of awaiting neurologic events before intervening surgically should not be adopted as a general clinical recommendation. One half of all neurologic events in the Veterans Administration trial were strokes that were unaccompanied by antecedent transient ischemia attack. As a result, and as has been documented in many clinical series, the incidence of warning transient ischemic attack in the presence of asymptomatic carotid stenosis prior to stroke is unusual and cannot be relied on as a warning for clinicians reluctant to consider endarterectomy in this patient population.

Conclusions

These randomized clinical trials on symptomatic and asymptomatic stenosis serve to underscore the validity of some prior retrospective analyses that demonstrated efficacy for operative intervention. Their importance, however, is derived from the multicenter and cooperative nature of their clinical methodology as well as the acknowledgment that any difference in clinical characteristics between treatment groups is unbiased. However, the results of these trials can not anticipate every clinical scenario presented in daily practice. Surgical judgment will continue to be required in analyzing the individual patient's risk factors as well as the morbidity and mortality of a particular surgical group in the performance of carotid endarterectomy. Finally, although percent stenosis has emerged as our currently most useful predictor of neurologic events, it is my opinion that other factors, individually or in combination, ultimately will prove to be of greater importance. As an example, among patients with asymptomatic high-grade stenosis in the medical group of the Veterans Administration trial [4], 20% of the population experienced all neurologic events whereas 80% completed the period of observation without developing neurologic symptomatology. This result suggests that percentage stenosis is a reasonable indicator of risk but certainly lacks the accuracy usually expected of clinical predictors. Further study should be directed toward identifying factors of importance in plaque morphology, the incidence of silent confirmed cerebral infarctions confirmed by computed tomography, the importance of collateral cerebral perfusion, and combinations of risk factors, including diabetes, hypertension, coronary artery disease, and others.

References and recommended reading

Papers of particular interest, published within the annual period of review, have been highlighted as:

- • Of special interest
- •• Of outstanding interest

1. •• NASCET Collaborators: **Beneficial Effect of Carotid Endarterectomy in Symptomatic Patients With High-Grade Carotid Stenosis.** *N Engl J Med* 1991, **325**:445–453.

This most influential randomized clinical trial clearly establishes the benefit of carotid endarterectomy in patients with recent transient ischemic attack and nondisabling stroke whose stenosis is 70% or greater.

2. •• European Carotid Surgery Trialists' Collaborative Group: **MRC European Carotid Surgery Trial: Interim Results for Symptomatic Patients With Severe (70-99%) or With Mild (0-29%) Carotid Stenosis.** *Lancet* 1991, **337**:1235–1243.

These trial results, announced almost simultaneously with those of the NASCET investigators (*N Engl J Med* 1991, 325:445–453), confirm the value of endarterectomy in patients with severe stenoses (70% to 99%).

3. •• VA Symptomatic Carotid Stenosis Group: **Carotid Endarterectomy and Prevention of Cerebral Ischemia in Symptomatic Carotid Stenosis.** *JAMA* 1991, **266**:3289–3294.

This confirmatory trial in symptomatic stenosis patients reduced the combined incidence of stroke and crescendo transient ischemic attack in patients with stenoses of 40% or less. Results were even more striking for stenoses of 70% or more.

4. •• Hobson RW, Weiss DG, Fields WS, Goldstone J, Moore WS, Towne JB, Wright CB, VA Cooperative Asymptomatic Carotid Artery Stenosis Study Group: **Efficacy of Carotid Endarterectomy for Asymptomatic Carotid Stenosis.** *N Engl J Med* 1993, **328**:221–227.

This article represents the first randomized clinical trial showing the efficacy of carotid endarterectomy in reducing combined neurologic events (transient ischemic attack, transient monocular blindness, and stroke) in patients with asymptomatic carotid stenosis.

5. Barnett HJM, Plum F, Walton JN: **Carotid Endarterectomy: An Expression of Concern.** *Stroke* 1984, **15**:941–943.
6. Easton JD, Sherman DG: **Stroke and Mortality Rate in Carotid Endarterectomy: 228 Consecutive Operations.** *Stroke* 1977, **8**:565–568.
7. Dyken ML, Pokras R: **The Performance of Endarterectomy for the Extracranial Arteries of the Head.** *Stroke* 1984, **15**:948–950.
8. Warlow C: **Carotid Endarterectomy: Does It Work?** *Stroke* 1984, **15**:1068–1076.
9. The EC/IC Bypass Study Group: **Failure of Extracranial-Intracranial Arterial Bypass to Reduce the Risk of Ischemic Stroke.** *N Engl J Med* 1985, **313**:1191–1200.
10. Veterans Administration Cooperative Study: **Role of Carotid Endarterectomy in Asymptomatic Carotid Stenosis.** *Stroke* 1986, **17**:534–539.
11. The Asymptomatic Carotid Atherosclerosis Study Group: **Study Design for Randomized Prospective Trial of Carotid Endarterectomy for Asymptomatic Atherosclerosis.** *Stroke* 1989, **20**:844–849.
12. Whisnant JP, Matsumoto M, Elveback LR: **The Effect of Anticoagulant Therapy on the Prognosis of Patients With Transient Cerebral Ischemic Attacks in a Community-Rochester Minnesota 1965-69.** *Mayo Clinic Proc* 1973, **48**:844–848.
13. Easton JD, Hart RG, Sherman DG, Kaste M: **Diagnosis and /Management of Ischemic Stroke: Part I. Threatened Stroke and Its Management.** *Curr Prob Cardiol* 1983, **8**:1–76.
14. Shaw DA, Venables GS, Cartlidge NEF, Bates D, Dickinson PH: **Carotid Endarterectomy in Patients With Transient Cerebral Ischemia.** *J Neurol Sci* 1984, **64**:45–53.
15. Fields WS, North RR, Hass WK, Galbraith JG, Wylie EJ, Ratinov G, Burns MH, MacDonald MC, Meyer JS: **Joint Study of Extracranial Arterial Occlusion as a Cause of Stroke: I. Organization of Study and Survey of Patient Population.** *JAMA* 1968, **203**:995–960.
16. Lynch TG, Hobson RW: **Noninvasive Cerebrovascular Diagnostic Techniques.** In *Vascular Surgery: Principles and Practice.* Edited by Wilson SE, Veith FJ, Hobson RW, Williams RA. New York: McGraw-Hill; 1987:105–134.
17. Roederer GO, Langlois YE, Jager KA, Primozlich JF, Beach KW, Phillips DJ, Strandness DE: **The Natural History of Carotid Arterial Disease in Asymptomatic Patients With Cervical Bruits.** *Stroke* 1984, **15**:605–613.
18. Hobson RW, Song IS, George AM, Weiss DG: **Arteriography for Asymptomatic Carotid Stenosis.** *Stroke* 1989, **20**:135.

19. SWANSON PD, *ET AL.*: A Cooperative Study of Hospital Frequency and Character of Transient Ischemic Attacks: II. Performance of Angiography Among Six Centers. *JAMA* 1977, 237:2202–2206.

20. CHAMBERS BR, NORRIS JW: The Case Against Surgery for Asymptomatic Carotid Stenosis. *Stroke* 1984, 15:964–967.

21. CHAMBERS BR, NORRIS JW: Outcome in Patients With Asymptomatic Neck Bruits. *N Engl J Med* 1986, 315:860–865.

22. BLACKSHEAR WM, *ET AL.*: Detection of Carotid Occlusive Disease by Ultrasonic Imaging and Pulsed Doppler Spectrum Analysis. *Surgery* 1979, 86:698–706.

23. RITTGERS SE, THORNHILL BM, BARNES RW: Quantitative Analysis of Carotid Artery Doppler Spectral Waveforms: Diagnostic Value of Parameters. *Ultrasound Med Biol* 1983, 9:255–264.

24. COMEROTA AJ, CRANLEY JJ, KATZ ML, COOK SE, SIPPEL PJ, HAYDEN WG, FOGARTY TJ, TYSON RR: Real-Time B-Mode Carotid Imaging: A Three Year Multicenter Experience. *Vasc Surg* 1984, 1:84–95.

25. HOBSON RW, BERRY SM, KATOCS AS, O'DONNELL JA, JAMIL Z, SAVITSKY JP: Comparison of Pulsed Doppler and Realtime B-Mode Echo Arteriography for Non-Invasive Imaging of the Extracranial Carotid Arteries. *Surgery* 1980, 87:286–293.

26. O'LEARY DH, CLOUSE ME, POTTER JE, WHEELER HG: The Influence of Noninvasive Tests on the Selection of Patients for Carotid Angiography. *Stroke* 1985, 16:264–267.

27. HILL JC, CARBONNEAU K, BALIGA PK: Safe Extracranial Vascular Evaluation and Surgery Without Preoperative Arteriography. *Ann Vasc Surg* 1990, 4:34.

28. AWAD I, MODIC M, LITTLE JR, FURLAN AJ, WEINSTEIN M: Focal Parenchymal Lesions in Transient Ischemic Attacks: Correlation of Computed Tomography and Magnetic Resonance Imaging. *Stroke* 1985, 17:399–403.

29. PERRONE P, *ET AL.*: CT Evaluation in Patients With Transient Ischemic Attack: Correlation Between Clinical and Angiographic Findings. *Eur Neurol* 1979, 18:217–221.

30. DYKEN MD: Carotid Endarterectomy Studies: A Glimmering of Science. *Stroke* 1986, 17:355–357.

31. COMMITTEE ON HEALTH CARE ISSUES, AMERICAN NEUROLOGICAL ASSOCIATION: Does Carotid Endarterectomy Decrease Stroke and Death in Patients With Transient Ischemic Attacks? *Ann Neurol* 1987, 22:72–76.

32. KARTCHNER MM, MCRAE LP: *The Clinical Use of Oculoplethysmography and Carotid Phonoangiography*. Edited by Baker WH. Mount Kisco: Futura; 1979.

33. CULLEN SJ, CORREA MC, CALDERON-ORTIZ M, WALBURN FJ, FAINES J: Clinical Sequelae in Patients With Asymptomatic Carotid Bruits. *Circulation* 1983, 68(suppl II):83–87.

34. MONETA GL, TAYLOR DC, NICHOLLS SC: Operative Versus Nonoperative Management of Asymptomatic High-Grade Internal Artery Stenosis: Improved Results With Endarterectomy. *Stroke* 1987, 18:1005–1010.

35. MOORE DJ, MILES RD, GOOLEY NA, SUMNER DS: Noninvasive Assessment of Stroke Risk in Asymptomatic and Nonhemispheric Patients With Suspected Carotid Disease. *Ann Surg* 1985, 202:491–504.

36. HEYMAN W, WILKINSON WE, HEYDEN S, HELMS MJ, BARTEL AG, KARP HR, TYROLER HA, HAMES CG: Risk of Stroke in Asymptomatic Persons With Cervical Arterial Bruits: A Population Study in Evans County, Georgia. *N Engl J Med* 1980, 302:838–841.

37. WOLF PA, KANNEL WB, SORLIE P, MCNAMARA P: Asymptomatic Carotid Bruit and the Risk of Stroke. *JAMA* 1981, 245:1442–1445.

38. THOMPSON JE, PATMAN RD, TALKINGTON CM: Asymptomatic Carotid Bruit: Long-Term Outcome in Patients Having Endarterectomy Compared With Unoperated Controls. *Ann Surg* 1978, 188:308–316.

39. MOORE WS, BOREN C, MALONE JM, GOLDSTONE J: Asymptomatic Carotid Stenosis: Immediate and Long-Term Results After Prophylactic Endarterectomy. *Am J Surg* 1979, 138:228–233.

40. ANDERSON RJ, HOBSON RW, PADBERG FT, PECORARO JP, DEGROOTE RD, JAMIL Z, LEE BC, BREITBART GB, FRANCO CD: Carotid Endarterectomy for Asymptomatic Carotid Stenosis: A Ten Year Experience With 120 Procedures in a Fellowship Training Program. *Ann Vasc Surg* 1991, 5:111–115.

41. BARNETT HJM, PLUM F, WALTON JN: Carotid Endarterectomy: An Expression of Concern. *Stroke* 1984, 15:941–943.

42. HOBSON RW, TOWNE JB: Carotid Endarterectomy for Asymptomatic Carotid Stenosis [Editorial]. *Stroke* 1989, 20:575–576.

43. THOMPSON JE: Don't Throw Out the Baby With the Bath Water [Editorial]. *J Vasc Surg* 1986, 4:543–546.

44. THE CASANOVA STUDY GROUP: Carotid Surgery Versus Medical Therapy in Asymptomatic Carotid Stenosis. *Stroke* 1991, 22:1229–1235.
• This randomized clinical trial showed no benefit for operative intervention in patients with asymptomatic carotid stenosis. However, the group of patients with stenoses of 90% or more and those progressing rapidly were referred for operation; the results of this trial were therefore inconclusive.

45. BARNETT HJM, HAINES SJ: Carotid Endarterectomy for Asymptomatic Stenosis. *N Engl J Med* 1993, 328:276–279.
• This major critique of the Veterans Administration trial on asymptomatic carotid stenosis (*N Engl J Med* 1993, 328:221–227) suggests that the study is invalidated because stroke alone was not significantly reduced. However, these reviewers reviewer failed to acknowledge the two-to-one trend in stroke reduction afforded by carotid endarterectomy, which should be kept in mind when evaluating the Veterans Administration data. In addition, the data from the Asymptomatic Carotid Atherosclerosis Study, soon to be published, will need to be reviewed before a final conclusion is reached.

46. TOWNE JB, WEISS DG, HOBSON RW: First Phase Report of Cooperative VA Asymptomatic Carotid Stenosis Study: Operative Morbidity and Mortality. *J Vasc Surg* 1990, 11:252–259.

47. BEEBE HG, CLAGETT GP, DEWEESE JA, *ET AL.*: Assessing Risk Associated With Carotid Endarterectomy. *Stroke* 1989, 20:314–315.

48. HERTZER NR, BEVEN EG, GREENSTREET RL, HUMPHRIES AW: Internal Carotid Back Pressures, Intraoperative Shunting, Ulcerated Atheromata, and the Incidence of Stroke During Carotid Endarterectomy. *Surgery* 1978, 83:306–312.

49. WHITNEY DG, KAHN EM, ESTES JW, JONES CE: Carotid Artery Surgery Without a Temporary Indwelling Shunt. *Arch Surg* 1980, 115:1393–1399.

50. JAVID H, OSTERMILLER WE, HENGESH JW, DYE WS, HUNTER JA, NAJAFI H, JULIAN OC: Carotid Endarterectomy for Asymptomatic Patients. *Arch Surg* 1971, 102:389–391.

Robert W. Hobson II, MD, Section of Vascular Surgery, Medical Science Building G-532, UMDNJ-New Jersey Medical School, 185 South Orange Avenue, Newark, NJ 07103-2714, USA.

Ischemic nephropathy as an indication for renal artery reconstruction in renovascular hypertension

Virginia S. Newman, MD, and Richard H. Dean, MD

Bowman Gray School of Medicine, Winston-Salem, North Carolina, USA

The utility of renal revascularization to control hypertension secondary to renal artery occlusive disease is widely recognized. However, revascularization for purposes of renal salvage, although performed successfully in many instances, is a more difficult issue, owing to the higher morbidity and mortality rates associated with operative intervention in an older patient population with significant comorbid conditions. It is therefore imperative to appropriately select patients who may benefit from revascularization, and the aim of our discussion is to aid in this selection process.

Current Opinion in General Surgery 1994:272–276

Early diagnosis of renovascular disease is of increasing importance, given that the disease is the most curable form of hypertension and one of the few potentially reversible causes of chronic renal failure. Although the true incidence is not known, renal insufficiency from occlusive disease is suspected to occur in as many as 26% of patients with renovascular hypertension [1].

Severe occlusive disease may lead to inadequate effective renal plasma flow and diminished excretory function of the kidney. Traditionally, study of the sequelae of renovascular occlusive disease has centered on the pathophysiology and management of the resultant renovascular hypertension. Recent reports, however, have emphasized the potential for simultaneous retrieval of excretory function in some patients with combined hypertension and renal insufficiency [2–5]. These observations have renewed awareness of this functional consequence of renal ischemia and have led to the coinage of the term *ischemic nephropathy.* By definition, ischemic nephropathy reflects the presence of anatomically severe occlusive disease of the extraparenchymal renal artery in a patient with excretory renal insufficiency.

Atherosclerotic renovascular stenosis comprises approximately 70% of renovascular pathology and represents a frequently bilateral and progressive process. Fibrodysplastic lesions, in particular, medical fibrodysplasia, make up the remaining 30% of cases [6]. Progression to a stenosis of greater than 70% or a lesion producing a gradient of at least 40 mm Hg has been shown to significantly reduce renal plasma flow, glomerular filtration rate, and urine flow rate [7]. Revascularization of such severely stenotic and even occluded renal arteries for renal salvage has now been reported in several series that show significant improvement in renal function and patient survival [8–16]. However, the current enthusiasm for revascularization of diseased renal arteries for this purpose must be tempered with good judgment. Patients with hypertension and chronic renal insufficiency secondary to atherosclerotic renovascular disease have multiple comorbid conditions because of the diffuse nature of atherosclerosis. Appropriate patient selection is therefore paramount to success in revascularization for renal salvage and is the focus of this discussion.

Three groups of patients are potential candidates for revascularization to improve renal function. The first group is represented by the patient with a normal or slightly elevated serum creatinine value who is found to have a poorly functioning or nonfunctioning kidney on diagnostic evaluation for renovascular hypertension. In this patient, overall renal function is maintained by the contralateral normal kidney, and the clinical question is whether to remove or to revascularize the nonfunctioning kidney. The second group is represented by the azotemic or dialysis-dependent patient who has extraparenchymal renovascular occlusive disease (ischemic nephropathy). In this patient, the clinical question is whether the probability of retrieving clinically significant function or significantly slowing the disease's progression justifies the risk of operation. The third group is represented by the patient with chronic renal insufficiency secondary to renovascular occlusive disease who experiences acute thrombosis of those diseased vessels, heralding oliguric or anuric re-

Abbreviation

EGFR—estimated glomerular filtration rate.

  ISBN 1-85922-671-X ISSN 1065–6243

nal failure. For this patient, the clinical questions are which diagnostic tool will be used to corroborate the diagnosis and what is the timing of intervention.

The nonazotemic patient

Hypertension in the nonazotemic patient with renal artery occlusion and a poorly functioning or nonfunctioning kidney can be treated equally well by revascularization or nephrectomy. However, the management of hypertension and the retrieval of function by revascularization would be superior if both of these end results could be predicted and assessed. The practical value of such predictions is obvious; as many as 35% of patients with mild contralateral occlusive lesions will progress to hemodynamically severe occlusive lesions within 5 years [17,18]. When such patients have undergone nephrectomy for renovascular hypertension and their contralateral disease has progressed, global renal function is threatened, and operative intervention must then be contemplated for severely azotemic, potentially dialysis-dependent renal failure patients. Moreover, the atherosclerotic occlusive disease in the remaining kidney may not develop in a recognizable manner or may develop at a site not amenable to surgical correction. On the other hand, a too aggressive attitude toward revascularization of the initially poorly functioning or nonfunctioning kidney, in which attempts are made to recover function at the lowest limits of retrievability, sometimes leads to revascularization of a kidney in which no functional response is achievable. In this instance, primary nephrectomy is simpler than revascularization and is equally effective in controlling hypertension. Removal of a nonfunctioning kidney does nothing to diminish excretory function. Indeed, subsequent improvement of blood pressure control with the concomitant elimination of high-dose diuretics and other medications that can adversely affect renal function may lead to improvement in function in the remaining kidney.

Many factors influence successful revascularization of poorly functioning kidneys. Although studies have not defined limits below which clinically important retrieval of function is impossible, they have identified preoperative variables that may predict a favorable response. The development of a collateral circulation to the chronically occluded kidney has been described and is considered an important prerequisite to restoration of renal function following repair [9,10,12]. A small but critical amount of blood flow can maintain the viability of renal parenchyma without demonstrable renal function. We reviewed the effect of revascularization on renal function in 64 patients who had a preoperative creatinine clearance by the affected kidney of less than or equal to 15 mL/min. Results of this study and our subsequent experience have led us to proceed with revascularization whenever the distal vessel is identified and appears normal by arteriography. Similarly, when at least 10% of total renal function comes from the poorly functioning kidney on isotope renography, we explore the distal vessel even when it is not visualized by arteriography. In about 40% of such cases, we find a normal distal vessel and proceed with revascularization. Nevertheless, if atherosclerotic lesions are present at the level of branches, we proceed with nephrectomy. Application of predictors, such as urinary hyperconcentration of nonreabsorbable solutes on split renal function studies and identification of a disease-free distal renal artery on angiography, should limit the frequency of inappropriate revascularization.

The azotemic patient

The severely azotemic patient with renovascular occlusive disease is closer to end-stage atherosclerosis than is the nonazotemic patient. Although retrieval of function has immediate practical significance, the hazard of aggravating renal failure to a dialysis-dependent level is obvious. Furthermore, placing the patient with dialysis dependence at potentially higher risk because of an inappropriate operation tempers enthusiasm for a nonselective approach to the management of these patients.

Initial experience with revascularization in these patients was reported by Morris *et al.* [19] in 1962. They described a salutory effect of revascularization on hypertension and renal function on eight azotemic patients with either severe bilateral renal artery occlusions or unilateral occlusive disease and absent contralateral kidney. Novick *et al.* [4] found a similar beneficial functional response to renal revascularization when bilateral lesions were corrected in azotemic patients. However, identifying and selecting the patients who may benefit from this procedure remains difficult because of the paucity of information available on the spectrum of clinical presentations and natural history of ischemic nephropathy. Circumstantial evidence suggests that renovascular disease is a more common cause of progressive renal failure in the atherosclerotic age group than previously recognized [20]. In a 1986 survey, 73% of end-stage renal disease patients were in the atherosclerotic age. In a report by Mailloux *et al.* [21], a presumed renovascular cause of end-stage renal disease increased in frequency from 6.7% during 1978 to 1981 to 16.5% during 1982 to 1985. The median age at onset of end-stage renal disease for that group was the oldest of all groups, falling in the seventh decade of life. Each of these clinical characteristics agree with the demographic data of our reported patient group with proven ischemic nephropathy [22]. In our group, all patients had at least moderate hypertension, the mean age was 63 years, and only 14% had diabetes mellitus. These data indicate that renovascular disease may be either the primary cause or a secondary accelerant of renal insufficiency in a larger proportion of patients with renal insufficiency than has been commonly recognized.

Using this premise as a guide, the authors currently screen all adult patients over the age of 50 years who have newly recognized renal insufficiency and hypertension. Renal duplex sonography is our preferred method for this preliminary screening, and our experience with this screening technique has been previ-

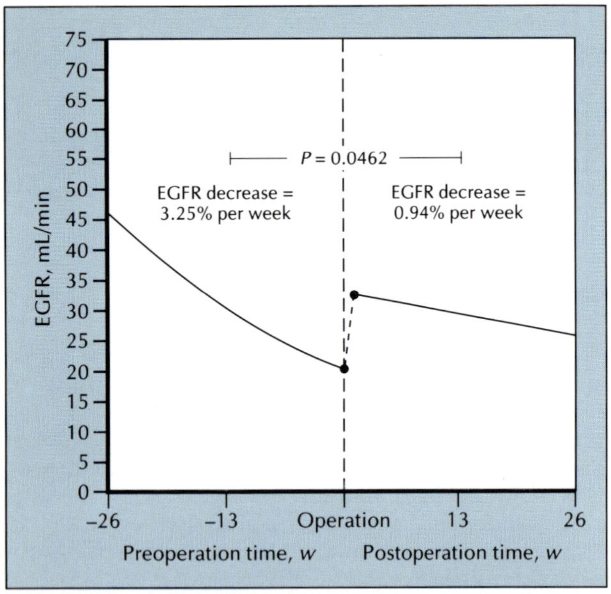

Fig. 1. Deterioration of estimated glomerular filtration rate (EGFR) per week during the 6 months before (n =50) and after (n = 32) renal revascularization. The immediate effect of operation on EGFR is also depicted. The P values for differences are determined using t-test for unpaired data. Note the improvement in the slope of decline in EGFR after operation. (*From* Dean *et al.* [22]; with permission.)

ously reported [23]. In that review, we found renal duplex sonography to have an overall accuracy of 96% for establishing the presence or absence of main renal artery occlusive disease. Because the term *ischemic nephropathy* implies the presence of global renal ischemia, we believe renal duplex sonography is an adequate method for initial screening of the renal insufficiency patient when it is performed by an experienced technician. Through this preliminary screening, we limit the use of arteriography to renal insufficiency patients with either positive renal duplex sonographic results or severe hypertension.

We have continued to rely on standard cut-film arteriography in patients with renal insufficiency who have clinical or duplex sonographic evidence of renovascular disease. In our experience, adequate assessment of the renal vasculature and juxtarenal aorta requires multiple injections when intra-arterial digital subtraction angiography is used. The use of a single, midstream flush aortogram requires no more contrast material than that required for such multiple intra-arterial digital subtraction studies. Additionally, standard arteriography provides information concerning cortical thickness and renal length as well as improved clarity for interpretation of the renal artery anatomy. The fact that arteriography in such patients with severe renal insufficiency, especially those with severe concomitant diabetes mellitus, can aggravate renal failure is widely recognized. Nevertheless, we believe this risk is justified in such patients who have severe or accelerated hypertension and in patients with positive renal duplex sonographic results. In these circumstances, the potential benefit derived from identification and correction of a functionally significant renovascular occlusive lesion exceeds the risk of arteriography.

The evolution of renal insufficiency in ischemic nephropathy was recently evaluated in a retrospective study of the estimated glomerular filtration rate (EGFR) and its rate of decline before and after revascularization in 58 patients [22]. Renal revascularization had a beneficial impact on both the rate of decline in EGFR and on EGFR itself when data for the entire group were analyzed collectively (Fig. 1). Of interest is that patients who experienced an immediate increase in glomerular filtration rate following surgery had an accelerated rate of functional decline preoperatively, approximately eight times the rate of progression seen in patients with renal failure from nonischemic etiologies (Fig. 2). The implication is that a rapidly deteriorating glomerular filtration rate should alert the physician to the potential presence of ischemic nephropathy and should argue for the likelihood of functional retrieval by revascularization after a conclusive diagnosis is made.

The observation that the salutory effect of surgery on the rate of deterioration was seen only in patients who experienced an immediate improvement in EGFR may have major clinical significance. First, the lesion may limit renal perfusion to a degree that it affects excretory function. Second, it may be the source of microscopic atheroembolization that destroys functioning renal parenchyma. Unfortunately, when the lesion was not producing significant reversible ischemia, as reflected by the absence of improvement in EGFR immediately following the operation, no improvement in the rate of decline in EGFR occurred after the operation (Fig. 3). This result indicates that when atheroembolism is the only potentially active pathophysiologic consequence of the lesion, its correction does not lead to clinically important deceleration of renal function decline.

The risk associated with renal revascularization in an azotemic patient is not inconsequential and merits comment. Overall operative experience with this group of patients is associated with a 6% to 9% operative mortality [24]. Approximately 80% to 90% of these patients have cardiac, cerebrovascular, or peripheral vascular manifestations of atherosclerosis [22,25•]. With such evidence of multifaceted, site-specific end-organ damage in this elderly population, the benefit afforded by a therapy with a relatively high operative mortality rate and a cumulative 1-year survival rate of only 78% must be questioned. Nevertheless, risk and survival should be placed into the context of the probability of survival without operation. In a study of the duration of survival following institution of dialysis, Mailloux *et al.* [21] found that end-stage renal disease caused by uncorrected renovascular disease was associated with the most rapid rate of death during follow-up. In their study, patients with renovascular disease had a median survival following initiation of dialysis of only 27 months and a 5-year survival of only 12%, which equates to an annual death rate in excess of 20%. Evidence suggests that revascularization of azotemic pa-

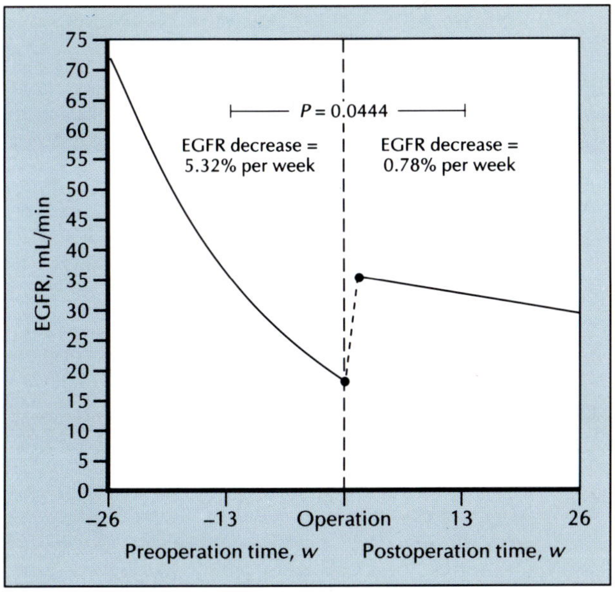

Fig. 2. Deterioration of estimated glomerular filtration rate (EGFR) per week during the 6 months before (n = 23) and after (n = 25) renal revascularization in a group of patients who received at least a 20% improvement in EGFR following operation. The immediate effect of operation on EGFR in this group is also depicted. The *P* values for differences are determined using *t*-test for unpaired data. Note the improvement in the slope of decline in EGFR after operation in this group. (*From* Dean *et al.* [22]; with permission.)

tients whose chronic renal insufficiency is caused by renovascular disease has the potential to improve renal function and prolong survival [15].

Yet, not all patients with azotemia and even bilateral renal artery stenosis benefit from revascularization. If the results of seven surgical series on revascularization in this patient population are combined, 55% of the patients demonstrate improvement of renal function, 31% experience no change, and 14% are made worse by the operation [26•]. Preoperative indicators that influence functional retrieval in this group are the severity of other occlusive lesions and the type of hypertension. Functionally severe, bilateral renal artery occlusions produce a particularly severe and difficult-to-control variety of hypertension. When such hypertension is present in combination with correctable bilateral stenoses and occlusions, revascularization should dramatically alleviate both the hypertension and the concomitant azotemia. In these patients, preoperative dependence on dialysis is not a negative factor for a successful outcome, even though some physicians do not believe that such revascularization can reverse long-standing dialysis dependence. This belief has little practical significance because these patients have little to lose from revascularization. They also have the greatest potential for retrieval of function and a chance for increased survival.

In contrast, absence of hypertension in the patient with renovascular occlusions and azotemia should argue against the probability that revascularization will improve renal function. Such lesions apparently are not of physiologic significance, because they do not produce an integral response to ischemia, namely, hypertension. Therefore, the clinician should hesitate to consider revascularization in an azotemic normotensive patient because the risk of aggravating renal failure outweighs the probability that function will be improved by such intervention.

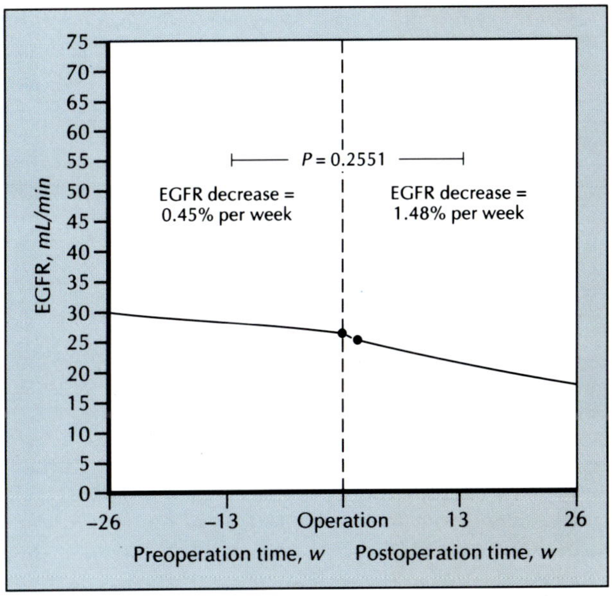

Fig. 3. Deterioration of estimated glomerular filtration rate (EGFR) per week during the 6 months before (n = 18) and after (n = 8) renal revascularization in a group of patients who received no significant immediate benefit in EGFR after operation. The *P* values for differences are determined using *t*-tests for unpaired data. Note the absence of improvement in the rate of deterioration of EGFR following operation in this group. (*From* Dean *et al.* [22]; with permission.)

The patient with acute occlusion

Finally, the patient with chronic occlusive disease and acute-onset oliguria or anuria must be considered. This acute onset is usually the consequence of acute thrombosis in the stenotic artery to a solitary kidney or to the only kidney with previous significant residual function. Most such patients will present with a history of hypertension, the severity of which has acutely accelerated, and the sudden development of oliguric renal failure. Diagnostic evaluation of any patient presenting with such signs should include angiography. Although the clinician was reticent in the past to perform angiography because of the nephrotoxic effect of the large amount of contrast material necessary for such an evaluation, the current use of "one-shot" aortography has greatly lessened the potential renal insult. A word of caution regarding interpretation of arteriograms in these patients is warranted. The absence of a nephrogram does not necessarily imply irretrievability of renal function. In a review of 31 patients who underwent surgical revascularization for prolonged anuria, Bilfinger *et al.* [27] noted no significant difference in renal function, blood pressure, or survival after renal reperfusion between patients with and those without nephrograms.

Although many physicians are tempted to react to the acute clinical presentation with immediate operation and attempted revascularization, a more carefully planned approach is superior. Because the acute event is usually at least 24 hours old and primarily represents reduction of perfusion to below the critical level for maintaining urinary output, preoperative correction of metabolic derangements is essential to reduce the risk of surgical intervention. Thus, the patient may require several days of dialysis or correction of other, more lethal, cardiac derangements before revascularization can be attempted. The physician should remember that renal failure can be controlled by hemodialysis while malignant hypertension and cardiac risk factors improve, and that the amount of retrievable renal function is not dependent on the timing of intervention. Indeed, successful revascularization has been reported after 42 days of anuria [28,29]. According to Hollenberg and Adams [30], a normal kidney relies on a high perfusion pressure and flow rate of 4 mL/min/g of tissue. Therefore, a significant drop in blood flow results in a reduction of filtrate production and a concomitant reduction in tubular work and oxygen consumption. In patients with acute occlusion, anuria reflects an inability to generate appreciable filtrate production rather than immediate and irreversible renal parenchymal damage. In a significant number of patients, urine flow is almost instantaneous after completion of the revascularization, and most patients require no further dialysis in the immediate postoperative period.

References and recommended reading

Papers of particular interest, published within the annual period of review, have been highlighted as:

- • Of special interest
- •• Of outstanding interest

1. Ying CY, Tifft CP, Gavras H, Chobanian AV: **Renal Revascularization in the Azotemic Hypertensive Patient Resistant to Therapy.** *N Engl J Med* 1984, **311**:1070–1075.
2. Scoble JE, Maher ER, Hamilton G, Dick R, Sweny P, Moorhead JF: **Atherosclerotic Renovascular Disease Causing Renal Impairment: A Case for Treatment.** *Clin Nephrol* 1989, **31**:119–122.
3. Bengtsson V, Borgentz SE, Norback B: **Surgical Treatment of Renal Artery Stenosis With Impending Anemia.** *Clin Nephrol* 1974, 2:222–229.
4. Novick AC, Pohl MA, Schreiber M, Gifford RY, Vidt DG: **Revascularization for Preservation of Renal Function in Patients With Atherosclerotic Renovascular Disease.** *J Urol* 1983, 129:907–911.
5. Bredenberg CE, Sampson LN, Ray FS, Cormier RA, Heintz S, Eldrup-Jorgensen J: **Changing Patterns in Surgery for Chronic Renal Artery Occlusive Diseases.** *J Vasc Surg* 1992, **15**:1018–1023.
6. Hovinga TK, de Jong PE, van der Hem GK, de Zee VW: **Relief of Renal Artery Stenosis: A Tool to Improve or Preserve Renal Function in Renovascular Disease?** *Nephrol Dial Transplant* 1990, **5**:481–488.
7. Jacobson HR: **Ischemic Renal Disease: An Overlooked Clinical Entity?** *Kidney Int* 1988, **34**:729–744.
8. Zinman L, Libertino JA: **Revascularization of the Chronic Totally Occluded Renal Artery with Restoration of Renal Function.** *J Urol* 1977, **8**:517.
9. Libertino JA, Zinman L, Breslin DJ, Swinton NW Jr, Legg MA: **Renal Artery Revascularization: Restoration of Renal Function.** *JAMA* 1980, **244**:1340–1342.
10. Lawrie GM, Morris GC Jr, DeBakey ME: **Long-Term Results of Treatment of the Totally Occluded Renal Artery in 40 Patients With Renovascular Disease.** *Surgery* 1988, **6**:953–959.
11. Novick AC: **Atherosclerotic Renovascular Disease.** *J Urol* 1981, **126**:567–572.
12. Dean RH, Lawson JD, Hollifield JW, Shack RB, Polterauer P, Rhamy RK: **Revascularization of the Poorly Functioning Kidney.** *Surgery* 1979, **85**:44–52.
13. Sicard GA, Etheredge EE, Mueser MN, Anderson CB: **Improved Renal Function After Renal Artery Revascularization.** *J Cardiovasc Surg* 1985, **26**:157–161.
14. Dean RH, Englund R, Dupont WD, Meacham PW, Plummer WD Jr, Perce R, Ezell C: **Retrieval of Renal Function by Revascularization: Study of Preoperative Outcome Predictors.** *Ann Surg* 1985, **202**:367–375.
15. Novick AC, Ziegelbaum M, Vidgt DG, Gifford RW Jr, Pohl MA, Goormastic M: **Trends in Surgical Revascularization for Renal Artery Disease: Ten Years' Experience.** *JAMA* 1987, **257**:498–501.
16. Hallet JW Jr, Fowl R, O'Brien PC, Bernatz PE, Pairoloro PC, Cherry KJ Jr, Hollier LH: **Renovascular Operations in Patients With Chronic Renal insufficiency: Do the Benefits Justify the Risk?** *J Vasc Surg* 1987, **5**:622–627.
17. Dean RH, Kieffer RW, Smith BM, Oates JA Norton JH, Hollifield JW, DuPont WD: **Renovascular Hypertension: Anatomic and Renal Function During Dry Therapy.** *Arch Surg* 1981, **116**:1408–1415.
18. Dean RH: **Renovascular Hypertension.** *Curr Probl Surg* 1985, **22**:1–67.
19. Morris GC Jr, DeBakey ME, Cooley DA: **Surgical Treatment of Renal Failure of Renovascular Origin.** *JAMA* 1962, **182**:609.
20. North Carolina Kidney Council: *Annual Report.* Raleigh: North Carolina Kidney Council; 1986.
21. Mailloux LU, Bellucci AG, Mossey RT, Napolitano B, Moore T, Wilkes BM, Bluestone PA: **Predictors of Survival in Patients Undergoing Dialysis.** *Am J Med* 1988, **84**:855–862.
22. Dean RH, Tribble RW, Hansen KJ, O'Neil E, Cravan TE, Redding JF: **Evolution of Renal Insufficiency in Ischemic Nephropathy.** *Ann Surg* 1991, **213**:446–456.
23. Hansen KJ, Tribble RW, Reavis SW, Canzanello VJ, Cravan TE, Plonk GW, Dean RH: **Renal Duplex Sonography: Evaluation of Clinical Utility.** *J Vasc Surg* 1990, **12**:227–236.
24. Libertino JA, Bosco PJ, Ying CY, Breslin DJ, Woods BO: **Renal Revascularization to Preserve and Restore Renal Function.** *J Urol* 1992, **147**:1485–1487.
25. • O'Neil E, Hansen KJ, Canzanello VJ, Pennell TC, Dean RH: **Prevalence of Ischemic Nephropathy in Patients with Renal Insufficiency.** *Am Surg* 1992, **58**:485–490.

Studies prevalence of ischemic nephropathy by using renal duplex sonography to assess the degree of renal artery occlusive disease in a select population of patients with renal insufficiency. Data suggest that a small but significant number of these patients do indeed have unsuspected ischemic nephropathy.

26. • Rimmer JM, Grennan FJ: **Atherosclerotic Renovascular Disease and Progressive Renal Failure.** *Ann Intern Med* 1993, **118**:712–719.

Excellent review of renovascular disease and renal failure with comparative analysis of surgical treatment and angioplasty for treatment in selected patients.

27. Bilfinger TV, Gore DC, Wolma FJ: **Renal Revascularization in Anuric Patients: Determinants of Outcome.** *South Med J* 1989, **82**:558–562.
28. Lacombe M: **Acute Non-traumatic Obstructions of the Renal Artery.** *J Cardiovasc Surg* 1992, **33**:163–168.
29. Pontremoli R, Rampoldi V, Morbidelli A, Fiorini F, Ranise A, Garibotto G: **Acute Renal Failure Due to Acute Bilateral Renal Artery Thrombosis: Successful Surgical Revascularization After Prolonged Anuria.** *Nephron* 1990, **56**:322–324.
30. Hollenberg NK, Adams NF: **The Renal Blood Supply in Oliguric States: When is a Kidney Ischemic? A Fundamental in Cardiology.** *Am Heart J* 1976, **91**:255–261.

Virginia S. Newman, MD, and Richard H. Dean, MD, Division of Surgical Sciences, Bowman Gray School of Medicine, Medical Center Boulevard, Winston-Salem, NC 27157, USA.

Index to subjects

Volume 2 1994

Abdominal injuries, 36–38, 47
Achalasia, esophageal, 117
Actinomycosis, 104–105
Acylated plasminogen-streptokinase activator complex see Anistreplase
Adaptation, physiological, of intestinal mucosa, 143–144
Adenocarcinoma see also Klatskin tumor
  of rectum, 85–93
  of stomach
    preoperative staging, 125–128
    surgery, 125
    survival rates, 126
Adenoma, diet in, 78
Adenosine diphosphate, 20
Adenosine triphosphate, 19–20
Advanced Pediatric Life Support, 43
Advanced Trauma Life Support, 44
Alteplase, 257–258, 261
Amputation, 228
Amylases, 173
Anal tuberculosis, 103–104
Anastomosis, surgical, 234
Angiography
  blunt injury, 32
  carotic stenosis, 267
  duodenal gastrinoma, 133
  neck injuries, 33
  penetrating wounds, 30–32
  vs. transesophageal echocardiography, 36
Angiotensin II, 151
Anistreplase, 257–258
Anorectal diseases, 78, 103–107
Anti-inflammatory agents, non-steroidal, 139
Antidiuretic hormones see Vasopressins
Antigens, 18, 239–240
Antireflux surgery, 117–118
Anuria, 274–275
Apoptosis, 247–249
APSAC see Anistreplase
ARDS see Respiratory distress syndrome, adult
Arginine, 26–28
Arterial occlusion
  physiopathology, 259
  surgery, 259–260
  thrombolytic therapy, 257–264
Arteriography see Angiography
Artificial respiration see Respiration, artificial
Ascites, pancreatic, 176
Asialoglycoprotein receptors, 19
Aspirin, 77–78
Athletic injuries, 106
ATP see Adenosine triphosphate
Azotemia see Uremia

Barium enema, 97–98
Biliary atresia, 168–172
Biliary tract, endoscopy, 203–204
Blood pressure, 31–32
Blood transfusion, autologous, 77
Blunt injuries see Wounds, nonpenetrating
Breast neoplasms, 217–223
  advanced, 220–221
  breast conserving therapy, 219–220
  drug therapy, 220
  early invasive, 219–220
  genetics, 217
  hormone therapy, 221
  mammography, 217–218
  noninvasive, 218–219
  radiotherapy, 219–220
  recurrence, 220
  screening for, 217–218

Carcinoembryonic antigen screening, 77, 98–99
Carcinoma
  esophageal, 113–116
  follicular, 55–56
  Huerthle cell, 56
  papillary, 53–55
    classification, 53
    iodine radioisotope scanning in, 55
    prognosis, 53–54
    thyroidectomy, 54–55
Carotid artery injuries, 33
Carotid stenosis
  angiography, 267
  asymptomatic, 266–269
  endarterectomy, 265–271
  and stroke, 267
  symptomatic, 265–266
Catheterization, in pancreatic pseudocyst, 175–176
Cell death, genetics, 247–249
Cells, cultured, mucosal healing models, 140–141
Cerebral ischemia, transient
  angiography, 267
  carotid endarterectomy in, 265–266
  computed tomography scans, 267
  occurrence, 265
Chemotherapy, adjuvant, 225
Cholangiocarcinoma, 159–160 see also Klatskin tumor
Cholangiopancreatography, endoscopic retrograde
  in common bile duct, 195–196, 203
  complications, 203
  in pancreatic pseudocyst, 174–176
Cholangioscopy, 206
Cholangitis, sclerosing, 156–160
  and cholangiocarcinoma, 159–160
  differential diagnosis, 157–158
  drug therapy, 157
  surgery, 158–160
Cholecystectomy, laparoscopic, 195–196, 203–206
Choledocholithiasis see Common bile duct calculi
Cholestasis, 164
Choristoma, 106
Chromosome mapping, 63
Clinical trials
  carotic endarterectomy, 265–271
  rectal neoplasms, combined therapy, 89
  thrombolytic agents, 262
Cloning, molecular, 64–65
Colectomy, laparoscopic, 196, 209–213
  cancer control, 208–210
  complications, 210
  cost-benefit analysis, 212
  hospital length of stay, 212

 ISBN 1-85922-671-X ISSN 1065–6243

intraperitoneal cancer staging, 210
quality of life, 212
tumor implantation, 209–210
Colonic neoplasms, recurrence, 95–96
Colonoscopy, 97
Colorectal neoplasms, 77–78
and aspirin, 77–78
autologous blood transfusion, 77
carcinoembryonic antigen screening, 77, 98–99
and constipation, 78
fecal occult blood testing, 79–83
genetics, 77
incidence, 94–95
laparoscopic colectomy in, 208
lymph node excision, 208–209
polyp removal, 77–78
postoperative follow-up, 94–103
prevention, 77–78
recurrence, postoperative, 94–97
screening, 77, 79–84
sigmoidoscopy, 83–84
staging, 95
Common bile duct calculi, laparoscopy, 195–196, 203–207
Constipation, 78
Cost-benefit analysis
of laparoscopic colectomy, 212
of thrombolytic therapy, 263
Critical illness
energy metabolism, 24
enteral nutrition, 25
nutritional management, 24–29
parenteral nutrition, 25
Crohn disease, 78, 103–104
Cytokines, 17, 250–251
Cytomegalovirus infections, 105

Diabetes mellitus, insulin-dependent
history, 179
islets of Langerhans transplantation, 183–184
occurrence, 179
pancreas transplantation, 180–183
Diarrheogenic tumor, 187
Diet, 78
Doxorubicin, 151, 224–225, 228
Duodenal obstruction, 123
Duodenal ulcer, 139
Duodenotomy, 134, 190

Eastern Cooperative Oncology Group, 89
Echocardiography, 35–36
Ectopic tissue see Choristoma
Electrocoagulation, 232
Embolism, 259
Emergency medical services, pediatric, 43–46
Empyema, pleural, 39
Endarterectomy, carotid, 265–269
Endoscopy, biliary, 203–204
Endothelins, 18
Energy metabolism, 24
Enteral nutrition, 25, 27
Epidermal growth factor-urogastrone, 141–142
Esophageal achalasia, 117
Esophageal diseases, minimal-access surgery, 117–119
Esophageal myotomy, 117
Esophageal neoplasms, 113–116
Esophageal resection, 113–116, 118
Esophagectomy, 113–114
Extracellular matrix proteins, 143
Extracorporeal membrane oxygenation, 10–12

Fasciitis, perineal necrotizing, 104
Fatty acids, in critical illness, 26–27
Fecal incontinence, surgery, 78
Fecal occult blood testing, 79–83, 97
Fibrinolysin, 257
Fibrinolytic agents see Thrombolytic agents
Fibroblast growth factors, 143
Floxuridine, 151–152
Fluorouracil, 89–90, 151
Folinic acid, 91
Foods, formulated, 27
Fournier's gangrene, 104
Fundoplication, laparoscopic, 118

Gastrin, 133
Gastrinoma
laparotomy, 70–71
localization, 187
metastasis, 70, 73, 190
occurrence, 69–70
surgery, 189–190
Gastrinoma, duodenal
endoscopy, 134
epidemiology, 132
laparotomy, 134
localization, 133–134
metastasis, 132
pancreatoduodenectomy, 71–72, 134
prognosis, 134–135
surgery, 134
ultrasonography, 127–128
in Zollinger-Ellison syndrome, 71, 131–132
Gastrinoma, pancreatic, 132
Gastrointestinal Tumour Study Group, 89
Gene therapy, in cancer, 249–251
Genes
knock-outs, 249
p53, 245–247
suppressor, tumor, 245
targeted disruption, 249
Wilms' tumor, 245
Genetics, biochemical, in cancer, 245–254
Glomerular filtration rate, 273
Glutamine, 26–27
Growth factors, in intestinal mucosa, 141–144
Guaiac test, 97

Hailey-Hailey disease, 103
Head injuries, in children, 46
Healing process, in intestinal mucosa, 138–146
growth factors, 141–143
matrix proteins, 143
models, 140–141
polyamine metabolism, 141
Helicobacter infections, 121–122
Helicobacter pylori, in peptic ulcer, 120–124
Hematoma, 106
Hemicholectomy, 211
Hemorrhage, in peptic ulcer, 122–123
Hemothorax, 39
Hernia, inguinal
laparoscopy, 195, 198–202
recurrence, 195, 201
surgery, types of, 198–199
Hernia, paraesophageal, surgery, 118
Hypertension, renovascular, 271–275

Ifosfamide, 224
Immune response, and nutrition, 26–27
Immunoscintigraphy, 98
Immunotherapy, cellular, 238–244

Indomethacin, 139
Inflammatory bowel diseases, 78, 139
Insulin-like growth factor I, 27–28
Insulinoma
  diagnosis, 186
  drug therapy, 187
  localization, 188
  surgery, 189
Interleukins, 250–251
Intestinal mucosa
  and growth factors, 141–144
  healing process, 138–146
  and non-steroidal anti-inflammatory agents, 139
Intestine, small, mucosal healing process, 138–146
Intubation, gastrointestinal, 25
Iodine radioisotope scanning, 55
Ischemic nephropathy, 271–275
Islets of Langerhans transplantation, 183–184

Kasai procedure see Portoenterostomy, hepatic
Ketone bodies, arterial ratio, in oxidation-reduction, 19–21
Kidney failure, chronic, 272–274
Kidney revascularization
  and glomerular filtration rate, 273
  mortality rate, 273
  prognosis, 273–274
  in renovascular hypertension, 271–272
  in uremic patients, 272–274
Killer cells, lymphokine-activated, 152–153, 241–242
Klatskin tumor, 161–167 see also Cholangiocarcinoma
  adjuvant therapy, 164
  diagnosis, 161–162
  differential diagnosis, 157
  palliative therapy, 164
  pathology, 161
  postoperative radiotherapy, 165
  staging, 162
  surgery, 162–164
  survival rates, 164–165
Knee injuries, 32

Lap belt ecchymosis, 47
Laparoscopy, 195–197
  antireflex, 118
  in blunt trauma, 38
  colectomy, 196, 209–213
  common bile duct calculi, 195–196, 204–206
  inguinal hernia, 195, 198–202
  in pediatric trauma, 46
  rectal excision, 235
  stomach neoplasm staging, 127
  trauma diagnosis, 36–38
Laparotomy, 70–71, 134
Leiomyoma, 105
Leucovorin, 91
Levamisole, 91
Lipoma, 106
Liquid ventilation, 12
Lithotripsy, 206
Liver, preoperative assessment, 17–23
Liver cirrhosis, diagnosis, 18–19
Liver diseases
  cytokines in, 17
  diagnosis, 17–19
  endothelins in, 18
  fibrin- and fibrinogen-related antigens in, 18
  magnetic resonance spectroscopy, 18
  methionine metabolism, 18
  vascular compliance, 18–19
  vasopressin clearance rate, 18
  vitronectin in, 18
Liver function tests, 17–19
Liver neoplasms
  biological therapy, 152–153
  blood supply, 151–152
  drug therapy, 151–154
  magnetic resonance imaging, 98
  non-surgical treatment, 151–155
  radiotherapy, targeted, 153
  secondary to colorectal neoplasms, 96
Liver transplantation
  arterial ketone body ratio, 20–21
  in biliary atresia, 170–171
  in sclerosing cholangitis, 158–159
Lung neoplasms, 96
Lymphadenectomy
  in colorectal carcinoma, 208–209
  for esophageal carcinoma, 114–115
  in stomach neoplasm metastasis, 128–129
Lymphocytes, tumor-infiltrating, 239–244

Magnetic resonance imaging, 98, 230
Major histocompatibility complex, 238
Mammography, 217–218
Mass screening
  breast neoplasms, 217–218
  carcinoembryonic antigens, 98–99
  colorectal neoplasms, 77, 79–84
Mastectomy, modified radical, 219
Mechanical ventilation see Respiration, artificial
Melanoma, tumor-specific T-cell antigens, 239–240
MEN-I see Neoplasms, multiple endocrine, type I
Mesna, 224
Metabolic clearance rate, 18
Methionine, 18
Methylene blue, 133–134
Microspheres, 151
Microsurgery, 232
Mitochondria, liver, 19
Mitomycin C, 152
Models, biological, intestinal mucosa healing process, 140–141
Molecular biology, in cancer, 245–254
Monophenol monooxygenase see Tyrosinase
MRI see Magnetic resonance imaging
Multiple endocrine neoplasms see Neoplasms, multiple endocrine
Myotomy, esophageal, 117

NAD+/NADH ratio, 19
National Polyp Study, 77
National Surgical Adjuvant Breast and Bowel Project, 90
Neck injuries, 33
Neoplasms
  cellular immunotherapy, 238–244
  gene therapy, 249–251
  genetics, 245–247
  metastasis
    from colorectal neoplasms, 96–97
    gastrinoma, 191
    therapy in liver, 151–155
  recurrence, 95
  seeding, 209–210
  staging, 125–128, 230
Neoplasms, multiple endocrine, 60–68
  type I, 60–62
    duodenal gastrinomas in, 132
    genetics, 60–62
    occurrence, 60

surgery, 72–73
tumor development, 61–62
in Zollinger-Ellison syndrome, 72–73, 192
type II, 62–66
gene mapping, 63
occurrence, 62–63
RET proto-oncogene, 65–66
Nephrectomy, 272
North Central Cancer Treatment Group, 89
NSAID see Anti-inflammatory agents, non-steroidal
Nuclear magnetic resonance, 18
Nucleotides, 26–27
Nutrition
in critical illness, 24–29
and immune response, 26–27
Nutritional requirements, 24–25

Octreotide, 177, 187–188
Oliguria, 274–275
Oncogenes, 245–247
Organ donors, 180
Ovarian neoplasms, 96–97
Oxidation-reduction see Redox
Oxygen, 7–8
Oxygenators, intravascular, 13

Pancreas transplantation
complications, 181
in diabetes mellitus type 1, 180–183
donor selection, 180
patient selection, 180
prognosis, 180–181
whole organ, 180–183
Pancreatic ascites, 176
Pancreatic fistula, 177
Pancreatic neoplasms, endocrine, 186–194
diagnosis, 186–187
drug therapy, 187–188
localization of, 188–189
metastasis, 190–191
occurrence, 186
surgery, 189–190
Pancreatic pseudocyst, 173–176
catheterization, 175–176
in children, 176
complications, 176
diagnosis, 173
management, 174–176
natural history, 173–174
surgery, 174–176
Pancreaticosplenectomy, 125
Pancreatoduodenectomy, 190
in duodenal gastrinoma, 71–72, 134
in Zollinger-Ellison syndrome, 71–72
Parenteral nutrition, total, 24–25
Pediatric Advanced Life Support, 43–44
Pediatric trauma, 41–49
Pelvic injuries, in children, 47
Pemphigus, benign familial, 103
Peptic ulcer
drug therapy, 121–122
etiology, 120
gastric outlet obstruction in, 123
helicobacter pylori in, 120–124
hemorrhage, 122–123
intractibility, 122
penetration, 123
perforation, 123
surgery, indications for, 122–123
Perfluorocarbons, 12
Peripheral vascular injuries, 30–34
Peritoneal lavage, 38, 45
Physical examination, postoperative, 97
Plasmin see Fibrinolysin
Plasminogin activator, recombinant tissue see Alteplase
Plasminogin activators, 257–259
Polyamines, 141
Polymerase chain reaction, 249
Polyps, intestinal, 77–78
Portoenterostomy, hepatic
in biliary atresia, 168–172
complications, 169–170
techniques, 170
Positive-pressure respiration, 9
Preoperative assessment, of liver function, 17–23
Proto-oncogenes, RET, 65–66

Radioimmunodetection, 98
Radioligand assay, 19
Radiotherapy, 153, 165
Receptors
asialoglycoprotein, 19
T-cell, 238–239, 241
Rectal neoplasms
preoperative staging, 230
radiotherapy, 85–93, 231–232
recurrence, 95–96
surgery, 85, 230–237
abdominoperineal resection, 234–235
anterior resection, 234
electrocoagulation, 232
extended resection, 235–236
laparoscopic excision, 235
local excision, 230–232
rectal excision, 232–233
transanal endoscopic microsurgery, 232
survival rates, 85
Rectum, rupture of, 106
Redox, 19–21
Redox tolerance test, 21
Renal artery obstruction, surgery
in nonuremic patients, 271–272
patient selection criteria, 271
in uremic patients, 272–274
Respiration, artificial, 9–10
adjunct therapy, 10
liquid ventilation, 12
positive-pressure respiration, 9
Respiratory distress syndrome, adult
drug therapy, 13
extracorporeal membrane oxygenation, 11–12
intravascular oxygenation, 13
oxygen consumption, 8
ventilatory pressure-volume relationships, 9
Respiratory distress syndrome, infant, 11–12
Respiratory failure
drug therapy, 13
extracorporeal life support, 10–12
intravascular oxygenation, 13
liquid ventilation, 12
management, 7–16
mechanical ventilation, 9–10
rt-PA see Alteplase

Sarcoma, soft tissue, 224–229
drug therapy, 224–226
radiotherapy, 226–227
surgery, 227–228
Semustine, 90
Septic severity, 25

Sigmoidoscopy, 83–84
Smoking, 121
Somatostatin, 188
Spectroscopy, magnetic resonance see Nuclear magnetic resonance
Sphincterotomy, laparoscopic, 205–206
Stomach neoplasms
  computed tomography, 127
  laparoscopy, 127
  lymphadenectomy, 128–129
  management, 125–130
  metastasis, 128
  occurrence, 125
  preoperative staging, 125–128
  surgery, 125, 128–129
  survival rates, 126
  ultrasonography, 126–128
Streptokinase, 257–258, 261
Stroke, 265–270
Surgery, antireflux, 117–118
Surgical mesh, 198–199, 201

T-lymphocytes
  antigen receptors, 238–239, 241
  and major histocompatibility complex, 238
  physiology, 238–239
  tumor-specific antigens, 239–240
Tamoxifen, 221
Thoracic injuries
  in children, 46
  diagnosis, 36
  thoracoscopy, 39
Thoracic outlet injuries, 33
Thoracoscopy, 38–39
Thrombolytic agents
  administration and dosage, 260–261
  clinical trials, 262
  pharmacodynamics, 257–259
Thrombolytic therapy, in arterial occlusion, 257–264
  cost-benefit analysis, 263
  prognosis, 261–264
  techniques, 260–261
Thrombosis, 259
Thyroid neoplasms, surgery, 53–59
Thyroidectomy
  complications, 56
  in papillary carcinoma, 54–55
  surgical techniques, 56–57
  for thyroid neoplasms, 53–59
Tissue culture, mucosal healing models, 140–141
Tomography, x-ray computed
  colorectal neoplasms, 98
  stomach neoplasm staging, 127
  transient cerebral ischemia, 267
Transesophageal echocardiography, 35–36
Transforming growth factors, 141–143
Transillumination, 133
Transplantation, liver, 20–21
Trauma see Wounds and injuries
Trefoil growth factors, 142
Tuberculosis, anal, 103–104
Tumor markers, biological, 99
Tumor necrosis factor, 153, 240–241
Tumor suppressor genes, 245
Tyrosinase, 240

Ultrasonography
  endoscopic
    duodenal gastrinoma localization, 133
    pancreatic endocrine tumor localization, 188
    rectal neoplasms, 98
    stomach neoplasm staging, 126–127
  intraoperative, 132
  pediatric trauma, 46
  penetrating wounds, 31–32
  preoperative rectal carcinoma staging, 230
  stomach neoplasm surgery, 127–128
Urokinase
  administration and dosage, 261
  clinical trials, 261–262
  pharmacodynamics, 257–258

Varicose veins, anorectal, 105
Vascular compliance, in liver diseases, 18–19
Vascular injuries
  angiography, 30–32
  penetrating wounds, 30–32
  peripheral, 30–34
  surgery, 32–33
  ultrasonography, 31–32
Vasopressins, 18
Venous injuries, 32–33
Ventilation, mechanical see Respiration, artificial
VIPoma see Diarrheogenic tumor
Vitronectin, 18

Wilms' tumor genes, 245
Wound healing see Healing process
Wounds, nonpenetrating, 32, 38
Wounds, penetrating
  angiography in, 30–32
  animal experiments, 31
  arterial blood pressure indices, 31–32
  laparoscopy in, 36–37
  thoracoscopy in, 39
  ultrasonography, 31–32
  vascular injuries, 30–32
Wounds and injuries
  in children, 41–49
    anatomical considerations, 41
    assessment of injuries, 45–46
    etiology, 43–44
    occurrence, 41
    prevention and control, 41–43
    radiography, 45
    rehabilitation, 43
    resuscitation, 44–45
    ultrasonography, 46
  diagnostic techniques, 35–40
    laparoscopy, 36–38
    thoracoscopy, 38–39
    transesophageal echocardiography, 35–36

Zollinger-Ellison syndrome
  diagnosis, 186–187
  duodenal gastrinoma in, 71, 131–132
  gastric acid hypersecretion, 187
  localization of, 189
  surgery, 69–76, 189–190
    indications for, 70
    laparotomy, 70–71
    multiple endocrine neoplasm type I, 72–73
    pancreatoduodenectomy, 71–72
    parietal cell vagotomy, 70

FREE POSTAGE! No stamp required if you live in the following countries:

AUSTRALIA, BELGIUM, BERMUDA, CYPRUS, DENMARK, FINLAND, FRANCE, GERMANY, HONG KONG, ICELAND, ISRAEL, ITALY, LUXEMBOURG, MONACO, THE NETHERLANDS, NEW ZEALAND, NORWAY, PORTUGAL, REPUBLIC OF IRELAND, SINGAPORE, SPAIN, SWEDEN, SWITZERLAND, THE UNITED ARAB EMIRATES, UNITED KINGDOM, UNITED STATES.

NO POSTAGE
NECESSARY
IF MAILED
IN THE
UNITED STATES

BUSINESS REPLY MAIL
FIRST CLASS MAIL PERMIT NO. 33925 PHILADELPHIA, PA

Postage Will Be Paid By Addressee

CURRENT SCIENCE
SUBSCRIPTIONS
20 N THIRD ST
PHILADELPHIA, PA 19106-9815

By air mail
Par avion

IBRS/CCRI NUMBER: PHQ-D/453/W

NE PAS AFFRANCHIR

NO STAMP REQUIRED

REPONSE PAYEE
GRANDE-BRETAGNE

CURRENT SCIENCE
34-42 CLEVELAND STREET
LONDON W1E 4QZ
GREAT BRITAIN

NO POSTAGE
NECESSARY
IF MAILED
IN THE
UNITED STATES

BUSINESS REPLY MAIL
FIRST CLASS PERMIT NO. 33925 PHILADELPHIA, PA

Postage Will Be Paid By Addressee

CURRENT SCIENCE
SUBSCRIPTIONS
20 N THIRD ST
PHILADELPHIA, PA 19106-9815